TECHNIQUES IN CORONARY ARTERY STENTING

TECHNIQUES IN CORONARY ARTERY STENTING

Antonio Colombo MD

Director, Cardiac Catheterization Laboratory
Centro Cuore Columbus, Milan,
Director, Invasive Cardiology,
San Raffaele Hospital, Milan, Italy and
Director, Investigational Angioplasty,
Lenox Hill Hospital, New York, New York, USA

Jonathan Tobis MD

Professor of Medicine
Director of Interventional Cardiology Research
UCLA School of Medicine
Division of Cardiology
Los Angeles, California
USA

MARTIN DUNITZ

© Martin Dunitz Ltd 2000

First published in the United Kingdom in 2000 by

Martin Dunitz Ltd
The Livery House
7–9 Pratt Street
London NW1 0AE

A CIP catalogue record for this book is available from the
British Library.

ISBN 1-85317-716-4

Distributed in the United States by:
Blackwell Science Inc.
Commerce Place, 350 Main Street
Malden, MA 02148, USA
Tel: 1-800-215-1000

Distributed in Canada by:
Login Brothers Book Company
324 Salteaux Crescent
Winnipeg, Manitoba, R3J 3T2
Canada
Tel: 204-224-4068

Distributed in Brazil by:
Ernesto Reichmann Distribuidora de Livros, Ltda
Rua Coronel Marques 335, Tatuape 03440-000
Sao Paulo
Brazil

Composition by Scribe Design, Gillingham, Kent
Printed and bound in Spain by Grafos S.A.

Contents

Contributors

Remo Albiero MD
Centro Cuore Columbus srl
Via M Buonarroti 48
20145 Milan
Italy

Antonio Colombo MD
Director, Cardiac Catheterization Lab
Centro Cuore Columbus
Via M Buonarroti 48
20145 Milan
Italy

George D Dangas MD
Washington Hospital Center, #4B-1
110 Irving Street, NW
Washington, DC 20010
USA

Steven L Goldberg MD
West Los Angeles VA Medical Center
Division of Cardiology
11031 Wiltshire Blvd
Los Angeles, CA 90073
USA

Joseph De Gregorio MD
Lenox Hill Hospital
Interventional Cardiology Group
9 Black Hall
100 E 77th Street
New York, NY 10021
USA

Shunji Kasaoka MD
Assistant Professor of Medicine
Yamaguchi University
Uhe
Japan

Carlo Di Mario MD
Centro Cuore Columbus srl
Via M Buonarroti 48
20145 Milan
Italy

Jeffrey Moses MD
Chief, Interventional Cardiology Group
Lenox Hill Hospital
9 Black Hall
100 E 77th Street
New York, NY 10021
USA

Issam Moussa MD
Director, Interventional Cardiology Research
Lenox Hill Hospital
9 Black Hall
100 E 77th Street
New York, NY 10021
USA

Bernhard Reimers MD
Ospedale Civile di Mirano
Laboratorio di Emodinamica
Via Luigi Mariutto, 13
30035 Mirano
Venezia
Italy

Jonathan M Tobis MD
Professor of Medicine
Director of Interventional Cardiology Research
UCLA School of Medicine
Room BL-394 CHS
Box 951717
Los Angeles, CA 90095-1717
USA

Preface

Our research collaboration, which forms the basis for this book, began in October 1992. At that time, there were several devices and techniques (laser photo ablation, directional atherectomy and rotational atherectomy) that had been developed to decrease restenosis associated with balloon angioplasty, but none of these appeared to make a dramatic impact. Stents for coronary artery disease were available in Europe, but the high incidence of subacute stent thrombosis inhibited their use except in emergency situations as a bail-out device during acute arterial closure. The trade-off of salvaging a dangerous situation in the catheterization laboratory for the possibility of subacute thrombosis and an out-of-hospital myocardial infarction was not a satisfactory alternative. To prevent stent thrombosis, an intense anticoagulation regimen was recommended; this included intravenous heparin after the procedure until the patient's prothrombin time became therapeutic with warfarin. This required several days in hospital and was associated with a high risk of bleeding from the groin and the possibility of surgical repair of the femoral artery.

In a parallel pathway, our research in intravascular ultrasound was providing new insights into the mechanism of action of the various angioplasty devices and increasing our knowledge of atherosclerotic disease. We reasoned that if we combined resources and used intravascular ultrasound to guide the multiple alternatives in coronary artery interventions we might maximize the result and improve the restenosis rate. Based on our experience with intravascular ultrasound following balloon angioplasty and directional atherectomy, we hypothesized that if we could obtain a lumen-to-vessel cross-sectional area of over 50%, we could debulk the plaque and lower restenosis. A complicated randomized trial was devised with multiple treatment arms using intravascular ultrasound in an iterative fashion to guide the procedure and to define the patient subgroups. As a last resort, if the desired result was not achieved in the aggressively treated ultrasound-guided group, then a stent could be placed. This

research protocol afforded us the opportunity of observing with intravascular ultrasound the results of coronary artery stenting as it was practiced at that time.

The primary observation was that, despite an excellent angiographic result, stents appeared by intravascular ultrasound to be inadequately deployed in over 80% of the cases. This was due to

(a) poor apposition of the stent struts against the arterial wall;
(b) an asymmetric deployment so that the lumen was not circular, which might predispose to turbulent flow;
(c) underexpansion of the stent struts.

Our response to these observations was to redilate the stents with higher pressure or a larger balloon. Subsequent intravascular ultrasound passes revealed dramatic improvement in the lumen cross-sectional area. Our approach to treating coronary artery lesions quickly shifted from the use of balloons or atherectomy devices to the almost exclusive use of stents. Not only were the immediate results improved, but the 6-month restenosis rate was also dramatically affected.

On the basis of these encouraging results, we began to think that the incidence of subacute thrombosis was not so much a problem of a metallic foreign body in the coronary artery, but more likely due to inadequate deployment when only angiographic guidance was used. It was at this time that an unfortunate twist of fate changed our approach to interventional procedures. A patient who had an excellent stent implantation as assessed by angiography and ultrasound developed a femoral artery bleed associated with warfarin therapy. He underwent vascular surgery to repair the artery but died from complications of the surgery. This unnecessary death prompted Antonio to stop using coumadin and post-procedure heparin if the result was successful by our ultrasound criteria. An antiplatelet regimen of aspirin and ticlopidine was used instead. Despite the removal of the aggressive anticoagulation regimen, subacute stent thrombosis plummeted to less than 1%, as did the attendant vascular complications. The length of hospitalization decreased from 4–5 days to 1 day. Not only were the immediate results excellent, but there was a significant reduction in the restenosis rate with intravascular ultrasound-guided stenting. We are sometimes asked, 'Was it the high-pressure inflations or the ticlopidine that made the difference?' Antonio's metaphorical response is typical of his wit and pragmatic approach to coronary interventions: 'Birds fly because they have wings *and* because they flap them!'

Since then, thousands of interventionalists have been trained in this technique of high-pressure balloon inflations and ultrasound guidance for stent insertion at multiple courses as well as visits through the Cuore Columbus in Milan, Italy. Our understanding of the process of coronary artery stenting has improved dramatically with the insights provided by intravascular ultrasound. New experience has been gained with multiple designs of stents and unusual clinical situations. This book is an attempt to describe that experience and share those insights with our colleagues.

Acknowledgements

There are many people to whom we are indebted for helping us develop and produce this book. Foremost we wish to express our appreciation for our colleagues and research associates who have been so productive in our laboratories. These include the authors of some of these chapters: Carlo DiMario for his expertise and personal charm, Steve Goldberg for his early and continued collaboration; Bernhard Reimers for his enthusiasm and analytic preciseness; Issam Moussa for his encyclopedic memory; Remo ALbiero for his fresh approach and helpful support; Joseph DeGregorio for his hard work and unyielding humor; Shunji Kasaoka for his tenacious analysis of endless data; and George Dangas for his important collaboration. Pat Hall, another transplant from the University of California, Irvine to Milan, was very influential in the early data analysis and his work has been incorporated throughout this book.

In addition, there are many people with whom we have collaborated over the years that were significant contributors to the common effort even though they are not listed as co-authors. These include our research associates from Japan who have been so diligent and have eased our burden: Shigeru Nakamura who first came to UC Irvine from Toho University and then worked in Milan; Takafumi Hiro from Yamaguchi University who taught us as much as we did him; Masahito Moriuchi who was the first fellow from Dr Saito's laboratory at Nihon University who was trained at UC Irvine, and Junko Honye who followed him; Tatsuro Akiyama from Dr Yamaguchi's department at Toho University and Yoshio Kobayashi from Osaka University who performed many of the statistical analyses; and Takehiro Yamashita from Hokkaido University who helped enormously in editing the figures.

It is also important to us to thank those individuals in the laboratory who gave so much of themselves so that the clinical procedures could run smoothly. These include Gina Tucci, the nursing director of the lab who never goes unnoticed during live case demonstrations; Massimo Ferraro the chief of technical support who 'gets the job done'; the wonderful cath lab nurses and technicians: Patrizia Briati, Marisa Caprino, Giovanna Busi, and Antonio Amato who work incredible hours with enthusiasm; and the secretaries and administrative assistants at Centro Cuore Columbus who provide such excellent support for the staff.

A special thanks goes to Giovanni Martini, the director of computer services at Centro Cuore Columbus, who produced many of the figures for this book.

At UC Irvine, my enduring gratitude goes to Beth Westberg, R.N. who helped maintain my equilibrium throughout the turmoil of this endeavour. The most important person in the production of this book was my administrative assistant, Kris Ekberg. She sacrificed many hours and even braved carpal tunnel syndrome to finish this book. We would also like to recognize the assistance of Alan Burgess and Clive Lawson, our editors, who have been most helpful in guiding this project.

To all of these people, and our families, we are deeply indebted for their kindness, support, and love.

Antonio Colombo
Jonathan Tobis

Chapter 1 Intravascular ultrasound imaging

Jonathan Tobis

This chapter provides background information for the interpretation of intravascular ultrasound (IVUS) images. Because observations of IVUS are critical to our understanding of the mechanisms and limitations of interventional techniques, it is important for interventional cardiologists to have a working knowledge of this methodology. Even if you do not use IVUS in your practice of angioplasty, it is worthwhile appreciating how the techniques of angioplasty have been affected by the insights of this unique imaging modality. For those readers who are interested in learning more about IVUS, there is a series of three videotapes, *IVUS Video Workshop*, which expands on the comments in this chapter. *IVUS Video Workshop* may be obtained from LMA Inc, PO Box 2515, Cupertino, CA 95015-2515, USA.

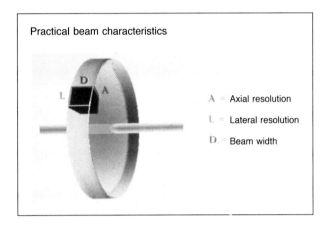

Figure 1.1 *The resolution of intravascular ultrasound images is described as the ability to discriminate two points along the radial axis or laterally along the circumference at any given depth.*

THERE ARE TWO BASIC TYPES OF IVUS CATHETERS: ROTATING MECHANICAL AND SYNTHETIC APERTURE

Between 1986 and 1988 several engineering groups were able to miniaturize piezoelectric transducers and deliver ultrasound energy to catheters that were approximately 1 mm in diameter.[1-6] There were three major designs of mechanical catheters: one in which the motor drive shaft rotated the transducer, another in which the shaft rotated a reflecting mirror, or a third in wich the shaft rotated both the transducer and the mirror in a fixed position at approximately 1800 revolutions per minute. The acoustic beam was directed perpendicular to the long axis of the catheter by reflecting against a metal mirror. The distance between the transducer and the mirror was set to diminish ring-down artefact created by the intense vibration when the transducer was stimulated. Another option was to place the transducer at an angle of 5–10° from the long axis. In all the catheters, a cone-shaped beam spreads out from the transducer (*Fig. 1.1*). The axial resolution of the image can be described in terms of the ability to differentiate two points along the radial axis, which depends on the depth of field and how the beam is focused. The other component of resolution is in the lateral axis or the ability to differentiate two distinct points around the circumference of the image at any given depth. For acoustic imaging, the resolution depends on the frequency of the catheter, but transducer technology and the electronics of the machine have a significant impact on image quality. For catheters operating at 25–30 MHz, the axial resolution is about 100 µm and the lateral resolution is 150 µm. The higher the frequency, the better the resolution but the smaller the depth of field that is visualized. There is also a trade-off between resolution with higher frequencies and increased reverberations from red blood cells within the lumen, which make it more difficult to distinguish the lumen from the intimal surface.[7]

The second general type of ultrasound catheter does not use a single transducer with mechanical rotation to sweep out a circumferential image; rather, it has 64 fixed transducer elements located around the circumference of the catheter tip.[8,9] The individual transducers are stimulated and the returning echoes are integrated by five miniaturized computer chips within the distal end of the catheter. The ultrasound information is focused by the electronic circuit according to the depth from the catheter. The advantages of this technology are:[10,11]

(a) the catheter tracks easily over a central core wire;
(b) there is no motion artefact resulting from non-uniform rotation, as may occur with the mechanical catheters; and
(c) the catheter is easily adaptable for combined imaging and therapeutic devices.

The image quality of the early synthetic aperture models was not equal to that of the mechanical devices. Recently, however, the transducers and electronics have significantly improved to rival the image quality of the mechanically rotating catheters. A more detailed description of the differences among catheters and their benefits and limitations can be found in a review by Bom and colleagues.[12]

The observations from IVUS imaging that are demonstrated in this book were obtained primarily with three mechanical rotating systems. Most of the histologic comparisons and the early work in interventional cardiology were performed between 1986 and 1993 with the InterTherapy® device. After 1994, the ultrasound studies were performed with the CVIS® device or the Hewlett–Packard machine.

IVUS IMAGES PROVIDE 'BREADLOAF' CUTS OF AN ARTERY

No matter which IVUS device is used, the images portrayed are perpendicular cross-sections of the artery along the length of the vessel as the catheter is advanced or withdrawn (*Fig. 1.2*). The catheters can be manually advanced over a guidewire and held in place while a particular segment of the artery is being interrogated, or the device can be attached to a mechanical pull-back sled that withdraws the catheter at a set rate, usually 0.5 or 1 mm/second. An average IVUS study takes approximately 1–3 minutes, depending on the type of information that one

Intracoronary ultrasound (30 MHz)

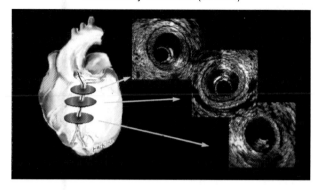

Figure 1.2 *Continuous intracoronary ultrasound images are obtained perpendicular to the long axis of the artery as the catheter is advanced or withdrawn within the lumen.*

attempts to obtain. The grayscale images provided are similar to a low-power microscopic cross-section of an artery. The interface of the lumen and the intima is often defined clearly enough to provide measurements of the lumen diameter and area. In addition, the plaque can frequently be identified separately from the adventitia so that the depth and cross-sectional area of the plaque can be outlined (*Fig. 1.3*). Several studies have demonstrated excellent correlations between ultrasound images and histologic preparations.[13–20] The lumen diameter and perimeter are usually easy to appreciate and measure with the trackball provided with the machine. If the boundary of the lumen is unclear, saline can be injected through the guiding catheter to clear the blood reflections from the lumen. As distinguished

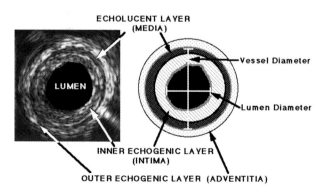

Figure 1.3 *The boundaries of a typical intravascular ultrasound image are compared with a schematic of the corresponding histologic structures.*

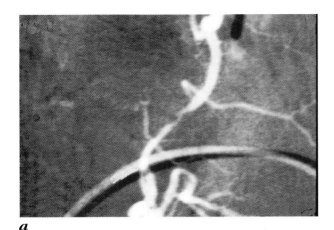
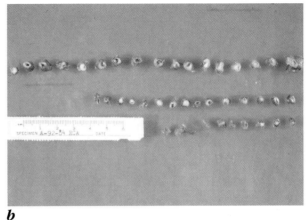

a   *b*

Figure 1.4 *(a) A digital subtraction angiogram of the right coronary artery reveals a tight stenosis in the mid portion. (b) The corresponding pathologic specimen obtained by cutting the artery in 5 mm segments from the ostium to the posterior descending and posterolateral branches.*

from the lumen, the diameter and area of the 'vessel' are defined in IVUS parlance as the outer boundary of the media–adventitia boundary. This definition has been chosen because it may be difficult to separate the plaque from the media on an IVUS image. The total plaque area is then obtained by subtracting the lumen area from the vessel area.

IVUS IMAGES PROVIDE DIRECT OBSERVATIONS IN VIVO OF ATHEROSCLEROTIC PATHOLOGY

Angiography has been, and will continue to be, the primary mode of imaging coronary artery disease and guiding interventional procedures. However, when we look at an angiogram, we often forget that it shows just the lumen of the vessel and does not directly show us the pathology, namely the atherosclerotic plaque. If the plaque impinges on the lumen then the indentation is used as a measure of the severity of the atherosclerosis. This method may lead to a false sense of security for several reasons. Because the lumen edges of an angiogram may have a smooth border, we assume that there is not a lot of disease in the vessel.[21] Pathologic studies demonstrate that the amount of atherosclerosis is underrepresented by angiography.[22–28] In *Fig. 1.4a* the angiogram of a right coronary artery (RCA) demonstrates severe stenosis in the mid-portion, but it was felt that the rest of the artery did not have significant

disease. Unfortunately, this patient did not survive an intervention of balloon angioplasty for the mid-RCA stenosis (this study was performed before stents became available). The corresponding pathologic cross-sections (see *Fig. 1.4b*) were taken every 5 mm along the length of the RCA and the posterior descending and posterior lateral branches. The diffuse nature of atherosclerosis is revealed in every cross-section.

Although this phenomenon was counter-intuitive for most angiographers, it became more readily accepted throughout the 1980s with the concept of vascular remodeling and compensatory dilatation that was proposed by Glagov and colleagues.[29] In their postmortem study of 125 left main coronary arteries, it was demonstrated that as the amount of atherosclerosis increased, the outer diameter of the vessel increased but the lumen remained constant until approximately 40% of the cross-sectional area was filled with plaque. At that point the outer dimension could not enlarge adequately to compensate for the increase in plaque area and so the lumen narrowed until it was finally recognized as diseased on angiography. As demonstrated in *Fig. 1.5*, the lumens from artery sections 1, 2, 3 and 4 would all appear to be the same on angiography, and all four would erroneously be considered normal. In distinction to angiography, IVUS looks beyond the lumen and reflects information directly about the pathology within the arterial wall. Thus, IVUS can distinguish normal from progressive stages of atherosclerosis in vivo.[8] IVUS studies confirm that arteries frequently expand radially as the plaque enlarges while

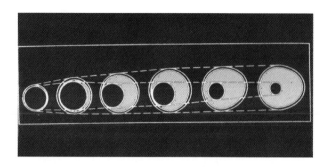

Figure 1.5 *Compensatory dilatation demonstrated schematically for a series of left main coronary arteries.*

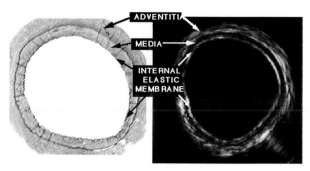

Figure 1.7 *A histologic presentation of a normal human coronary artery (left) is compared with the intravascular ultrasound image obtained in vitro at the same cross-section.*

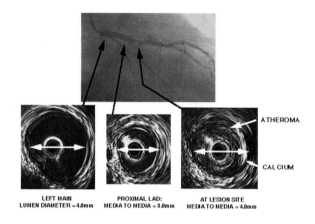

Figure 1.6 *Compensatory dilatation observed in vivo with intravascular ultrasound imaging.*

of IVUS images and corresponding histologic cross-sections demonstrate that the first reflection in a normal artery is due to the presence of the internal elastic membrane. In a normal human artery the endothelium is only one cell layer thick and is not a significant contributor to the ultrasound image. As intimal hyperplasia develops, the reflections from the collagen matrix help to compose the first ultrasound ring. The middle echolucent layer appears black on the ultrasound image because it corresponds to the smooth muscle cells of the media. At the periphery there is a second echogenic layer composed of the reflections from the external elastic membrane and the large collagen content of the adventitia.

AS INTIMAL PROLIFERATION PROGRESSES, ULTRASOUND IMAGES REFLECT THE CHANGE IN ELASTIC TISSUE AND COLLAGEN

maintaining the lumen cross-sectional area so that adequate blood flow is provided (*Fig. 1.6*).

CORRELATION BETWEEN IVUS AND HISTOLOGY: NORMAL HUMAN CORONARY ARTERIES HAVE A THREE-LAYER APPEARANCE

On IVUS imaging, a normal human coronary artery has a three-layer appearance consisting of an inner echoreflective (or white) ring, an echolucent (or black) middle zone, and an echogenic outer white band (*Fig. 1.7*).[30] Ultrasound waves are reflected from collagen and elastin fibers and are not reflected well from smooth muscle cells. Side-by-side comparisons

In our comparison studies, IVUS images and corresponding histologic cross-sections were analyzed in over 300 non-selected autopsy specimens. As the human artery gets older, the thickness of the intima increases (*Fig. 1.8*).[30] All males over the age of 13 demonstrate intimal hyperplasia. Fibrous tissue in the intimal matrix is a good echo reflector; it frequently shows a speckled black and white pattern. A small amount of intimal hyperplasia makes it easier to distinguish media from the plaque.[31,32] The ability to distinguish the layers of an artery with IVUS depends not only on the amount of intimal thickness but also on whether the internal elastic membrane is present

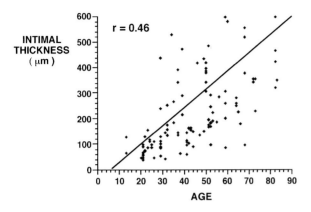

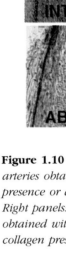

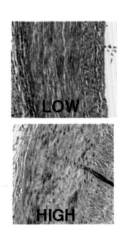

Figure 1.8 *Graph of age vs. intimal thickness from an unselected autopsy series.*

Figure 1.10 *Left panels: histologic cross sections of two arteries obtained with elastin stains demonstrating the presence or absence of the internal elastic membrane. Right panels: histologic cross sections of two arteries obtained with trichrome stains to identify the amount of collagen present in the media.*

and on the ratio of smooth muscle cells to collagen within the media.[33,34] With increasing age, the amount of internal elastic membrane diminishes, although there is wide variability, and is partly dependent on the amount of plaque that is present (*Fig. 1.9*). With increasing age there is also more deposition of collagen within the muscular media layer (*Fig. 1.10*). In the trichrome stains in *Fig. 1.10* (right panels), media muscle cells stain red and collagen stains blue. The panels on the left are stained for elastin to identify the internal elastic membrane. As the plaque matures and becomes calcified, there may be destruction of the media layer at the base of the plaque.[35,36] These variables have a direct influence on the ability to perceive a three-layer appearance on an ultrasound

image. As intimal hyperplasia develops, a three-layer appearance can be seen if the media is echolucent or if the internal elastic membrane is still present. However, if both the internal elastic membrane is absent and there is destruction of the media or increased collagen content in the media, then only a two-layer appearance is seen on the ultrasound image (*Fig. 1.11*).

These factors can affect the appearance of the ultrasound image along the length of an artery or even within the same cross-section. As shown in *Fig. 1.12*,

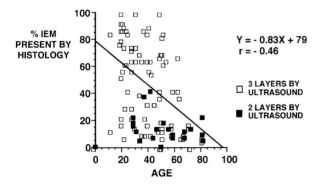

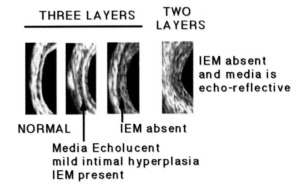

Figure 1.9 *Graph of age vs. the circumferential percent of internal elastic membrane (IEM) present on histologic cross sections.*

Figure 1.11 *Intravascular ultrasound images of different patterns which produce two or three apparent layers to the artery wall. IEM, internal elastic membrane.*

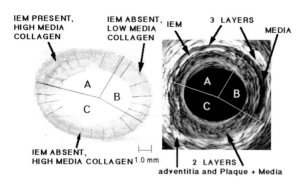

Figure 1.12 *Variation in the two or three layer appearance of an intravascular ultrasound image (right) compared with the corresponding histologic cross-section (left). IEM, internal elastic membrane.*

there is a three-layer appearance in segment A due to the presence of the internal elastic membrane, even though the media is not very echolucent because of the high content of collagen. In segment B, the internal elastic membrane is absent, but there still is a three-layer appearance because the media in that segment has a low content of collagen and therefore appears black, separating the echogenic adventitia from the less echogenic intimal plaque. In segment C, there is both destruction of the internal elastic membrane and a high content of collagen in the media, and so only two layers are visualized. The echogenicity of adventitia is usually higher than that of plaque (unless calcium is present), so that the outline of the plaque can still be seen at the boundary with the adventitia. For research purposes there is some distinction made between measurements of the plaque, which are outlined at the inner boundary of the media and measurements of the plaque plus media, which are outlined at the external elastic membrane (i.e. at the interface of the adventitia). These distinctions are rather esoteric and are not particularly relevant for the clinician who wants to know the size of the lumen, grossly the amount of plaque, and the media-to-media dimensions of the vessel. How these measurements are used in coronary interventions is discussed later.

IVUS PROVIDES INFORMATION ABOUT PLAQUE COMPOSITION

When IVUS images are analyzed side by side with the histologic samples of the tissue from which they have

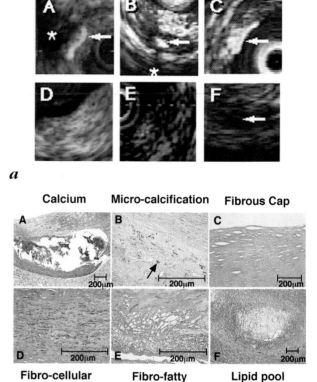

Figure 1.13 *Six histologic types of plaque (b) are compared with their corresponding representation by intravascular ultrasound imaging (a).*

been obtained, there are certain descriptive patterns that may be helpful in distinguishing the type of tissue that is present.[37] The process of identifying the composition of the plaque by the ultrasound picture pattern is called tissue characterization.[38–40] As demonstrated in *Fig. 1.13*, when histologic tissues are segregated into six general types (calcification, microcalcification, fibrous acellular tissue, fibrous cellular tissue, fibrous fatty tissue and fatty tissue), the corresponding ultrasound pictures demonstrate the following characteristics:

(a) calcium has the unique characteristic of being intensely echoreflective at the initial interface with drop-out of echoes peripherally; this is termed 'shadowing' (see *Fig. 1.13A*);

(b) microcalcification can be identified as a very small area, 0.1–0.2 mm in diameter with intense echoreflections and a small radiating arc of shadowing behind it (see *Fig. 1.13B*);

(c) a fibrous acellular capsule appears on ultrasound as an intense echoreflection, which may be equal to or greater than the adventitia echogenicity, but is distinguished from calcification because there is no shadowing behind it (see *Fig. 1.13C*).

The next three categories show a more mixed pattern:

(d) mixed cellularity interspersed within fibrous tissue is depicted on ultrasound images as a homogenous black and white speckled pattern with moderate echogenicity (see *Fig. 1.13D*);

(e) as fatty elements increase within the plaque, the echogenicity decreases, as reflected in the fibrous fatty plaque seen in *Fig. 1.13E*, which has more black or echolucent areas within the echogenic fibrous tissue;

(c) a large deposition of lipid within the body of the plaque is more likely to be represented by a homogenous echolucent zone (see *Fig. 1.13F*).

IVUS IS SENSITIVE FOR IDENTIFYING CALCIUM BUT IS LESS RELIABLE FOR DISTINGUISHING FIBROUS PLAQUES FROM FATTY PLAQUES

Most investigators report a high sensitivity with IVUS for identifying calcium as a hyperechogenic area with shadowing.[41–43] Unfortunately, the ability of IVUS to distinguish fibrous tissue from fatty tissue is less exact, with sensitivity of the order of 50% (*Table 1.1*).[44] This is more evident when ultrasound images are interpreted independently than when histology and ultrasound images are viewed side by side in a

Table 1.1
Sensitivity of intravascular ultrasound for detection of plaque components

	Ultrasound descriptors		
Histologic class	Echogenic with shadow	Echogenic without shadow	Hypo-echogenic
Calcified	91%	9%	0%
Fibrous	0%	50%	50%
Fatty	0%	60%	40%

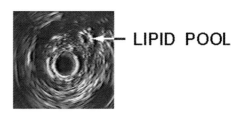

Figure 1.14 *Tissue characterization. Drop out of echoes within a plaque due to lipid accumulation demonstrated by intravascular ultrasound imaging.*

non-blinded manner. Atherosclerotic plaques often have a mixed tissue composition of lipid and fibrous tissue, and IVUS technology is simply not sensitive enough at the current time to make those fine distinctions. It would be beneficial if IVUS images could accurately identify those plaques that have a thin fibrous capsule and a lipid-rich core that is ripe for rupture (*Fig. 1.14*).[45,46] Unfortunately, the sensitivity for identifying these plaques is limited at present and we have not used this information to treat a plaque pre-emptively solely on the basis of the tissue components of a lipid core.

IVUS MACHINES PRODUCED BY DIFFERENT MANUFACTURERS MAY PORTRAY THE SAME CROSS-SECTION DIFFERENTLY

Aficionados of IVUS are sometimes confused by differences in interpretation or quantitative measurements reported in the literature. To a large extent, many of these inconsistencies can be explained by differences in the machines that were used for these studies. To assess this variability, we analyzed in a blinded manner the IVUS images of the same arterial sections in vitro from machines of four different companies and compared these images with histologic sections.[47] There can be a significant difference in the image presentation, recognition of a two- or three-layer appearance of the artery, the amount of plaque present, and the composition of the plaque as interpreted from these images (*Fig. 1.15*). These observations were made in 1994, and the technology of several of these devices has improved dramatically since then. *Figure 1.16* demonstrates the quality of a current synthetic aperture ultrasound device. There is

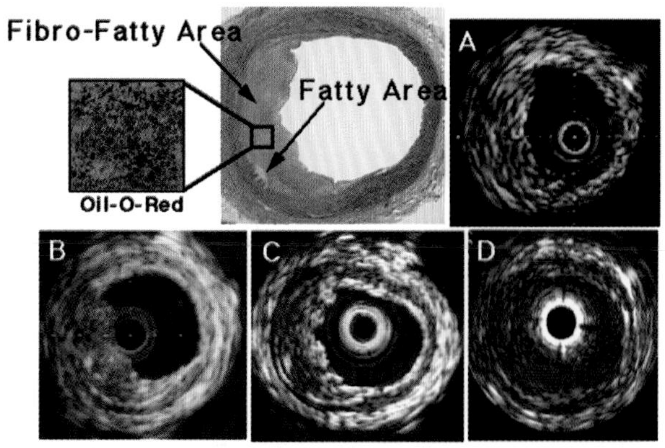

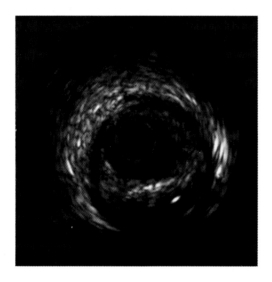

Figure 1.15 *The same cross-sectional area of plaque was imaged in vitro by four different intravascular ultrasound machines.*

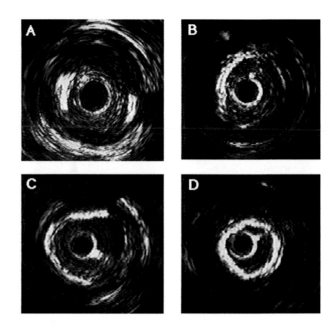

Figure 1.17 *Different patterns of coronary artery calcification represented by intravascular ultrasound as intense white reflections with shadowing peripherally.*

Figure 1.16 *An intravascular ultrasound image obtained with a synthetic aperture device in 1998.*

significant improvement in resolution and ability to recognize plaque boundary, media, and tissue components.

IVUS IDENTIFIES CALCIUM ON A MICROANATOMIC SCALE

One important observation of IVUS is the recognition of a higher prevalence of plaque calcification than is appreciated by angiography.[48–50] Angiography identifies calcium at the site of a stenosis in only 15% of cases

whereas some degree of calcium is seen by ultrasound in up to 85% of these stenoses. The high sensitivity for depicting calcified areas of plaque has been useful in demonstrating the various anatomical positions of calcium throughout the length of an artery.[51,52] As shown in *Fig. 1.17*, calcified areas of intense echogenicity with shadowing frequently occur at the base of the plaque but may subtend a variable circumference. *Figure 1.17d* shows calcified plaque at the lumen–plaque interface. These types of plaque are very resistant to balloon dilatation alone and impede stent expansion. When calcification is seen at the lumen–plaque interface, a technique such as rotational atherectomy is usually necessary. Understanding the composition and biomechanical hardness of the plaque may be very useful when deciding what type of interventional device should be used.

IVUS IS SENSITIVE FOR THE LENGTH OF ARC OF CALCIFIED PLAQUE BUT NOT ITS DEPTH

The sensitivity of intravascular ultrasound for identifying calcium is a double-edged sword. In a histologic comparison study in which the amount of calcium was

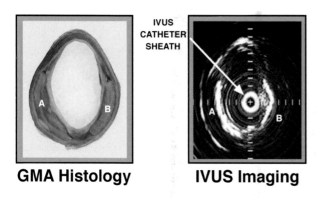

GMA Histology   **IVUS Imaging**

Figure 1.18 *A calcified artery was imaged by intravascular ultrasound (IVUS) (right panel) then embedded in plastic to obtain accurate histologic cross sections without tearing artifacts. GMA, glycomethyl methacrylate.*

accurately preserved by embedding the plaques in a plastic (methyl methacrylate), IVUS was shown to be sensitive for identifying the presence of calcium and for measuring the calcified plaque length of arc.[53] In *Fig. 1.18*, the calcified plaque stains blue; IVUS is accurate in showing the length of arc around the circumference of the individual calcified plaque segments. However, because calcium reflects ultrasound so well, it inhibits penetration distally and is incapable of accurately revealing the depth of the plaque. As seen in *Fig. 1.19*, although the plaque in the histology section on the right is twice as large as the plaque in the first panel, the ultrasound images cannot distinguish a difference in the depth of these calcified plaques. IVUS underestimates the area of plaque on average by 39%.

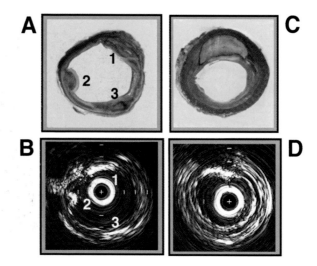

Figure 1.19 *Histologic sections of plastic embedded calcified arteries (a, c) compared with their corresponding intravascular ultrasound images (b, d).*

intervals for histologic analysis and half the arteries were burned to an ash to measure the residual calcium phosphate. The results demonstrated that, although IVUS and ultrafast CT are similarly sensitive for identifying the presence of calcium, IVUS underestimates the amount of calcium compared to ultrafast CT (*Fig. 1.20*). On the other hand, ultrafast CT underestimates the volume of fibro-fatty plaque as compared with intravascular ultrasound which correlates more closely with histology.

IVUS AND ELECTRON BEAM COMPUTED TOMOGRAPHY ARE COMPARABLE IN THEIR SENSITIVITY FOR IDENTIFYING CALCIUM

Although fluoroscopy or cine angiography underestimates the presence of calcium, electron beam computed tomography (ultrafast CT) is very sensitive for identifying calcium in atherosclerotic plaques.[54–58] In an in vitro study performed to determine how IVUS compares with ultrafast CT for identifying calcium and plaque, 20 atherosclerotic arterial samples were imaged in vitro by IVUS and then placed in a chest phantom and imaged by ultrafast CT.[58] Half of the arteries were sectioned at 1 mm

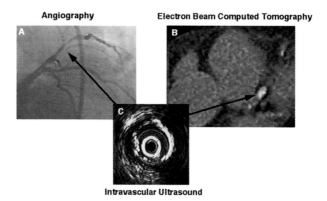

Angiography   **Electron Beam Computed Tomography**

Intravascular Ultrasound

Figure 1.20 *A comparison of three imaging modalities for identification of plaque dimensions and amount of calcium.*

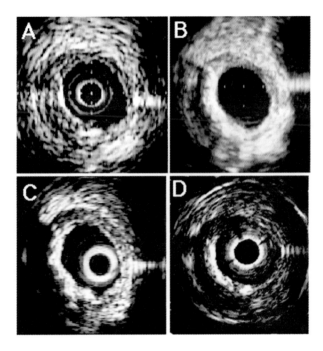

Figure 1.21 *The same cross-section of an artery in vitro was imaged by four intravascular ultrasound machines. The identification and quantification of the amount of calcified plaque is very variable.*

THE REPRESENTATION OF CALCIUM IS ALSO MACHINE DEPENDENT

Just as different machines portray plaque composition and plaque cross-sectional area differently, the identification of calcified plaque as well as the volume of calcified plaque varies with the type of intravascular

Necrotic Lipid Pool

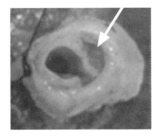 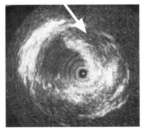

Figure 1.22 *An area of plaque filled with lipid or necrotic tissue can be confused with a calcified area with peripheral shadowing.*

ultrasound machine used.[44,47] In *Fig. 1.21a* the same arterial cross-section was imaged by four different ultrasound machines. The intensity of the echo reflection from calcium and the amount of peripheral shadowing are quite different in these four pictures. On a quantitative basis (see *Fig. 1.21b*), there is also a statistically different estimation of calcified cross-sectional area of plaque among the four devices.

Occasionally, a necrotic or lipid pool can be misinterpreted as a calcified plaque because of the intense echo reflections from the fibrous capsule and dropout of echoes caused by the large amount of lipid or necrotic liquid material within the plaque. The distinction is that there is a small amount of echo reflection from the fibrous tissue at the base of the plaque (*Fig. 1.22*). This type of plaque, although it appears to be calcified, would actually respond very nicely to expansion and stent insertion. On the other hand, a procedure such as atherectomy that would remove the fibrous plaque might be complicated by the release of a large amount of thrombogenic material from the lipid pool.

FRESH THROMBUS HAS TYPICAL CHARACTERISTICS THAT CAN BE IDENTIFIED BY IVUS

IVUS has been useful for identifying thrombus in vivo when it may not be suspected by angiography.[59] The tissue characteristics that are helpful in identifying thrombus are:

(a) the presence of a mobile mass of echoes within the lumen or an echoreflective cord waving in the blood flow; or
(b) scintillating reflections (i.e. echoes that appear to sparkle even with the catheter in a stationary position).

These types of presentation are most commonly seen with fresh thrombus. It is much more difficult to diagnose a mural thrombus because the thrombus becomes organized and more adherent to the wall of the artery. Occasionally, a small layered echo structure along the wall or in an ulcerated plaque will move, consistent with a mural thrombus. Angioscopy is more sensitive than IVUS for identifying the presence of thrombus in stable or unstable angina.[60–63] Since the recognition of thrombus by IVUS is often dependent on its motion, it is hard to

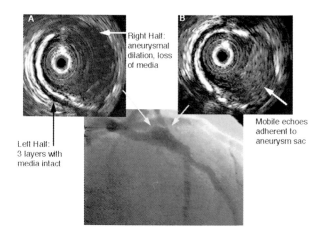

Figure 1.23 *An aneurysmally dilated artery with a mural thrombus identified by intravascular ultrasound imaging.*

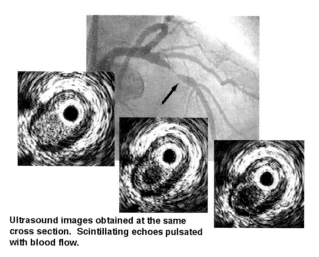

Figure 1.24 *Intravascular ultrasound representation of recent thrombus.*

demonstrate what thrombus looks like in a single-frame ultrasound image. *Figures 1.23* and *1.24* show representative examples of how a thrombus appears in a stop frame mode. A videotape format is necessary to appreciate the dramatic nature of the mobile mass of echoes. In general, the interpretation of any IVUS image is significantly enhanced when seen in real-time video format.

The angiogram in *Fig. 1.23* is from a patient who presented with an acute myocardial infarction. Instead of finding an occluded vessel we were surprised to see patent arteries but a large aneurysm in the proximal left anterior descending artery (LAD). We were about to dilate a distal intermediate stenosis when we decided to do pre-intervention ultrasound imaging. The ultrasound study in *Fig. 1.23a* revealed an unusual arterial architecture. The left half of the artery had a three-layer ultrasound appearance consistent with a thin rim of intima, media, and adventitia. Between 12 o'clock and 6 o'clock there was loss of the three-layer appearance with aneurysmal dilatation owing to absence of the media in this part of the artery. Of note on the ultrasound images was the lack of any significant lumen narrowing or atherosclerosis. The ultrasound image of the aneurysm at the mid-section (*Fig. 1.23b*) showed the same wall architecture but, in addition, between 2 o'clock and 5 o'clock there was a mobile mass of echoes adherent to the aneurysm sac. This mass of echoes fluctuated with pulsatile blood flow.

Another distinguishing characteristic of echoes from a thrombus is that they cannot be washed away by an injection of saline through the guiding catheter. Our conclusion, after seeing these images, was that the patient's myocardial infarction was probably due to an embolic event from the thrombus in the aneurysm. Therefore, rather than dilating the intermediate lesion in the distal vessel, we elected to treat him with heparin and long-term warfarin therapy.

The case demonstrated in *Fig. 1.24* is a dramatic presentation of intraluminal thrombus.[59] The patient had presented a few days earlier with an acute myocardial infarction and had been treated with intravenous streptokinase. At the time of the angiogram the patient was asymptomatic. The angiogram revealed thrombolysis in myocardial infarction (TIMI) grade 3 flow, but there was also a significant residual stenosis in the proximal LAD. Although there did not appear to be any intraluminal defect on angiography IVUS imaging revealed the presence of bright, sparkling echoes in a mass-like structure between 6 o'clock and 9 o'clock just distal to the lesion. The mass of echoes cleared and recurred in association with the pulsatile blood flow, as demonstrated in the series of three ultrasound images that were obtained at the same position without moving the ultrasound catheter. Directional atherectomy was performed and histology confirmed that this structure was a thrombus.

SPONTANEOUS RUPTURE OF 'THE UNSTABLE PLAQUE' HAS BEEN OBSERVED IN VIVO BY IVUS

One desirable aspect of tissue characterization with IVUS would be the capacity to diagnose an unstable plaque. An unstable plaque has been described as a plaque with a large lipid component covered by a thin fibrous cap.[64,65] It has been hypothesized that one common method of plaque progression is spontaneous rupture of the fibrous capsule and thrombus formation as blood mixes with the thrombogenic lipid core.[66–68] This mechanism is also proposed as the cause of most acute myocardial infarctions if the thrombus is not impeded by lytic enzymes. Although plaque rupture occurs only sporadically, this phenomenon has been documented in vivo.[45,46] *Figure 1.25* shows the angiogram and IVUS image of the proximal left main artery in a patient who was being studied for consideration of angioplasty of the LAD. The ultrasound images in real time showed a mobile thrombus in the lumen of the left main artery; the thrombus was attached to a plaque with an echolucent core consistent with lipid. The plaque was not hemodynamically significant since it only subtended 30% of the available cross-sectional area, yet it had ruptured spontaneously. This IVUS observation is consistent with the suggestion that this is a sporadic but recurrent event in the progression of atherosclerosis as well as the immediate precipitating cause of acute ischemic syndromes.[68]

ARE 'SOFT ECHOES' EQUIVALENT TO 'SOFT TISSUE'? AN ULTRASOUND ASSESSMENT OF BIOMECHANICAL PROPERTIES IN ATHEROSCLEROTIC PLAQUE

The limitations in our ability to characterize the components of atherosclerotic plaque accurately led to some confusion in nomenclature. As distinct from calcified tissue, which is accurately represented by ultrasound as intense echo reflections with peripheral shadowing, the term 'soft echoes' has been used to refer to less echogenic plaques. Our concern is that the use of the term 'soft echoes' could be misinterpreted as suggesting that the plaque itself is soft. Although it may be softer than calcium, it is still hard

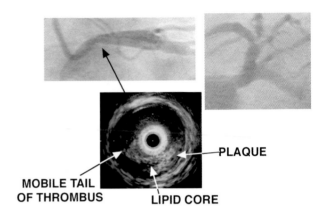

Figure 1.25 *Intravascular ultrasound identification of a vulnerable plaque with mobile tail of thrombus emanating from the lipid core.*

and may respond differently to interventional devices than truly soft lipid-filled plaque. When assessing arterial samples in vitro, we have always been struck by how firm the tissue feels. To test the biomechanical properties of plaque, 33 plaques were imaged with ultrasound and then placed in a unidirectional compression ergometer to measure the stress–strain relationship. Force was applied from the ergometer and the displacement of the tissue was measured at static equilibrium.[69] This study demonstrated that calcified plaque has a distinctive stiffness constant that is different from that of other types of plaque. However, there is significant overlap between plaques that were identified as fibrous (i.e. echogenic without shadowing) or fatty (i.e. hypoechogenic).

Given the limitations of resolution of intravascular ultrasound imaging at the present time, we feel comfortable using a nomenclature that distinguishes calcified from non-calcified plaque. But one must be cautious because non-calcified plaques are not necessarily 'soft' when we apply a balloon or atherectomy device. In general, non-calcified fibrotic plaques respond well to directional atherectomy. Another way of describing the images is to use the direct echo descriptors without any subjective interpretation:

(a) echogenic tissue with shadowing;
(b) echogenic without shadowing; or
(c) hypoechogenic plaque.

In general, these descriptors correspond to calcified tissue, non-calcified fibrous tissue, and fibrous tissue mixed with an increased lipid content.

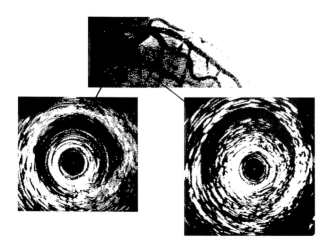

Figure 1.26 *'Napkin ring' stenosis: intravascular ultrasound identified a short significant stenosis in the mid LAD that was not appreciated by angiography.*

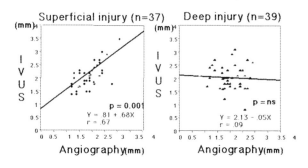

Figure 1.27 *Correlation between angiograms and intravascular ultrasound images when the treated lesion sites are segregated according to the presence of superficial or deep injury.*

A COMPARISON OF ANGIOGRAPHY AND IVUS – OR WHY ISN'T ANGIOGRAPHY GOOD ENOUGH?

Several in vitro and clinical studies have demonstrated that IVUS and angiographic measurements of lumen diameter correlate well when there is minimal disease or if the lumen is circular.[70] However, angiography can be misleading, especially when there is an overlap of vessels or if a short stenosis is present. *Figure 1.26* provides evidence for what has been called a 'napkin ring' stenosis.[71] This is a very short stenosis, only 1–2 mm in length, such that even in multiple angiographic projections, contrast is in front of or behind the stenosis; this makes the stenosis appear less significant than it is. On the angiogram of this patient, who was symptomatic, it appears that a mild stenosis is present in the proximal LAD. On IVUS imaging the real stenosis is in the mid-LAD where the ultrasound catheter is wedged into the speckled reverberations of plaque. The mid-LAD was treated with balloon angioplasty with relief of the patient's symptoms.

Angiography may also be misleading if the lumen topography is irregular. This frequently occurs after balloon dilatation where dissections may cause an overestimation of the benefit of angioplasty.[72–76] *Figure 1.27* summarizes the analysis of ultrasound measurements of lumen diameter compared with angiography following balloon dilatation. The lesions were separated on the basis of the ultrasound images

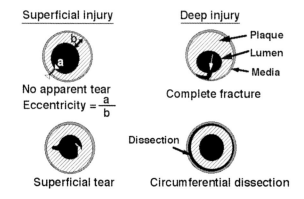

Figure 1.28 *Descriptors of plaque morphology by IVUS following balloon dilatation.*

into a group that had minimal tears or stretching of the artery (superficial injury) and a group that had more extensive dissection through to the media (deep injury) (*Fig. 1.28*). In the group with only stretching or minimal tears (superficial injury) there is a good correlation between angiography and IVUS diameter measurements, but in the group where there are extensive tears that extend to the media (deep injury), the correlation between ultrasound and angiography is much more disparate.[77] This discrepancy can be explained by the fact that contrast fills the dissection behind the plaque and makes it appear as if the diameter of the lumen is greater than what is measured by ultrasound imaging from within the vessel.

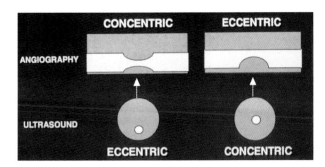

Figure 1.29 *A schematic drawing to demonstrate how angiography and ultrasound can present different descriptions of whether a lesion is eccentric or concentric.*

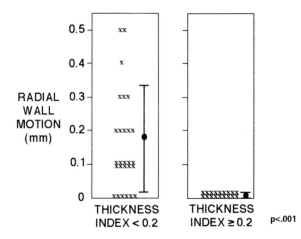

Figure 1.30 *The distensibility of the arterial wall depends on the relative thickness of the involved wall segment.*

Magnification and scaling errors reveal another major difference between angiography and IVUS in quantitative analysis.[78,79] With angiography, there are significant magnification assumptions when using the guiding catheter as the ruler. A 2.7 mm guide catheter represents only 11 pixels in a matrix of 640 × 480 pixels. Measurements of an artery edge can easily be off by 1 or 2 pixels, which for an artery between 1 and 4 mm is nearly 10% of the ruler. With IVUS imaging, the 'ruler' is inherent to the image and is based on the speed of sound in tissue at 37°C. These observations suggest that quantitative coronary angiography has been given too much credence. It is like trying to make a three-decimal-place accuracy out of a technique whose scale may be off by several tenths of a millimeter. We should not confuse the reproducibility that computerized measurements provide with accuracy in representing complex luminal topography.

Another area where there is disagreement between ultrasound and angiography is in the description of plaque eccentricity.[6,8,80] An angiogram that is described as showing a concentric lesion may, in fact, appear to be eccentric on cross-sectional imaging with ultrasound because the plaque itself is not visualized on the angiogram (*Fig. 1.29*). Conversely, an eccentric plaque by angiography may appear to be concentric on cross-sectional imaging with ultrasound. This discordance between angiography and ultrasound for the description of plaque eccentricity occurs in approximately 20% of lesions. This observation undermines the validity of this angiographic descriptor as a predictor of responses to coronary interventions.

ARTERIAL WALL DISTENSIBILITY IS A FUNCTION OF PLAQUE THICKNESS

One of the more curious observations provided by IVUS is the assessment of wall movement during systole and diastole.[81,82] During the cardiac cycle, the normal arterial wall moves by 5–15% of the diameter of the vessel (*Fig. 1.30*). As intimal thickness progresses, arterial distensibility decreases. When the plaque thickness is greater than 20% of the diameter of the vessel, that segment of artery wall does not move in response to pressure changes during the cardiac cycle. If a plaque is eccentric, ultrasound reveals that the uninvolved portion of the arterial wall continues to expand. If the intimal hyperplasia is concentric and the thickness is greater than 20% of the diameter, then the plaque has minimal or no motion until balloon dilatation is performed (see below on the mechanism of balloon angioplasty).

COMPLICATIONS OF IVUS

IVUS imaging has a low risk of complications provided certain precautions are observed. Although IVUS imaging is relatively atraumatic compared to balloon angioplasty and other devices, it must be remembered that it is still an invasive procedure and can create dissections, either from the guidewire or the ultrasound catheter. The IVUS catheter may also traumatize a stent, especially a coiled stent if a strut is caught by the plastic catheter.[83] In a self-reporting registry series of 2207 IVUS examinations, the most common problem was spasm or ischemia.[84] The incidence of spasm was 3.2% in non-transplant patients. This is most often seen when the catheter is advanced into a distal segment of the artery or when the catheter is passed through a tight stenosis before an intervention, thus restricting distal blood flow. This problem is quickly reversed by removing the catheter and infusing intracoronary nitroglycerin. After balloon angioplasty, the IVUS catheter can pick up a flap, especially if the guidewire is repositioned and has entered the false lumen. The treatment for this complication has been repeat balloon dilatation or insertion of a stent. However, acute myocardial infarction and death have been reported as resulting from this complication, which emphasizes that all operators need to be sensitive to these potential problems.

In the IVUS registry, major complications were reported most commonly when IVUS was used during coronary interventions as opposed to diagnostic procedures. The incidence of non-fatal myocardial infarction or emergency bypass surgery was approximately 0.2%, although in half of the cases it was unclear whether the complication was due to the ultrasound examination or the angioplasty itself. This registry information was obtained before the wide availability of stents.

One way of avoiding these complications is never to push the ultrasound catheter when there is resistance to its passage. This often happens when the short monorail catheters are advanced through a tortuous segment of vessel. Another clue that the ultrasound catheter is not passing smoothly is if separation of the catheter away from the guidewire in the aorta can be seen or if the guiding catheter backs out while the operator tries to advance the ultrasound catheter. The central lumen over-the-wire catheters are less traumatic and track the wire better. In models in which the wire is retracted and then reinserted through the distal end of the plastic sheath (such as the CVIS 2.9 Fr Microview), there is the potential for wire trauma during re-emergence of the guidewire from the distal end. Owing to these concerns for safety, our preference has been to use the 3.2 Fr monorail despite its larger size instead of the 2.9 Fr catheter.

IVUS imaging in transplant patients is a separate category that deserves special attention.[85,86] The denervated arteries in transplant patients are much more prone to spasm from the mechanical stimulation of the ultrasound device than other arteries are. Furthermore,

the arteries are less responsive to intracoronary nitroglycerin or calcium channel blockers, which makes the spasm potentially much more prolonged and may produce significant ischemia with profound hemodynamic compromise. In a series of 304 transplant arteries that were studied with IVUS imaging at the University of California, Los Angeles, the incidence of spasm with or without ST segment elevation on electrocardiogram was 19%. In addition, there were two patients who had a dissection that required balloon dilatation to compress the tear. Outside this series, we are aware of an unreported case of severe retrograde dissection with massive anterior wall infarction in a transplant patient that required a second transplant to salvage this life-threatening complication.

NEW DIRECTIONS IN IVUS IMAGING

Over the past few years, all the IVUS manufacturers have made significant progress in image quality. One of the major innovations has been the use of digital storage capabilities. In this mode, not only are the ultrasound images downloaded to videotape for later review, but the images are also immediately available for review from the computer hard drive. This preserves image quality, which is often lost in the process of analog conversion. The images are also immediately available for the operator to scroll through the database and select the images of interest. Specific frames can then be stored in separate memory. The digital format also enhances the ability to make on-line measurements. The digital images can be downloaded to removable compact disks, which can store multiple imaging runs. The digital format also facilitates the storage of measurements and formatting reports in a database; these can incorporate representative images as well as the measurements.

Another significant advance has been in the area of ultrasound catheter design. The catheters continue to be miniaturized. A 2.6 Fr monorail device has recently been released with a 40 MHz transducer. In addition, several of the companies have been working on an ultrasound imaging core which is 0.46 mm (0.018 inches) in diameter. This catheter, which is the size of a guidewire, could then be introduced through standard balloons for imaging both before and after interventional procedures. We may also see a resurgence of interest in devices that combine ultrasound imaging capabilities with interventional techniques. Although Yock and colleagues[87] produced a directional atherectomy catheter that incorporated ultrasound imaging for guidance, the development of this device was put on hold because of the decreased use of directed atherectomy by the interventional community. Now that plaque debulking has recaptured the imagination of some interventionalists, we may see a resurgence of interest in a combined atherectomy catheter with ultrasound guidance to enhance our ability to direct the device into the plaque and away from the free wall of the artery.

CORONARY INTERVENTIONS: IVUS INSIGHTS ON MECHANISMS OF ACTION

BALLOON ANGIOPLASTY

In vitro IVUS studies reveal plaque is torn at its thinnest segment or adjacent to a calcified zone

In vitro studies using IVUS before and after balloon dilatation of atherosclerotic segments help to identify the mechanism of action of balloon angioplasty. Histologic studies show that the plaque is frequently torn at its thinnest segment; if the plaque is calcified, the tear usually occurs at the junction of fibrous tissue and the calcified portion.[88–97] Compared with histologic assessment, IVUS has the benefit of being able to image the artery before balloon dilatation as well as after it.[15] IVUS images before and after balloon dilatation show that the lumen enlarges as a result of plaque tear and separation of the torn ends (*Fig. 1.31*). In addition, a new echolucent zone behind the plaque corresponds to dissection of the artery where the plaque is separated from the media. Occasionally, when larger balloons are used, the entire plaque may be rotated free from the media owing to torsional forces that leave an entire ring of dissection around the circumference of the plaque. These dissections do not necessarily result in collapse of the plaque into the artery because it may be supported at its proximal and distal ends to the vessel wall.

IVUS imaging after balloon dilatation in vivo reveals new insights compared to angiography

When IVUS imaging was initially applied to patients who had balloon angioplasty, some of the observa-

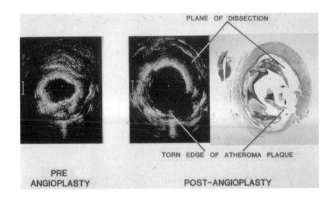

Figure 1.31 *A comparison of intravascular ultrasound images before (left panel) and after (middle panel) balloon angioplasty in vitro compared with the same histologic cross-section (right panel).*

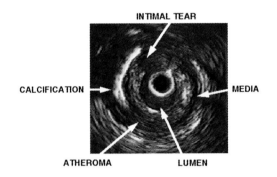

Figure 1.32 *Intravascular ultrasound image obtained in vivo following angiographically successful balloon angioplasty. The plaque is torn at the edge between fibrous and calcified tissue.*

tions were quite unexpected.[72,98] As opposed to the angiographic results, which suggested that a large lumen had been obtained, the usual finding with IVUS was that only a relatively small tear had occurred in the plaque with separation of the torn ends (*Fig. 1.32*). One was immediately impressed with the large amount of residual plaque that remained following balloon dilatation.[99] These observations helped our understanding of how easily restenosis could occur by elastic recoil and mild intimal proliferation. After seeing IVUS images, one wondered how balloon dilatation yielded as high a degree of long-term success as it did. It also suggested that animal studies that showed that restenosis was due primarily to intimal hyperplasia were misleading and that the major component of restenosis was probably due to elastic recoil and remodeling of the artery and less to intimal hyperplasia.[100,101] These hypotheses were later supported by serial clinical studies following directional atherectomy, which demonstrated that two-thirds of restenosis was due to adventitial contraction or 'negative remodeling' and only one-third of restenosis was explained by intimal proliferation.[102]

The second major observation on the mechanism of balloon dilatation was the change in the lumen area from systole to diastole once the plaque had been fractured by the balloon. Although the volume of plaque had not been altered by balloon dilatation, the lumen cross-sectional area was dramatically increased by pulsatile blood flow in diastole. The plaque acts as a scar that immobilizes the wall of the artery. By cutting the plaque, balloon dilatation permits increased mobility of the arterial wall in response to the change in lumen pressure, thus increasing blood flow.[75]

(c) a full-thickness tear with separation of the torn ends and a dissection behind the plaque extending for a variable length around the circumference of the artery;
(d) a dissection of 270° or more with separation of the plaque from the arterial wall, not necessarily causing collapse of the lumen depending on how the plaque is supported proximally and distally;
(e) a stretching effect without fracture of the plaque in a concentric plaque; and
(f) a stretching effect of balloon dilatation without fracture in an eccentric plaque where only the free wall is stretched.

It was initially hypothesized that these morphologic patterns might have a significant influence on restenosis, but further experience in several studies has not shown that plaque morphology following balloon dilatation influences restenosis (see Chapter 4).

There are six ultrasound patterns of morphologic response to percutaneous transluminal coronary angioplasty

The response to balloon dilatation can be separated arbitrarily into six patterns based on the presence and extent of plaque tears, dissection or stretching (*Fig. 1.33*).[98,103] These morphologic patterns can be briefly described as:

(a) a partial tear of the plaque not extending out to the media;
(b) a full-thickness tear of the plaque without dissection;

Ultrasound observations after percutaneous transluminal coronary angioplasty: appreciation of the plaque burden

There are two other noteworthy observations in IVUS imaging following balloon dilatation. The first is that at the level of a treated stenosis there is a large residual plaque burden with an average cross-sectional area of 8 mm². This mean residual plaque represents 62% of the total vessel cross-sectional area (defined as the area within the boundary of the media). Although it has always been recognized that balloon

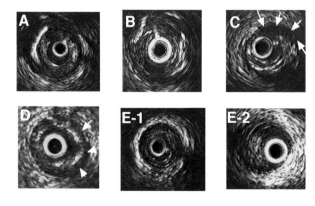

Figure 1.33 *Six different morphologic responses to balloon dilatation as represented by intravascular ultrasound imaging in vivo.*

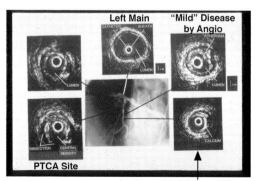

Figure 1.34 *The first human IVUS coronary study with InterTherapy catheter 1968.*

dilatation does not remove any plaque, it was instructive to visualize in vivo the minimal effect of balloon dilatation despite a successful angiographic response.

The second quantitative observation was that in the so-called normal angiographic segment, the mean plaque burden measured by IVUS equals 35% of the vessel cross-sectional area.[98,104] The images in *Fig. 1.34* are from the first human intracoronary study performed with an InterTherapy IVUS catheter in 1988.[37] After balloon dilatation in the proximal LAD, the ultrasound images from the angiographically normal section of the mid LAD demonstrate a circular lumen with normal dimensions due to compensatory dilatation, but the amount of plaque or calcium in the wall of the artery is not appreciated by angiography.[105–107] These observations in vivo are consistent with the pathologic studies of Glacov and colleagues.[29]

These insights provided by IVUS had a significant impact on the way that we, as interventional cardiologists, interpreted angiograms. We began to estimate a greater degree of atherosclerosis even when there was only minimal indentation on the angiogram. When we review an angiogram now, we project in the mind's eye what the likely pathology would be by IVUS and understand the extensive plaque thickening that is required before even a minimal lesion is seen by angiography. This is one of the subtle learning processes that influences our interpretation of an interventional procedure and affects our decision-making process during our interventions, as discussed in later sections.

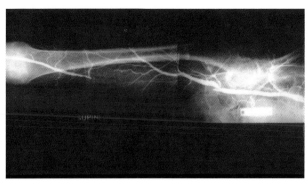

a

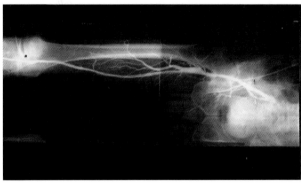

b

Figure 1.35 *Peripheral angiograms of a superficial femoral artery demonstrate a 22 cm long occlusion (a) and successful recanalization and balloon dilatation (b).*

IVUS reveals the mechanism of recanalization for chronic total obstructions

Chronic total arterial occlusions can be some of the most challenging obstructions to treat. Whether in the periphery or in the coronary circulation, the obstructions are usually calcified and resistant to probing with a guidewire. Even if a guidewire passes through the chronic occlusion, standard forms of therapy, such as balloon dilatation or rotational atherectomy, have a high rate of restenosis.[108] Stent deployment in these obstructions has improved the acute and long-term results.[109] Observations with IVUS help us understand the difficulties in treating chronic total occlusions. We have studied over 100 patients with chronic total occlusions of the superficial femoral artery.[110] These occlusions may be as long as 30 cm before the artery reconstitutes, usually at the level of the abductor canal (*Fig. 1.35*). These obstructions can be mechanically

probed with a guidewire and catheter, initially from an antegrade approach from the common femoral artery. If necessary, the patient can be placed in a prone position and a retrograde puncture of the popliteal artery can be used to probe the occluded segment. After mechanically re-establishing a channel through the occluded segment, an IVUS catheter can be advanced over a guidewire in the newly created lumen. In the majority of the cases we see a double lumen with the IVUS device passing through the newly created lumen between the plaque and the media (*Fig. 1.36*).[111] These observations indicate that the pathway of recanalization usually does not pass through the center of the plaque to find the old lumen, but instead travels along the side of the artery until the plaque thins out or a distal dissection permits re-entry into the distal lumen.[112]

To test this hypothesis, an in vitro series of experiments was performed using completely occluded human arteries obtained following amputation.[113] A

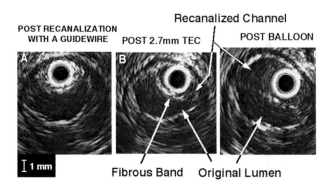

POST RECANALIZATION WITH A GUIDEWIRE POST 2.7mm TEC Recanalized Channel POST BALLOON

Fibrous Band   Original Lumen

Figure 1.36 *Intravascular ultrasound images following recanalization of a chronic total occlusion in a superficial femoral artery reveals the pathway that the recanalization guidewire has taken. TEC, transluminal extraction catheter.*

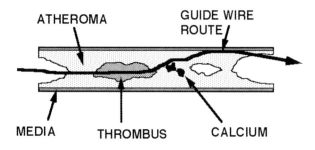

ATHEROMA   GUIDE WIRE ROUTE

MEDIA   THROMBUS   CALCIUM

Figure 1.38 *Schematic representation of the pathway of least resistance for guidewires attempting to recanalize occluded arteries as interpreted from the intravascular ultrasound images.*

guidewire and catheter were passed from the proximal to the distal segment with successful re-entry of the guidewire at the distal end. To document the pathway of recanalization, a silk suture was tied to the distal end of the guidewire, the guidewire was withdrawn and the silk suture was tied in place after being pulled back throughout the length of the recanalized segment. The arterial segments were then prepared for histology and cut in a serial breadloaf fashion. The histologic sections revealed that, instead of the guidewire going through the center of the plaque to re-establish a channel, the majority of the guidewires entered a dissection plane between the plaque and media, similar to the position found with IVUS cross-sectional analysis in vivo (*Fig. 1.37*).

These observations suggest that the main mechanism of recanalization of chronically occluded arteries is for the guidewires and catheters to take the pathway of least resistance around calcified or fibrotic plaque (*Fig. 1.38*). Instead of going through the central portion of the plaque, the guidewires enter the natural dissection plane between the plaque and media. This is the plane that is used in surgical dissections, such as the removal of plaque during carotid endarterectomies. Instead of surgical blunt dissection with forceps, the interventionalist performs a blunt dissection with a guidewire and catheter. The guidewire may continue along this plane for 1–30 cm before it perforates the artery, re-enters the lumen distally, or continues to stay in the dissection plane until a guidewire (antegrade or retrograde) enters the true distal lumen. In this context, the high rate of restenosis in chronic total occlusions with balloon dilatation or rotational atherectomy is understandable since the plaque is pushed to the side by the new channel but is susceptible to elastic recoil. Stent deployment in this setting has a lower rate of restenosis because it maintains the integrity of the new lumen and inhibits the elastic recoil from the adventitia and media.

DIRECTIONAL ATHERECTOMY

The high rate of restenosis with directional atherectomy is due to its similarity to balloon dilatation

IVUS has provided significant insights into the mechanism of action of directional coronary atherectomy

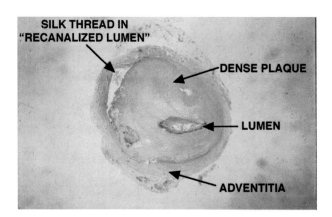

SILK THREAD IN "RECANALIZED LUMEN"

DENSE PLAQUE

LUMEN

ADVENTITIA

Figure 1.37 *Histologic cross section of an occluded tibial artery used to identify the pathway of recanalization of chronic total occlusions.*

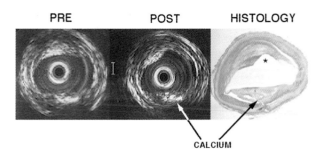

Figure 1.39 *In vitro intravascular ultrasound images before and after directional atherectomy compared with the same cross-section of the artery after histologic preparation.*

(DCA) and helps us to understand why the restenosis rate of early trials, such as CAVEAT, were so high.[114-127] In vitro studies have demonstrated that IVUS is as accurate as histology in identifying the amount of material that is removed by DCA (*Fig. 1.39*).[128] When the angiographic results of DCA are compared with those of IVUS, some important lessons of this technology are revealed.[129] *Figure 1.40* shows a severe stenosis in the mid-LAD, which was successfully treated with DCA. The ultrasound image shows that the catheter before DCA has been wedged into the plaque. This emphasizes that the lower limit of lumen measurements by IVUS is the size of the catheter (about 1.0 mm in diameter). Angiography is more accurate for measuring minimal lumen diameter before an intervention; however, IVUS permits us to measure the plaque cross-sectional area bounded by the media both before and after an intervention. After atherectomy, the lumen in *Fig. 1.40* is significantly enlarged, but if the diameter of the vessel is measured from media to media, the vessel is significantly enlarged by stretching, as occurs with balloon dilatation. *Figure 1.41* shows a successful DCA by angiography; IVUS again reveals that a significant amount of the plaque has been removed, but not the two calcified segments of plaque at 9 o'clock and 3 o'clock.[130]

Figure 1.42 represents another example of a successful angiographic result with DCA, but in this case the ultrasound study demonstrates that only a very small amount of plaque has been removed despite multiple passes. This example emphasizes that angiography may overestimate the debulking or atherectomy component of DCA. It should be noted that DCA with IVUS guidance is performed in an iterative fashion;[131] after an adequate number of cuts with the DCA device, IVUS is performed and the DCA

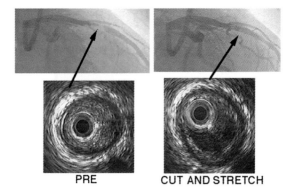

Figure 1.40 *Angiograms and associated intravascular ultrasound images obtained before and after directional atherectomy. The angiograms demonstrate lumen improvement but the ultrasound images reveal the mechanism is a combination of balloon stretching of the vessel as well as removal of part of the plaque.*

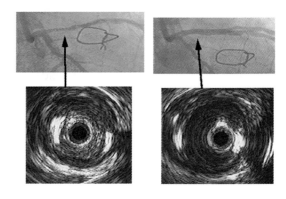

Figure 1.41 *Successful directional atherectomy by angiography and by ultrasound. Note that the calcified plaques at the 3-o'clock and 9-o'clock positions have not been removed.*

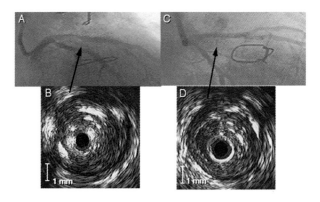

Figure 1.42 *Successful directional atherectomy by angiography but inadequate plaque removal demonstrated by intravascular ultrasound images.*

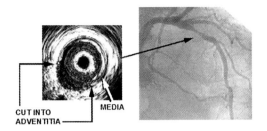

Figure 1.43 *Intravascular ultrasound imaging may reveal excessive removal of tissue during directional atherectomy procedures.*

device is reinserted and directed to the quadrants that reveal residual plaque by IVUS. In addition, if IVUS reveals that a section of plaque has been removed from the artery wall and only the media and adventitia remain, then the DCA device is directed away from those quadrants.[132]

Figure 1.43 shows that, unlike angiography, IVUS can identify when the media or adventitia has been removed by DCA. This method of IVUS-guided DCA therefore improves the safety of the procedure as well as maximizing the amount of material that is removed. Despite this attempt to maximize plaque removal, the observations from IVUS imaging reveal that the cutting effect of DCA accounts for 60% of the new lumen, whereas the stretching effect accounts for approximately 40% of the new lumen (*Fig. 1.44*). In the CAVEAT trial,[115] IVUS imaging was not used and it is likely that even a greater amount of plaque

was left behind than was appreciated by angiography.[116] The stretching effect would have been even more significant in this study which may help explain why the restenosis rate was 50% as opposed to 57% by balloon angioplasty alone. With this new awareness, other DCA trials were designed to be more aggressive. In the OARS trial,[133] directional atherectomy was optimized and the restenosis rate was significantly reduced to 29%. In the ABACAS trial,[134] IVUS imaging was used to guide the atherectomy so that a residual plaque cross-sectional area of 47% was left. This resulted in a restenosis rate of 21%. These observations have led to a renewed interest in debulking before stenting (see Chapter 19).

EXCIMER LASER ANGIOPLASTY

IVUS reveals that excimer laser therapy removes only a minimal amount of atherosclerotic tissue

Between 1989 and 1993 there was much enthusiasm for excimer laser angioplasty, despite the fact that there were no randomized controlled trials to demonstrate any improved efficacy beyond balloon angioplasty alone.[135-140] Based on our observations with IVUS imaging, we were not so optimistic about the benefit of the excimer laser devices as they were currently configured.[141] *Figure 1.45* demonstrates the result of an excimer laser angioplasty plus balloon dilatation that was considered to be a successful result in the era before stents. *Figure 1.46* demonstrates an angiogram of a diffusely diseased LAD following excimer laser treatment. The ultrasound images reveal only small nicks in the circumferential

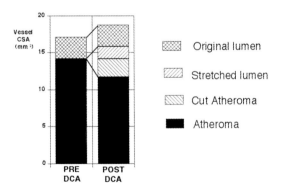

Figure 1.44 *Summary of mean vessel and atheroma areas before and following directional coronary atherectomy. CSA, cross sectional area.*

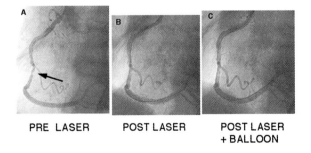

PRE LASER   POST LASER   POST LASER + BALLOON

Figure 1.45 *A successful excimer laser angioplasty as documented by angiography.*

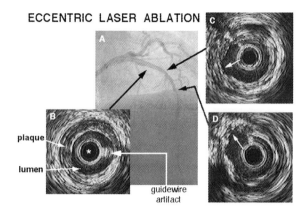

ECCENTRIC LASER ABLATION

Figure 1.46 *Following a successful laser angioplasty, intravascular ultrasound reveals that only a minimal amount of plaque has been removed.*

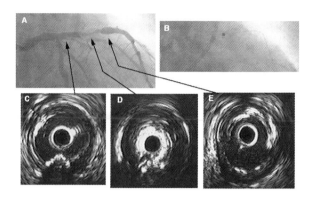

Figure 1.47 *The laser catheter could not be advanced through this mid LAD lesion. Intravascular ultrasound imaging reveals intense calcification at the lumen plaque interface (panel d).*

plaque, thus demonstrating that only a minimal amount of the tissue has been removed (approximately 10% of the cross-sectional area). The implication is that only a minimal amount of ablation actually occurs with the excimer laser device and that most of the lumen enlargement is due to a stretching effect of the balloon.[142,143] The expectation, based on IVUS imaging, that the restenosis rate would be similar to that following balloon angioplasty was eventually demonstrated in clinical trials.[144,145]

Figure 1.47 reveals another example of how IVUS imaging was useful in understanding the mechanism of action of excimer laser catheters. In this mid-LAD lesion, the excimer laser catheter could not be advanced despite maximum energy and number of laser pulses. After the excimer laser was removed, IVUS revealed that the stenosis had a calcified capsule completely encircling the interface with the lumen (see *Fig. 1.47d*). In our experience, excimer laser therapy was never effective in ablating calcified plaque. Initial reports that excimer laser therapy could treat calcified lesions were presumably based on misinterpretation of the angiograms. An angiogram that shows calcium at the lesion site does not necessarily mean that the calcium is at the luminal side of the plaque.[146,147] It is much more likely in these cases that the calcium is at the base of the plaque and therefore does not interact with the laser pulses. These microanatomic distinctions of plaque morphology cannot be obtained from angiograms. We concluded from these IVUS observations that excimer laser catheters are not effective in treating atherosclerotic plaques. Future developments may demonstrate other areas in which lasers may be

efficacious, such as treating the fibrous tissue of in-stent restenosis.

ROTATIONAL ATHERECTOMY

Rotational atherectomy is the only technique that consistently removes calcified plaque

Unlike some of the technologies discussed above, in which IVUS has demonstrated a discrepancy between the supposed mechanism of action and the actual effects of the device, rotational atherectomy has been shown by intravascular ultrasound imaging to be extremely effective in removing calcified plaque (*Fig. 1.48*).[148,149] Whether or not rotational atherectomy will

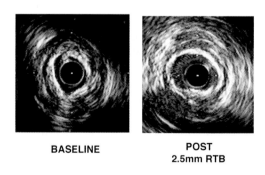

BASELINE   POST
2.5mm RTB

Figure 1.48 *Intravascular ultrasound images of a dense fibrocalcific plaque before and after treatment with a 2.5 mm diameter rotational atherectomy burr. RTB, rotablator.*

be demonstrated to be effective in reducing restenosis with adjuvant balloon dilatation or with coronary stents remains to be demonstrated in prospective randomized trials.[150-152] The initial results of the STRATAS trial,[158] which compared an aggressive strategy of a high burr-to-artery ratio (0.8) versus a lower ratio (0.6) plus balloon angioplasty, indicate that the aggressive strategy did not confer any additional benefit.[154] However, in the presence of severely calcified plaques, it is our experience that effective coronary stenting cannot be achieved unless rotational atherectomy is first performed so that the calcified capsule of the plaque is effectively removed (see Chapter 14). It is not known whether the primary effect of this device is to debulk the plaque or to change the compliance of the lesion by removing the calcified capsule to permit greater expansion of the stent. Nevertheless, coronary artery stenting is more easily performed in heavily calcified arteries following rotational atherectomy.

The microanatomic position of calcium is critical in its effect on the biomechanical properties of the plaque

Calcium can be distributed at the base of the plaque or within the body of the plaque and may subtend variable degrees of arc around the circumference (see *Fig. 1.17*). These plaques can still be treated with direct stent insertion because the fibrous portion of the plaque is more compliant to the expanding pressure of the balloon and stent. However, when a circumferential calcified matrix exists at the lumen–plaque interface, there is marked resistance to balloon expansion, and a stent cannot be adequately deployed in this setting. The position and extent of calcium can be observed with IVUS before the intervention. Pre-intervention imaging may be one of the most important uses of IVUS and may strongly influence the interventional strategy or the decision of which device to use.[155,155] Another 'rule of thumb' that may be useful during procedures is that if the ultrasound catheter cannot be advanced through a stenotic area, it is likely that the plaque capsule is calcified. When this occurs, we frequently perform rotational atherectomy before predilatation or stent placement. This rule does not apply if there are other technical reasons for not being able to pass the ultrasound catheter, such as severe tortuosity or retroflexion of the vessel, such as in a circumflex artery.

The purpose of reviewing this experience of ultrasound imaging with multiple interventional techniques is to demonstrate the benefits of understanding the mechanism of action of these devices by using a cross-sectional imaging technology that visualizes and quantifies the plaque in vivo before and after the device is used. The remainder of this chapter emphasizes how this information has been incorporated into our clinical practice and how it has led to the development of enhanced stent deployment.

IVUS-GUIDED CORONARY INTERVENTIONS

In October 1992 we embarked on an ambitious research project to determine whether IVUS guidance of angioplasty and atherectomy could diminish restenosis. At that time, owing to a high subacute thrombosis rate, the use of stents was reserved for bailout situations when an artery was compromised following balloon dilatation. Our concept was that to decrease the rate of restenosis after angioplasty, plaque burden would need to be decreased to less than 50% of the available cross-sectional area of the vessel. If this decrease could be achieved with a combination of atherectomy and balloon dilatation, we hypothesized that the incidence of restenosis would be diminished. IVUS was an ideal way to guide these repetitive interventions because it was the only method that could quantify the cross-sectional area of the plaque and the vessel. The plan was to use any combination of rotational atherectomy, DCA or balloon dilatation to achieve a lumen cross-sectional area greater than 50% of the total vessel cross-sectional

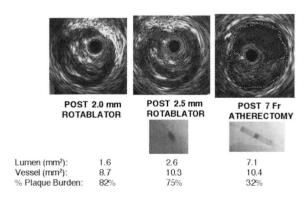

	POST 2.0 mm ROTABLATOR	POST 2.5 mm ROTABLATOR	POST 7 Fr ATHERECTOMY
Lumen (mm²):	1.6	2.6	7.1
Vessel (mm²):	8.7	10.3	10.4
% Plaque Burden:	82%	75%	32%

Figure 1.49 *Sequential interventions using different devices under intravascular ultrasound guidance to maximize the lumen cross-sectional area.*

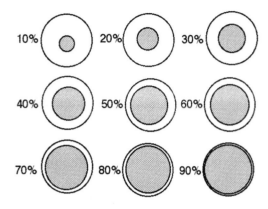

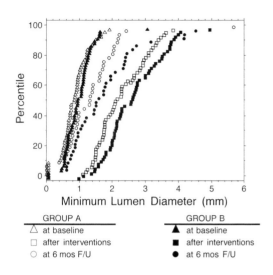

Figure 1.50 *Cross-sectional intravascular ultrasound images representing different percentages of lumen area relative to total cross-sectional area (bounded by the media).*

Figure 1.52 *Cumulative percentile results of angiographic minimum lumen diameter in the control group A and the intravascular ultrasound treated group B.*

area (*Fig. 1.49*). The decision to use 50% as the cut-off was our best guess based on previous observations with IVUS. IVUS showed us that, after balloon angioplasty, the mean lumen area was only 35% of the vessel cross-sectional area and that, after aggressive atherectomy, the mean lumen cross-sectional area reached 45% of the vessel cross-sectional area. *Figure 1.50* schematically represents what a cross-sectional ultrasound image of an artery would look like for each decile of lumen-to-vessel ratio.

The study protocol (*Fig. 1.51*) was a randomized design of all patients treated with balloon dilatation, Rotablator, or DCA according to the operator's preference. After the operator thought the procedure had

been successful by angiographic criteria, IVUS imaging was performed. The patients assigned to group A had no further intervention. In patients assigned to group B, if the residual lumen was < 50% after initial treatment, then further interventions could be performed until the operator thought that no further benefit was likely to be obtained. Only at that point could a stent be used to try to maximize the lumen area to achieve the study protocol guideline of a lumen > 50% of the vessel cross-sectional area.

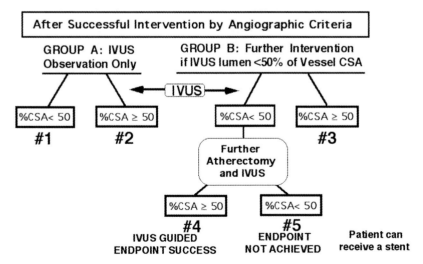

Figure 1.51 *Schematic outline of protocol for an intravascular ultrasound guided study.*

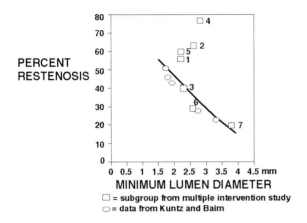

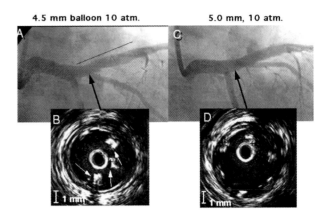

Figure 1.53 *A graph of percent of patients with restenosis in the different subgroups from the multiple intervention IVUS guided study plotted along with data from previous angioplasty studies of restenosis.*

Figure 1.54 *Intravascular ultrasound images demonstrate incomplete stent apposition despite an excellent angiographic result.*

Despite our enthusiasm for using ultrasound as a means for guiding these multiple interventional procedures, the follow-up angiographic results demonstrated that there was no difference in the lumen diameter in the control group A versus the IVUS-guided group B (*Fig. 1.52*). In addition, when the final minimum lumen diameter of the subgroups was plotted against the percentage restenosis (*Fig. 1.53*), the group with the most aggressive ultrasound-guided interventions (subgroup 4) had the highest restenosis rate, at 75%. Despite this disappointing result, another observation during this study was to have a much more profound effect on interventional cardiology. As noted in *Fig. 1.53*, the subgroups 6 and 7, which had the lowest restenosis rate, were the ones in which stents were inserted, especially after debulking with IVUS guidance (subgroup 7). These results with aggressive IVUS-guided stenting were so impressive that we abandoned this study protocol and began to place stents in all acceptable lesions. In addition, there were three major observations recognized by IVUS during this study that had a significant impact on the way stents were subsequently deployed.

IVUS OBSERVATIONS OF CORONARY ARTERY STENTS: ANGIOGRAPHY OVERESTIMATES THE INTRASTENT LUMEN

Our primary concern in 1992–1993 was the high rate of subacute stent thrombosis, which inhibited the widespread use of coronary stents.[156–170] Our initial observations of coronary stents with IVUS led us to

an alternative explanation of why subacute stent thrombosis occurred.

The first observation by IVUS was that there often was incomplete stent apposition against the arterial wall.[171] Despite the use of a large balloon and a successful angiographic result, IVUS showed that the stent struts were not fully apposed to the arterial wall and were stranded in the middle of the lumen (*Fig. 1.54*). By using a larger balloon, the stent struts were appropriately positioned against the arterial plaque.

The second observation was that a number of stents were asymmetrically deployed (*Fig. 1.55*). At the time we thought this might create turbulent flow and be another initiating factor for subacute stent thrombosis. On the basis of these ultrasound observations, we would redilate with either a larger

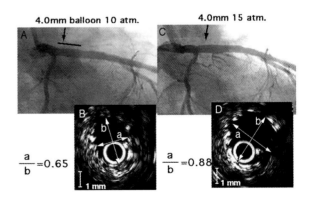

Figure 1.55 *Intravascular ultrasound images show an eccentric lumen in cross-section despite an apparent full expansion by angiography.*

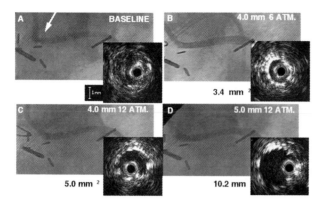

Figure 1.56 *Sequential angiograms and intravascular ultrasound images of a saphenous vein graft during stent deployment demonstrate how IVUS is used to guide the procedure and maximize the stent lumen cross-sectional area.*

balloon or at higher pressures to attempt to get a more symmetrical distribution of lumen shape.[172]

The third observation provided by IVUS imaging was that many stents were inadequately expanded despite what appeared to be an appropriate angiographic result. The baseline study (*Fig. 1.56*) reveals an ostial stenosis of a saphenous vein graft, which is significant both by angiography and by ultrasound. Following inflation of the stent with a 4 mm balloon at 6 atmospheres (which at the time was the recommended pressure) the angiographic result is significantly improved; however, the ultrasound cross-sectional lumen area is only 3.4 mm². By using higher pressures (12 atmospheres) with the same balloon we were able to increase the dimensions to 5 mm². By using a larger balloon and higher pressure the final result was 10.2 mm². This use of IVUS-guided stent deployment increased the residual lumen cross-sectional area by 300% from 3.4 mm² to 10.2 mm².

These types of observations with IVUS led us to believe that the high incidence of subacute stent thrombosis was perhaps not primarily due to any inherent thrombogenicity of the metal and the presence of a foreign body in the artery, but to inadequate deployment with an insufficient lumen cross-sectional area resulting in diminished flow or turbulence, which promotes thrombosis.

Coronary artery stenting with IVUS guidance but without coumadin

When the Palmaz–Schatz and Gianturco–Roubin stents were first released, an attempt was made to

diminish the catastrophic sequelae of subacute stent thrombosis by using an aggressive anticoagulation regimen.[164,173–175] This included heparinization following the procedure until an adequate elevation of the prothrombin time could be obtained with coumadin. This prolonged the hospital stay and produced major bleeding complications at the site of the arterial puncture.[176] The impetus to insert stents without coumadin therapy came from the death of a patient who had had a successful stent implantation but who died as a result of bleeding complications from the groin and subsequent surgery to repair the artery. Given the results of our ultrasound observations of the large lumen area that could be obtained with IVUS guidance, we cautiously withheld coumadin from our stented patients and slowly began to diminish the time of heparin treatment following the procedure. In addition, the antiplatelet regimen of aspirin was augmented with ticlopidine. The results of the study were published in 1995 and had a significant impact on the way that coronary artery stenting has been performed since.[177]

During this study, 359 patients (452 lesions) were treated with 864 Palmaz–Schatz stents using angiographic guidance initially. Successful stent deployment was obtained in 438 lesions (97%) and IVUS was subsequently performed in 420 lesions. In 402 lesions, a successful result was obtained according to our angiographic and IVUS criteria. The 6-month cumulative incidence of stent thrombosis was only 1.4% despite the absence of coumadin therapy or heparin after the procedure.

A summary of the clinical events using this protocol is provided in *Table 1.2*. The initial incidence of MI, bypass surgery, death or repeat percutaneous transluminal coronary angioplasty (PTCA) was extremely low, at a total of 5.4%, and was a significant improvement on any coronary interventional

Table 1.2

Intravascular ultrasound guided Palmaz–Schatz stent implants: initial experience – clinical events

$n = 474$	Early (< 1 mo)	Late (1–6 mos)	Cumulative (> 8 mos)
MI	3.6%	1.0%	4.6%
CABG	3.4%	3.6%	7.0%
Death	1.0%	1.3%	2.3%
Repeat PTCA	2.1%	12.7%	13.7%
MACE	5.4%	17.3%	22.6%

technique that had been reported at that time. Without the use of an aggressive anticoagulation regime, the vascular complication rate was significantly reduced to 0.6%. The hospital stay was decreased from an average of 5 days with coumadin therapy to 1 day after the procedure. Moreover, the final minimum lumen diameter was markedly improved to 3.39 mm compared with the results that were obtained without ultrasound guidance, such as the STRESS or BENESTENT trials, in which the mean final minimum lumen diameter in the stent group was 2.45 mm and 2.48 mm, respectively.[175,178,179] The overall angiographic restenosis rate at 6 months was 20%, and for single stents it was 14% which was significantly lower than the figure of 29% reported in the STRESS trial.

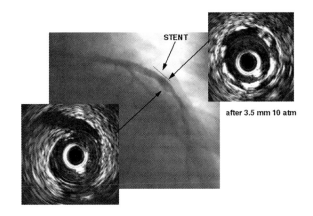

Figure 1.57 *Focal vessel rupture demonstrated by angiography and intravascular ultrasound occurred distal to this Palmaz–Schatz stent because the expansion balloon was longer than the stent.*

Our learning curve for IVUS-guided stenting

Significant insights were also gained in the initial phases by the use of different dilatation strategies. As demonstrated in *Table 1.3*, the first 60 patients in phase 1 were treated with a high balloon-to-vessel ratio (1.2:1) but with a mean pressure of only 12 atmospheres. The mean final percentage stenosis was a dramatic –8% with only one significant complication of vessel rupture. The next 300 patients in phase 2 were treated with higher pressures (a mean of 15 atmospheres) and, although a slight improvement in the final percentage stenosis was attained, this was achieved at the expense of an increase in complications and vessel ruptures of 3.4%.

On the basis of these data, the technique was altered to using a smaller balloon-to-vessel ratio of only 1.0 but with a higher mean pressure of 16 atmospheres. Although the final percentage stenosis was less (+5%), the complication rate was significantly improved, at 0.7%.

In retrospect we believe that part of the reason for the complication rate was that, at the time these early studies were being performed, the high-pressure balloons were compliant and were longer than the Palmaz–Schatz stents. Therefore the artery proximal and distal to the stent was subjected to both a high pressure and a large balloon. Arterial ruptures (*Fig. 1.57*), were only seen outside of the stent struts or if a calcified lesion was extremely resistant (this occurred before our current approach of debulking calcified lesions). These complications have dimin-

Table 1.3
Effect of different dilatation strategies

n = 501	Phase 1 (40)	Phase 2 (299)	Phase 3 (162)	p value
Balloon/vessel ratio*	1.3 ± 0.2	1.2 ± 0.2	1.0 ± 0.1	<0.0001
Maximum pressure (atm)†	12.3 ± 2.6	15.0 ± 2.8	16.0 ± 2.8	<0.0001
Percentage final stenosis*	-8 ± 17	-10 ± 15	1 ± 10	<0.0001
Vessel rupture or major dissection*	1 (3%)	8 (3.4%)	1 (0.7%)	=0.10

* Phase 3 compared to phase 1 or 2;   † phase 1 compared to phase 2 or 3

ished as stent and balloon technology have matured and as our experience with treating different lesion subsets has evolved.

Current IVUS criteria for successful stent deployment: a moving target

There has never been a randomized clinical outcome trial to establish the best IVUS criteria for optimal stent deployment as determined by incidence of subacute stent thrombosis or restenosis. When we initially conceptualized how large a stent should be, we asked, 'How large should this artery be if it were not diseased?' We knew by IVUS that atherosclerosis was diffuse and that even the so-called angiographically normal artery segment had an average of 35% of the vessel cross-sectional area filled with plaque. We reasoned that we should try to get the stented lumen cross-sectional area $\geq 60\%$ of the proximal vessel area as measured by IVUS at the media–plaque boundary. Another hypothesis was that the stented lumen should be as large as the reference lumen. But any definition has complexity: do we use the lumen proximal or distal to the stent or an average as the reference? What if it is at a bifurcation? What about long lesions where the vessel tapers? How large does the stent have to be to avoid subacute stent thrombosis and to diminish restenosis?

The incidence of achieving the IVUS criteria of success depends strongly on the quantitative definition of a successful result. In a retrospective analysis, we looked at 682 consecutive patients with 921 lesions who had IVUS-guided stenting (*Table 1.4*). Five different IVUS criteria for an optimal result were reviewed (*Table 1.5*). No patient was excluded from this analysis, which included native arteries and vein grafts (3%). The indications for stenting were representative of a non-selected population (*Table 1.6*), as was the variable types of stents that were employed (*Table 1.7*). The angiographic and pertinent proce-

Table 1.4

Intravascular ultrasound guided stenting

Patients	n = 682
Age	58 ± 10
Male	594 (87%)
Multivessel disease	330 (48%)
Unstable angina	196 (29%)
Ejection fraction	57 ± 11

Between March 30, 1993 and June 30, 1995, 682 consecutive patients with 921 lesions had intravascular ultrasound-guided coronary stenting

Table 1.5

Five different intravascular ultrasound criteria for success

- Intrastent MLCSA > 9 mm²
- Intrastent MLCSA > 90% of average reference lumen cross-sectional area
- Intrastent MLCSA > 80% of average reference lumen cross-sectional area
- Intrastent MLCSA > 90% of distal reference lumen cross-sectional area

MLCSA, minimum lumen cross-sectional area

Table 1.6

Intravascular ultrasound guided stenting. Indications for stenting (April 1993–June 1995)

	Number (%)
Stented lesions	1096
Elective	666 (61)
Restenosis	97 (9)
Suboptimal PTCA	112 (10)
Dissection	77 (7)
Acute closure	33 (3)
Chronic occlusion	94 (9)
Acute MI	5 (1)
Lesion ID on IVUS	12 (1)

Table 1.7

Intravascular ultrasound guided stenting

Stent type	Number	%
Palmaz–Schatz stent	599	65
Gianturco–Roubin stent	78	8
Wiktor stent	69	8
AVE stent	26	3
Cordis stent	18	2
Wallstent	48	5
Combination	77	9

Table 1.8

Intravascular ultrasound guided stenting. Angiographic and procedural characteristics

Lesion	n = 921
Reference diameter (mm)	3.20 ± 0.55
< 3 mm	35%
> 3 mm	65%
Minimum lumen diameter (mm)	0.94 ± 0.55
Percentage diameter stenosis	69 ± 18
Lesion length (mm)	10.43 ± 7.11
Stents per lesion	1.6 ± 1
Balloon/artery ratio	1.14 ± 0.16
Balloon inflation pressure (atm)	16 ± 3

dural characteristics are shown in *Table 1.8*. The stents were deployed at relatively high pressures with large balloons (balloon-to-artery ratio 1.14 ± 0.16)

with an attempt to expand the stented lumen maximally. Despite the care taken to maximize the stent lumen, the frequency of achieving the different IVUS criteria of success varied between 23% and 79% (*Fig. 1.58*). The incidence of subacute thrombosis was much lower (1%) than the incidence of not meeting our optimized IVUS criteria (21% to 41%); clearly these criteria do not set a lower limit or threshold below which stent thrombosis will occur.

The more interesting question is whether meeting these IVUS criteria is associated with a lower restenosis rate. *Figure 1.59* shows the incidence of angiographic restenosis according to the different IVUS criteria. There was a significant difference in restenosis rate only for those lesions in which the lumen cross-sectional area was more than 9 mm² or when the intrastent lumen area was more than 70% of the largest balloon nominal cross-sectional area. How can we explain these findings? The multiple variables that are associated with restenosis are described in greater detail in Chapter 4. One of the strongest predictors is the final minimum lumen

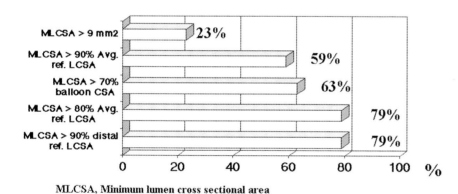

MLCSA, **Minimum lumen cross sectional area**

Figure 1.58 *Frequency of achieving various intravascular ultrasound criteria.*

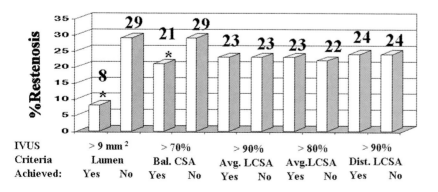

* **p < 0.05** for lesions that met vs lesions that did not meet criteria

Figure 1.59 *Angiographic restenosis according to different intravascular ultrasound criteria.*

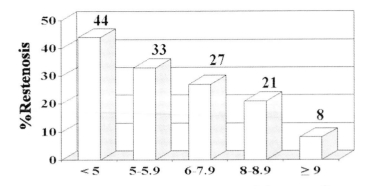

Figure 1.60 *Restenosis according to final minimum lumen cross-sectional area.*

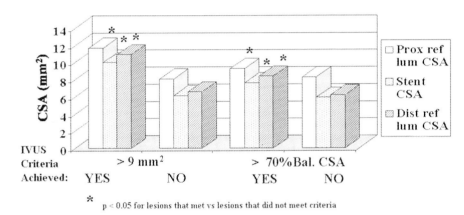

Figure 1.61 *Intrastent and reference IVUS measurements according to different criteria.*

*
p < 0.05 for lesions that met vs lesions that did not meet criteria

cross-sectional area by IVUS (*Fig. 1.60*); the strongest predictor of achieving a stented lumen cross-sectional area >9 mm^2 is the reference lumen diameter and the balloon-to-vessel ratio. In other words, a larger stented lumen is achievable in bigger arteries, and these arteries are likely to have a lower restenosis rate. This is demonstrated in *Fig. 1.61* where the proximal and distal reference lumen measurements are shown along with the minimum stented lumen area. The reference lumens in these lower restenosis groups were significantly larger in those lesions that met the criteria than in the lesions in which the IVUS criteria were not achieved.

In summary, among the different IVUS criteria that have been proposed as the measure of a successful stent result, only the absolute lumen area > 9 mm^2 correlated with a lower restenosis rate (8%). This criterion was not often achieved (23%) and was obtained in larger vessels and with a high balloon-to-vessel ratio (> 1.2:1). Moreover, the criteria that are based on the ratio of stent lumen to distal or average reference lumen cross-sectional area were more likely to be met in smaller vessels. Despite the fact that these strict IVUS criteria were met, if the lesions

were located in smaller vessels they had similar restenosis rates to those lesions that did not meet the IVUS criteria.

THE MUSIC TRIAL CRITERIA FOR SUCCESSFUL STENTING

The MUSIC trial was a prospective study of the use of IVUS-guided stenting using strict criteria for a successful result.[181] The MUSIC trial established stringent IVUS criteria and asked operators to optimize stents so that the stented lumen was ≥ 90% of the average reference cross-sectional area (*Table 1.9*). If the minimal in-stent lumen area was ≥ 9.0 mm^2 then the in-stent minimum lumen area had to be ≥ 80% of the average reference lumen areas but > 90% of the proximal reference lumen area. In addition, the stent had to be symmetrically expanded and fully apposed to the arterial wall for the entire length of the stent. Using these strict criteria only approximately 50% of

Table 1.9
The MUSIC criteria

1 Complete apposition of the stent over its entire length
2 In-stent minimal LA ≥ 90% of the average reference LA or ≥ 100% of LA of the reference segment with the lowest LA
3 In-stent LA of proximal stent entrance ≥ 90% of proximal reference LA
4 Symmetric stent expansion defined by LDmin/LDmax ≥ 0.7
5 In case minimal in-stent reaches ≥ 9.0 mm²: In-stent minimal LA ≥ 80% of the average reference LA or ≥ 90% of LA of the reference segment with the lowest LA In-stent LA of proximal stent entrance ≥ 90% of proximal reference LA

LA = lumen area; LD = lumen diameter.

stented lesions were successfully optimized, despite the use of large balloons and high pressures. Despite the inability to achieve these strict criteria in most of the patients, the 6-month results showed improvements over non-IVUS-guided stenting. Major cardiac events, as well as restenosis, were determined in 161 patients who received a single Palmaz–Schatz stent in a de novo coronary lesion. The incidence of restenosis was only 7%.[183] Target lesion revascularization was performed with repeat PTCA in only 4% of the patients. In comparison with other series of coronary artery stenting, IVUS guidance using these strict criteria appears to significantly reduce the restenosis rate and need for subsequent PTCA.

Restenosis is multifactorial and the operator cannot control factors such as the lesion length and size of the artery. What we try to do within these constraints is to use IVUS to optimize stent deployment (i.e. to maximize the stented lumen cross-sectional area without excessive trauma to the vessel). Our current practice is outlined here. Subsequent chapters describe how this is accomplished for different lesion subsets.

GENERAL TECHNIQUE OF IVUS-GUIDED STENT OPTIMIZATION

1. Use pre-intervention IVUS to choose the device: balloon dilatation, rotational, or directional atherectomy.

2. Try to debulk calcified or large plaque burdens.

3. Either before intervention or after the initial device, use IVUS to measure the media-to-media diameter proximal and distal to the lesion. Choose a balloon of this average diameter to expand the stent at 12–16 atmospheres. Our mean pressure is 14 atmospheres.

4. Use IVUS to check the final result. Make sure the struts are well apposed, the stent covers the lesion, and that the lumen cross-sectional area is 'optimized' (i.e. as large as the distal reference cross-sectional area using the recommended balloon size and pressure) or that the stented lumen is ≥ 55% of the average reference vessel cross-sectional area.

5. There is no single IVUS criterion of success; rather it is a process of choosing your devices and balloons to maximize the stent lumen cross-sectional area for the given vessel size. It is this approach to stenting that improves success, maximizes minimum lumen diameter, and diminishes restenosis.

The technique of larger balloons and higher pressure inflations to deploy coronary artery stents without subsequent anticoagulation was rapidly adopted by most interventional cardiologists. Subsequent papers demonstrated a marked reduction in subacute stent thrombosis, vascular complications and patient stay.[187–189] Several authors also reported excellent results using this balloon dilatation strategy without IVUS-guidance to assess their results.[188–190] It now appears that IVUS imaging is not necessary to obtain a low incidence of subacute stent thrombosis.[190,191] There are still other potential advantages of using IVUS during stent deployment, the most significant of which is the influence of ultrasound guidance on restenosis, which is discussed in Chapter 4.

REFERENCES

1. Yock PG, Linker DT, Angelsen BAJ. Two-dimensional intravascular ultrasound: technical development and initial clinical experience. *J Am Soc Echocardiogr* 1989; **2**: 296–304.

2. Mallery JA, Tobis JM, Griffith J et al. Assessment of normal and atherosclerotic arterial wall thickness with an intravascular ultrasound imaging catheter. *Am Heart J* 1990; **119**: 1392–1400.

3. Yock PG, Johnson EL, Linker DT. Intravascular ultrasound: development and clinical potential. *Am J Card Imaging* 1988; **2**: 185–193.

4. Gussenhoven EJ, Essed CE, Lancee CT et al. Arterial wall characteristics determind by intravascular ultrasound imaging: an in vitro study. *J Am Coll Cardiol* 1989; **14**: 947–952.

5. Pandian NG, Kreis A, Weintraub A et al. Real-time intravascular ultrasound imaging in humans. *Am J Cardiol* 1990; **65**: 1392–1396.

6. Potkin BN, Bartorelli AL, Gessert JM et al. Coronary artery imaging with intravascular high-frequency ultrasound. *Circulation* 1990; **81**: 1575–1585.

7. Yamada EG, Fitzgerald PJ, Sudhir K, Hargrave VK, Yock PG. Intravascular ultrasound imaging of blood: the effect of hematocrit and flow on backscatter. *J Am Soc Echocardiogr* 1992; **5**: 385–392.

8. Nissen SE, Grines CL, Gurley JC et al. Application of a new phased-array ultrasound imaging catheter in the assessment of vascular dimensions: in vivo comparison to cine-angiography. *Circulation* 1990; **81**: 660–666.

9. Hodgson JMcB, Graham SP, Sheehan H et.al. Percutaneous intravascular ultrasound imaging: validation of a real time synthetic aperture array catheter. *Am J Card Imag* 1998; **5**: 65.

10. Cacchione JG, Reddy K, Richards F et al. Combined intra-vascular ultrasound/angioplasty balloon catheter: initial use during PTCA. *Cathet Cardiovasc Diagn* 1991; **24**: 99–101.

11. Mudra H, Klauss V, Blasini R et al. Ultrasound guidance of Palmaz–Schatz intracoronary stenting with a combined intravascular ultrasound balloon catheter. *Circulation* 1994; **90**: 1252–1261.

12. Bom Nicolaas, Lancee CT, Gussenhoven EJ et al. Basic principles of intravascular ultrasound imaging. In: Tobis JM, Yock PD, eds. *Intravascular Ultrasound Imaging*. New York: Churchill Livingstone, 1992, 7–15.

13. Nishimura RA, Edwards WD, Warnes CA et al. Intravascular ultrasound imaging: in vitro validation and pathologic correlation. *J Am Coll Cardiol* 1990; **16**: 145–154.

14. Moriuchi M, Tobis JM, Mahon D et al. The reproducibility of intravascular ultrasound imaging in vitro. *J Am Soc Echocardiogr* 1990; **3**: 444–450.

15. Tobis JM, Mallery JA, Gessert J et al. Intravascular ultrasound cross-sectional arterial imaging before and after balloon angioplasty in vitro. *Circulation* 1989; **80**: 873–882.

16. Borst C, Savalle LH, Smits PC et al. Imaging of post-mortem coronary arteries by 30 MHz intravascular ultrasound. *Int J Card Imaging* 1991; **6**: 239–246.

17. Di Mario C, The SH, Madretsma S et al. Detection and characterization of vascular lesions by intravascular ultrasound: an in vitro study correlated with histology. *J Am Soc Echocardiogr* 1992; **5**: 135–146.

18. Peters RJ, Kok WE, Havenith MG et al. Histopathologic validation of intracoronary ultrasound imaging. *J Am Soc Echocardiogr* 1994; **7**: 230–241.

19. Wenguang L, Gussenhoven WJ, Zhong Y et al. Validation of quantitative analysis of intravascular ultrasound images. *Int J Card Imaging* 1991; **6**: 247–253.

20. Anderson MH, Simpson IA, Katritsis D et al. Intravascular ultrasound imaging of the coronary arteries: an in vitro evaluation of measurement of area of the lumen and atheroma characterisation. *Br Heart J* 1992; **68**: 276–281.

21. Nissen SE, Gurley JC, Grines CL et al. Intravascular ultrasound assessment of lumen size and wall morphology in normal subjects and patients with coronary artery disease. *Circulation* 1991; **84**: 1087–1099.

22. Arnett EN, Isner JM, Redwood DR et al. Coronary artery narrowing in coronary heart disease: comparison of cineangiographic and necropsy findings. *Ann Intern Med* 1979; **91**: 350–356.

23. Vlodaver Z, Frech R, Van Tassel RA, Edwards JE. Correlation of the antemortem coronary arteriogram and the postmortem specimen. *Circulation* 1973; **47**: 162–169.

24. Vlodaver Z, Edwards JE. Pathology of coronary atherosclerosis. *Prog Cardiovasc Dis* 1971; **14**: 256–274.

25. Waller BF, Roberts WC. Amount of narrowing by atherosclerotic plaque in 44 nonbypassed and 52 bypassed major epicardial coronary arteries in 32 necropsy patients who died within 1 month of aortocoronary bypass grafting. *Am J Cardiol* 1980; **46**: 956–962.

26. Waller BF. Anatomy, histology, and pathology of the major epicardial coronary arteries relevant to echocardiographic imaging techniques. *J Am Soc Echocardiogr* 1989; **2**: 232–252.

27. Waller BF, Pinkerton CA, Slack JD. Intravascular ultrasound: a histological study of vessels during life. The new 'gold standard' for vascular imaging. *Circulation* 1992; **85**: 2305–2310.

28. Warnes CA, Roberts WC. Comparison at necropsy by age group of amount and distribution of narrowing by atherosclerotic plaque in 2995 five-mm long segments of 240 major coronary arteries in 60 men aged 31 to 70 years with sudden coronary death. *Am Heart J* 1984; **108**: 431–435.

29. Glagov S, Weisenberg E, Zarins CK, Stankunavicius R, Kolettis GJ. Compensatory enlargement of human atherosclerotic coronary arteries. *N Engl J Med* 1987; **316**: 1371–1375.

30. Maheswaran B, Leung CY, Gutfinger DE et al. Intravascular ultrasound appearance of normal and mildly diseased coronary arteries: correlation with histologic specimens. *Am Heart J* 1995; **130**: 976–986.

31. Fitzgerald PJ, Goar FG, Connolly RJ et al. Intravascular ultrasound imaging of coronary arteries. Is three layers the norm. *Circulation* 1992; **86**: 154–158.

32. Siegel RJ, Chae JS, Maurer G, Berlin M, Fishbein MC. Histopathologic correlation of the three-layered intravascular ultrasound appearance of normal adult human muscular arteries. *Am Heart J* 1993; **126**: 872–878.

33. Porter TR, Radio SJ, Anderson JA, Michels A, Xie F. Composition of coronary atherosclerotic plaque in the intima and media affects intravascular ultrasound measurements of intimal thickness. *J Am Coll Cardiol* 1994; **23**: 1079–1084.

34. Porter TR, Sears T, Xie F et al. Intravascular ultrasound study of angiographically mildly diseased coronary arteries. *J Am Coll Cardiol* 1993; **22**: 1858–1865.

35. Isner JM, Donaldson RF, Fortin AH, Tischler A, Clarke RH. Attenuation of the media of coronary arteries in advanced atherosclerosis. *Am J Cardiol* 1986; **58**: 937–939.

36. Gussenhoven EJ, Frietman PA, The SH et al. Assessment of medial thinning in atherosclerosis by intravascular ultrasound. *Am J Cardiol* 1991; **68**: 1625–1632.

37. Tobis JM, Mallery J, Mahon D et al. Intravascular ultrasound imaging of human coronary arteries in vivo. Analysis of tissue characterizations with comparison to in vitro histological specimens. *Circulation* 1991; **83**: 913–926.

38. Linker DT, Kleven A, Groenningsaether A, Yock PG, Angelsen BAJ. Tissue characterization with intra-arterial

ultrasound: special promise and problem. *Int J Card Imag* 1991; **6**: 255–263.

39. Rasheed Q, Dhawale PJ, Anderson J, Hodgson JM. Intracoronary ultrasound-defined plaque composition: computer-aided plaque characterization and correlation with histologic samples obtained during directional coronary atherectomy. *Am Heart J* 1995; **129**: 631–637.

40. Keren G, Leon MB. Characterization of atherosclerotic lesions by intravascular ultrasound: possible role in unstable coronary syndromes and in interventional therapeutic procedures. *Am J Cardiol* 1991; **68**: 85B-91B.

41. Linker DT, Yock PG, Groenningsaether A et al. Analysis of backscattered ultrasound from normal and diseased arterial wall. *Int J Card Imaging* 1989; **4**: 177–185.

42. Fitzgerald PJ, Ports TA, Yock PG. Contribution of localized calcium deposits to dissection after angioplasty: an observational study using intravascular ultrasound. *Circulation* 1992; **86**: 64–70.

43. Friedrich GJ, Moes NY, Muhlberger VA et al. Detection of intralesional calcium by intracoronary ultrasound depends on the histologic pattern. *Am Heart J* 1994; **128**: 435–441.

44. Hiro T, Leung CY, Russo RJ et al. Variability in tissue characterization of atherosclerotic plaque by intravascular ultrasound: a comparison of four intravascular ultrasound systems. *Am J Card Imaging* 1996; **10–4**: 209–218.

45. Zamorano J, Erbel R, Ge J et al. Spontaneous plaque rupture visualized by intravascular ultrasound. *Eur Heart J* 1994; **15**: 131–133.

46. Park JB, Tobis JM. Spontaneous plaque rupture and thrombus formation in the left main coronary artery documented by intravascular ultrasound. *Cathet Cardiovasc Diagn* 1996; **40–44**: 358–360.

47. Hiro T, Leung CY, Russo RJ et al. Variability of a three-layered appearance in intravascular ultrasound coronary images: a comparison of morphometric measurements with four intravascular ultrasound systems. *Am J Card Imaging* 1996; **10–4**: 219–227.

48. Mintz GS, Douek P, Pichard AD et al. Target lesion calcification in coronary artery disease: an intravascular ultrasound study. *J Am Coll Cardiol* 1992; **20**: 1149–1155.

49. Rosenfield K, Losordo DW, Ramaswamy K et al. Three-dimensional reconstruction of human coronary and peripheral arteries from images recorded during two-dimensional intravascular ultrasound examination. *Circulation* 1991; **84**: 1938–1956.

50. Nissen SE, Gurley JC, Booth DC, DeMaria AN. Intravascular ultrasound of the coronary arteries: current applications and future directions. *Am J Cardiol* 1992; **69**: 18H-29H.

51. Mintz GS, Potkin BN, Cooke R et al. Intravascular ultrasound imaging in a patient with unstable angina. *Am Heart J* 1992; **123**: 1692–1694.

52. Fitzpatrick LA, Severson A, Edwards WD, Ingram RT. Diffuse calcification in human coronary arteries. Association of osteo-pontin with atherosclerosis. *J Clin Invest* 1994; **94**: 1597–1604.

53. Kostamaa H, Donovan J, Kasaoka S et al. Calcified plaque cross sectional area in human arteries: correlation between intravascular ultrasound and un-decalcified histology. *Am Heart J* 1999; **137**: 482–488.

54. Wang S, Detrano RC, Secci A et al. Detection of coronary calcification with electron-beam computed tomography: evaluation of interexamination reproducibility and comparison of three image-acquisition protocols. *Am Heart J* 1996; **132**: 550–558.

55. Wong ND, Detrano RC, Abrahamson D et al. Coronary artery screening by electron beam computed tomography. Facts, controversy, and future. *Circulation* 1995; **92**: 632–636.

56. Mahaisavariya P, Detrano R, Kang X et al. Quantitation of in vitro coronary artery calcium using ultrafast computed tomography. *Cathet Cardiovasc Diagn* 1994; **32**: 387–393.

57. Wong ND, Vo A, Abrahamson D et al. Detection of coronary artery calcium by ultrafast computed tomography and its relation to clinical evidence of coronary artery disease. *Am J Cardiol* 1994; **73**: 223–227.

58. Gutfinger DE, Leung CY, Hiro T et al. In vitro atherosclerotic plaque and calcium quantitation by intravascular ultrasound and electron-beam computed tomography. *Am Heart J* 1996; **131**: 899–906.

59. Chemarin-Alibelli MJ, Pieraggi MT, Elbaz M et al. Identification of coronary thrombus after myocardial infarction by intracoronary ultrasound compared with histology of tissues sampled by atherectomy. *Am J Cardiol* 1996; **77**: 344–349.

60. Yock PG, White CJ, Fitzgerald PJ, Ramee SR. Advances in intravascular imaging: angioscopy and ultrasound. In: *Textbook of Interventional Cardiology* 1991; Update 2: 15–27.

61. Feld S, Ganim M, Carell ES et al. Comparison of angioscopy, intravascular ultrasound imaging and quantitative coronary angiography in predicting clinical outcome after coronary intervention in high risk patients. *J Am Coll Cardiol* 1996; **28**: 97–105.

62. Siegel RJ, Chae JS, Forrester JS, Ruiz CE. Angiography, angioscopy, and ultrasound imaging before and after percutaneous balloon angioplasty. *Am Heart J* 1990; **120**: 1086–1090.

63. Teirstein PS, Schatz RA, Denardo SJ, Jensen EE, Johnson AD. Angioscopic versus angiographic detection of thrombus during coronary interventional procedures. *Am J Cardiol* 1995; **75**: 1083–1087.

64. Davies MJ. Pathology of arterial thrombosis. *Br Med Bull* 1994; **50**: 789–802.

65. Davies MJ, Richardson PD, Woolf N et al. Risk of thrombosis in human atherosclerotic plaques: role of extracellular lipid, macrophage, and smooth muscle cell content. *Br Heart J* 1993; **69**: 377–381.

66. Ambrose JA, Winters SL, Arora RR et al. Coronary angiographic morphology in myocardial infarction: a link between the pathogenesis of unstable angina and myocardial infarction. *J Am Coll Cardiol* 1985; **6**: 1233–1238.

67. Falk E, Shah PK, Fuster V. Coronary plaque disruption. *Circulation* 1995; **92**: 657–671.

68. Fuster V. Elucidation of the role of plaque instability and rupture in acute coronary events. *Am J Cardiol* 1995; **76**: 24C–33C.

69. Hiro T, Leung CY, de Guzman S et al. Are soft echoes really soft? Intravascular ultrasound assessment of mechanical properties in human atherosclerotic tissue. *Am Heart J* 1997; **133**: 1–7.

70. Nakamura S, Mahon DJ, Maheswaran B et al. An explanation for discrepancy between angiographic and intravascular ultrasound measurements after percutaneous transluminal coronary angioplasty. *J Am Coll Cardiol* 1995; **25**: 633–639.

71. Ehrlich S, Honye J, Mahon D et al. Unrecognized stenosis by angiography documented by intravascular ultrasound imaging. *Cathet Cardiovasc Diagn* 1991; **23**: 198–201.

72. Potkin BN, Keren G, Mintz GS et al. Arterial responses to balloon coronary angioplasty: an intravascular ultrasound study. *J Am Coll Cardiol* 1992; **20**: 942–951.

73. Moriuchi M, Saito S, Honye J et al. intravascular ultrasound imaging in human peripheral and coronary arteries in vivo. *Jpn Circ J* 1992; **56**: 578–585.

74. Yock PG, Fitzgerald PJ, Linker DT, Angelsen BAJ. Intravascular ultrasound guidance for catheter-based coronary interventions. *J Am Coll Cardiol* 1991; **17**: 39B–45B.

75. Fitzgerald PJ, Yock PG. Mechanisms and outcomes of angioplasty assessed by intravascular ultrasound imaging. *J Clin Ultrasound* 1993; **21**: 579–588.

76. Hausmann D, Sudhir K, Fitzgerald P et al. Contrast-enhanced intravascular ultrasound: validation of a new technique for delineation of the vessel wall boundary. *J Am Coll Cardiol* 1994; **23**: 981–987.

77. Nakamura S, Mahon DJ, Maheswaran B et al. An explanation for discrepancy between angiographic and intravascular ultrasound measurements after percutaneous transluminal coronary angioplasty. *J Am Coll Cardiol* 1995; **25**: 633–639.

78. Hausmann D, Lundkvist AJ, Friedrich G et al. Lumen and plaque shape in atherosclerotic coronary arteries assessed by in vivo intracoronary ultrasound. *Am J Cardiol* 1994; **74**: 857–863.

79. Hausmann D, Lundkvist AJ, Friedrich GJ et al. Intracoronary ultrasound imaging: intraobserver and interobserver variability of morphometric measurements. *Am Heart J* 1994; **128**: 674–680.

80. Waller BF. The eccentric coronary atherosclerotic plaque: morphologic observations and clinical relevance. *Clin Cardiol* 1989; **12**: 14–20.

81. Sudhir K, MacGregor JS, Barbant SD et al. Assessment of coronary conductance and resistance vessel reactivity in response to nitroglycerin, ergonovine and adenosine: in vivo studies with simultaneous intravascular two-dimensional and doppler ultrasound. *J Am Coll Cardiol* 1993; **21**: 1261–1268.

82. Reddy KG, Suneja R, Nair RN et al. Measurement by intracoronary ultrasound of in vivo arterial distensibility within atherosclerotic lesions. *Am J Cardiol* 1993; **72**: 1232–1237.

83. Nicosia A, van der Giessen WJ, Airiian SG et al. Is intravascular ultrasound after coronary stenting a safe procedure? Three cases of stent damage attributable to ICUS in a tantalum coil stent. *Cathet Cardiovasc Diagn* 1997; **40**: 265–270.

84. Hausmann D, Erbel R, Alibelli-Chemarin MJ et al. The safety of intracoronary ultrasound. A multicenter survey of 2207 examinations. *Circulation* 1995; **91**: 623–630.

85. Klauss V, Ackermann K, Spes CH et al. Coronary plaque morphologic characteristics early and late after heart transplantation: in vivo analysis with intravascular ultrasonography. *Am Heart J* 1997; **133**: 29–35.

86. Tuzcu EM, Hobbs RE, Rincon G et al. Occult and frequent transmission of atherosclerotic coronary disease with cardiac transplantation. Insights from intravascular ultrasound. *Circulation* 1995; **91**: 1706–1713.

87. Fitzgerald PJ, Belef M, Connolly AJ et al. Design and initial testing of an ultrasound-guided directional atherectomy device. *Am Heart J* 1995; **129**: 593–598.

88. Block PC, Myler RK, Stertzer S, Fallon JT. Morphology after transluminal angioplasty in human beings. *N Engl J Med* 1981; **305**: 382–385.

89. Block PC. Mechanism of transluminal angioplasty. *Am J Cardiol* 1984; **53**: 69C-71C.

90. Block PC, Baughman KL, Pasternak RC, Fallon JT. Transluminal angioplasty: correlation of morphologic and angiographic findings in an experimental model. *Circulation* 1980; **61**: 778–785.

91. Farb A, Virmani R, Atkinson JB, Kolodgie FD. Plaque morphology and pathologic changes in arteries from patients dying after coronary balloon angioplasty. *J Am Coll Cardiol* 1990; **16**: 1421–1429.

92. Soward AL, Essed CE, Serruys PW. Coronary arterial findings after accidental death immediately after successful percutaneous transluminal coronary angioplasty. *Am J Cardiol* 1985; **56**: 794–795.

93. Mizuno K, Kurita A, Imazeki N. Pathological findings after percutaneous transluminal coronary angioplasty. *Br Heart J* 1984; **52**: 588–590.

94. Lyon RT, Zarins CK, Lu CT et al. Vessel, plaque, and lumen morphology after transluminal balloon angioplasty. Quantitative study in distended human arteries. *Arteriosclerosis* 1987; **7**: 306–314.

95. Waller BF. Morphologic correlates of coronary angiographic patterns at the site of percutaneous transluminal coronary angioplasty. *Clin Cardiol* 1988; **11**: 817–822.

96. Waller BF, Gorfinkel HJ, Rogers FJ et al. Early and late morphologic changes in major epicardial coronary arteries after percutaneous transluminal coronary angioplasty. *Am J Cardiol* 1984; **53**: 42C–47C.

97. Waller BF. Pathology of transluminal balloon angioplasty used in the treatment of coronary heart disease. *Hum Pathol* 1987; **18**: 476–484.

98. Honye J, Mahon DJ, Jain A et al. Morphological effects of coronary balloon angioplasty in vivo assessed by intravascular ultrasound imaging. *Circulation* 1992; **85**: 1012–1025.

99. Hodgson JM, Reddy KG, Suneja R et al. Intracoronary ultrasound imaging: correlation of plaque morphology with angiography, clinical syndrome and procedural results in patients undergoing coronary angioplasty. *J Am Coll Cardiol* 1993; **21**: 35–44.

100. Nobuyoshi M, Kimura T, Nosaka H et al. Restenosis after successful percutaneous transluminal coronary angioplasty: serial angiographic follow-up of 229 patients. *J Am Coll Cardiol* 1988; **12**: 616–623.

101. Nobuyoshi M, Kimura T, Ohishi H et al. Restenosis after percutaneous transluminal coronary angioplasty: pathologic observations in 20 patients. *J Am Coll Cardiol* 1991; **17**: 433–439.

102. Kimura T, Kaburagi S, Tamura T et al. Remodeling of human coronary arteries undergoing coronary angioplasty or atherectomy. *Circulation* 1997; **96**: 475–483.

103. Gerber TC, Erbel R, Gorge G et al. Classification of morphologic effects of percutaneous transluminal coronary angioplasty assessed by intravascular ultrasound. *Am J Cardiol* 1992; **70**: 1546–1554.

104. Ge J, Erbel R, Gerber T et al. Intravascular ultrasound imaging of angiographically normal coronary arteries: a prospective study in vivo. *Br Heart J* 1994; **71**: 572–578.

105. Gerber TC, Erbel R, Gorge G et al. Extent of atherosclerosis and remodeling of the left main coronary artery determined by intravascular ultrasound. *Am J Cardiol* 1994; **73**: 666–671.

106. Ge J, Erbel R, Zamorano J et al. Coronary artery

remodeling in atherosclerotic disease: an intravascular ultrasonic study in vivo. *Coron Artery Dis* 1993; **4**: 981–986.

107. Zamorano J, Erbel R, Ge J et al. Vessel wall changes in the proximal non-treated segment after PTCA. An in vivo intracoronary ultrasound study. *Eur Heart J* 1994; **15**: 1505–1511.

108. Ellis SG, Vandormael MG, Cowley MJ et al. Coronary morphologic and clinical determinants of procedural outcome with angioplasty for multivessel coronary disease. Implications for patient selection. Multivessel Angioplasty Prognosis Study Group. *Circulation* 1990; **82**: 1193–1202.

109. Goldberg SL, Colombo A, Maiello L et al. Intracoronary stent insertion after balloon angioplasty of chronic total occlusions. *J Am Coll Cardiol* 1995; **26**: 713–719.

110. Gordon IL, Conroy RM, Tobis JM et al. Determinants of patency after percutaneous angioplasty and atherectomy of occluded superficial femoral arteries. *Am J Surg* 1994; **168**: 115–119.

111. Schryver TE, Popma JJ, Kent KM et al. Use of intracoronary ultrasound to identify the 'true' coronary lumen in chronic coronary dissection treated with intracoronary stenting. *Am J Cardiol* 1992; **69**: 1107–1108.

112. Tobis JM, Miranda CP, Deutsch L et al. The mechanism of peripheral recanalization by laser-assisted thermal angioplasty: confirmation by intravascular sonography. *Am J Roentgenol* 1990; **155**: 1100–1102.

113. Tobis J, Smolin M, Mallery J et al. Laser-assisted thermal angioplasty in human peripheral artery occlusions: mechanism of recanalization. *J Am Coll Cardiol* 1989; **13**: 1547–1554.

114. Pavlides GS, Hauser AM, Grines CL et al. Clinical, hemodynamic, electrocardiographic and mechanical events during nonocclusive, coronary atherectomy and comparison with balloon angioplasty. *Am J Cardiol* 1992; **70**: 841–845.

115. Topol EJ, Leya F, Pinkerton CA et al. A comparison of directional atherectomy with coronary angioplasty in patients with coronary artery disease. The CAVEAT Study Group. *N Engl J Med* 1993; **329**: 221–227.

116. Matar FA, Mintz GS, Pinnow E et al. Multivariate predictors of intravascular ultrasound end points after directional coronary atherectomy. *J Am Coll Cardiol* 1995; **25**: 318–324.

117. Popma JJ, Mintz GS, Satler LF et al. Clinical and angiographic outcome after directional coronary atherectomy. A qualitative and quantitative analysis using coronary arteriography and intravascular ultrasound. *Am J Cardiol* 1993; **18**: 55E–64E.

118. Kuntz RE, Hinohara T, Safian RD et al. Restenosis after directional coronary atherectomy. Effects of luminal diameter and deep wall excision. *Circulation* 1992; **86**: 1394–1399.

119. Garratt KN, Holmes DRJ, Bell MR et al. Restenosis after directional coronary atherectomy: differences between primary atheromatous and restenosis lesions and influence of subintimal tissue resection. *J Am Coll Cardiol* 1990; **16**: 1665–1671.

120. Baim DS, Hinohara T, Holmes D et al. Results of directional coronary atherectomy during multicenter preapproval testing. The US Directional Coronary Atherectomy Investigator Group. *Am J Cardiol* 1993; **72**: 6E–11E.

121. O'Brien ER, Alpers CE, Stewart DK et al. Proliferation in primary and restenotic coronary atherectomy tissue. Implications for antiproliferative therapy. *Circ Res* 1993; **73**: 223–231.

122. Hinohara T, Robertson GC, Selmon MR et al. Restenosis after directional coronary atherectomy. *J Am Coll Cardiol* 1992; **20**: 623–632.

123. Hinohara T, Rowe MH, Robertson GC et al. Effect of lesion characteristics on outcome of directional coronary atherectomy. *J Am Coll Cardiol* 1991; **17**: 1112–1120.

124. Johnson DE, Braden L, Simpson JB. Mechanism of directed transluminal atherectomy. *Am J Cardiol* 1990; **65**: 389–391.

125. Johnson DE, Hinohara T, Selmon MR et al. Primary peripheral arterial stenoses and restenoses excised by transluminal atherectomy: a histopathologic study. *J Am Coll Cardiol* 1990; **15**: 419–425.

126. Popma JJ, De Cesare NB, Pinkerton CA et al. Quantitative analysis of factors influencing late lumen loss and restenosis after directional coronary atherectomy. *Am J Cardiol* 1993; **71**: 552–557.

127. Fishman RF, Kuntz RE, Carrozza JPJ et al. Long-term results of directional coronary atherectomy: predictors of restenosis. *J Am Coll Cardiol* 1992; **20**: 1101–1110.

128. Nakamura S, Mahon DJ, Leung CY et al. Intracoronary ultrasound imaging before and after directional coronary atherectomy: in vitro and clinical observations. *Am Heart J* 1995; **129**: 841–851.

129. Umans VA, Baptista J, Di Mario C et al. Angiographic, ultrasonic, and angioscopic assessment of the coronary artery wall and lumen area configuration after directional atherectomy: the mechanism revisited. *Am Heart J* 1995; **130**: 217–227.

130. Hong MK, Wong SC, Mintz GS et al. A modified directional atherectomy catheter for resection of calcified atherosclerotic plaques. *Coron Artery Dis* 1995; **6**: 335–339.

131. Kimura BJ, Fitzgerald PJ, Sudhir K et al. Guidance of directed coronary atherectomy by intracoronary ultrasound imaging. *Am Heart J* 1992; **124**: 1365–1369.

132. Suneja R, Nair RN, Reddy KG et al. Mechanisms of angiographically successful directional coronary atherectomy: evaluation by intracoronary ultrasound and comparison with transluminal coronary angioplasty. *Am Heart J* 1993; **126**: 507–514.

133. Simonton CA, Leon MB, Baim DS et al. 'Optimal' directional coronary atherectomy: final results of the Optimal Atherectomy Restenosis Study (OARS). *Circulation* 1998; **97**: 332–339.

134. Sumitsuji S, Suzuki T, Hosokawa H et al. Vessel and plaque change in 3 and 6 months follow-up after aggressive directional coronary atherectomy in Adjunctive Balloon Angioplasty following Coronary Atherectomy Study (ABACAS). *Circulation* 1997; **I-408** (abstract).

135. Bittl JA, Sanborn TA. Excimer laser-facilitated coronary angioplasty. Relative risk analysis of acute and follow-up results in 200 patients. *Circulation* 1992; **86**: 71–80.

136. Bittl JA, Sanborn TA, Tcheng JE et al. Clinical success, complications and restenosis rates with excimer laser coronary angioplasty. The Percutaneous Excimer Laser Coronary Angioplasty Registry. *Am J Cardiol* 1992; **70**: 1533–1539.

137. Karsch KR, Haase KK, Voelker W et al. Percutaneous coronary excimer laser angioplasty in patients with stable and unstable angina pectoris. Acute results and incidence

of restenosis during 6–month follow-up . *Circulation* 1990; **81**: 1849–1859.

138. Litvack F, Eigler NL, Margolis JR et al. Percutaneous excimer laser coronary angioplasty. *Am J Cardiol* 1990; **66**: 1027–1032.

139. Bittl JA, Kuntz RE, Estella P et al. Analysis of late lumen narrowing after excimer laser-facilitated coronary angioplasty. *J Am Coll Cardiol* 1994; **23**: 1314–1320.

140. Litvack F, Eigler N, Margolis J et al. Percutaneous excimer laser coronary angioplasty: results in the first consecutive 3,000 patients. The ELCA Investigators. *J Am Coll Cardiol* 1994; **23**: 323–329.

141. Honye J, Mahon DJ, Nakamura S et al. Intravascular ultrasound imaging after excimer laser angioplasty. *Cathet Cardiovasc Diagn* 1994; **32**: 213–222.

142. Buchwald AB, Werner GS, Unterberg C et al. Restenosis after excimer laser angioplasty of coronary stenoses and chronic total occlusions. *Am Heart J* 1992; **123**: 878–885.

143. Mintz GS, Kovach JA, Javier SP et al. Mechanisms of lumen enlargement after excimer laser coronary angioplasty. An intravascular ultrasound study. *Circulation* 1995; **92**: 3408–3414.

144. Brinker JA. Laser angioplasty: the great 'light' hope. *Am J Cardiol* 1992; **70**: 1605–1606.

145. Vandormael M, Reifart N, Preusler W et al. Comparison of excimer laser angioplasty and rotational atherectomy with balloon angioplasty for complex lesions: ERBAC study final results (abstract). *J Am Coll Cardiol* 1994; **Suppl**: 57A.

146. Israel DH, Marmur JD, Sanborn TA. Excimer laser-facilitated balloon angioplasty of a nondilatable lesion. *J Am Coll Cardiol* 1991; **18**: 1118–1119.

147. Cook SL, Eigler NL, Shefer A et al. Percutaneous excimer laser coronary angioplasty of lesions not ideal for balloon angioplasty. *Circulation* 1991; **84**: 632–643.

148. Mintz GS, Potkin BN, Keren G et al. Intravascular ultrasound evaluation of the effect of rotational atherectomy in obstructive atherosclerotic coronary artery disease. *Circulation* 1992; **86**: 1383–1393.

149. Kovach JA, Mintz GS, Pichard AD et al. Sequential intravascular ultrasound characterization of the mechanisms of rotational atherectomy and adjunct balloon angioplasty. *J Am Coll Cardiol* 1993; **22**: 1024–1032.

150. Warth DC, Leon MB, O'Neill W et al. Rotational atherectomy multicenter registry: acute results, complications and 6–month angiographic follow-up in 709 patients. *J Am Coll Cardiol* 1994; **24**: 641–648.

151. Ellis SG, Popma JJ, Buchbinder M et al. Relation of clinical presentation, stenosis morphology, and operator technique to the procedural results of rotational atherectomy and rotational atherectomy-facilitated angioplasty. *Circulation* 1994; **89**: 882–892.

152. Bertrand ME, Lablanche JM, Leroy F et al. Percutaneous transluminal coronary rotary ablation with Rotablator (European experience). *Am J Cardiol* 1992; **69**: 470–474.

153. Whitlow PL, Cowley MJ, Kuntz RE et al. Study To determine Rotablator And Transluminal Angioplasty Strategy (STRATAS): acute results. *Circulation* 1996; **Suppl I**: 435.

154. Mintz GS, Pichard AD, Kovach JA et al. Impact of preintervention intravascular ultrasound imaging on transcatheter treatment strategies in coronary artery disease. *Am J Cardiol* 1994; **73**: 423–430.

155. Gerritsen GP, Gussenhoven EJ, The SH et al. Intravascular ultrasonography before and after intervention: in vivo comparison with angiography. *J Vasc Surg* 1993; **18**: 31–40.

156. Herrmann HC, Buchbinder M, Clemen MW et al. Emergent use of balloon-expandable coronary artery stenting for failed percutaneous transluminal coronary angioplasty. *Circulation* 1992; **86**: 812–819.

157. Haude M, Erbel R, Straub U et al. Results of intracoronary stents for management of coronary dissection after balloon angioplasty. *Am J Cardiol* 1991; **67**: 691–696.

158. Kiemeneij F, Laarman GJ, van der Wieken R, Suwarganda J. Emergency coronary stenting with the Palmaz–Schatz stent for failed transluminal coronary angioplasty: results of a learning phase. *Am Heart J* 1993; **126**: 23–31.

159. Fischman DL, Savage MP, Leon MB et al. Effect of intracoronary stenting on intimal dissection after balloon angioplasty: results of quantitative and qualitative coronary analysis. *J Am Coll Cardiol* 1991; **18**: 1445–1451.

160. George BS, Voorhees WD, Roubin GS et al. Multicenter investigation of coronary stenting to treat acute or threatened closure after percutaneous transluminal coronary angioplasty: clinical and angiographic outcomes. *J Am Coll Cardiol* 1993; **22**: 135–143.

161. Roubin GS, Cannon AD, Agrawal SK et al. Intracoronary stenting for acute and threatened closure complicating percutaneous transluminal coronary angioplasty. *Circulation* 1992; **85**: 916–927.

162. Strauss BH, Serruys PW, de Scheerder IK et al. Relative risk analysis of angiographic predictors of restenosis within the coronary wall stent. *Circulation* 1991; **84**: 1636–1643.

163. Serruys PW, Strauss BH, Beatt KJ et al. Angiographic follow-up after placement of a self-expanding coronary-artery stent. *N Engl J Med* 1991; **324**: 13–17.

164. Schatz RA, Baim DS, Leon M et al. Clinical experience with the Palmaz–Schatz coronary stent. Initial results of a multicenter study. *Circulation* 1991; **83**: 148–161.

165. Maiello L, Colombo A, Gianrossi R et al. Coronary stenting for treatment of acute or threatened closure following dissection after coronary balloon angioplasty. *Am Heart J* 1993; **125**: 1570–1575.

166. Nath FC, Muller DW, Ellis SG et al. Thrombosis of a flexible coil coronary stent: frequency, predictors and clinical outcome. *J Am Coll Cardiol* 1993; **21**: 622–627.

167. Agrawal SK, Ho DS, Liu MW et al. Predictors of thrombotic complications after placement of the flexible coil stent. *Am J Cardiol* 1994; **73**: 1216–1219.

168. Sutton JM, Ellis SG, Roubin GS et al. Major clinical events after coronary stenting. The multicenter registry of acute and elective Gianturco–Roubin stent placement. The Gianturco–Roubin Intracoronary Stent Investigator Group. *Circulation* 1994; **89**: 1126–1137.

169. Bilodeau L, Hearn JA, Dean LS, Roubin GS. Prolonged intracoronary urokinase infusion for acute stent thrombosis. *Cathet Cardiovasc Diagn* 1993; **30**: 141–146.

170. Haude M, Erbel R, Issa H et al. Subacute thrombotic complications after intracoronary implantation of Palmaz–Schatz stents. *Am Heart J* 1993; **126**: 15–22.

171. Goldberg SL, Colombo A, Nakamura S et al. Benefit of intracoronary ultrasound in the deployment of Palmaz–Schatz stents. *J Am Coll Cardiol* 1994; **24**: 996–1003.

172. Nakamura S, Colombo A, Gaglione A et al. Intracoronary ultrasound observations during stent implantation. *Circulation* 1994; **89**: 2026–2034.

173. Schatz RA, Goldberg S, Leon M et al. Clinical experience with the Palmaz–Schatz coronary stent. *J Am Coll Cardiol* 1991; **17**: 155B–159B.

174. Savage MP, Fischman DL, Schatz RA et al. Long-term angiographic and clinical outcome after implantation of a balloon-expandable stent in the native coronary circulation. Palmaz–Schatz Stent Study Group. *J Am Coll Cardiol* 1994; **24**: 1207–1212.

175. Serruys PW, de Jaegere P, Kiemeneij F et al. A comparison of balloon-expandable-stent implantation with balloon angioplasty in patients with coronary artery disease. Benestent Study Group. *N Engl J Med* 1994; **331**: 489–495.

176. Cohen DJ, Krumholz HM, Sukin CA et al. In-hospital and one-year economic outcomes after coronary stenting or balloon angioplasty. Results from a randomized clinical trial. Stent Restenosis Study Investigators. *Circulation* 1995; **92**: 2480–2487.

177. Colombo A, Hall P, Nakamura S et al. Intracoronary stenting without anticoagulation accomplished with intravascular ultrasound guidance. *Circulation* 1995; **91**: 1676–1688.

178. Fischman DL, Leon MB, Baim DS et al. A randomized comparison of coronary-stent placement and balloon angioplasty in the treatment of coronary artery disease. Stent Restenosis Study Investigators. *N Engl J Med* 1994; **331**: 496–501.

179. Macaya C, Serruys PW, Ruygrok P et al. Continued benefit of coronary stenting versus balloon angioplasty: one-year clinical follow-up of Benestent trial. Benestent Study Group. *J Am Coll Cardiol* 1996; **27**: 255–261.

180. Moussa I, Moses J, Di Mario C et al. Does the specific intravascular ultrasound criterion used to optimize stent expansion have an impact on the probability of stent restenosis? *Am J Cardiol* 1999; **83**: 1012–1017.

181. de Jaegere P, Mudra H, Almagor Y et al. In-hospital and 1-month clinical results of an international study testing the concept of IVUS guided optimized stent expansion alleviating the need of systemic anticoagulation (abstract). *J Am Coll Cardiol* 1996; **27**: 137A.

182. Mudra H, Sunamura M, Figulla H et al. *J Am Coll Cardiol* 1997; **29**: 171A.

183. Russo RJ, Schatz RA, Sklar MA et al. Ultrasound guided coronary stent placement without prolonged systemic anticoagulation (abstract). *J Am Coll Cardiol* 1995; 50A.

184. Alfonso F, Rodriguez P, Phillips P et al. Clinical and angiographic implications of coronary stenting in thrombus-containing lesions (abstract). *J Am Coll Cardiol* 1997; **29**: 725–733.

185. Sukin CA, Baim DS, Caputo RP et al. The impact of optimal stenting techniques on cardiac catheterization laboratory resource utilization and costs. *Am J Cardiol* 1997; **79**: 275–280.

186. Mudra H, Regar E, Klauss V et al. Serial follow-up after optimized ultrasound-guided deployment of Palmaz–Schatz stents. In-stent neointimal proliferation without significant reference segment response. *Circulation* 1997; **95**: 363–370.

187. Sankardas MA, McEniery PT, Aroney CN, Bett JHN. Elective implantation of intracoronary stents without intravascular guidance or subsequent warfarin. *Cathet Cardiovasc Diagn* 1995; **37**: 355–359.

188. Karrillon GJ, Morice MC, Benveniste E et al. Intracoronary stent implantation without ultrasound guidance and with replacement of conventional anticoagulation by antiplatelet therapy. 30–day clinical outcome of the French Multicenter Registry. *Circulation* 1996; **94**: 1519–1527.

189. Goods CM, Al-Shaibi KF, Yadav SS et al. Utilization of the coronary balloon-expandable coil stent without anticoagulation or intravascular ultrasound. *Circulation* 1996; **93**: 1803–1808.

190. Serruys PW, Emanuelsson H, van der Giessen W et al. Heparin-coated Palmaz–Schatz stents in human coronary arteries. Early outcome of the Benestent-II Pilot Study. *Circulation* 1996; **93**: 412–422.

191. Tobis JM, Colombo A. Do you need IVUS guidance for coronary stent deployment? *Cathet Cardiovasc Diagn* 1996; **37**: 360–361.

Chapter 2 **A comparison of current stents**

Antonio Colombo and Jonathan Tobis

Over the past 5 years our laboratory has been asked to evaluate many of the new stents in preparation for clinical release. The purpose of developing these new stents is to overcome some of the limitations of the original stent designs. The most important feature of a stent is its capacity to provide sufficient scaffolding to the vessel wall. A necessary but secondary feature is the deliverability of the stent to the target site. Although problems with delivering the stent create immediate difficulty for the operator, inadequate vessel scaffolding is the more significant problem for the patient. A final attribute of a good stent is that it should be able to achieve the first two goals while employing a minimal amount of metal. For each clinical and anatomical situation, there are stent characteristics that are more desirable than others. Despite a legitimate goal for each company to provide 'a stent for all seasons', we believe it is important to tailor the stent to the requirements of the lesion. We are frequently asked which single stent we prefer. This is not an easy question to answer because technology advances in a leap-frog manner. What we might recommend today could be obsolete 6 months from now. In addition, certain stents are better suited for different anatomic locations. With this disclaimer clearly in mind, this chapter attempts to summarize our experience with many of the stents that we have tested. The reader should appreciate that these data were derived over different time periods and were not obtained from randomized controlled studies. We have grouped the lesions into those in vessels of similar size and those of similar length, but there is always the possibility of unappreciated bias that could influence the results. Some of the newer flexible stents were used for the more difficult lesion subsets, and this will influence the relative restenosis rates. With these precautionary statements providing the ground rules, we present the following comparison of the stents that we have tested.

ALL STENTS GLOBAL DATA

There are many decisions that enter into the choice of which stent to use for a specific lesion. These include lesion length, tortuosity, vessel size, and lesion location. Certainly one of the major concerns is the restenosis rate, since the ability to get the stent to the lesion and achieve an immediately successful result can be significantly tempered by a high rate of recurrence. With the provisos described in the introduction in mind, the global restenosis rate for 11 of the stents with which we have the most experience is shown in *Fig. 2.1*. The data are presented in ascending order of restenosis. The interpretation of the data should be influenced by the subset analysis that follows. Since the reference vessel size is a strong contributor to restenosis (see Chapter 4), the average reference vessel size for each of the stents is shown in *Fig. 2.2* in ascending order. It is apparent that the Gianturco–Roubin II stent and the Arterial

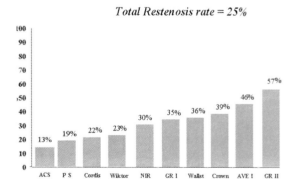

Figure 2.1 *Restenosis rate for all lesions according to stent type 1993–1998.*

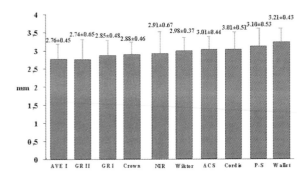

Figure 2.2 *Average reference vessel size for each stent type.*

DIVIDING LESIONS ACCORDING TO LENGTH AND VESSEL WIDTH

Perhaps a fairer way of looking at restenosis data is to group the lesions according to the size of the vessel and the length of the lesion. For the purpose of this analysis, a large vessel is defined as the mean of the angiographic proximal and distal lumen diameters ≥ 3.0 mm; a small vessel is considered to be < 3.0 mm. A long lesion is defined as ≥ 20 mm in length, whereas a short lesion is defined as < 20 mm in length. In this 2×2 matrix, there are four subgroups:

(a) large vessels with short lesions, in which the overall restenosis rate was 16%;

Vascular Engineering (AVE) stent have been used more commonly in smaller vessels that are more difficult to approach with some of the other stents. On the other hand, the Palmaz–Schatz stent and the Wallstent have been used in larger arteries or vein grafts. The percentage of times that a particular stent has been chosen to treat vessels smaller than 3 mm is shown in *Fig. 2.3*. Several of the stents with higher restenosis rates, such as the Gianturco–Roubin I stent, the Gianturco–Roubin II stent, the AVE stent, the BeStent and the Crown stent, were also stents that were more frequently chosen to treat smaller vessels, and this influences their restenosis rate. Randomized trials in which similar lesion characteristics are treated with different stents are needed to determine if there are real distinctions in restenosis rates.

Large vessels – short lesions

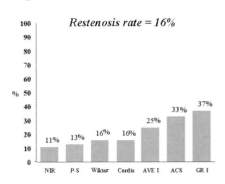

Figure 2.4 *Restenosis rate of different stents when placed in large vessels with short lesions.*

Large vessels – long lesions

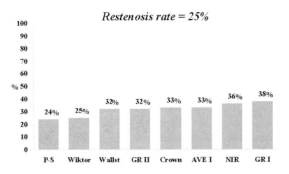

Figure 2.5 *Restenosis rate of different stents when placed in large vessels with long lesions.*

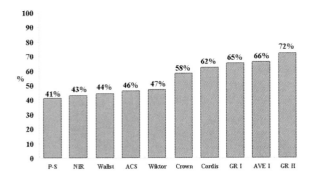

Figure 2.3 *Percent of lesions treated in arteries smaller than 3 mm for each stent type.*

Small vessels – short lesions

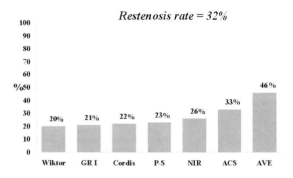

Figure 2.6 Restenosis rate of different stents when placed in small vessels with short lesions.

Small vessels – long lesions

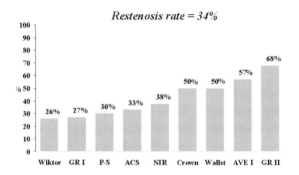

Figure 2.7 Restenosis rate of different stents when placed in small vessels with long lesions.

Table 2.1
Percentage of metal surface area: a comparison among different stents

Type stent	% metal surface area
AVE	8.4%
ACS Multilink	9%
Wiktor	9%
Gianturco–Roubin	10%
Palmaz–Schatz	15%
Cordis	15%
Coronary Wallstent	15%
Peripheral Wallstent	26%

a comparison among some of the more common stents for the percentage of metal surface area.

DESCRIPTION OF THE INDIVIDUAL STENTS

PALMAZ–SCHATZ SLOTTED TUBULAR DESIGN

The Palmaz–Schatz stent (*Fig. 2.8*) was one of the first available devices, and we have therefore had the most experience with it. Even with the onslaught of multiple stents with improvements in design that facilitate trackability, there are certain lesion subsets for which we still find that the strength of the

(b) large vessels with long lesions, in which the overall restenosis rate was 25%;
(c) small vessels with short lesions, in which the overall restenosis rate was 32%; and
(d) small vessels with long lesions, in which the restenosis rate was the highest at 34%.

The restenosis rates for the individual stents in these four group subsets are provided in *Figs 2.4, 2.5, 2.6* and *2.7*.

Of the potential influences that design has on stent function, the percentage of metal surface area coverage has been felt to be a significant factor for immediate and long-term results.[1] *Table 2.1* provides

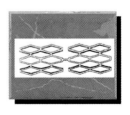

Manufacturer		J&J Cordis
Structure		Slotted tube
Material		Stainless Steel
Strut thickness	*(mm)*	0.07
Metal / Artery	*(%)*	20
Recoil	*(%)*	6
Foreshortening	*(%)*	8
Radiopacity		low
Markers		no
Lengths	*(mm)*	15
Diameters	*(mm)*	3.0....4.0

Figure 2.8 Palmaz–Schatz 153

Table 2.2
Palmaz–Schatz™

Patients 890		*Lesions 1059*	
Stents/lesion	= 1.4	Average ref. vess. size	= 3.10 ± 0.53
Thrombosis	= 1.5%	Large vessels (615 les)	= 3.46 ± 0.42
Procedural success	= 98%	Small vessels (423 les)	= 2.66 ± 0.27
		Large vs small (%)	= 59 vs 41

Palmaz–Schatz slotted tube is very effective. *Table 2.2* summarizes our experience in 1059 lesions from 890 patients. Despite the bulky nature of the Palmaz–Schatz stent, a 98% procedural success rate was achieved. This high success rate was due in part to removing the stent from the delivery system and hand crimping it on a high-pressure balloon to lower the profile. To increase the ability to get the stent to distal lesions or through tortuous vessels, the articulation was occasionally cut and a half stent was mounted alone on a balloon.[2] Alternatively, when stent delivery was not a problem but plaque prolapse through the articulation was, the articulation was folded over to approximate the scaffolding ends without removing the stent from the delivery system.[3] A further description of these techniques is provided in Chapter 6.

Our overall restenosis rate with the Palmaz–Schatz stent has been 19%. These data are subdivided into the four subgroups in *Table 2.3*. The angiographic restenosis rate varied between 13% for large vessels with short lesions and 30% for small vessels with long lesions. An example of a long-term successful stent insertion using the 15 mm Palmaz–Schatz stent is provided in *Fig. 2.9*. Although the articulation strut was placed in the Palmaz–Schatz stent to provide increased flexibility, it was frequently observed that a common site for in-stent restenosis was at the articulation. This concern was addressed by a modification of the Palmaz–Schatz stent to a spiral design (*Fig. 2.10*). Although this stent provided more support at the articulation site, the new design increased the rigidity of the stent and made it more difficult to track through tortuous portions of the artery.

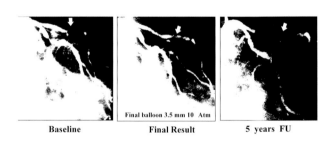

Baseline	Final Result	5 years FU

Figure 2.9 *Five-year follow-up of a stent placed in the mid-left anterior descending coronary artery demonstrates long-term patency.*

Table 2.3
Palmaz–Schatz™

Nr of lesions elegible for FU	= 1032
Lesions with FU	= 619 (61%)
Global restenosis rate	= 19%

Large short 280 (Rest. 13%)	Large long 93 (Rest. 24%)	Small short 171 (Rest. 23%)	Small long 72 (Rest. 30%)

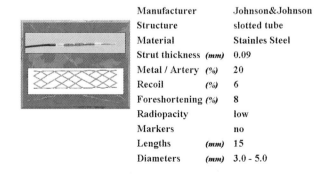

Manufacturer	Johnson&Johnson
Structure	slotted tube
Material	Stainles Steel
Strut thickness *(mm)*	0.09
Metal / Artery *(%)*	20
Recoil *(%)*	6
Foreshortening *(%)*	8
Radiopacity	low
Markers	no
Lengths *(mm)*	15
Diameters *(mm)*	3.0 - 5.0

Figure 2.10 *Palmaz–Schatz 154 spiral design.*

Table 2.4

Gianturco–Roubin I™

Patients 123		*Lesions 166*	
Stents/lesion	= 1.5	Average ref. vess. size	= 2.85 ± 0.48
Thrombosis	= 3%	Large vessels (55 les)	= 3.37 ± 0.32
Procedural success	= 99%	Small vessels (104 les)	= 2.57 ± 0.28
		Large vs small (%)	= 35 vs 65

Table 2.5

Gianturco–Roubin I™

Nr of lesions elegible for FU   = 160
Lesions with FU   = 124 (77%)
Global restenosis rate   = 35%

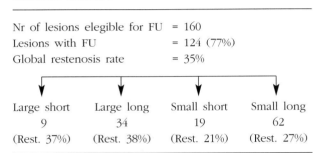

Large short	Large long	Small short	Small long
9	34	19	62
(Rest. 37%)	(Rest. 38%)	(Rest. 21%)	(Rest. 27%)

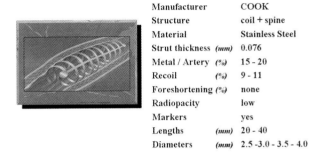

Manufacturer		COOK
Structure		coil + spine
Material		Stainless Steel
Strut thickness	*(mm)*	0.076
Metal / Artery	*(%)*	15 - 20
Recoil	*(%)*	9 - 11
Foreshortening	*(%)*	none
Radiopacity		low
Markers		yes
Lengths	*(mm)*	20 - 40
Diameters	*(mm)*	2.5 -3.0 - 3.5 - 4.0

Figure 2.11 *Gianturco–Roubin II.*

Despite the technical limitations of this design, subsequent randomized clinical trials demonstrated that the Palmaz–Schatz stent performed as well as other slotted tube stents[4,5] and better than the Gianturco–Roubin II stent[6] as an antirestenosis device.

GIANTURCO–ROUBIN COILED STENT

The original Gianturco–Roubin stent provided more flexibility than the Palmaz–Schatz stent. However, the clam-shell design did not maintain continuous radial support of the artery. Although this design was very useful as a bail-out device for tacking up significant dissections, the lack of structural support appeared to influence the overall restenosis rate. It must be cautioned that this stent was used more commonly in smaller vessels because of its increased flexibility. However, after matching for vessel size and lesion length, this stent was still associated with a higher restenosis rate than the Palmaz–Schatz stent.[7] Our results with the Gianturco–Roubin stent are provided in *Table 2.4*, and the restenosis rates in the four subsets are provided in *Table 2.5*.

In an attempt to address the concerns of the first design, the Gianturco–Roubin II stent was developed with a coiled structure and a continuous spine to provide more longitudinal support and prevent separation of the coils (*Fig. 2.11*). Compared to the original design, the Gianturco–Roubin II stent is improved in that it has greater trackability and radial strength, a lower profile balloon delivery system and a greater ability to prevent stent uncoiling. The Gianturco–Roubin II stent performs admirably in terms of its flexibility and ability to reach distal lesions in small vessels with a 98% procedural success rate (*Table 2.6*). However, in our experience, the angiographic restenosis rate has been disappointing. The overall restenosis rate is 57% and is as high as 68% in the toughest subgroup of small vessels and long lesions (*Table 2.7*). These results are consistent with the results of the recently completed randomized trial comparing the Gianturco–Roubin II stent to the Palmaz–Schatz stent [6] In this trial, angiographic restenosis was 43% for the Gianturco–Roubin II and 19% for the Palmaz–Schatz stent. The explanation for this high restenosis rate in the Gianturco–Roubin II stent is not clear, but it may be due to several factors, such as a higher ratio of stent length to lesion length, inappropriate stent upsizing, and, potentially, the coating that is used on the stent. A clinical example of the Gianturco–Roubin II stent is provided in *Fig. 2.12*.

Table 2.6

Gianturco–Roubin II™

Patients 52		Lesions 100	
Stents/lesion	= 1.4	Average ref. vess. size	= 2.77 ± 0.48
Thrombosis	= 3%	Large vessels (24 les)	= 3.36 ± 0.31
Procedural success	= 99%	Small vessels (60 les)	= 2.53 ± 0.30
		Large vs small (%)	= 29 vs 71

Table 2.7

Gianturco–Roubin II™

Nr of lesions elegible for FU = 99
Lesions with FU   = 65 (66%)
Global restenosis rate   = 57%

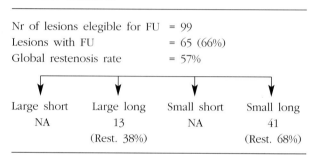

Large short	Large long	Small short	Small long
NA	13	NA	41
	(Rest. 38%)		(Rest. 68%)

The baseline angiogram in the left anterior oblique view (see *Fig. 2.12a*) and right anterior oblique view (see *Fig. 2.12b*) shows several sequential lesions in the mid-right coronary artery. These were treated with three 20 mm Gianturco–Roubin II stents. These were inflated with a 4 mm balloon to 20 atmospheres. The angiogram in *Fig. 2.12c* demonstrates the radiopacity of the stent before contrast filling.

THE NIR STENT

The NIR stent is a balloon-expandable, uniform cellular meshwork that is characterized by moderate longitudinal flexibility and low profile before expansion. A description of the NIR 7-cell and 9-cell stents is provided in *Figs 2.13* and *2.14*. After expansion, the NIR stent has high radial support and minimal recoil owing to its unique rectangular strut design. This design provides significant plaque scaffolding, but the stent delivery is somewhat hampered by its limited flexibility. Despite these concerns, the NIR stent had a procedural success rate of 99% (*Table 2.8*). The restenosis rate in the various subsets is also acceptable, although it is slightly higher than that found in some of the other stents. The restenosis rate in the easiest lesion subset of large vessels with short lesions was only 20%. These results are consistent

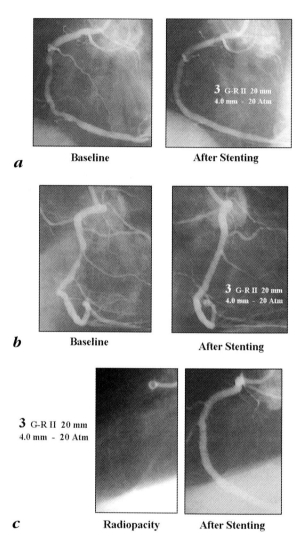

Figure 2.12 *Sequential lesions in the right coronary artery treated with the Gianturco–Roubin II stent. (a) Images before and after stenting in the left anterior oblique projection. (b) Images before and after stenting in the right anterior oblique projection. (c) Radiograph without contrast injection demonstrates the radiopacity of the G–R II stent.*

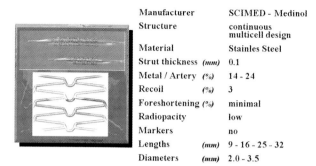

Manufacturer		SCIMED - Medinol
Structure		continuous multicell design
Material		Stainles Steel
Strut thickness	*(mm)*	0.1
Metal / Artery	*(%)*	14 - 24
Recoil	*(%)*	3
Foreshortening	*(%)*	minimal
Radiopacity		low
Markers		no
Lengths	*(mm)*	9 - 16 - 25 - 32
Diameters	*(mm)*	2.0 - 3.5

Figure 2.13 *NIR 7-cell.*

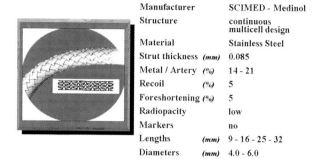

Manufacturer		SCIMED - Medinol
Structure		continuous multicell design
Material		Stainless Steel
Strut thickness	*(mm)*	0.085
Metal / Artery	*(%)*	14 - 21
Recoil	*(%)*	5
Foreshortening	*(%)*	5
Radiopacity		low
Markers		no
Lengths	*(mm)*	9 - 16 - 25 - 32
Diameters	*(mm)*	4.0 - 6.0

Figure 2.14 *NIR 9-cell.*

Table 2.8

NIR™ stent

Patients 246		Lesions 348	
Stents/lesion	= 1.2	Average ref. vess. size	= 3.00 ± 0.53
Thrombosis	= 0.6%	Large vessels (155 les)	= 3.41 ± 0.35
Procedural success	= 99%	Small vessels (150 les)	= 2.58 ± 0.32
		Large vs small (%)	= 51 vs 49

with the results of the NIRVANA trial,[5] which compared the NIR stent to the Palmaz–Schatz stent in simple lesions. In this trial, angiographic restenosis at 9 months was 20% for the NIR stent and 22% for the Palmaz–Schatz stent. However, in the more complicated lesion subset of small vessels with short lesions, the restenosis rate was 38% (*Table 2.9*).

A clinical example of a NIR stent in a tortuous vessel is provided in *Fig. 2.15*. A 16 mm NIR stent was able to negotiate the sharp bends in this obtuse

marginal artery. The significant scaffolding support provided after inflation with a 3.5 mm balloon at 14 atmospheres is demonstrated, both acutely and at the 6-month follow-up study.

The number of cells in the NIR stents refers to the number of units that make up the circumference of the stent. For the same diameter of balloon expan-

Table 2.9

NIR™ stent

Nr of lesions elegible for FU = 343
Lesions with FU = 232 (68%)
Global restenosis rate = 30%

Large short	Large long	Small short	Small long
84	14	97	8
(Rest. 20%)	(Rest. 14%)	(Rest. 38%)	(Rest. 25%)

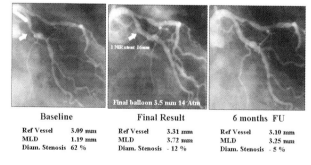

	Baseline	Final Result	6 months FU
Ref Vessel	3.09 mm	3.31 mm	3.10 mm
MLD	1.19 mm	3.72 mm	3.25 mm
Diam. Stenosis	62 %	- 12 %	- 5 %

Figure 2.15 *Successful treatment of a tortuous circumflex artery with the NIR stent. MLD, minimum lumen diameter.*

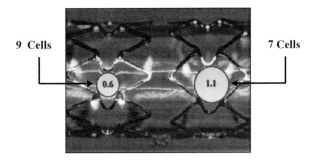

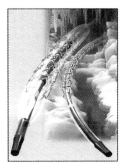

Figure 2.16 *Comparison of the intra-cell cross-sectional space available in the NIR 7-cell versus the 9-cell stent.*

Figure 2.18 *NIR on Activa.*

Manufacturer		SCIMED Medinol
Structure		Cont. multicellular
Material		Stainless Steel
Strut thickness	*(mm)*	0.085
Metal / Artery	*(%)*	14.5 *(7 cells)* - 17 *(9 cells)*
Recoil	*(%)*	5
Foreshortening	*(%)*	5
Radiopacity		Low
Markers		No
Lengths	*(mm)*	9, 16, 25, 32
Diameters	*(mm)*	2.5 .....4.0; 7-9 Cells

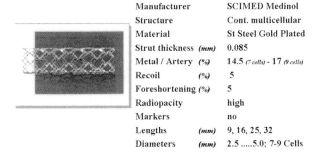

Manufacturer		SCIMED Medinol
Structure		Cont. multicellular
Material		St Steel Gold Plated
Strut thickness	*(mm)*	0.085
Metal / Artery	*(%)*	14.5 *(7 cells)* - 17 *(9 cells)*
Recoil	*(%)*	5
Foreshortening	*(%)*	5
Radiopacity		high
Markers		no
Lengths	*(mm)*	9, 16, 25, 32
Diameters	*(mm)*	2.5 .....5.0; 7-9 Cells

Figure 2.17 *NIR Royal.*

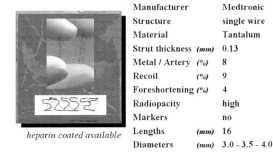

heparin coated available

Manufacturer		Medtronic
Structure		single wire
Material		Tantalum
Strut thickness	*(mm)*	0.13
Metal / Artery	*(%)*	8
Recoil	*(%)*	9
Foreshortening	*(%)*	4
Radiopacity		high
Markers		no
Lengths	*(mm)*	16
Diameters	*(mm)*	3.0 - 3.5 - 4.0

Figure 2.19 *Wiktor.*

sion, the area between struts is larger in the 7-cell stent than with the 9-cell stent. A comparison of the cell diameter available for a balloon to pass through the NIR 7-cell stent compared with the NIR 9-cell stent is shown in *Fig. 2.16*. With nine cells to go around the circumference of the vessel, the intrastrut diameter through which a balloon or a second stent to a side branch must pass is only 0.6 mm. With seven cells making up the circumference of the stent, the diameter between struts is 1.1 mm. The NIR Royal stent has been developed to increase radiopacity by plating this stainless steel stent with gold (*Fig. 2.17*). A recent alteration of the NIR stent is called the NIR on Activa™, which places the stainless steel NIR 7-cell stent or 9-cell stent on a low profile Activa™ balloon (*Fig. 2.18*). This lower profile significantly increases its capacity to reach small vessels in tortuous lesions. In addition, the Activa™ balloon is a high-pressure

balloon so that the stent can be delivered and expanded maximally with the same balloon.

WIKTOR STENT

The Wiktor stent (*Fig. 2.19*) has a coiled, sine-wave design. It is made out of tantalum to provide high radiopacity. Owing to its high visibility, no markers are necessary to help position the stent. However, the disadvantage of the high radiopacity is that it may be difficult to assess the degree of residual stenosis by angiography. As with all coiled stents, the design improves the flexibility and permits the stent to pass through tortuous segments and into distal lesions. The negative aspect of this design is that the stents can be uncoiled, especially if used in complex lesions such as those with bifurcations where the stent has

Table 2.10
Wiktor™ stent

Patients 90		Lesions 140	
Stents/lesion	= 1.5	Average ref. vess. size	= 2.98 ± 0.37
Thrombosis	= 3.5%	Large vessels (71 les)	= 3.36 ± 0.34
Procedural success	= 93%	Small vessels (64 les)	= 2.58 ± 0.31
		Large vs small (%)	= 53 vs 47

Table 2.11
Wiktor™ stent

Nr of lesions elegible for FU	= 131
Lesions with FU	= 89 (68%)
Global restenosis rate	= 23%

Large short	Large long	Small short	Small long
30	20	24	15
(Rest. 16%)	(Rest. 25%)	(Rest. 20%)	(Rest. 26%)

Stenting a Tortuous Vessel (I)

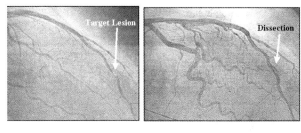

Baseline   **After Balloon Angioplasty**

a

Stenting a Tortuous Vessel (II)

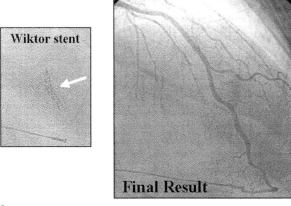

b

Figure 2.20 *Use of the Wiktor stent to treat a dissection following balloon angioplasty of the distal left anterior descending coronary artery.*

to be recrossed with another balloon or a separate stent. In our experience, the overall procedural success rate is 93%, which is somewhat less than with the other stents (*Table 2.10*). The overall restenosis rate is acceptable at 23%, and it varies between 16% for the low-risk subsets and 26% for the high-risk subsets (*Table 2.11*). These results are consistent with a recently reported large study of the Wiktor stent in which the restenosis rate was 20%.[8] A clinical example of the flexibility of the Wiktor stent is provided in *Fig. 2.20*. A dissection developed in this lesion in the distal left anterior descending artery (LAD) following balloon dilatation, and this was successfully approached and supported with the Wiktor stent. The clinical use of a long Wiktor-i stent (*Fig. 2.21*) is shown in *Fig. 2.22*. This chronic total occlusion of the right coronary artery was supported nicely with a 30 mm flexible Wiktor-i stent without straightening out the bends in the artery, which could create new stenoses at the hinge points.

WALLSTENT

In 1986, the Wallstent became the first stent to be clinically tested.[9] It is structurally very different from most of the other stents that are commonly used today (*Fig. 2.23*). The stent is produced as a multiple wire braid, which has the unique property of self-expanding once the protective sheath is removed. There is approximately 20% foreshortening as the stent expands, which makes it more difficult to

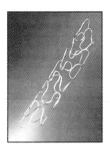

Manufacturer		Medtronic
Structure		Single wire
Material		Tantalum
Strut thickness	*(mm)*	0.13
Metal / Artery	*(%)*	9
Recoil	*(%)*	7
Foreshortening	*(%)*	4
Radiopacity		high
Markers		no
Lengths	*(mm)*	20-30-38
Diameters	*(mm)*	2.5....4.0

Figure 2.21 *Wiktor-i*

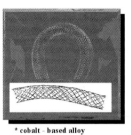

* cobalt - based alloy

Manufacturer		Schneider
Structure		multiple wire braid
Material		Elgiloy *
Strut thickness	*(mm)*	0.10
Metal / Artery	*(%)*	14
Recoil	*(%)*	n.a.
Foreshortening	*(%)*	20
Radiopacity		moderate
Markers		no
Lengths	*(mm)*	15 - 50
Diameters	*(mm)*	4.0 - 6.0

Figure 2.23 *Wallstent*

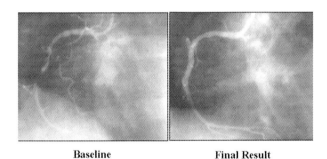

Baseline   Final Result

Figure 2.22 *Use of a 30 mm long flexible Wiktor-i stent to treat a long lesion in the mid-right coronary artery.*

position the stent precisely. One of the beneficial characteristics is its high flexibility, despite its long length. This permits the stent to approach long lesions in vein grafts or in large vessels without side branches, such as the right coronary artery.

Our experience with the Wallstent is provided in *Tables 2.12* and *2.13*. Unlike other stents, the

Wallstent was applied only for long lesions in which one would expect a higher restenosis rate. The overall restenosis rate was 36%, but it was as high as 50% in the subset of small vessels less than 3 mm in diameter with long lesions. The recently completed WINS study[10] demonstrated equivalency between the Wallstent and the Palmaz–Schatz stent in saphenous vein grafts. Angiographic restenosis at 6 months was 38.6% for the Wallstent and 40.8% for the PS stent. Unlike the balloon-expandable stents, which tend to have some degree of recoil, the Wallstent may continue to expand after implantation (*Fig. 2.24*). In this example, a diffusely diseased portion of the left anterior descending artery was treated with a peripheral Wallstent 51 mm in length and 6 mm in diameter. At the time of deployment, the lumen diameter was 2.5 × 2.7 mm. However, at 6-month follow-up, the stent had expanded significantly with a diameter of 5 mm by intravascular ultrasound (see *Fig. 2.24b*). There was significant growth of intimal tissue within the stent, so that the residual lumen appeared adequate at 2.2 mm. The subacute stent thrombosis rate of 1.8% is no different from that of other stents in our series, despite the fact that the peripheral

Table 2.12
Wallstent™

Patients 83		Lesions 96	
Stents/lesion	= 1.1	Average ref. vess. size	= 3.21 ± 0.43
Thrombosis	= 1.2%	Large vessels (54 les)	= 3.56 ± 0.34
Procedural success	= 97%	Small vessels (42 les)	= 2.65 ± 0.32
		Large vs small (%)	= 56 vs 44

Table 2.13
Wallstent™

Nr of lesions elegible for FU = 75
Lesions with FU   = 55 (77%)
Global restenosis rate   = 36%

Large short NA	Large long 28 (Rest. 32%)	Small short NA	Small long 27 (Rest. 50%)

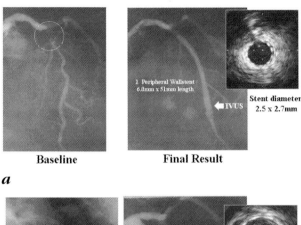

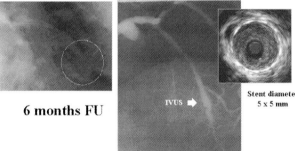

Figure 2.24 *(a) A long peripheral wallstent was placed in the left anterior descending coronary artery. (b) The IVUS exam obtained six months later reveals that the stent struts have expanded from 2.5 to 5.0 mm in diameter. Despite this extensive auto-expansion, the lumen is filled with significant neointimal hyperplasia so that the angiogram does not demonstrate the aneurysmal dilatation.*

Wallstent has a much larger metal surface area. This observation favors the argument that subacute stent thrombosis is not due to inherent thrombogenicity of the metal as much as to the lumen cross-sectional area and flow within the vessel.

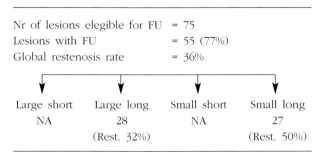

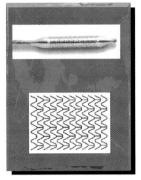

Manufacturer		ACS
Structure		Etched tube
Material		Stainless Steel
Strut thickness	*(mm)*	0.06
Metal / Artery	*(%)*	7 - 15
Recoil	*(%)*	6
Foreshortening	*(%)*	5
Radiopacity		low
Markers		no
Lengths	*(mm)*	15 - 25 - 35
Diameters	*(mm)*	3.0 - 4.0

Figure 2.25 *ACS Multilink.*

ACS MULTILINK STENT

The ACS Multilink stent has a slotted tubular meshwork design and is made of rings connected at multiple sites by longitudinal bridges (*Fig. 2.25*). The stent has significant flexibility with excellent plaque coverage. The stent is made from stainless steel and does not have any markers, which limits the radiopacity and makes it difficult to expand the stent precisely with a high-pressure balloon after deployment. The Multilink stent was released for clinical use in the USA in the autumn of 1997 after a randomized trial showed safety and efficacy comparable to those of the Palmaz–Schatz stent.[4]

Our experience with the Multilink is shown in *Tables 2.14* and *2.15*. The stent performed very well in terms of its ability to reach the lesion, with a 100% procedural success rate. The overall restenosis rate was impressively low at 13%. The 15 mm stent was most readily available and this stent was used in shorter lesions, which could account for the lower restenosis rate. In addition, directional atherectomy was frequently used in association with this stent, which may also account for the lower restenosis rate in our series.

An example of a Multilink stent deployed in a left main artery lesion is provided in *Fig. 2.26*. This 46-year-old woman with stable angina and a positive stress test had a stenosis in the distal left main artery involving the ostium of the LAD and the circumflex artery. This was treated by placing an intra-aortic balloon pump prophylactically and then performing directional atherectomy with a 7 Fr device. Eleven cuts were made in the distal left main and proximal ostium of the LAD. A 15 mm long ACS Multilink stent was placed in the distal left main artery and was

Table 2.14
ACS Multilink™

Patients 68		Lesions 103	
Stents/lesion	= 1.2	Average ref. vess. size	= 3.16 ± 0.47
Thrombosis	= 1%	Large vessels (54 les)	= 3.43 ± 0.40
Procedural success	= 100%	Small vessels (37 les)	= 2.77 ± 0.22
		Large vs small (%)	= 59 vs 41

Table 2.15
ACS Multilink™

Nr of lesions elegible for FU = 103
Lesions with FU   = 77 (75%)
Global restenosis rate   = 13%

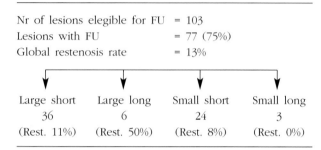

Large short	Large long	Small short	Small long
36	6	24	3
(Rest. 11%)	(Rest. 50%)	(Rest. 8%)	(Rest. 0%)

expanded with a 4 mm balloon to 18 atmospheres. The final minimum lumen diameter was 3.6 mm. The artery did not show any evidence of restenosis on the 4-month follow-up study (see *Fig. 2.26b*).

Despite the excellent long-term results with the Multilink stent, this device has two main limitations:

(a) the delivery balloon is very compliant and extends well beyond the stent edges, which may predispose to edge dissections after deployment; and
(b) the large profile of the delivery system and the inability to visualize the stent on fluoroscopy increase the risk of accidental stent dislodgment in complex lesions.

To remedy these limitations, a modified Multilink stent design was introduced – the Duet stent. The Duet stent is a next generation Multilink stent with enhanced strut width, radiopacity, radial strength, and flexibility. It is mounted on a low-profile, high-pressure stent delivery system. A prospective multi-center registry was performed in 270 patients with single de novo lesions of less than 25 mm in length. The procedural success rate was 99.6%, the stent thrombosis rate was 1.1%, and the angiographic restenosis rate at 6 months was acceptable, at 22%.[11]

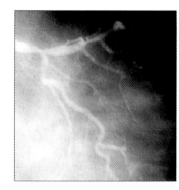
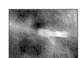

DCA 7 F : 11 cuts
with IABP support

Baseline

a

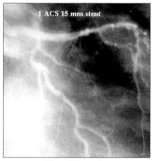
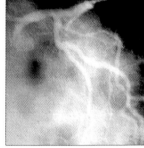

1 ACS 15 mm stent

Final Result   **4 month Follow-Up**

b

Figure 2.26 *(a) The stenosis in the distal left main coronary artery extended into the ostium of the LAD. This was treated with directional atherectomy followed by placement of a 15 mm long Multilink stent (b). DCA, directional coronary atherectomy; IABP, intra-aortic balloon pump.*

AVE MICROSTENT

The Arterial Vascular Engineering (AVE) Company has produced a series of stent designs with unique capabilities. The original design, called the AVE I

Table 2.16

AVE stents™

Patients 104		Lesions 196	
Stents/lesion	= 1.2	Average ref. vess. size	= 2.85 ± 0.48
Thrombosis	= 2.6%	Large vessels (64 les)	= 3.32 ± 0.30
Procedural success	= 99%	Small vessels (108 les)	= 2.56 ± 0.32
		Large vs small (%)	= 37 vs 63

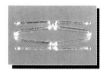

Milan experience   :   198 implantations

151 implantations for failed positioning of other stents.

* *Disadvantages : migration of subunits ; incomplete plaque scaffolding.*

Figure 2.27 *AVE Microstent I.*

Table 2.17

AVE stents

Nr of lesions elegible for FU	= 194
Lesions with FU	= 132 (68%)
Global restenosis rate	= 45%

Large short	Large long	Small short	Small long
35	3	67	9
(Rest. 40%)	(Rest. 0%)	(Rest. 48%)	(Rest. 56%)

Microstent, had subunits that were 3 mm long and were laser bonded together; this produced significant flexibility (*Fig. 2.27*). The subunits were formed by a sinusoidal coil that provided significant radial support. Our experience covers 196 implantations of the AVE I Microstent. The stent was used in 151 cases when other stents failed to reach the lesion site. Despite the difficulty of the lesion subsets, the procedural success rate was 99% (*Table 2.16*). The Microstent has the unique capacity of permitting deployment in extremely distal segments or through the struts of other stents when no other stents will pass. The early design, however, had some difficulties with migration of subunits and incomplete plaque scaffolding resulting in prolapse of tissue through the stent struts. These factors probably account for the higher overall restenosis rate of 45% (*Table 2.17*).

As a result of these observations, several modifications to the stent design were made for the AVE II Microstent (*Fig. 2.28*). The performance of this design was compared to the Palmaz–Schatz stent in a multicenter, randomized trial that included 661 patients.[12] In this trial, angiographic restenosis at 6 months was 24.8% for the AVE stent and 22.9% for the Palmaz–Schatz stent.

Further design refinements led to the GFX model (*Fig. 2.29*). In the AVE GFX stent, the sinusoidal subunits have been shortened to 2 mm, which significantly improves the flexibility. At the same time, the

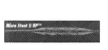

Manufacturer		AVE
Structure		sinusoidal bonded crowns
Material		**Stainless Steel**
Strut thickness	*(mm)*	**0.15 - 0.20**
Metal / Artery	*(%)*	**14**
Recoil	*(%)*	**8**
Foreshortening	*(%)*	**5**
Radiopacity		**moderate**
Markers		**no**
Lengths	*(mm)*	**9-12-18-24-30-39**
Diameters	*(mm)*	**2.5 - 3.0 - 3.5 - 4.0**

Figure 2.28 *AVE Micro II.*

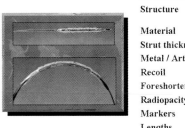

Manufacturer		AVE
Structure		Ellipto - rectangular
Material		Stainless Steel
Strut thickness	*(mm)*	0.13
Metal / Artery	*(%)*	20
Recoil	*(%)*	4
Foreshortening	*(%)*	2 -5
Radiopacity		moderate
Markers		no
Lengths	*(mm)*	8-12-18-24-30-40
Diameters	*(mm)*	2.5 - 3.0 - 3.5 - 4.0

Figure 2.29 *AVE GFX.*

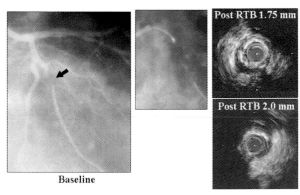

Baseline

a

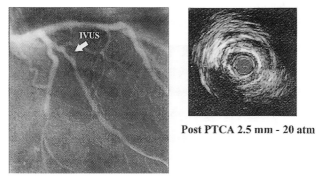

Post PTCA 2.5 mm - 20 atm

b

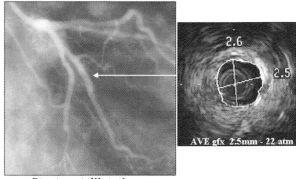

**Stent post dilatation
2.5 mm - 22 atm**

c

amount of metal is increased, which provides greater support and diminishes plaque prolapse. A clinical example of the flexibility and strength of the AVE GFX stent is provided in *Fig. 2.30*. In this calcified, obtuse marginal lesion, the artery was prepared with rotational atherectomy using a 1.75 mm burr and a 2.0 mm burr (see *Fig. 2.30a*). A high-pressure balloon inflation was performed at 20 atmospheres with a 2.5 mm balloon to dilate the lesion before stent deployment (see *Fig. 2.30b*). The stent was then deployed in this small calcified artery and inflated with a 2.5 mm balloon at 22 atmospheres, which yielded a lumen of 2.5 × 2.6 mm, as documented by intravascular ultrasound (see *Fig. 2.30c*).

The flexibility and trackability of the AVE II Microstent is demonstrated in *Fig. 2.31*. The diffusely diseased right coronary artery (RCA) was prepared with rotational atherectomy, incrementally using a 1.25 mm burr to a 2.0 mm burr. A 30 mm Crown stent was placed in the artery in an attempt to pass it to the distal segment. The Crown stent would not make the bend at the acute margin and had to be deployed in the mid-RCA. A 39 mm long AVE II Microstent was then chosen and passed through the initially deployed Crown stent and around the acute margin to the distal RCA. A second 39 mm AVE II Microstent was also passed through the Crown stent and positioned between the other two stents.

THE PURA VARIO STENT

The PURA Vario stent (*Fig. 2.32*) has a slotted meshwork design and is made of stainless steel. It has low radiopacity and there are no markers on the stents. It comes in lengths varying from 10 mm to

Figure 2.30 *AVE GFX in a calcified lesion. (a) This heavily calcified obtuse marginal artery was prepared for stenting with rotational atherectomy. (b) High-pressure balloon dilatation at 20 atmospheres with a 2.5 mm balloon. (c) Stent deployment at high pressures in a small vessel. RTB, rotablator.*

40 mm, and the joints provide a moderate amount of flexibility associated with adequate radial support. Procedural success rate is high at 98% and the overall restenosis rate is only 16% (*Tables 2.18* and *2.19*).[13]

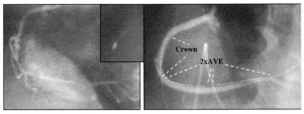

**30mm Crown did not reach distal lesion
that was easily crossed by 2 AVE stents**

Baseline, RTB 1.25-2.0mm   Proximal 30mm Crown, distal 2x39mm AVEII

Figure 2.31 *Demonstration of the flexibility and trackability of the AVE stent.*

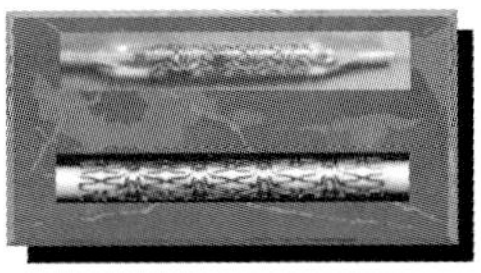

Manufacturer		DEVON
Structure		slotted tube with curved links
Material		Stainless Steel
Strut thickness	*(μm)*	0.10
Metal / Artery	*(%)*	24
Recoil	*(%)*	< 2.5
Foreshortening	*(%)*	5
Radiopacity		low
Markers		no
Lengths	*(mm)*	10-16-22-28-34-40
Diameters	*(mm)*	3.0 - 5.0

Figure 2.32 *PURA Vario.*

Table 2.18
PURA Vario™ stent

Patients 80		Lesions 110	
Stents/lesion	= 1.2	Average ref. vess. size	= 3.13 ± 0.51
Thrombosis	= 2%	Large vessels (55 les)	= 3.43 ± 0.36
Procedural success	= 98%	Small vessels (31 les)	= 2.60 ± 0.25
		Large vs small (%)	= 64 vs 36

Table 2.19
PURA Vario™ stent

Nr of lesions elegible for FU = 108
Lesions with FU = 68 (63%)
Global restenosis rate = 16%

Large short	Large long	Small short	Small long
31	5	15	4
(Rest. 16%)	(Rest. 20%)	(Rest. 7%)	(Rest. 25%)

A clinical example of the use of the PURA Vario stent during multivessel stenting is provided in *Fig. 2.33*. The right coronary artery in this patient had a chronic total occlusion in its mid-portion with left to right collaterals. Following dilatation with a 3 mm balloon, the extent of the distal vessel became apparent; however, there was a significant residual shelf at the entrance to the occlusion (see *Fig. 2.33a*). A 16 mm long PURA Vario stent was deployed on a

3.5 mm balloon at 12 atmospheres. The final result, shown in *Fig. 2.33b*, demonstates adequate perfusion to the distal vessel in this diffusely diseased artery. Our attention was then directed to the lesion in the mid-LAD, which was treated with two PURA Vario stents. These were also delivered on a 3.5 mm balloon and deployed at 16 atmospheres (see *Fig. 2.33c*).

CROWN STENT

The Crown stent is a newer slotted tubular meshwork design produced by Johnson and Johnson (*Fig. 2.34*). It comes in lengths between 15 mm and 30 mm but does not have an articulation as did the original Johnson and Johnson stent. Although the Crown stent is not as flexible as some of the other stent designs, it provides excellent scaffolding support and the procedural success rate was 100% in selected lesions (*Table 2.20*). In addition, the stent is mounted on a high pressure balloon with some retention property and a balloon length which matches the stent length in order to lower the risk of persistent trauma.

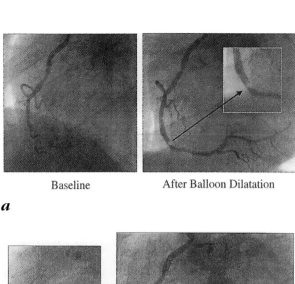

Baseline   After Balloon Dilatation

a

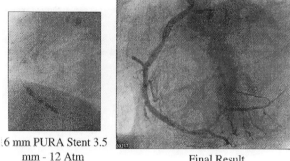

.6 mm PURA Stent 3.5 mm - 12 Atm   Final Result

b

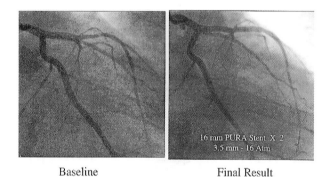

16 mm PURA Stent X 2 3.5 mm - 16 Atm

Baseline   Final Result

c

Figure 2.33 *The PURA-Vario stent used for multivessel disease. (a) An occluded mid-right coronary artery that was mechanically reopened and treated with balloon dilatation. A residual shelf remained. (b) A 16 mm long PURA-Vario stent was deployed at 12 atmospheres on a 3.5 mm balloon. (c) The lesion in the mid LAD was then treated with two stents.*

The global restenosis rate was acceptable at 28%; however, this stent was used more often in long lesions, which could explain the higher restenosis

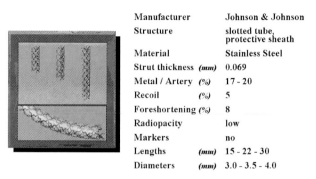

Manufacturer		Johnson & Johnson
Structure		slotted tube, protective sheath
Material		Stainless Steel
Strut thickness	*(mm)*	0.069
Metal / Artery	*(%)*	17 - 20
Recoil	*(%)*	5
Foreshortening	*(%)*	8
Radiopacity		low
Markers		no
Lengths	*(mm)*	15 - 22 - 30
Diameters	*(mm)*	3.0 - 3.5 - 4.0

Figure 2.34 *Crown.*

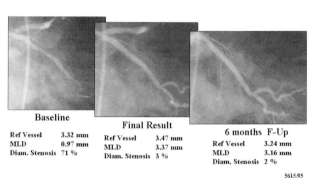

Baseline

Ref Vessel	3.32 mm
MLD	0.97 mm
Diam. Stenosis	71 %

Final Result

Ref Vessel	3.47 mm
MLD	3.37 mm
Diam. Stenosis	3 %

6 months F-Up

Ref Vessel	3.24 mm
MLD	3.16 mm
Diam. Stenosis	2 %

5615/95

Figure 2.35 *Deployment of a 30 mm long Crown stent in the obtuse marginal artery. There is no significant restenosis at six-month follow-up. The rigidity of the stent tends to straighten out the vessel. MLD, minimal lumen diameter.*

rate (*Table 2.21*). A clinical example of deployment of the Crown stent is shown in *Fig. 2.35*. This diffusely diseased obtuse marginal vessel was treated with a 30 mm long Crown stent, which maintained excellent lumen patency at the 6-month follow-up. This strong plaque support is useful in calcified lesions (*Fig. 2.36*). This diseased segment of the proximal and mid-LAD was prepared with sequential Rotablator burrs between 1.25 mm and 2.0 mm. A 30 mm long Crown stent was then passed with its protective sheath. The entrance to the diagonal branch was maintained by passing an ACE 2.0 mm balloon through the side struts of the stent. Simultaneous inflations were then performed as the Crown stent was expanded with a 3.5 mm balloon at 20 atmospheres.

Table 2.20

Crown™ stent

Patients 49		*Lesions 74*	
Stents/lesion	= 1.2	Average ref. vess. size	= 2.97 ± 0.49
Thrombosis	= 0%	Large vessels (29 les)	= 3.41 ± 0.29
Procedural success	= 100%	Small vessels (36 les)	= 2.61 ± 0.30
		Large vs small (%)	= 45 vs 55

Table 2.21

Crown™ stent

Nr of lesions elegible for FU = 74
Lesions with FU = 50 (68%)
Global restenosis rate = 28%

Large short	Large long	Small short	Small long
11	4	25	2
(Rest. 9%)	(Rest. 0%)	(Rest. 40%)	(Rest. 0%)

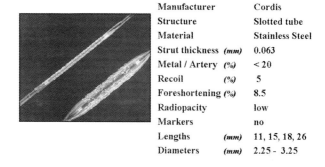

Manufacturer		Cordis
Structure		Slotted tube
Material		Stainless Steel
Strut thickness	*(mm)*	0.063
Metal / Artery	*(%)*	< 20
Recoil	*(%)*	5
Foreshortening	*(%)*	8.5
Radiopacity		low
Markers		no
Lengths	*(mm)*	11, 15, 18, 26
Diameters	*(mm)*	2.25 - 3.25

Figure 2.37 *Mini crown.*

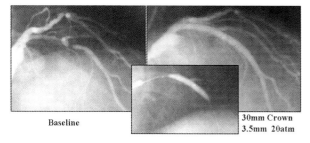

Baseline

30mm Crown
3.5mm 20atm

- Calcified lesion treated with 1.25-2.0mm Rotablator.
- Stent Struts crossed with 2.0mm ACE balloon.

Figure 2.36 *30 mm long Crown stent used in a calcified artery to provide greater structural support. The insert shows a 2.0 mm ACE crossing through the struts of the Crown stent to dilate the diagonal branch.*

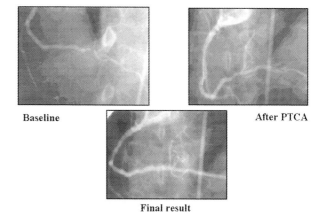

Baseline

After PTCA

Final result

Figure 2.38 *Use of the mini Crown stent to treat a bifurcation lesion in a small posterior descending vessel.*

Most stents are designed to reach maximum structural integrity at a diameter of 3 mm. This may not provide optimum support for smaller vessels. The Mini-crown stent (*Fig. 2.37*) was developed to address this concern of adequate stent support for smaller vessels. This stent also has a stainless steel, slotted tubular design, but it comes in sizes that provide optimum support between 2.25 mm and 3.25 mm. A clinical example of the use of the Mini-crown

stent for a distal vessel is provided in *Fig. 2.38*. There was a subtotal occlusion of the distal RCA at the bifurcation with the posterior descending artery (PDA). Two Mini-crown stents passed easily into this small artery and provided excellent support for the

Table 2.22

Cordis™ stent

Patients 46		Lesions 58	
Stents/lesion	= 1.2	Average ref. vess. size	= 3.01 ± 0.51
Thrombosis	= 3.4%	Large vessels (22 les)	= 3.46 ± 0.38
Procedural success	= 93%	Small vessels (36 les)	= 2.73 ± 0.26
		Large vs small (%)	= 38 vs 62

Table 2.23

Cordis™ stent

Nr of lesions elegible for FU = 56
Lesions with FU = 36 (64%)
Global restenosis rate = 22%

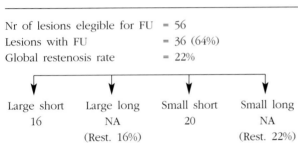

Large short	Large long	Small short	Small long
16	NA	20	NA
	(Rest. 16%)		(Rest. 22%)

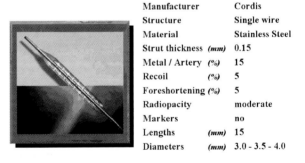

Manufacturer		Cordis
Structure		single sinusoidal helical coil
Material		Tantalum
Strut thickness	*(mm)*	0.127
Metal / Artery	*(%)*	15
Recoil	*(%)*	< 10
Foreshortening	*(%)*	10
Radiopacity		high
Markers		no
Lengths	*(mm)*	15
Diameters	*(mm)*	3.0 - 3.5 - 4.0

Figure 2.39 *Cordis.*

diffusely diseased distal RCA and PDA. There was no restenosis at the 6-month follow-up angiogram.

CORDIS STENTS

The Cordis stent has a single sinusoidal helical coil of tantalum with a strut thickness of 0.13 mm (*Fig. 2.39*). This provides excellent radiopacity, and no markers are required. The benefits of this stent, as with other coil stents, is that it is very flexible and can be implanted in tortuous vessels. However, this stent also suffers from the same problems as the other coil stents, namely, significant plaque prolapse. In addition, coiled stents may be deformed after they are expanded. Restenosis can be concealed by the excessive radiopacity of the tantalum material. Our clinical experience with the Cordis stent is shown in *Tables 2.22* and *2.23*. The global restenosis rate was acceptable at 22%; however, the majority of our experience with this stent was with the 15 mm long version, and so it was used in shorter lesions, which have a propensity to lower restenosis rate.

The next design by Cordis is the Crossflex, which consists of a single-wire, sinusoidal, stainless steel coil (*Fig. 2.40*). Park and colleagues[14] reported a single-center experience with this stent in 209

Manufacturer		Cordis
Structure		Single wire
Material		Stainless Steel
Strut thickness	*(mm)*	0.15
Metal / Artery	*(%)*	15
Recoil	*(%)*	5
Foreshortening	*(%)*	5
Radiopacity		moderate
Markers		no
Lengths	*(mm)*	15
Diameters	*(mm)*	3.0 - 3.5 - 4.0

Figure 2.40 *Crossflex.*

patients with 226 lesions. Follow-up angiography was performed in 82% of eligible lesions and clinical follow-up in all patients at 11 months. Angiographic restenosis was reported in 16.3% of lesions and target lesion revascularization in 7.2% of patients. The newest design is called the Crossflex Laser Cut (LC) (*Fig. 2.41*), which has excellent tracking and flexi-

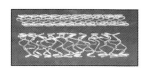

Manufacturer		Cordis
Structure		Slotted tube
Material		Stainless Steel
Strut thickness	*(mm)*	0.14
Metal / Artery	*(%)*	14
Recoil	*(%)*	< 3
Foreshortening	*(%)*	4 - 8
Radiopacity		moderate
Markers		no
Lengths	*(mm)*	18, 27
Diameters	*(mm)*	3.0 - 4.0

Figure 2.41 *Crossflex LC.*

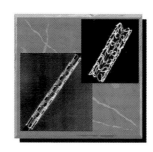

Manufacturer		Medtronic
Structure		Serpentine struts
Material		stainless steel
Strut thickness	*(mm)*	0.075
Metal / Artery	*(%)*	12 - 18
Recoil	*(%)*	minimal
Foreshortening	*(%)*	none
Radiopacity		low
Markers		yes
Lengths	*(mm)*	15 - 25 - 35
Diameters	*(mm)*	3.0 - 5.5

Figure 2.42 *BeStent.*

Table 2.24
BeStent™ stent

Patients 57		*Lesions 70*	
Stents/lesion	= 1.4	Average ref. vess. size	= 2.91 ± 0.40
Thrombosis	= 0%	Large vessels (19 les)	= 3.37 ± 0.23
Procedural success	= 100%	Small vessels (38 les)	= 2.68 ± 0.22
		Large vs small (%)	= 33 vs 67

bility. In addition, this stent can be crossed easily to place a second stent for difficult bifurcation lesions (see *Fig. 10.11*).

THE BESTENT

The BeStent is now manufactured by Medtronic Inc. The structure has a slotted tubular design of serpentine struts that are made of stainless steel. The strut thickness is 0.075 mm (*Fig. 2.42*). The stent comes in variable lengths between 15 mm and 35 mm with a uniform design that has no welding points. The stent has excellent longitudinal flexibility associated with high radial strength. Despite the long length, there is no shortening during expansion and the stent has a very low profile, even with hand crimping.

Our clinical experience with the BeStent in shown in *Tables 2.24* and *2.25*. The high flexibility is shown by the procedural success rate of 100%. Although the number of cases is limited, the global restenosis rate was 28%, but it was higher in the long lesion, small vessel subset. A clinical example of a BeStent is shown in *Fig. 2.43*. The baseline angiogram shows a

Table 2.25
BeStent™ stent

Nr of lesions elegible for FU	= 70
Lesions with FU	= 57 (81%)
Global restenosis rate	= 28%

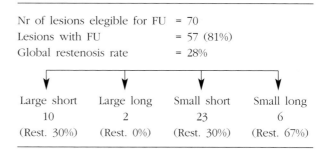

Large short	Large long	Small short	Small long
10	2	23	6
(Rest. 30%)	(Rest. 0%)	(Rest. 30%)	(Rest. 67%)

tight focal stenosis at the origin of the LAD. This was treated by directional atherectomy and then placement of a 15 mm long BeStent, which was expanded on a 4 mm balloon at 18 atmospheres (see *Fig. 2.43b*). The 6-month follow up angiogram (see *Fig. 2.43c*) demonstrates that the ostium of the LAD is widely patent. There is some mild tortuosity and minimal luminal narrowing at the distal left main artery (arrowhead); however, the patient was asymptomatic and had no evidence of ischemia on stress testing. Debulking the plaque before stenting may have diminished restenosis in this ostial LAD, but it may also have traumatized the distal left main artery.

Atherectomy + BeStent on ostial LAD (I)

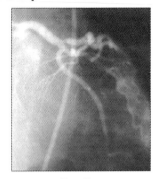

Baseline

a

Atherectomy + BeStent on ostial LAD (II)

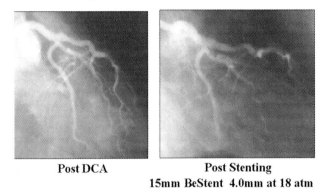

Post DCA   **Post Stenting**
15mm BeStent 4.0mm at 18 atm

b

Atherectomy + BeStent on ostial LAD (III)

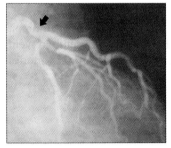

6 Months Follow - Up

c

Figure 2.43 *A BeStent was placed in this ostial LAD lesion after directional atherectomy. The six-month follow-up image (c) reveals no restensosis.*

The use of the BeStent is also being evaluated in small vessels (< 3.0 mm in diameter) as compared to balloon angioplasty in a French multicenter prospective randomized trial (the BESMART trial).[15]

JOMED STENTS

The JOMED International Company in Sweden has made several unusual stent designs for particular lesion subsets. For standard lesions there is the JoStent+plus (*Fig. 2.44*) and for lesions that require more flexibility or that are in bends, there is the JoStent flex (*Fig. 2.45*). The JoStent-S is designed for placement at side branch bifurcations (*Fig. 2.46*). This slotted tubular stent is made of stainless steel and is unusual in having large strut spaces placed around the central portion of the stent. The width of these larger strut spaces is 3.5 mm, which permits easier passage of a balloon or stent into the side branch. (The NIR side stent also comes in a design

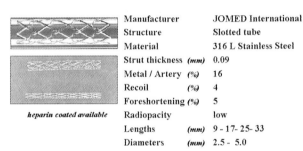

heparin coated available

Manufacturer		JOMED International
Structure		Slotted tube
Material		316 L Stainless Steel
Strut thickness	*(mm)*	0.09
Metal / Artery	*(%)*	16
Recoil	*(%)*	4
Foreshortening	*(%)*	5
Radiopacity		low
Lengths	*(mm)*	9 - 17- 25- 33
Diameters	*(mm)*	2.5 - 5.0

Figure 2.44 *Jostent plus.*

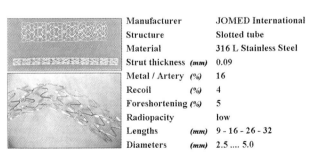

heparin coated available

Manufacturer		JOMED International
Structure		Slotted tube
Material		316 L Stainless Steel
Strut thickness	*(mm)*	0.09
Metal / Artery	*(%)*	16
Recoil	*(%)*	4
Foreshortening	*(%)*	5
Radiopacity		low
Lengths	*(mm)*	9 - 16 - 26 - 32
Diameters	*(mm)*	2.5 .... 5.0

Figure 2.45 *JoStent Flex.*

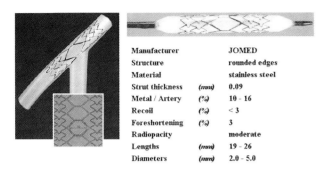

Manufacturer		JOMED
Structure		rounded edges
Material		stainless steel
Strut thickness	*(mm)*	0.09
Metal / Artery	*(%)*	10 - 16
Recoil	*(%)*	< 3
Foreshortening	*(%)*	3
Radiopacity		moderate
Lengths	*(mm)*	19 - 26
Diameters	*(mm)*	2.0 - 5.0

Figure 2.46 *JoStent S. JoStent side branch.*

Manufacturer		JOMED International
Structure		Slotted tube
Material		316 L Stainless Steel
Strut thickness	*(mm)*	0.09
Metal / Artery	*(%)*	10 - 16
Recoil	*(%)*	< 3
Foreshortening	*(%)*	5
Radiopacity		low
Lengths	*(mm)*	17 - 28
Diameters	*(mm)*	2.5....5.0

heparin coated available

Figure 2.48 *JoStent asymmetric side branch.*

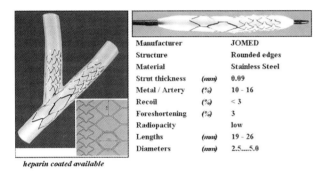

Manufacturer		JOMED
Structure		Rounded edges
Material		Stainless Steel
Strut thickness	*(mm)*	0.09
Metal / Artery	*(%)*	10 - 16
Recoil	*(%)*	< 3
Foreshortening	*(%)*	3
Radiopacity		low
Lengths	*(mm)*	19 - 26
Diameters	*(mm)*	2.5....5.0

heparin coated available

Figure 2.47 *JoStent B. JoStent bifurcation.*

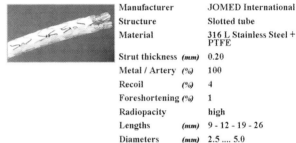

Manufacturer		JOMED International
Structure		Slotted tube
Material		316 L Stainless Steel + PTFE
Strut thickness	*(mm)*	0.20
Metal / Artery	*(%)*	100
Recoil	*(%)*	4
Foreshortening	*(%)*	1
Radiopacity		high
Lengths	*(mm)*	9 - 12 - 19 - 26
Diameters	*(mm)*	2.5 .... 5.0

Figure 2.49 *JoStent coronary stent graft.*

that has a large side strut to permit passage of balloons to treat bifurcation lesions.) Another variety of stent that JOMED has made for bifurcations is the JoStent B (*Fig. 2.47*). This stent has the large spaced struts in the proximal portion. The proximal larger struts are then placed at the bifurcation and the distal segment supports the main branch of the artery, but the larger side struts permit passage of a second stent through the first one. A variation of this stent for bifurcations is the JoStent asymmetric side branch (*Fig. 2.48*). This stent has the large strut hole placed in the proximal portion, but not at the end of the stent as in the JoStent B. However, the large stent struts permit the passage of another balloon or stent through them into the side branch. This design provides more support for the artery proximal to the bifurcation.

JOMED also produces a covered stent made out of polytetrafluoroethylene (PTFE) (*Fig. 2.49*). The purpose of the plastic-covered stent is to inhibit restenosis. This would be especially useful in vein grafts or long segments of the native coronary arteries without side branches, such as the right coronary artery. In addition, this stent has been used in emergency situations to cover a ruptured arterial section (see *Fig. 15.13*) and for coronary aneurysms that could have the predisposition to rupture or form a thrombus.[16] An example of a coronary aneurysm that was treated with a PTFE-covered stent is provided in *Fig. 2.50*. This patient returned for a 6-month follow-up control study after treatment of a chronic total occlusion. A half Palmaz–Schatz stent had been placed in the obtuse marginal artery and dilated with a 3.5 mm balloon at 12 atmospheres. This aneurysm was

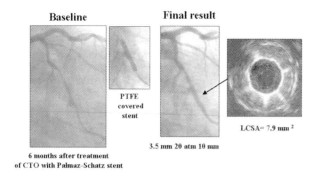

Baseline — Final result

PTFE covered stent

LCSA= 7.9 mm²

3.5 mm 20 atm 10 mm

6 months after treatment of CTO with Palmaz-Schatz stent

Figure 2.50 *An aneurysm occurred in this obtuse marginal artery six months after treatment of a chronic total occlusion. To exclude the possibility of rupture, a PTFE covered stent was deployed. The ultrasound image demonstrates the intense reflection from the plastic material. The radial spokes are caused by reverberations from the metal struts on the stent. LCSA, lumen cross sectional area. CTO, chronic total occlusion.*

treated by placing a PTFE-covered stent, which was dilated at 20 atmospheres using a 10 mm long balloon with a diameter of 3.5 mm. Intravascular ultrasound showed that the final lumen cross-sectional area was 7.9 mm². The PTFE stent provides an unusual intravascular ultrasound pattern. The initial reflection from the PTFE material is very intense with some radial spokes from the metal support struts. There is a secondary harmonic reverberation, which makes it appear as if there is a relatively echolucent space behind the plastic-covered stent. This can be misleading, but this same image pattern is seen even when an aneurysm is not present. It is due to the intense reverberation from the plastic itself.

The potential benefit of PTFE-covered stents in saphenous vein grafts may be based on achieving two objectives:

(a) lowering the rate of distal embolization by sequestering the friable material behind the stent; and

(b) reducing restenosis by providing a physical barrier to neointimal hyperplasia.[17] Our preliminary experience with PTFE-covered stents supports the short-term safety of this device in terms of the incidence of distal embolization and stent thrombosis.[18] However, data on long-term outcome await the results of an ongoing randomized study comparing the PTFE-covered JOMED stent to the bare JOMED stent (The RECOVERS trial).

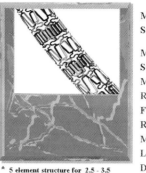

Manufacturer	Biocompatibles
Structure	Interlocking arrowheads
Material	Stainless Steel
Strut thickness *(mm)*	0.075
Metal / Artery *(%)*	14
Recoil *(%)*	2
Foreshortening *(%)*	< 2
Radiopacity	low
Markers	no
Lengths *(mm)*	15 - 28
Diameters *(mm)*	2.5 -4.0

* 5 element structure for 2.5 - 3.5
6 element structure for 3.0 - 8.0

Figure 2.51 *DivYsio.*

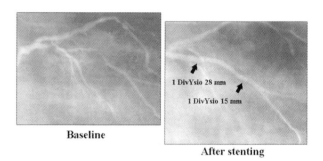

1 DivYsio 28 mm

1 DivYsio 15 mm

Baseline

After stenting

Figure 2.52 *DivYsio stents for diffuse disease in a tortuous artery.*

DIVYSIO STENT

The DivYsio stent (*Fig. 2.51*), made by Biocompatibles Inc., has an unusual structural design of interlocking arrowheads. The stent is made out of stainless steel and comes in a wide range of lengths and diameters. The DivYsio stent has excellent flexibility for tracking lesions in small vessels and diffuse disease (*Fig. 2.52*). Despite the severe tortuosity and diffuse nature of the disease in this large obtuse marginal branch, the lesion was nicely covered by two DivYsio stents. The efficacy of this stent is being tested in comparison to the Multilink stent in a prospective randomized trial (the DISTINCT trial).

BARD XT STENT

The Bard XT stent is a very versatile stent that has been developed by Bard Inc. (*Fig. 2.53*). This stent uses a sinusoidal wave segment, which is bonded to

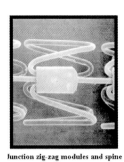

Manufacturer		BARD
Structure		Modular zigzag
Material		Stainless Steel
Strut thickness	*(mm)*	0.15
Metal / Artery	*(%)*	13-20
Recoil	*(%)*	5
Foreshortening	*(%)*	none
Radiopacity		low
Markers		yes, spine
Lengths	*(mm)*	6-11-15-19-24-34
Diameters	*(mm)*	2.5....4.0

Junction zig-zag modules and spine

Figure 2.53 *Bard XT.*

Pre - mounted on a dedicated dual balloon

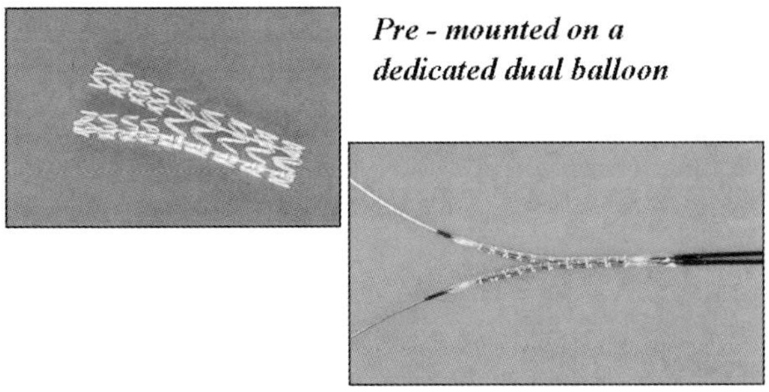

Figure 2.55 *Bard Bifurcate XT.*

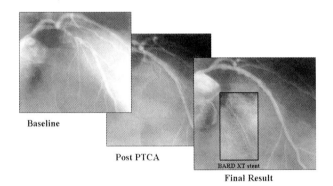

Baseline

Post PTCA

BARD XT stent

Final Result

Figure 2.54 *A Bard XT was placed in this LAD to treat a long dissection following balloon dilatation. The insert reveals the radiopacity of the backbone of the XT stent.*

a spine that connects all of the modular crowns. The stent is made out of stainless steel with a strut thickness of 0.15 mm, which gives it moderate radiopacity.

An example of the Bard XT stent in clinical use is shown in *Fig. 2.54*. The LAD has a long diffuse area of narrowing that extends proximally and distally from the first septal perforator. Following balloon dilatation there is a dissection distally as well as loss of the septal perforator. The Bard XT stent was placed, with resolution of the dissection. There was good flow throughout the artery although the septal perforator still could not be visualized. The backbone of the stent struts is radiopaque, as demonstrated in the insert on the final result angiogram. The clinical efficacy of this stent has been demonstrated in comparison to the Palmaz–Schatz stent in a large prospective randomized trial of 649 patients.[19]

Bard Inc. has also been experimenting with a bifurcation stent with two legs extending from a proximal, larger trunk (*Fig. 2.55*). The stent is premounted on two dedicated balloons, which are then passed over two guidewires placed across the bifurcation. The expectation is that the two legs will extend into the bifurcation branches and the carina of the proximal stent will fit into the carina of the bifurcation. Unfortunately, the clinical feasibility of passing this stent has been less than satisfactory, probably owing to crossing of the guidewires.

SUMMARY OF COMPARISON OF STENTS

Figure 2.56 ranks 15 stents on a subjective scale for ability to track over a guidewire and cross a tight lesion through a tortuous vessel. *Figure 2.57* compares these stents in terms of their ability to cover the lesion adequately and prevent plaque prolapse. With these two scales as an admittedly subjective analysis, we provide the following recommendations as to our preferences for stent selection for specific lesion subsets.

DISCRETE LESIONS

Proximal discrete lesions that are not located on a bend > 45° and that have no significant tortuosity in the proximal segment can be treated with several different types of stents. The slotted tubular design is our preference because of the increased lesion coverage, low recoil, and the low risk of plaque prolapse

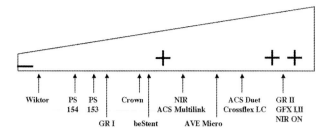

Figure 2.56 *Schematic scale of the ability of several stents to track over a guidewire and cross a lesion.*

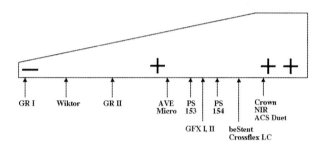

Figure 2.57 *Schematic scale of the ability of several stents to provide adequate scaffolding for a treated lesion.*

with this stent design. These lesions respond well to the Palmaz–Schatz stent, Crown stent, NIR stent, ACS Multilink stent, BeStent, or PuraVario stent. The newer varieties of slotted tubular stents have several beneficial features over the classic Palmaz–Schatz stent. These include rounded edges at the free ends of each strut, the absence of a transverse bridge connecting the struts, which decreases the crimped profile, the absence of the articulation bridge, and the availability of different designs and thicknesses for vessels larger or smaller than 3.5 mm.

TORTUOUS LESIONS

Slotted tubular stents tend to straighten out the vessel and may be too rigid for very tortuous vessels. We prefer a stent that is more flexible and will conform better to the original anatomy. One option for treating tortuous lesions is to use coiled stents such as the

Wiktor-i stent (which is similar to the original Wiktor stent but has tighter waves) or the Crossflex II stent (which is similar to the original Crossflex stent but has welding between the coils). The Gianturco–Roubin II stent conforms very nicely and is very flexible but has a high restenosis rate. Another alternative is to use the AVE II Microstent or the AVE GFX stent. Although the AVE I Microstent is flexible and can reach tortuous segments, the wire thickness is significant (0.20 mm) and the gaps created by each 3 mm segment may result in tissue prolapse. The more recent GFX stent has an oval wire thickness of 0.012 mm and each stent segment is 2 mm in length. This improves flexibility and diminishes tissue prolapse. The ACS Multilink stent, despite having a slotted tubular design, has unique flexibility, which makes it suitable for lesions on a bend or in tortuous arteries.

OSTIAL LESIONS

As described in Chapter 11, ostial lesions should be divided between aorto-ostial and coronary ostial stenoses. For aorto-ostial lesions, the slotted tubular design provides the necessary radial support and visibility to facilitate the treatment of this lesion subset. For vessels of diameter ≥ 4 mm, the Palmaz biliary stent is preferred because it couples high radial support with adequate visibility on fluoroscopy. For aorto-ostial lesions located in vessels smaller than 4 mm in diameter, the spiral articulated Palmaz–Schatz stent has adequate radial support and fair radiopacity. We have also had good results with the NIR stent and especially the NIR Royale stent which is more radiopaque.

For lesions that are located in a coronary ostium, such as the proximal LAD or circumflex artery, a variety of stents can be used, although the presence of a proximal marker or adequate radiopacity of the stent are favorable features since precise placement of the stent is critical.

BIFURCATION LESIONS

The most important element in treating a bifurcation lesion is to decide, before the procedure, whether both branches of the bifurcation need to be stented or if only the major branch needs a stent while the other branch can be dilated through the deployed stent. Our preference is to place a single stent in the main branch and to dilate the side branch (see

Chapter 10). However, an exception to this statement is the situation in which both branches are reasonably large (≥ 3.5 mm). In such cases, it is preferable to debulk the bifurcation using directed atherectomy into one branch or, preferably, both branches of the bifurcation. We have tried a variety of stents for treating bifurcation lesions, and our recommendations for this complex lesion subset are likely to change in the future.

Currently, we prefer the newer slotted tubular stents or the AVE GFX stent since these provide both flexibility and increased ease of crossing the stent to treat the side branch. The AVE GFX stent provides several advantages when both branches of a bifurcation require a so-called kissing bifurcational stent. The GFX stent is free of sharp edges, it has good radial support, lesion coverage is similar to that of slotted tubular stents, it is moderately visible (an important element in dealing with bifurcation lesions), and it can be recrossed fairly easily, even by another stent. This last issue is important because it is possible, after deployment of kissing stents at a bifurcation, that a dissection may arise distal to one of the stents, which could require the placement of a stent distal to the stents deployed at the bifurcation.

Another option that we have found useful in treating bifurcations is the Multilink stent on a low-profile delivery system. This stent is well secured on the balloon and has strut openings which can be dilated up to 4 mm permitting the passage of another stent if necessary. For bifurcation lesions, the Crossflex LC appears to combine the flexibility of a coiled stent with the radial support of the sinusoidal designs (see *Fig. 10.11*).

LESIONS IN THE LEFT MAIN ARTERY

Treatment of lesions in the left main artery frequently involves the combined challenges of an aorto-ostial lesion with a bifurcation lesion. Our preferred stent selection is a slotted tubular design or the AVE GFX stent. The problem with stenting unprotected lesions in the left main artery is that stent restenosis may present with sudden death (see Chapter 12). For this reason we prefer to perform atherectomy to debulk the lesion before stenting so as to minimize the risk of restenosis. It is preferable to have a stent with significant radial support as well as adequate radiopacity to enable the stent to be precisely placed either at the aorto-ostial junction or at the bifurcation of the LAD and circumflex if the lesion extends as far as that.

CALCIFIED LESIONS

Since calcified lesions are more resistant than non-calcified lesions, it is important to have a stent with minimal recoil and strong radial support. For these reasons we tend to choose a slotted tubular stent for calcified lesions. We also recommend using rotational atherectomy, sometimes combined with directional atherectomy, to debulk the plaque before stent insertion. Among the slotted tubular stents that have been useful in these situations is the Palmaz–Schatz stent, especially with the spiral articulation. The NIR stent or the PURA Vario stent have also been used successfully. Non-slotted tubular stents that have been effective include the AVE II Microstent, the AVE GFX stent and the Crossflex stent. The ACS Multilink stent is also useful, especially if the lesion has been effectively debulked; however, if a large calcified plaque burden remains, the Multilink stent may not have the radial strength to obtain an optimal lumen area.

CHRONIC TOTAL OCCLUSIONS

There are two main issues to be considered when dealing with the choice of stent for treating chronic total occlusions:

(a) the amount of plaque mass in these lesions tends to be large; and
(b) it is not unusual for the passage through the occluded segment to occur by creating a false lumen in a dissection plane between the plaque and media, with distal re-entry into the true lumen.

Both of these considerations may result in the need for stenting a long segment of the vessel. The Palmaz–Schatz stent has been shown to be more beneficial than balloon angioplasty in the treatment of chronic total occlusions. The restenosis rate in the SICCO study[20] was 32% with the Palmaz–Schatz stent and 74% with PTCA alone. In addition to the various slotted tubular stents that provide adequate radial support in this setting, the Wallstent needs to be considered, especially when dealing with large vessels and diffuse disease such as occlusions in the right coronary artery. Other stents that are effective for chronic total occlusions are the AVE Micro and GFX series and the newer ACS DUET stent.

LESIONS IN VESSELS SMALLER THAN 3.0 MM IN DIAMETER

When treating lesions in small vessels, we are confronted with a number of problems, including difficult access and high restenosis rates. Until recently, there were no stents that were made specifically to be expanded in small vessels. Most stents do not obtain optimal radial support until the diameter is greater than 3.0 mm. A number of stents have now been developed to address this situation. Stents such as the Mini-crown stent, the 5-cell NIR stent, the small-vessel BeStent and the small-vessel PURA Vario A stent are designed to fit vessels with diameters < 3.0 mm. Long-term follow-up data are only now being acquired for these new stents. However, our initial impression is that these stents provide good flexibility for reaching distal lesions in small vessels. Whatever stent is chosen, we feel it is important to use intravascular ultrasound to ascertain the precise size of the vessel (see Chapter 9). Often, the vessel size as measured media to media on ultrasound is larger than expected by angiography, and the artery will accept a larger balloon to expand the stent and optimize the lumen cross-sectional area.

SAPHENOUS VEIN GRAFTS

Lesions located in saphenous vein grafts frequently involve the combination of diffuse disease in relatively large vessels. In light of these factors, we consider the Wallstent to be the most suitable device for lesions in saphenous vein grafts. Although the initial reports of this stent were unsatisfactory, with a 7.6% mortality and a 24% incidence of complete occlusion, subsequent use of this stent has shown improved results. The Wallstent is difficult to position precisely; however, its flexibility, self-expansive radial strength, and variable lengths make it an excellent choice for treating diffuse disease in vein grafts. If a lesion in a saphenous vein graft involves the aorto-ostial junction, then our preference is to use a Palmaz biliary stent, which provides both excellent radial support and good visibility. Plastic-covered stents, such as the JOMED device with PTFE, may be especially useful in treating saphenous vein grafts since there are no side branches to be concerned with and the inner plastic coating may decrease intimal proliferation. For more focal lesions in saphenous vein grafts, the Palmaz–Schatz, Crown, or NIR stents are also good choices. Another problem that is unique to stenting saphenous vein grafts is the risk

Table 2.26
Summary of stents for specific lesions

	Discrete	Long	Calcified	Ostial	Bifurcation	Dissection	Tortuosity	Vein graft	Small vessel
Crown	+++	++	+++	++	+	+	−	++	−
Mini Crown	++	+	++	++	++	+	+	−	+++
Crossflex	+	−	+	−	++	++	++	−	−
Crossflex LC	++	++	++	+	+	+	+	+	−
NIR 9 cells	++	++	+++	++	−	−	−	++	−
NIR 7 cells	+++	++	++	++	+	+	+	+	−
NIR 5 cells	+	+	+	−	++	+	+	−	+++
AVE GFX	++	++	++	+	+++	+++	+++	+	+
ACS Multilink	++	++	−	+	+	+	−	+	−
ACS Duet	+++	++	+++	+++	+	+	+	+	−
GR II	−	−	−	−	+	++	+++	−	+
Wiktor	+	+	−	−	++	+	−	−	−
BeStent	++	++	+	++	+	−	−	+	−
Mini BeStent	+	+	+	+	+	+	+	−	+++
Wallstent	−	++	−	−	−	−	−	++	−
PTFE covered	+++	−	++	++	−	−	−	+++	−
DivYsio	+++	++	++	+	+	+	+	+	−

(−) = Not recommended; (+) = good; (++) = very good; (+++) = excellent

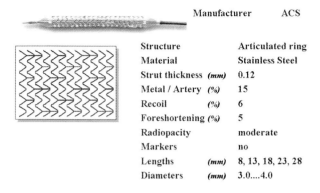

Manufacturer		ACS
Structure		Articulated ring
Material		Stainless Steel
Strut thickness	*(mm)*	0.12
Metal / Artery	*(%)*	15
Recoil	*(%)*	6
Foreshortening	*(%)*	5
Radiopacity		moderate
Markers		no
Lengths	*(mm)*	8, 13, 18, 23, 28
Diameters	*(mm)*	3.0....4.0

Figure 2.58 *ACS Duet.*

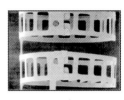

Manufacturer		Navius
Structure		Multiple radial bands
Material		Stainless Steel
Strut thickness	*(mm)*	0.025
Metal / Artery	*(%)*	37.5
Recoil	*(%)*	0
Foreshortening	*(%)*	0
Radiopacity		low
Markers		no
Lengths	*(mm)*	8 - 16
Diameters	*(mm)*	2.0 ... 4.0

Figure 2.59 *Accuflex.*

of distal embolization. In our experience there is no particular stent that is more likely to limit this complication. If the angiographic appearance suggests a large thrombus load, we frequently infuse abciximab and may perform transluminal extraction catheter atherectomy or use an AngioJet before stenting.

ACUTE VESSEL CLOSURE

The original application for coronary artery stenting was the clinical situation of an acute or threatened closure following balloon dilatation. The stents that have been used most extensively in this situation are the Gianturco–Roubin I stent and the Palmaz–Schatz stent. More recently, high success rates have been reported, even in complex anatomy or with long dissections, using the Gianturco–Roubin II stent or the AVE II Microstent. The ideal stent for treating a dissection during impending closure should be premounted (possibly on a high-pressure balloon) and easy to deliver even in complex anatomy; it should have reasonable lesion coverage and be available in different lengths. Several of the newer stents match these requirements, including the Gianturco–Roubin II stent, the AVE II Microstent, the AVE GFX stent and the Crossflex II stent. When treating dissections, it may become necessary to place a short stent distally through the stent that is deployed first. This may occur when a residual distal dissection is not evident at the time of the first stent implantation. The AVE II Microstent, the AVE GFX stent and the Mini-crown stent on a low profile delivery system are appropriate choices for this situation. In this clinical setting it is frequently helpful to use either intravascular ultrasound or fractional flow reserve,

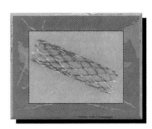

Manufacturer		PAS
Structure		Slotted tube
Material		Nitinol
Strut thickness	*(mm)*	0.177
Metal / Artery	*(%)*	36
Recoil	*(%)*	3 - 6
Foreshortening	*(%)*	11
Radiopacity		moderate
Markers		no
Lengths	*(mm)*	7 - 15
Diameters	*(mm)*	3.0 - 6.0

Figure 2.60 *ACT one.*

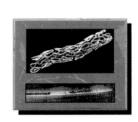

Manufacturer		Angiodynamics
Structure		single wire long. spine
Material		Platinum- Iridium
Strut thickness	*(mm)*	0.127
Metal / Artery	*(%)*	1 - 10
Recoil	*(%)*	7
Foreshortening	*(%)*	12
Radiopacity		high
Markers		no
Lengths	*(mm)*	15 - 25 - 35
Diameters	*(mm)*	3.0 - 6.0

Figure 2.61 *AngioStent.*

or both, to have a better appreciation of the clinical significance of the dissection and to determine whether it is necessary to place a second stent.

CONCLUSION

As stent technology has improved, coronary interventionalists have an ever-increasing number and variety

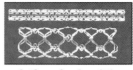

a platform for β emitting radioactive stent

Manufacturer		Cordis
Structure		Slotted tube
Material		Stainless Steel
Strut thickness	*(mm)*	0.075
Metal / Artery	*(%)*	14
Recoil	*(%)*	< 5
Foreshortening	*(%)*	8
Radiopacity		low
Markers		no
Lengths	*(mm)*	15, 25
Diameters	*(mm)*	3.0 ....4.0

Figure 2.62 *BX stent.*

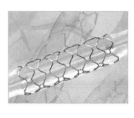

Manufacturer		Cardio Vascular
Structure		Uniform cellular mesh
Material		Stainless Steel
Strut thickness	*(mm)*	0.09
Metal / Artery	*(%)*	11
Recoil	*(%)*	5
Foreshortening	*(%)*	12
Radiopacity		low
Markers		no
Lengths	*(mm)*	17 - 27
Diameters	*(mm)*	3.0....4.0

Figure 2.65 *Enforcer.*

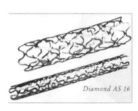

Manufacturer		PHYTIS
Structure		Slotted tube
Material		Stainless Steel
Strut thickness	*(mm)*	0.06
Metal / Artery	*(%)*	n.a.
Recoil	*(%)*	4
Foreshortening	*(%)*	< 10
Radiopacity		moderate
Markers		no
Lengths	*(mm)*	9 -16
Diameters	*(mm)*	3.0....5.0

Figure 2.63 *Diamond AS.*

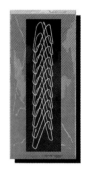

Manufacturer		Global
Structure		Single wire
Material		Stainless Steel
Strut thickness	*(mm)*	0.175
Metal / Artery	*(%)*	11 - 15
Recoil	*(%)*	5 - 9
Foreshortening	*(%)*	0
Radiopacity		low
Markers		no
Lengths	*(mm)*	12,16, 20, 24, 30, 40
Diameters	*(mm)*	2.5....4.5

Figure 2.66 *Freedom.*

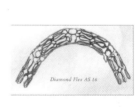

Manufacturer		PHYTIS
Structure		Slotted tube
Material		Stainless Steel
Strut thickness	*(mm)*	0.08
Metal / Artery	*(%)*	n.a.
Recoil	*(%)*	4
Foreshortening	*(%)*	< 10
Radiopacity		moderate
Markers		no
Lengths	*(mm)*	16
Diameters	*(mm)*	3.0....6.0

Figure 2.64 *Diamond AS Flex.*

Manufacturer		Inflow Dymamics		
Structure		Slotted tube		
Material		Stainless Steel		
Strut thickness	*(mm)*	0.075	Foreshortening *(%)*	5
Metal / Artery	*(%)*	12	Radiopacity	low high for gold plated
Recoil	*(%)*	5		
			Markers	no
			Lengths *(mm)*	7,9,11,15,23
			Diameters *(mm)*	2.5 ..... 5.0

Figure 2.67 *In Flow.*

of stents from which to choose. It is important to keep in mind that we want to select a stent that provides the greatest support for the patient's safety. Appropriate stent selection is important to achieve an optimal minimum lumen diameter with as low a risk as possible. *Table 2.26* provides a summary of the stents that we recommend for specific lesions. This table also contains some newer designs that we consider to be 'third-generation' stents. These stents include the NIR-ON stent, the ACS DUET stent (*Fig. 2.58*), the Crossflex LC stent, and the GFX II stent. These stents have the following critical properties:

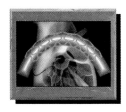

Manufacturer		Uni - Cath
Structure		Slotted tube
Material		Stainless Steel
Strut thickness	*(mm)*	n.a.
Metal / Artery	*(%)*	16
Recoil	*(%)*	0
Foreshortening	*(%)*	5-8
Radiopacity		low
Markers		no
Lengths	*(mm)*	17 - 27 - 37
Diameters	*(mm)*	2.5....4.0

Figure 2.68 *IRIS.*

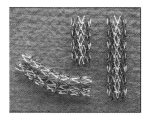

Manufacturer		PAS
Structure		Slotted tube
Material		Nitinol
Strut thickness	*(mm)*	0.05
Metal / Artery	*(%)*	23
Recoil	*(%)*	6
Foreshortening	*(%)*	0
Radiopacity		moderate
Markers		no
Lengths	*(mm)*	15- 20- 30- 40
Diameters	*(mm)*	2.75...... 4.0

Figure 2.71 *Paragon.*

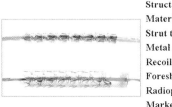

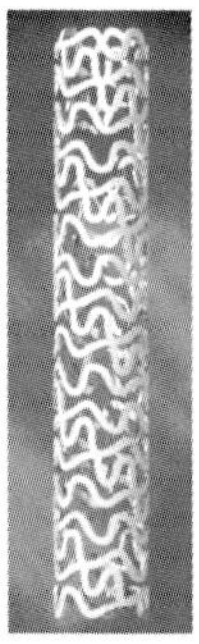

Manufacturer		AMG
Structure		Slotted tube
Material		Stainless Steel
Strut thickness	*(mm)*	0.095
Metal / Artery	*(%)*	8 - 11
Recoil	*(%)*	2
Foreshortening	*(%)*	0
Radiopacity		Moderate
Markers		No
Lengths	*(mm)*	9 - 17- 28
Diameters	*(mm)*	2.5 ..... 4.5

Figure 2.69 *MAC Stent.*

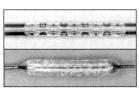

Manufacturer		Spectranetics
Structure		Slotted tube
Material		Stainless Steel
Strut thickness	*(mm)*	0.12
Metal / Artery	*(%)*	18
Recoil	*(%)*	2
Foreshortening	*(%)*	< 5
Radiopacity		moderate
Markers		no
Lengths	*(mm)*	9 - 16 - 25 - 35
Diameters	*(mm)*	2.5 .... 5.0

Figure 2.72 *R Stent.*

Manufacturer		AMG
Structure		Slotted tube
Material		Stainless Steel
Strut thickness	*(mm)*	0.085
Metal / Artery	*(%)*	n.a
Recoil	*(%)*	2
Foreshortening	*(%)*	0
Radiopacity		low
Markers		no
Lengths	*(mm)*	10, 16, 28
Diameters	*(mm)*	2.5 .... 4.5

Figure 2.70 *OMEGA Stent.*

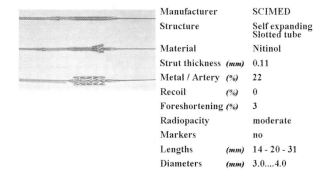

Manufacturer		SCIMED
Structure		Self expanding Slotted tube
Material		Nitinol
Strut thickness	*(mm)*	0.11
Metal / Artery	*(%)*	22
Recoil	*(%)*	0
Foreshortening	*(%)*	3
Radiopacity		moderate
Markers		no
Lengths	*(mm)*	14 - 20 - 31
Diameters	*(mm)*	3.0....4.0

Figure 2.73 *Radius.*

(a) the loaded stent has a very low profile that compares well with the profile of PTCA balloons;

(b) the mechanism for attaching the stent to the balloon is very effective, which diminishes the chance of losing the stent during delivery or withdrawal;

(c) the stents are mounted on moderate to high pressure balloons; and

(d) the radiopacity is good, especially for the three last-named stents.

These qualities combine to permit us to entertain

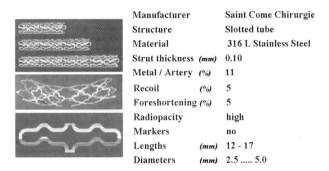

Manufacturer		Saint Come Chirurgie
Structure		Slotted tube
Material		316 L Stainless Steel
Strut thickness	*(mm)*	0.10
Metal / Artery	*(%)*	11
Recoil	*(%)*	5
Foreshortening	*(%)*	5
Radiopacity		high
Markers		no
Lengths	*(mm)*	12 - 17
Diameters	*(mm)*	2.5 ..... 5.0

Figure 2.74 *The 'M' Stent.*

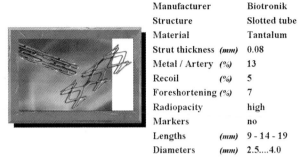

Manufacturer		Biotronik
Structure		Slotted tube
Material		Tantalum
Strut thickness	*(mm)*	0.08
Metal / Artery	*(%)*	13
Recoil	*(%)*	5
Foreshortening	*(%)*	7
Radiopacity		high
Markers		no
Lengths	*(mm)*	9 - 14 - 19
Diameters	*(mm)*	2.5....4.0

Figure 2.77 *TENSUM.*

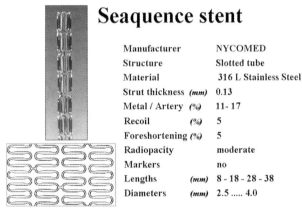

Seaquence stent

Manufacturer		NYCOMED
Structure		Slotted tube
Material		316 L Stainless Steel
Strut thickness	*(mm)*	0.13
Metal / Artery	*(%)*	11- 17
Recoil	*(%)*	5
Foreshortening	*(%)*	5
Radiopacity		moderate
Markers		no
Lengths	*(mm)*	8 - 18 - 28 - 38
Diameters	*(mm)*	2.5 ..... 4.0

Figure 2.75 *Seaquence stent.*

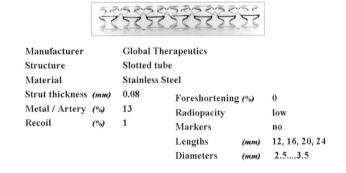

Manufacturer	Terumo	Recoil	*(%)*	5
Structure	Four diamond connected	Foreshortening	*(%)*	5
		Radiopacity		low
Material	Stainless steel	Markers		no
Strut thickness *(mm)*	0.075	Lengths	*(mm)*	20
Metal / Artery *(%)*	18	Diameters	*(mm)*	3.0 - 3.5

Figure 2.78 *Terumo stent.*

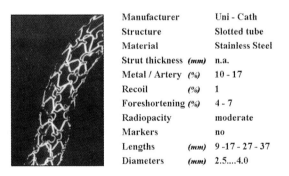

Manufacturer		Uni - Cath
Structure		Slotted tube
Material		Stainless Steel
Strut thickness	*(mm)*	n.a.
Metal / Artery	*(%)*	10 - 17
Recoil	*(%)*	1
Foreshortening	*(%)*	4 - 7
Radiopacity		moderate
Markers		no
Lengths	*(mm)*	9 -17 - 27 - 37
Diameters	*(mm)*	2.5....4.0

Figure 2.76 *Spiral Force.*

Manufacturer		Global Therapeutics
Structure		Slotted tube
Material		Stainless Steel
Strut thickness	*(mm)*	0.08
Metal / Artery	*(%)*	13
Recoil	*(%)*	1

Foreshortening	*(%)*	0
Radiopacity		low
Markers		no
Lengths	*(mm)*	12, 16, 20, 24
Diameters	*(mm)*	2.5....3.5

Figure 2.79 *V-Flex.*

the possibility that lesions may be treated with 'primary stenting', (i.e. it may not be necessary to predilate a lesion – these stents could be delivered and expanded at high pressures as the initial treatment, which might decrease the incidence of dissection that may occur during predilatation). Stent design is a rapidly changing field that will continue to witness significant progress in the years to come. Other new stent designs are illustrated in *Figs 2.59* to *2.80*, along with a brief description of their characteristics.

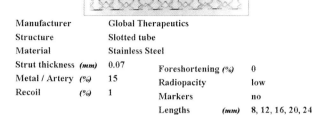

Manufacturer	Global Therapeutics		
Structure	Slotted tube		
Material	Stainless Steel		
Strut thickness *(mm)*	0.07	Foreshortening *(%)*	0
Metal / Artery *(%)*	15	Radiopacity	low
Recoil *(%)*	1	Markers	no
		Lengths *(mm)*	8, 12, 16, 20, 24
		Diameters *(mm)*	2.5....3.5

Figure 2.80 *V-Flex plus.*

REFERENCES

1. Rogers C, Edelman ER. Endovascular stent design dictates experimental restenosis and thrombosis. *Circulation* 1995; **91**: 2995–3001.
2. Colombo A, Goldberg SL, Almagor Y et al. A novel strategy for stent deployment in the treatment of acute or threatened closure complicating balloon coronary angioplasty. Use of short or standard (or both) single or multiple Palmaz–Schatz stents. *J Am Coll Cardiol* 1993; **22**: 1887–1891.
3. Moussa I, Moses J, Colombo A. A method to eliminate articulation from the Palmaz–Schatz stent delivery system. *Cathet Cardiovasc Diagn* 1997; **40**: 212–216.
4. Carrozza JP Jr, Hermiller JB Jr, Linnemeier TJ et al. Quantitative coronary angiographic and intravascular ultrasound assessment of a new nonarticulated stent: report from the Advanced Cardiovascular Systems Multilink stent pilot study. *J Am Coll Cardiol* 1998; **31**: 50–56.
5. Baim DEA. NIRVANA: NIR Vascular Advanced North American Trial. *Circulation* 1999; in press.
6. Lansky AJ, Popma JJ, Hanzel GS et al. Predictors of late clinical outcome after Gianturco–Roubin II stent use. Final results of the GR II randomized clinical trial. *Circulation* 1998; **98**: 3478.
7. Moussa I, Tobis JM, Moses JW et al. A matched comparsion between the Palmaz–Schatz stent and the Gianturco–Roubin stent: angiographic and clinical follow-up results (abstract).

Eur Heart J 1997; **18**: P1002.
8. Martinez Elbal L, López Mínguez JR, Alonso M et al. Wiktor coronary stent for elective placement with an antiaggregation regimen. WINE study. *Rev Esp Cardiol* 1998; **51**: 450–457.
9. Sigwart U, Puel J, Mirkovitch V et al. Intravascular stents to prevent occlusion and restenosis after transluminal angioplasty. *N Engl J Med* 1987; **316**: 701–706.
10. Safian RD, Kaplan B, Schreiber T et al. Final results of the randomized Wallstent endoprosthesis in saphenous vein graft trial (WINS) (abstract). *J Am Coll Cardiol* 1999; **33**: 37A.
11. Kereiakes DJ, Midei M, Hermiller J et al. Procedural and late outcomes following Multi-Link DUET coronary stent deployment: final report for the US Registry (abstract). *J Am Coll Cardiol* 1999; **33**: 95A.
12. Heuser R, Kuntz R, Lansky A et al. Six-month clinical and angiographic results of the SMART trial (abstract). *J Am Coll Cardiol* 1998; **31**: 64A.
13. Reimers B, Moussa I, Kobayashi Y et al. Immediate results with the newly designed Pura-Vario coronary stent. *Am J Cardiol* 1997; **80**: 130.
14. Park SJ, Park SW, Lee CW et al. Immediate results and late clinical outcomes after new CrossFlex coronary stent implantation. *Circulation* 1998; **98**: 4480.
15. Koning R, Khalife K, Gilard M et al. Clinical events and angiographic results of the first 142 patients randomized in the BESMART study (abstract). *J Am Coll Cardiol* 1999; **33**: 95A.
16. Di Mario C, Caprari M, Santoli C et al. Transcatheter repair of a large coronary pseudoaneurysm using ultrasound guidance and vein-covered stents. *G Ital Cardiol* 1997; **27**: 701–705.
17. Elsner M, Britten M, Auch-Schwelk W et al. Distribution of neointimal proliferation in human coronary arteries treated with PTFE stent grafts (abstract). *J Am Coll Cardiol* 1999; **33**: 17A.
18. Moussa I, Inglese L, Di Mario C et al. Immediate and short-term results of the implantation of PTFE covered stents in saphenous vein grafts (abstract). *Eur Heart J* 1998; **19**: P2822.
19. Carrozza JP, Kereiakes D, Caputo RP et al. Final acute, 30-day, and 6-month clinical and angiographic outcome from the multicenter randomized EXTRA trial comparing the operator-mounted XT and Palmaz–Schatz coronary stents. *Circulation* 1998; **98**: 3474.
20. Sirnes PA, Golf S, Myreng Y et al. Stenting in Chronic Coronary Occlusion (SICCO): a randomized, controlled trial of adding stent implantation after successful angioplasty. *J Am Coll Cardiol* 1996; **28**: 1444–1451.

Chapter 3 Subacute stent thrombosis: chronology of stent implantation technique and pharmacologic therapy

Issam Moussa

INTRODUCTION

It has been clear from the initial report of stent implantation in humans[1] that acute and subacute thrombosis was a major limitation. In the European multicenter registry of the self-expanding Wallstent,[2] thrombosis occurred in 24% of patients despite vigorous anticoagulation. In the multicenter clinical trial of the Palmaz–Schatz stent,[3] the anticoagulation regimen consisted of aspirin (325 mg daily) and dipyridamole (75 mg tid), which were begun 24–48 hours before stenting. All patients were treated with low-molecular-weight dextran 40 (100 ml per hour intravenously), beginning 2 hours before stent deployment and continued for a total dose of 1 liter. Heparin was given during the procedure to maintain the partial thromboplastin time at 2–2.5 times control and continued for 24 hours after the procedure. The first 67 patients in this series were not treated with warfarin and had a thrombosis rate of 11.9%. The subsequent patients were treated with warfarin to keep the prothrombin time at 16–18 seconds for 1 month. The overall stent thrombosis rate was 5% at a mean time of 6 days after the procedure. The incidence of stent thrombosis and vascular complications remained high in the first two prospective randomized clinical trials that compared elective stenting to percutaneous transluminal coronary angiography.[4,5] Stent thrombosis occurred in 3.5% of patients in both the Belgium–Netherlands Stent Investigations Trial (BENESTENT) I and the Stent Restenosis Study (STRESS) trials and major bleeding complications occurred in 4.6% and 7.4% of patients, respectively. The incidence of stent thrombosis was even higher when stenting was used for bail-out indications despite full anticoagulation. Herrmann and colleagues[6] reported subacute stent thrombosis in 16.6% of patients and myocardial infarction (MI), coronary artery bypass grafts, or death in 27.8% of patients undergoing bail-out stenting. Other studies of bail-out stenting with anticoagulation and low-pressure stent deployment showed similar results.[7,8]

INSIGHTS FROM THE EVOLUTION IN STENT IMPLANTATION TECHNIQUE AND PHARMACOLOGIC THERAPY

The high rate of stent thrombosis and bleeding complications associated with the initial use of stents and warfarin prompted investigators to re-evaluate the technique of stent implantation and the pharmacological regimen used post-stenting.

Intravascular ultrasound (IVUS) observations after stent implantation[9,10] demonstrated that the traditional stent implantation technique that had been in clinical use (stent expansion using ≤ 10 atmospheres of pressure) may result in an acceptable angiographic appearance, but 80% of stents were underexpanded when interrogated by IVUS. In addition, it was demonstrated that the use of larger balloons or higher inflation pressures, or both, led to improved stent expansion in most of these lesions. These preliminary observations led to the hypothesis that stent thrombosis was primarily a consequence of stent underexpansion and that optimal stent expansion with IVUS guidance might decrease stent thrombosis without the need for anticoagulation.

With respect to the pharmacological regimen, new data suggested that arterial thrombosis was a platelet-dependent event.[11,12,13] Therefore, efforts were directed at examining the role of a new antiplatelet agent, ticlopidine, which has been in clinical use since the early 1980s. This agent irreversibly blocks the binding of fibrinogen to platelets, an effect that appears to be 85% effective against inhibiting platelet aggregation. These effects peak in 3 days and persist for ≥ 10 days after withdrawal of treatment.

The following discussion reviews the key studies that evaluated the role of stent implantation technique and antiplatelet therapy to gain insight into the magnitude of the contribution of both measures to making coronary stenting a safer and more effective modality for treating obstructive coronary artery disease.

IS TICLOPIDINE ALONE EFFECTIVE WHEN USED AFTER THE 'TRADITIONAL' STENT IMPLANTATION TECHNIQUE?

As opposed to coumadin, there is no prospective randomized trial that tested the efficacy of ticlopidine in the era of 'traditional' stent implantation technique. The only study that reported the use of ticlopidine after 'traditional' stent implantation was published by Barragan and colleagues[14] in 1994. In this study, 238 patients had stent implantation in 244 arteries employing the traditionally used technique at that time (no data about balloon size or inflation pressure were provided). All patients were given 500 mg/day ticlopidine (started 3 days before stenting) and a bolus dose of 10,000 IU of heparin during the procedure, then 100–1500 IU per hour for 20 hours. Following removal of the arterial sheath, they were given subcutaneous heparin for 1 week and ticlopidine (500 mg/day) for 3–6 months. The overall stent thrombosis rate at 30 days was 4.2% (3.5% for elective stenting and 7.9% for bail-out stenting). Clinical events were death in five patients (2%), Q-wave MI in three patients (1.2%), and non-Q-wave MI in two patients (1.7%). Peripheral vascular complications occurred in 4.6% of patients.

The results of this study demonstrate that the use of ticlopidine alone after 'traditional' stent implantation reduces stent thrombosis to a level that still is not clinically acceptable. This conclusion is supported by the fact that the incidence of stent thrombosis after elective stenting in that study (3.5%) was the same as the stent thrombosis rates reported in the STRESS and BENESTENT I trials, which used coumadin and aspirin after traditional stent implantation.

If we hypothesize that IVUS never existed and we were to continue stent implantation using relatively undersized and underinflated balloons, the stent thrombosis rate and vascular complications with ticlopidine might be lower than they are with coumadin. However, this rate of stent thrombosis would still have clinical relevance and may have impeded the wide application of this device.

THE EFFICACY OF ANTIPLATELET THERAPY AFTER OPTIMAL STENT EXPANSION USING IVUS GUIDANCE

Based on the observation of a high frequency of stent underexpansion following the traditional stenting technique, a prospective registry was initiated in March 1993[15] to test the hypothesis that stent thrombosis was primarily due to stent underexpansion and that appropriate stent expansion using IVUS guidance may reduce stent thrombosis. In this registry, 359 consecutive patients undergoing Palmaz–Schatz stent implantation were enrolled. A total of 321 patients who had adequate stent expansion were treated with antiplatelet therapy (252 patients treated with aspirin and ticlopidine and 69 patients treated with aspirin alone). Stent thrombosis at 30 days occurred in 0.9% of patients (0.8% in patients treated with ticlopidine and aspirin and 1.4% in patients treated with aspirin alone).

The main difference between this study and previous studies in which ticlopidine had been used was the introduction of an aggressive stent expansion strategy and the combination of ticlopidine and aspirin. This study suggested that the use of antiplatelet therapy leads to a significant reduction in stent thrombosis when appropriate stent expansion is achieved under IVUS guidance.

THE EFFICACY OF ASPIRIN ALONE VERSUS ASPIRIN AND TICLOPIDINE AFTER IVUS-GUIDED STENT IMPLANTATION

After it had been shown that antiplatelet therapy was safe and effective following IVUS-guided stent implantation, the question that arose was whether ticlopidine offers an additional protective effect to aspirin alone.

A small prospective randomized study[16] involving 226 patients with 294 lesions undergoing IVUS-guided coronary stenting was performed. In this study, 103 patients were randomized to aspirin alone (325 mg/day) and 123 patients received a combination of aspirin and ticlopidine (ticlopidine 250 mg bd orally for 1 month). At 1 month, the rate of stent thrombosis was 2.9% in the aspirin-alone group and 0.8% in the combined ticlopidine and aspirin group (p = 0.2). Cumulative major clinical events after successful stenting occurred in 3.9% of patients in the aspirin group and in 0.8% in the combined ticlopidine and aspirin group (p = 0.1). There were no medication side effects in the aspirin group; in the combined group, side effects occurred in three patients (p = 0.2). In this study, the group treated with aspirin alone had a trend toward a higher incidence of stent thrombosis than the group treated with aspirin and ticlopidine, and this difference translated into three episodes of death caused by stent thrombosis in patients assigned to aspirin alone. These differences did not reach statistical significance, but the study was terminated owing to the occurrence of these three deaths.

Further data on the use of aspirin alone after IVUS-guided stenting came from a retrospective analysis involving 801 consecutive patients.[17] In this study, patients were assigned to receive either aspirin therapy alone (264 patients with 348 lesions) or a combination of ticlopidine and aspirin (537 patients with 737 lesions). At 1 month, there was no difference in the aspirin group compared with the combined ticlopidine and aspirin group in the rate of any stent thrombosis (1.9% versus 1.9%; p = 1), subacute stent thrombosis (1.9% versus 1.3%; p = 0.5), cumulative major adverse clinical events (1.9% versus 2.0%; p = 1), or peripheral vascular complications (0.5% versus 0.2%, p = 0.3). Side effects occurred only in 1.9% of patients in the combined ticlopidine and aspirin group (p = 0.04). However, in this study patients receiving aspirin alone had fewer traditional risk factors for stent thrombosis than the patients in the combined ticlopidine and aspirin group. Two additional points should be noted with respect to the above studies: IVUS guidance was performed in the majority of patients, but not in all, and achieving optimal stent expansion by IVUS was not a prerequisite for receiving antiplatelet therapy.

To examine the relation between IVUS guidance and the protective role of aspirin alone, more rigorous multicenter prospective registries were initiated. The first was the MUSIC Registry,[18] which was a prospective multicenter study that was designed to test the safety of aspirin alone after IVUS-guided stent implantation. This registry included 133 patients who underwent optimal placement of a single Palmaz–Schatz stent accomplished with IVUS guidance in de novo coronary lesions followed by aspirin > (100 mg/day). Stent thrombosis occurred in 2 patients (1.3%), both of whom were treated successfully with repeat balloon angioplasty.

The second was the West-2 Registry,[19] which included 165 patients with stable or unstable angina with a single de novo lesion in a vessel with a diameter > 2.75 mm. Aspirin alone was used in 124 patients (75%) who met the criteria of optimal stent expansion by IVUS. The other patients either did not have IVUS for technical reasons (14 patients, 8.5%) or did not meet criteria of optimal stent expansion (27 patients, 16.5%) and therefore received a combination of aspirin and ticlopidine. Stent thrombosis occurred in two patients (1.2%). However, it is of interest to note that thrombosis occurred in 1 patient who did not have IVUS interrogation because of the occurrence of cardiac tamponade and subsequent surgical exploration. This patient had stent thrombosis 6 days post-procedure. The second patient who had stent thrombosis was receiving aspirin and ticlopidine. None of the patients who had optimal stent expansion and was receiving aspirin alone had stent thrombosis.

The collective body of evidence to date suggests that when optimal expansion during stent implantation is attained using IVUS guidance, aspirin alone is effective against thrombosis. However, it must be emphasized that optimal stent deployment cannot be achieved in all lesions despite the use of IVUS guidance and large balloon sizes. Our studies have shown that suboptimal stent deployment occurs in about 33% of unselected cases despite the use of IVUS. Therefore, additional protection against stent thrombosis (besides aspirin) appears justified.

WHAT IS THE BEST PHARMACOLOGIC REGIMEN AFTER CONTEMPORARY STENTING WITHOUT IVUS GUIDANCE?

After it had been demonstrated that the use of aspirin and ticlopidine (or aspirin alone) was safe and effective when stents were optimally expanded using IVUS guidance, several investigators tested the possibility of using combined antiplatelet therapy after optimal stent implantation with only angiographic guidance. Registries and prospective randomized trials were performed.

The French Registry[20] reported outcomes in 2900 patients who underwent successful stent implantation in 30 centers. The overall incidence of subacute thrombosis was 1.8% of patients. It is difficult to evaluate the relative contribution of stenting technique in this particular study because the technique changed over the duration of the study and because the details were not reported. However, an interesting observation is that stent thrombosis occurred in 10% of patients in whom final stent expansion was performed with balloons ≤ 2.5 mm in diameter. One explanation is that this represents a subgroup of patients with small vessels in whom undersized balloons were used for stent expansion.

Using the Gianturco–Roubin stent, Goods and colleagues[21] reported on 216 patients selected out of 369 patients who underwent stent implantation followed by aspirin (325 mg/day) and ticlopidine (250 mg bd orally) for 1 month. Eligibility for inclusion was based on adequate coverage of intimal dissections, absence of residual filling defects, and normal thrombolysis in myocardial infarction (TIMI) grade 3 flow in the stented vessel. Stents implanted had a stent-to-vessel ratio of 1.17:1 and were expanded using a mean inflation pressure of 15 atmospheres. At 1 month follow-up, stent thrombosis occurred in two patients (0.9%). Vascular access site complications occurred in four patients (1.9%) and bleeding that required blood transfusion occurred in four patients (1.9%).

The Intracoronary Stenting and Antithrombotic Regimen (ISAR) trial[22] was a prospective randomized trial that enrolled 517 patients after successful placement of a Palmaz–Schatz stent expanded using a balloon-to-artery ratio of 1.13:1 and mean inflation pressure of 16 atmospheres. The pharmacologic regimen consisted of ticlopidine plus aspirin in 257 patients and intravenous heparin, phenprocoumon, and aspirin in 260 patients. The primary cardiac end-point was a composite measure of cardiac death, MI, coronary artery bypass surgery, or repeated angioplasty. Of the patients assigned to antiplatelet therapy, 1.6% reached a primary cardiac end-point, as opposed to 6.2% of those assigned to anticoagulant therapy. Occlusion of the stented vessel occurred in 0.8% of the antiplatelet therapy group and in 5.4% of the anticoagulant therapy group. Hemorrhagic complications occurred only in the anticoagulant therapy group (6.5%).

These data suggest that when an angiographically guided contemporary stenting technique is used (i.e.

stents are expanded using high inflation pressure or high balloon-to-vessel ratio with moderate inflation pressure) the combination of ticlopidine and aspirin is more effective than aspirin and coumadin.

IS ASPIRIN OR TICLOPIDINE ALONE AS EFFECTIVE AS THE COMBINATION AFTER CONTEMPORARY STENTING WITHOUT IVUS GUIDANCE?

After demonstrating the efficacy of combined aspirin and ticlopidine after angiographically optimal stent implantation, the next question was: could aspirin alone or ticlopidine alone yield similar results to aspirin and ticlopidine?

Goods and colleagues[23] reported a retrospective comparison between 46 selected patients who received aspirin alone versus 338 selected patients who received aspirin plus ticlopidine after successful implantation of the Gianturco–Roubin stent. The stents implanted had a stent-to-vessel ratio of 1.17:1 and were expanded using an inflation pressure of 15 atmospheres. During 1-month follow-up, stent thrombosis occurred in three patients in the aspirin alone group (6.5%) versus three patients in the aspirin plus ticlopidine group (0.9%) ($p = 0.02$).

The STARS trial[24] compared the efficacy of various pharmacological regimens on the incidence of stent thrombosis after angiographic optimal Palmaz–Schatz stent implantation (in-stent residual diameter stenosis of < 10%). In this study, a total of 1655 patients (1780 lesions) were randomized to aspirin alone, aspirin plus coumadin, or aspirin plus ticlopidine. The incidence of stent thrombosis, target vessel revascularization, and Q-wave MI within 30 days was significantly lower for aspirin plus ticlopidine (0.6%) than it was for either aspirin plus coumadin (2.5%) or aspirin alone (3.8%) ($p = 0.001$). Patients who were recruited into this trial but had suboptimal final results were followed in the STARS Registry.[25] This registry included 267 patients (336 lesions), of whom 35% had more than two stents, 29% had severe dissection or slow flow, 26% had dissection after stenting, and 10% had a residual percentage diameter stenosis > 10%. The post-stenting pharmacological regimen consisted of aspirin in 99% of patients, ticlopidine in 69%, coumadin in 34%, enoxaparin in 10%, and abciximab in 9%, with various combinations. Stent thrombosis in this cohort occurred in 3% of patients.

Barragan and colleagues[26] reported a prospective registry of ticlopidine alone started 2 days before stent implantation and continued for 1 month afterwards. At 1-month follow-up, stent thrombosis had occurred in 1% of patients. Of special note, this study presents a unique opportunity to measure the relative contribution of improved stenting technique and the addition of ticlopidine to the post-stenting pharmacological regimen. The incidence of stent thrombosis in this study is significantly lower than that reported by the same group in 1994,[14] when ticlopidine was used after traditional stenting and stent thrombosis occurred in 4.2% of patients. The combination of these two studies suggests that the use of a more aggressive stent expansion strategy in the more recent series contributed significantly to the reduction in stent thrombosis.

When an angiographically guided contemporary stenting technique is used (i.e. stents are expanded using high inflation pressure or high balloon-to-vessel ratio with moderate inflation pressure) aspirin alone is inferior to the combination of ticlopidine and aspirin in preventing stent thrombosis. Although ticlopidine alone may be protective against stent thrombosis, there are data to suggest that the combination of the two agents may be more effective than ticlopidine alone.[27]

THE EFFICACY OF HEPARIN-COATED STENTS

The only large trial testing the efficacy of heparin-coated Palmaz–Schatz stents was BENESTENT II.[28] However, the combination of aspirin and ticlopidine was used in this study as well. Therefore, the efficacy of heparin-coated stents in reducing stent thrombosis independently from the use of antiplatelet agents has not yet been demonstrated.

DOES IVUS GUIDANCE OFFER AN ADVANTAGE OVER ANGIOGRAPHIC GUIDANCE OF CORONARY STENTING FOR THE PREVENTION OF THROMBOSIS?

Two large prospective randomized trials are in progress to compare the effect of IVUS guidance with the effect of angiographic guidance on stent throm-

bosis and restenosis. Preliminary data from the AVID trial[29] in the first 136 patients receiving post-stenting aspirin and ticlopidine randomized to angiographic guidance or IVUS guidance showed no significant difference in stent thrombosis at 1 month (2.9% versus 1.5%). Similarly, the 1-month outcome in the first 100 patients in the Optimization with ICUS to Reduce Stent Restenosis (OPTICUS) trial[30] showed a similar incidence of major adverse coronary events between the IVUS group and the angiography group.

When coronary stents are implanted using contemporary techniques in patients treated with a combination of aspirin and ticlopidine, IVUS guidance does not have an added protective effect to diminish stent thrombosis. However, one situation in which IVUS guidance does provide an additive safety effect is when aspirin alone is used post-stenting.

THE EMERGING ROLE OF CLOPIDOGREL AS AN ALTERNATIVE TO TICLOPIDINE

Clopidogrel is a thienopyridine derivative that inhibits platelet aggregation by blocking adenosine 5'-diphosphate (ADP) from binding to its platelet receptor. This prevents the integration of fibrinogen to the glycoprotein IIb/IIIa complex.[31] Although both ticlopidine and clopidogrel prevent platelet aggregation evoked by shear stress, experimental studies suggest that clopidogrel is more effective than either aspirin or ticlopidine in preventing high shear stress-dependent coronary stent thrombosis.[32]

Furthermore, clopidogrel has a favorable safety profile and, unlike ticlopidine, it has not been associated with serious hematological side effects. Routine hematological monitoring is mandatory with ticlopidine therapy to ensure early detection of these potentially lethal events. The incidence of neutropenia with ticlopidine is proportional to the duration of treatment (up to 2.4%); it may resolve with drug cessation in most cases, but not in all.[11] Another serious side effect of ticlopidine is thrombotic thrombocytopenic purpura (TTP). A recent review[33] documented 60 cases of TTP among patients treated with ticlopidine with an associated mortality rate of 33%. In this review, 12 patients developed TTP after receiving ticlopidine for 3 weeks or less after stent implantation. Other common, but less serious adverse effects reported to accompany ticlopidine use are gastrointestinal symptoms.

Clopidogrel was developed because it did not show bone marrow toxicity in tissue culture and animal models. In the large CAPRIE trial,[34] the incidence of severe neutropenia with long-term use was only 0.05%, which was similar to the rate seen with aspirin (0.04%). In addition, the proportions of patients with severe rash and diarrhea while on clopidogrel in this trial were less than those reported with ticlopidine but twice as high as those reported with aspirin. Therefore, the combination of a favorable safety profile and a proven clinical antiplatelet effect makes clopidogrel an attractive alternative to ticlopidine for use after coronary stent implantation.

To determine the efficacy of clopidogrel and aspirin in comparison with ticlopidine and aspirin after stent deployment, we retrospectively evaluated these two regimens in all patients undergoing stent implantation in Lenox Hill Hospital, New York, USA.[35] Between September 1996 and June 1998, 2057 patients underwent coronary stent implantation. A total of 368 patients were excluded from this analysis owing to the use of warfarin or platelet IIb/IIIa receptor antagonists or because of an unsuccessful procedure. The final study population consisted of patients who underwent coronary stenting followed by treatment with ticlopidine and aspirin (TA group; n = 1406) and patients who underwent coronary stenting followed by treatment with clopidogrel and aspirin (CA group; n = 283 patients). At 1 month, there was no difference in incidence of stent thrombosis (1.5% versus 1.4%; p = 1.0) or major adverse cardiac events (3% versus 2%; p = 0.85) between the TA and CA groups. The probability of any side effect (neutropenia, diarrhea, rash) was significantly lower in the CA group (5% versus 10%; p = 0.006; relative risk 0.53; confidence interval 0.32–0.86).

These data suggest that clopidogrel may be an effective pharmacological regimen after coronary stent implantation. Furthermore, the simpler dosing regimen, the absence of neutropenia, and the lower frequency of other side effects make it a safe alternative to ticlopidine. Randomized trials will be needed to test the validity of these findings

PREDICTORS OF STENT THROMBOSIS

Owing to the heterogeneity among different studies evaluating predictors of stent thrombosis (primarily with respect to the post-stenting pharmacologic regimen), a distinction has to be made between studies performed in the era of warfarin use with traditional stent technique and studies performed in the era of antiplatelet therapy with contemporary deployment techniques.

TRADITIONAL STENT IMPLANTATION WITH ANTICOAGULATION THERAPY

Several factors were identified that increased the risk of stent thrombosis in this era. Agrawal and colleagues[36] reported that the predictors of stent thrombosis using the flexible coil stent were residual dissections, persistent filling defects, small stent size (< 2.5 mm), and multiple stents. Nath and coleagues[37] reported that lesion eccentricity, bail-out stenting, unstable angina, and subtherapeutic anticoagulation were factors predisposing to stent thrombosis using a similar stent design.

CONTEMPORARY STENT IMPLANTATION WITH ANTIPLATELET THERAPY

We studied 997 consecutive patients who had stent implantation in 1332 lesions and were subsequently treated only with antiplatelet therapy.[38] Subacute stent thrombosis (SST) occurred in 17 patients (1.3%). When we separated patients with SST from patients without SST according to the indication for coronary stenting (*Table 3.1*) we did not see any significant

Table 3.1

Sub-Acute Stent Thrombosis (SST) Analysis. Study Population

	No SST Group *982 patients*	*SST Group* *17 patients*	*p* *value*
Age	58 ± 9	58 ± 9	NS
Male	88%	87%	NS
EF	57 ± 11	49 ± 15	0.005
Prior MI	55%	87%	0.01
Multivessel dis.	49%	47%	NS
Unstable angina	20%	33%	NS

difference even in the group who had coronary stenting performed for acute or threatened vessel closure. This is different from what was reported in the early experience with the use of ticlopidine.[14] Optimal stent expansion and full coverage of dissection are the most likely explanations for this lower rate of stent thrombosis in this high-risk clinical subset traditionally plagued with prohibitive rates of stent occlusion.

When we analysed the two groups (no SST and SST) according to the type of stent used, only the combination of different types of stents had an impact on the incidence of stent thrombosis. The use of a combination of stents was prevalent in 7% of lesions that did not develop SST compared to a prevalence of 24% in lesions that developed SST. The fact that lesions treated with stent combinations have a higher incidence of stent thrombosis may not be a cause-and-effect relationship but may be due to the propensity to use different stents in very complex anatomical settings where the first type of stent has failed and other stents are used to overcome technical difficulties. Based on a multiple logistic regression analysis, the two clinical variables associated with a higher risk for SST were a low baseline ejection fraction ($p = 0.005$) and stenting an artery supplying an infarcted area ($p = 0.01$) (*Table 3.2*). Among the procedural variables, the presence of an angiographic complication such as a significant residual dissection and persistent slow flow following stenting are the most important variables associated with the risk of SST. An example of an angiographic complication not resolved by stenting which progressed to SST is shown in *Fig. 3.2.*

Several other investigators have studied predictors of stent thrombosis. Unstable angina before intervention was not found to be predictive of stent thrombo-

sis in most studies.[22,24,26,38] With respect to baseline angiographic characteristics, it has been suggested that the presence of thrombus may increase the subsequent risk of stent thrombosis.[39] However, recent reports have discredited this traditional risk factor and stenting has become a common first-line treatment in acute MI.[40] In addition, unlike the era of traditional stenting, small vessel size is no longer considered to be an independent predictor of stent thrombosis.[24,26,38,39,41] With respect to procedural factors, stent implantation for a bail-out indication is not predictive of stent thrombosis[26,38,39] unless the angiographic problem is not resolved at the end of the procedure. The balloon-to-vessel ratio is also an important factor that may reflect the appropriateness of stent expansion.[26,38] This factor was clearly illustrated in the French Registry, where stent thrombosis was 10% when balloons ≤ 2.5 mm were used, 2.3% when balloons of 3.0 mm were used, and 1% when balloons ≥3.5 mm were used. The presence of a significant dissection or slow flow at the end of the procedure is also predictive of thrombosis.[24,38,39] However, recent data question the axiom that any angiographic dissection needs to be covered by a stent.[42] IVUS evaluation or doppler interrogation have been proposed as tools to evaluate the clinical significance of a dissection.

CASE STUDIES

CASE 1

A 72-year-old white man was admitted with a diagnosis of unstable angina. Cardiac catheterization revealed a left ventricular ejection fraction (LVEF) of 25% and triple-vessel disease. The circumflex artery had a total occlusion in the proximal segment (*Fig. 3.1a*). After recanalization, 3 AVE stents were implanted with a total length of 48 mm: the most distal was 2.5 mm in diameter and 6 mm long, the second was 3.0 mm in diameter and 24 mm long, and the most proximal was 4.0 mm in diameter and 18 mm long. The final minimal lumen cross-sectional area was 4.5 mm² in the distal stented segment and 6.9 mm² in the proximal segment. The patient was put on ticlopidine and aspirin, but he discontinued ticlopidine because of a skin rash. The patient returned 2 days after the procedure with an evolving MI. Cardiac catheterization revealed stent thrombosis (see *Fig. 3.1b*). Abciximab was administered and the vessel was reopened with balloon dilataton. IVUS interrogation revealed plaque prolapse inside the

Table 3.2
Sub-Acute Stent Thrombosis (SST) Analysis. Indication for stenting

	No SST Group 1315 patients	SST Group 17 patients	p value
Elective	65%	58%	NS
Restenosis	9%	0	NS
Suboptimal	10%	18%	NS
Threatened or acute closure	10%	12%	NS
CTO	7.6%	12%	NS
Acute MI	0.4%	0	NS

Baseline   3 x 30 mm balloon after recanalization   2 AVE stents

a

After balloon dilation and Reopro, IVUS reveals tissue flap protruding through AVE stent

b

c

Figure 3.1 *Subacute stent thrombosis after treatment of a chronic total occlusion of the circumflex/obtuse marginal artery. (a) Angiogram at baseline and after treatment with balloon dilatation and placement of two AVE stents. (b) Angiographic appearance 12 hours later. After the subacute occlusion was reopened with balloon dilatation, intravascular ultrasound revealed a tissue flap protruding through the AVE stent. (c) Treatment of the plaque protrusion with a NIR 7-cell stent.*

Baseline   Post multiple stenting

a

8 days after

b

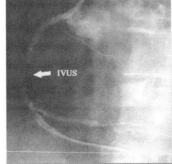

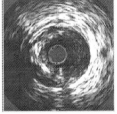

Plaque prolapse

c

Figure 3.2 *Subacute stent thrombosis following the use of multiple coiled stents. After reestablishing blood flow, IVUS imaging revealed prolapse of plaque through the stent coils.*

proximal AVE stent so a NIR stent was implanted at that site (see *Fig. 3.1b* and *3.1c*). Subsequently, the patient did well with no further events.

This case exemplifies several of the predisposing factors that have been identified for producing subacute stent thrombosis. The patient had a low ejection fraction, which would predispose to a slower flow state. In addition, the length of the stenosis and stented segment was long, which would predispose to restenosis, and the artery lumen size was small. The distal segment was only 2.5 mm in diameter by angiography and had a minimum lumen cross-sectional area of only 4.5 mm² by intravascular ultrasound. Although the patient was placed on a combination of ticlopidine and aspirin, he could not tolerate the ticlopidine because of the skin rash. Moreover, at the time of the episode of SST, IVUS imaging revealed a tissue flap in the proximal portion of the circumflex artery that had prolapsed through the AVE stent. Although the size of the tissue prolapse would not appear to be significant enough to cause thrombosis in a normal patient, it might serve as a nidus for thrombosis in a patient with low flow, in a small distal vessel, who could not take ticlopidine.

CASE 2

A 50-year-old man was admitted with progressive exertional angina. Cardiac catheterization revealed a LVEF of 60% and two-vessel disease. The right coronary artery had several stenoses: a lesion involving both the posterior descending artery and the posterolateral branch, and a mid-lesion (*Fig. 3.2a*). Two Wiktor stents were implanted by a 'kissing' technique at the bifurcation with residual dissection distal to the stent in the posterolateral branch but with TIMI grade 3 flow. The mid-lesion was treated with two Gianturco–Roubin I stents (each 20 mm). The total length of stents was 70 mm. All stents were dilated with a 3.5 mm balloon inflated to 18 atmospheres (see *Fig. 3.2a*). The patient was discharged on ticlopidine and aspirin. The patient returned 8 days post-procedure with chest pain and was found to have stent thrombosis (see *Fig. 3.2b*). IVUS was performed immediately after re-establishing blood flow to the distal vessel. The IVUS study shown in *Fig. 3.2c* demonstrates significant tissue prolapse through the Gianturco–Roubin stent. An additional Palmaz–Schatz stent was implanted inside the Gianturco–Roubin stent and a second

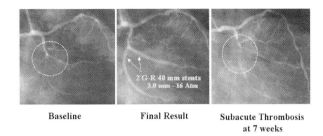

| Baseline | Final Result | Subacute Thrombosis at 7 weeks |

Figure 3.3 *Subacute stent thrombosis at a bifurcation lesion between the obtuse marginal and circumflex artery. The relatively late development of subacute stent thrombosis at seven weeks would be due, in part, to aggressive neointimal hyperplasia within the Gianturco–Roubin II stents.*

Palmaz–Schatz stent was implanted distal to the Gianturco–Roubin stent to cover a dissection. The predisposing factors in this case were a long dissection and significant tissue prolapse. The extensive length of stent also predisposes to restenosis.

CASE 3

A 65-year-old white man was admitted with unstable angina. Cardiac catheterization revealed a LVEF of 55% and two-vessel disease. The circumflex artery had severe proximal stenoses involving the first, second, and third obtuse marginal artery (*Fig. 3.3*). Two 3.0 mm Gianturco–Roubin II stents (each 40 mm long) were implanted in the mid-circumflex artery and the second obtuse marginal artery. Both were expanded with a 3.0 mm balloon inflated at 10 atmospheres. The patient was treated with asprin and ticlopidine. At 7 weeks, the patient returned with acute onset of chest pain. Coronary angiography showed evidence of stent thrombosis in the proximal circumflex artery.

In this case example it is less clear why the patient developed SST. The patient had good flow with a normal LVEF. An adequate sized balloon was chosen and the final angiographic result appeared appropriate, although the results were not confirmed with IVUS imaging. In this case, the onset of subacute stent thrombosis 7 weeks after the procedure makes us think that the patient may have had aggressive restenosis, which has been reported with the Gianturco–Roubin II stent. The aggressive restenosis may then have proceeded to a slow flow state and subsequent thrombosis. As in the previous cases, since IVUS was not performed, it is possible that inadequate scaffolding by the Gianturco–Roubin II stent permitted tissue prolapse.

SUMMARY

The subject of stent thrombosis illustrates that in biology there is often more than one factor to explain a certain observation. The available data in humans clearly demonstrate the multifactorial nature of this process. Impaired blood flow caused by poor left ventricular function, dissection, or stent underexpansion and the presence of a foreign body may initiate platelet activation, which in turn leads to thrombus formation. The data indicate that prevention of stent thrombosis starts with appropriate stent expansion; if this is achieved then antiplatelet therapy will be effective in reducing stent thrombosis. IVUS has provided the insight into understanding the importance of stent expansion and has taught us that one deployment technique does not fit all situations. The appropriate use of this imaging technology will continue to expand our knowledge in this rapidly evolving field. Newer antiplatelet regimens may enhance the safety of catheter-based coronary interventions. These issues are particularly critical in high-risk patients where one might have to accept a suboptimal result or where an intrinsic high thrombosis risk is unavoidable.

REFERENCES

1. Sigwart U, Puel J, Mirkovitch V et al. Intravascular stents to prevent occlusion and restenosis after transluminal angioplasty. *N Engl J Med* 1987; **316**: 701–706.
2. Serruys PW, Strauss BH, Beatt KJ et al. Angiographic follow-up after placement of a self-expanding coronary artery stent. *N Engl J Med* 1991; **324**: 13–17.
3. Schatz RA, Baim DS, Leon M et al. Clinical experience with the Palmaz–Schatz coronary stent. Initial results of a multicenter study. *Circulation* 1991; **83**: 148–161.
4. Serruys P, Jaegere P, Kiemeneij F et al. A comparison of balloon expandable stent implantation with balloon angioplasty in patients with coronary artery disease. *N Engl J Med* 1994; **331**: 489–495.
5. Fischman D, Leon M, Baim D et al. A randomized comparison of coronary stent placement and balloon angioplasty in the treatment of coronary artery disease. *N Engl J Med* 1994; **331**: 496–501.
6. Herrmann NC, Buchbinder M, Clemen MW et al. Emergent use of balloon expandable coronary artery stenting for failed percutaneous transluminal coronary angioplasty. *Circulation* 1992; **86**: 812–819.
7. Roubin GS, Cannon AD, Agrawal SK et al. Intracoronary stenting for acute or threatened closure complicating percutanuous transluminal coronary angioplasty. *Circulation* 1992; **85**: 916–927.
8. George BS, Voorhees WD, Roubin GS et al. Multicenter investigation of coronary stenting to treat acute or threatened closure after percutanuous transluminal coronary angioplasty: clinical and angiographic outcomes. *J Am Coll Cardiol* 1993; **22**: 135–143.
9. Nakamura S, Colombo A, Gaglione A et al. Intracoronary ultrasound observations during stent implantation. *Circulation* 1994; **89**: 2026–2034.
10. Goldberg SL, Colombo A, Nakamura S et al. The benefit of intracoronary ultrasound in the deployment of Palmaz–Schatz stents. *J Am Coll Cardiol* 1994; **24**: 996–1003.
11. Saltiel E, Ward A. Ticlopidine: a review of its pharmacodynamic and pharmacokinetic properties, and therapeutic efficacy in platelet dependent disease states. *Drugs* 1987; **34**: 222–262.
12. Hass WK, Easton JD, Adams HP et al for the Ticlopidine Aspirin Stroke Study Group. A randomized trial comparing ticlopidine hydrochloride with aspirin for the prevention of stroke in high risk patients. *N Engl J Med* 1989; **321**: 501–507.
13. Hardisty RM, Powling MJ, Nokes TJC. The action of ticlopidine on human platelets: studies on aggregation, secretion, calcium mobilization, and membrane glycoproteins. *Thromb Haemost* 1990; **64**: 105–155.
14. Barragan P, Sainsous J, Silvestri M et al. Ticlopidine and subcutaneous heparin as an alternative regimen following coronary stenting. *Cathet Cardiovasc Diagn* 1994; **32**: 133–138.
15. Colombo A, Hall P, Nakamura S et al. Intracoronary stenting without anticoagulation accomplished with intravascular ultrasound guidance. *Circulation* 1995; **91**: 1676–1688.
16. Hall P, Nakamura S, Maiello L et al. A randomized comparison of combined ticlopidine and aspirin therapy versus aspirin therapy alone after successful intravascular ultrasound-guided stent implantation. *Circulation* 1996; **93**: 215–222.
17. Albiero R, Hall P, Itoh A et al. Results of a consecutive series of patients recieving only antiplatelet therapy after optimized stent implantation: comparison of ASA alone versus combined ticlopidine and aspirin therapy. *Circulation* 1997; **95**: 1145–1156.
18. de Jaegere P, Mudra H, Figulla H et al for the MUSIC study investigators. Intravascular ultrasound-guided optimized stent deployment. Immediate and 6 months clinical and angiographic results from the Multicenter Ultrasound Stenting in Coronaries Study (MUSIC Study). *Eur Heart J* 1998; **19**: 1214–1223.
19. Serruys PW, van der Giessen W, Garcia E et al for the West-2 Investigators. Clinical and angiographic results with the Multilink stent implanted under intravascular ultrasound guidance (West-2 study). *J Invas Cardiol* 1998; **10 (suppl B)**: 20B–27B.
20. Karrillon GJ, Morice MC, Benveniste E et al. Intracoronary stent implantation without ultrasound guidance and with

replacement of conventional anticoagulation by antiplatelet therapy. *Circulation* 1996; **94**: 1519–1527.

21. Goods C, Al-Shaibi K, Yadav S et al. Utilization of the coronary balloon-expandable coil stent without anticoagulation or intravascular ultrasound. *Circulation* 1996; **93**: 1803–1808.

22. Schomig A, Neumann FJ, Kastrati A et al. A randomized comparison of antiplatelet and anticoagulant therapy after the placement of coronary artery stents. *N Engl J Med* 1996; **334**: 1084–1089.

23. Goods C, Al-Shaibi K, Liu M et al. Comparison of aspirin alone versus aspirin plus ticlopidine after coronary artery stenting. *Am J Cardiol* 1996; **78**: 1042–1044.

24. Leon MB, Baim DS, Popma JJ et al. A clinical trial comparing three antithrombotic drug regimens after coronary-artery stenting. Stent Anticoagulation Restenosis Study Investigators. *N Engl J Med* 1998; **339**: 1665–1671.

25. Leon MB, Cutlip D, Fitz Patrick M et al. Acute results and one year outcomes of the Stent Anticoagulation Regimen Study (STARS) Registry. *Circulation* 1997; **96**: 3315.

26. Barragan P, Sainsous J, Silvestri M et al. Coronary artery stenting without anticoagulation, aspirin, ultrasound guidance, or high balloon pressure: prospective study of 1,051 consecutive patients. *Cathet Cardiovasc Diagn* 1997; **42**: 367–373.

27. Rupprecht HJ, Darius H, Borkowsky U et al. Comparison of antiplatelet effects of aspirin, ticlopidine, or their combination after stent implantation. *Circulation* 1998; **97**: 1046–1052.

28. Serruys P, Emanuelsson H, van der Giessen W et al on behalf of the Benestent-II Study Group. Heparin-coated Palmaz–Schatz stents in human coronary arteries. Early outcome of the Benestent-II pilot study. *Circulation* 1996; **93**: 412–422.

29. Russo RJ, Teirstein PS, for the AVID investigators. Angiography versus intravascular ultrasound-directed stent placement (abstract). *Circulation* 1996; **94**: 1536.

30. Mudra H, Henneke KH, Kanig A et al. Interim results of the OPTICUS randomized stent restenosis study (abstract). *Circulation* 1997; **96**: 3259.

31. Mills DC, Puri R, Hu CJ et al. Clopidogrel inhibits the binding of ADP analogues to the receptor mediating inhibition of platelet adenylate cyclase. *Arterioscler Thromb* 1992; **12**: 430–436.

32. Makkar R, Eigler N, Kaul S et al. Clopidogrel, a novel platelet ADP receptor antagonist inhibits aspirin and ticlopidine resistant stent thrombosis (abstract). *J Am Coll Cardiol* 1997; **29 (suppl A)**: 353A.

33. Bennett CL, Weinberg PD, Rosenberg Ben-Dror K et al. Thrombotic thrombocytopenic purpura associated with ticlopidine. *Ann Intern Med* 1998; **128**: 541–544.

34. A randomized, blinded, trial of Clopidogrel versus aspirin in patients at risk for ischemic events (CAPRIE). CAPRIE Steering Committee. *Lancet* 1996; **348**: 1329–1339.

35. Moussa I, Oetgen M, Roubin GS et al. The effectiveness of clopidogrel and aspirin versus ticlopidine and aspirin in preventing stent thrombosis after coronary stent implantation. *Circulation* 1999; **99**: 2364–2366.

36. Agrawal S, Ho D, Liu M et al. Predictors of thrombotic complications after placement of the flexible coil stent. *Am J Cardiol* 1994; **73**: 1216–1221.

37. Nath C, Muller D, Ellis S et al. Thrombosis of a flexible coil coronary stent: frequency predictors and clinical outcome. *J Am Coll Cardiol* 1993; **21**: 622–627.

38. Moussa I, Di Mario C, Reimers B et al. Subacute stent thrombosis in the era of intravascular ultrasound-guided coronary stenting without anticoagulation: frequency, predictors and clinical outcome. *J Am Coll Cardiol* 1997; **29**: 6–12.

39. Schomig A. Particular benefit from antiplatelet therapy for patients at high risk for adverse cardiac events after coronary stent placement. Analysis of a prospective risk stratification protocol in the ISAR-Trial. *Circulation* 1996; **94**: 1501.

40. Stone GW, Brodie BR, Griffin JJ et al. Prospective, multicenter study of the safety and feasibility of primary stenting in acute myocardial infarction: in-hospital and 30–day results of the PAMI stent pilot trial. Primary Angioplasty in Myocardial Infarction Stent Pilot Trial Investigators. *J Am Coll Cardiol* 1998; **31**: 23–30.

41. Roberts DK, Arthur A, Bellinger RL et al. Reduced anticoagulation protocol for stenting (RAPS) in smaller coronary vessels using intravascular ultrasound guidance: 30 day procedural results (abstract). *J Am Coll Cardiol* 1996; **27**: 393A.

42. Kobayashi, N, De Gregorio, J, Adamian, M et al. New approaches to evaluate coronary dissections post coronary intervention: all dissections are not malignant (abstract). *J Am Coll Cardiol* 1999; **33**: 71A.

Chapter 4   Angiographic and ultrasound descriptors of in-stent restenosis

Shunji Kasaoka and Jonathan Tobis

The problem of restenosis has always been the Achilles' heel for interventional procedures. Although intracoronary stenting has dramatically lowered the rate of restenosis compared with balloon angioplasty, in-stent restenosis continues to be an important clinical problem.[1-9] In an attempt to understand the causes of restenosis, there have been many studies that describe the predictors of restenosis.[10-13] The different conclusions among these studies may derive from differences in patient population as well as from the techniques and type or number of stents used. The following analysis reviews our database of 1706 patients, in which 2343 lesions were treated between April 1993 and April 1997. This review consists of all our patients who received stents without anticoagulation during this period. The purpose of the study was to evaluate the clinical, angiographic, and ultrasound predictors of in-stent restenosis.

Restenosis was defined as > 50% diameter narrowing of any portion of the stented segment compared to the average of the proximal and distal segments on an angiogram performed within 6 months after stent insertion. Angiographic follow-up was obtained at a mean of 5.5 ± 2.5 months in 1149 patients (67%) with 1633 stented lesions (70%). The baseline clinical, angiographic, and procedural characteristics of the study patients are shown in *Table 4.1* and *Table 4.2*. There were minimal differences in the baseline clinical angiographic or procedural characteristics between the groups of patients who did or did not receive follow-up angiography, which suggests that the lesions analysed are representative of the entire patient population. Unlike most published randomized trials, this population is not selected and consists of all the patients (except those cases where in-stent restenosis was the target lesion) treated at the Columbus Hospital in Milan, Italy. For descriptive purposes, the patients were classified into two groups; 871 patients (1224 lesions) without restenosis and 278 patients (409 lesions) with restenosis.

STENT IMPLANTATION PROCEDURE

This analysis is based on stents that were deployed without anticoagulation therapy.[13] The Palmaz–Schatz stent was the stent most commonly used (46%). Other stents included the NIR stent (10%), the Gianturco–Roubin stent (8%), the Arterial Vascular Engineering (AVE) Microstent (7%), the Wiktor stent (5%), the Wallstent (5%), the Multilink stent (4%), and the Cordis stent (2%). A combination of stents was used in 9% of lesions. After intracoronary stent implantation, angiographic optimization was performed by using high-pressure balloon dilatations to achieve a satisfactory angiographic result with < 20% residual stenosis by visual estimate. After the angiographic result was considered acceptable such that the procedure would ordinarily be terminated, intravascular ultrasound (IVUS) was performed. IVUS imaging was obtained in 904 patients (79%) with 1248 lesions (76%). Alternatively, IVUS imaging was obtained before any intervention or after the first pre-dilatation in 218 lesions (13%). The measured IVUS lumen area was used to choose the balloon for expanding the stent. Based on our previous observations with IVUS imaging of stents,[15] it was noted that the area achieved within the expanded stent is, on average, only 70% of the expected balloon area. From these observations, a table was generated so that the chosen balloon would provide an expanded stent lumen equal to the proximal reference lumen area as measured by IVUS. If IVUS imaging was not available, a balloon diameter was chosen that was equal to or up to 0.5 mm larger than the angiographic reference lumen diameter. All patients were scheduled for repeat coronary angiography at 6 months after stent insertion, or earlier if symptoms or exercise tolerance tests suggested restenosis. Total stent length was defined as the sum of the length of all stents implanted for each lesion.

Table 4.1

Baseline characteristics in the group with and the group without follow-up angiography

	With follow-up angiography n (%)	Without follow-up angiography n (%)	p value
Number of patients	1149	557	
Number of lesions	1633	710	
Age, yr	58 ± 10	59 ± 10	0.006
Male	1013 (88)	478 (87)	NS
Risk factors			
Hypercholesterolemia	654 (57)	277 (50)	0.007
Active smoker	376 (33)	182 (33)	NS
Diabetes	150 (13)	70 (13)	NS
Hypertension	473 (41)	251 (45)	NS
Prior myocardial infarction	624 (54)	317 (57)	NS
Prior angioplasty	115 (10)	61 (11)	NS
Prior CABG	122 (11)	51 (9)	NS
Ejection fraction, %	59 ± 11	57 ± 12	0.002
Unstable angina	333 (29)	170 (31)	NS
Multivessel disease	624 (55)	295 (53)	NS
Indication for stenting			
Elective	1090 (67)	428 (61)	0.003
Chronic occlusion	157 (10)	75 (11)	NS
Suboptimal angioplasty	145 (9)	60 (8)	NS
Dissection	102 (6)	71 (10)	0.001
Restenosis	93 (6)	50 (7)	NS
Acute vessel closure	31 (2)	14 (2)	NS
Acute myocardial infarction	5 (1)	5 (1)	NS
Treated vessel			
LAD	796 (49)	333 (47)	NS
LCX	318 (19)	135 (19)	NS
RCA	445 (27)	202 (28)	NS
LM	23 (1)	13 (2)	NS
SVG	51 (3)	27 (4)	NS
Modified AHA/ACC lesion type			
A	67 (4)	45 (7)	0.02
B1	479 (30)	224 (33)	NS
B2	684 (43	268 (39)	NS
C	368 (23)	147 (21)	NS
Number of stents per lesion	1.5 ± 0.9	1.5 ± 1.1	NS
Single stent	1096 (67)	491 (69)	NS
Palmaz–Schatz stent	752 (50)	345 (53)	NS
IVUS guidance	1246 (77)	444 (65)	<0.0001
Angiographic RLD (mm)	3.1 ± 0.5	3.0 ± 0.5	NS
Final MLD (mm)	3.1 ± 0.6	3.1 ± 0.5	NS
Lesion length (mm)	11 ± 7	11 ± 7	NS
Total stent length (mm)	26 ± 16	25 ± 17	NS

CABG = coronary artery bypass graft, LAD = left anterior descending coronary artery, LCX = left circumflex coronary artery, LM = left main coronary artery, MLD = minimal lumen diameter, RCA = right coronary artery, RLD = reference lumen diameter, SVG = saphenous vein graft

Table 4.2
Clinical, angiographic, and procedural characteristics in the restenosis or no restenosis groups

	No restenosis n (%)	Restenosis n (%)	p value
Number of patients	871	278	
Number of lesions	1224	409	
Age, yr	58 ± 9	59 ± 10	0.008
Male	776 (89)	237 (85)	NS
Risk factors			
Hypercholesterolemia	479 (55)	175 (63)	0.028
Active smoker	301 (35)	75 (27)	0.017
Diabetes	99 (11)	51 (18)	0.003
Hypertension	359 (41)	114 (41)	NS
Prior myocardial infarction	477 (55)	147 (53)	NS
Prior angioplasty	84 (10)	31 (11)	NS
Prior CABG	81 (9)	41 (15)	0.011
Unstable angina	243 (28)	90 (32)	NS
Follow-up duration, mo	5.5 ± 2.4	5.3 ± 2.9	NS
Treated vessels			
LAD	611 (50)	185 (45)	NS
LCX	225 (18)	93 (23)	NS
RCA	339 (28)	106 (26)	NS
LM	20 (2)	3 (1)	NS
SVG	29 (2)	22 (5)	0.002
Modified AHA/ACC lesion types			
A	53 (4)	14 (4)	NS
B1	382 (32)	97 (24)	0.004
B2	515 (43)	169 (42)	NS
C	247 (21)	121 (30)	<0.0001
Chronic occlusion	114 (9)	43 (11)	NS
Dissection	63 (5)	39 (10)	0.002
Ostial lesion	85 (7)	34 (8)	NS
Bifurcation	272 (23)	107 (27)	NS
Restenotic lesion	68 (6)	25 (6)	NS
Number of stents per lesion			
Mean ± SD	1.4 ± 0.8	1.6 ± 1.0	<0.0001
1 stent	853 (70)	243 (60)	0.0001
2 stents	252 (20)	99 (24)	NS
≥3 stents	119 (10)	67 (16)	0.0002
Total stent length (mm)	24 ± 15	31 ± 19	<0.0001
Palmaz–Schatz stent	617 (54)	135 (38)	<0.0001
IVUS guidance	952 (78)	296 (72)	0.026

CABG = coronary artery bypass graft, IVUS = intravascular ultrasound, LAD = left anterior descending coronary artery, LCX = left circumflex coronary artery, LM = left main coronary artery, RCA = right coronary artery, SVG = saphenous vein graft

QUANTITATIVE ANGIOGRAPHIC ANALYSIS

Quantitative coronary angiographic analysis was performed using digital calipers or quantitative coronary angiography by experienced angiographers who were not involved in the stent procedure. Angiographic measurements were obtained during diastole. The lesions were measured from an optically magnified image in a single, matched 'worst' view using the guiding catheter as the reference object for magnification calibration. Previous studies have shown that digital calipers correlate closely with computer-assisted methods with a low interobserver and intraobserver variability.[16,17] Minimum lumen diameter, reference lumen diameter (proximal and distal to the lesion or the stent), and percentage diameter stenosis before and after stent implantation and at follow-up were measured.

INTRAVASCULAR ULTRASOUND EQUIPMENT AND MEASUREMENTS

From April 1993 until November 1993, coronary arteries were imaged with a 3.9 Fr monorail ultrasound system with a 25 MHz transducer-tipped catheter. A Cardiovascular Imaging System (CVIS) machine with a 3.2 Fr catheter was used after November 1993. Images were initially obtained with a manual pull-back system, but from July 1994 a mechanical pull-back device at a speed of 0.5 mm/second was always employed. The ultrasound catheter was advanced distal to the stent, and images were recorded on super VHS videotape while the imaging catheter was withdrawn. Off-line quantitative measurements from videotape playback were performed during the procedure. The lumen cross-sectional area was measured at the proximal and distal reference sites and at the most narrowed point within the stent.

STATISTICAL ANALYSIS

Statistical analysis was performed with commercially available software programs (Statview 4.5 and JMP 3.1). Values were expressed as mean ± standard deviation. Differences between groups were evaluated by chi-square analysis or Fisher exact test for categoric variables and Student's t-test for continuous variables. P values < 0.05 were considered significant.

Univariate logistic regression analysis was used to select the clinical, angiographic or IVUS predictors of angiographic restenosis. Univariate predictors of angiographic restenosis with a p value < 0.2 were entered into a multivariate logistic model. A backward elimination was used to select independent predictors. A p value < 0.05 was required for all variables to be included in the final multivariate stepwise model. The odds ratios and 95% confidence intervals are presented in the tables for the final

multivariate model. The odds ratio (OR) was calculated as:

$$OR = e^{(bX)}$$

where b is the estimate and X is the unit measurement for continuous variables. For minimum lumen diameter and reference lumen diameter, the unit of measurement was taken as 1 mm, for stent length it was 10 mm, for cross-sectional area it was 1 mm², and for age it was 10 years. An odds ratio > 1 means an increase in predicted risk of restenosis for the variable listed.

COMPARISON OF PATIENTS WITH AND WITHOUT FOLLOW-UP ANGIOGRAPHY

Table 4.1 compares the two groups with and without follow-up angiography. The patients without follow-up angiography were older and had a lower ejection fraction and a higher incidence of hypercholesterolemia, dissection, and type A lesions than the group with follow-up angiography. They also had a lower incidence of IVUS guidance. However, there were no differences in the number of stents per lesion, angiographic reference lumen diameter, final minimum lumen diameter, lesion length, and total stent length between the two groups.

ANGIOGRAPHIC AND PROCEDURAL CHARACTERISTICS

The angiographic incidence of in-stent restenosis was documented in 278 patients (24%) with 409 lesions (25%). The age of patients in the restenosis group was slightly higher (59 ± 10 versus 58 ± 9 years, p = 0.008) (see *Table 4.2*). There was no difference in follow-up duration between the no-restenosis group and the restenosis group. However, the restenosis group had a greater frequency of hypercholesterolemia (63% versus 55%, p = 0.028), diabetes mellitus (18% vs. 11%, p = 0.003), and previous coronary bypass (15% vs. 9%, p = 0.011), but fewer active smokers (27% versus 35%, p = 0.017). There was a higher incidence of saphenous vein graft (5% versus 2%, p = 0.002), type C lesions (30% versus 21%, p <

Table 4.3

Angiographic and IVUS measurements in the restenosis or no restenosis groups

	No restenosis	Restenosis	p value
Angiographic			
Number of lesions	1224	409	
Lesion length (mm)	11 ± 7	12 ± 8	0.0008
Reference diameter (mm)	3.1 ± 0.5	2.8 ± 0.5	<0.0001
Pre MLD (mm)	0.9 ± 0.6	0.8 ± 0.5	0.004
Final MLD (mm)	3.2 ± 0.6	2.9 ± 0.5	<0.0001
Pre %DS	70 ± 17	70 ± 17	NS
Final %DS	0.0 ± 13	3.1 ± 14	<0.0001
Acute gain (mm)	2.2 ± 0.7	2.0 ± 0.7	<0.0001
Intravascular ultrasound			
Number of lesions	952	296	
Proximal Ref. L-CSA (mm^2)	9.4 ± 3.4	8.1 ± 2.7	<0.0001
Distal Ref. L-CSA (mm^2)	7.5 ± 3.2	6.1 ± 2.3	<0.0001
Stent L-CSA (mm^2)	8.0 ± 2.6	6.5 ± 2.1	<0.0001

Acute gain = Final MLD - Pre MLD, MLD = minimal lumen diameter, Ref. L-CSA = reference lumen cross-sectional area, %DS = percent diameter stenosis

0.0001), and dissection (10% versus 5%, $p = 0.002$) in the restenosis group. The restenosis group also had a greater frequency of multiple stents (40% versus 30%, $p = 0.0001$) and a longer total stent length (31 ± 19 mm versus 24 ± 15 mm, $p < 0.0001$). Palmaz–Schatz stents were used more frequently in the no-restenosis group than in the restenosis group (54% versus 38%, $p < 0.0001$). IVUS guidance was used in 952 lesions (78%) in the no-restenosis group, compared to 296 lesions (72%) in the restenosis group ($p = 0.026$).

ANGIOGRAPHIC ANALYSIS

The angiographic results are provided in *Table 4.3*. Lesion length in the restenosis group was longer than in the no-restenosis group (12 ± 8 mm versus 11 ± 7 mm, $p = 0.0008$). Angiographic reference lumen diameter (2.8 ± 0.5 mm versus 3.1 ± 0.5 mm, $p < 0.0001$) and final minimum lumen diameter (2.9 ± 0.5 mm versus 3.2 ± 0.5 mm, $p < 0.0001$) were significantly smaller in the restenosis group than in the no-restenosis group. There was no difference in percentage diameter stenosis before the stent procedure between the two groups; however, the no-restenosis group had a significantly lower percentage diameter

stenosis after the stent procedure (0 ± 13% versus 3.1 ± 14%, $p < 0.0001$). There was a significant inverse correlation between the final minimum lumen diameter and the in-stent restenosis rate ($p < 0.0001$) (*Fig. 4.1a*).

IVUS ANALYSIS

The no-restenosis group had a larger proximal or distal reference lumen cross-sectional area than the restenosis group (see *Table 4.3*). The final stent lumen cross-sectional area in the no-restenosis group (8.0 ± 2.6 mm^2) was greater than in the restenosis group (6.5 ± 2.1 mm^2, $p < 0.0001$). There was an inverse correlation between the stent lumen cross-sectional area and the in-stent restenosis rate ($p < 0.0001$) (see *Fig. 4.1b*).

EFFECT OF NUMBER OR LENGTH OF STENTS ON RESTENOSIS

As shown in *Fig. 4.2a*, there was a significant correlation between the number of stents and the in-stent

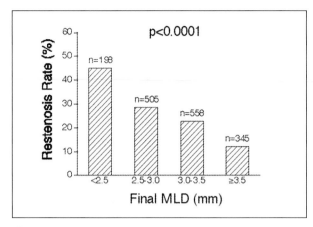

a

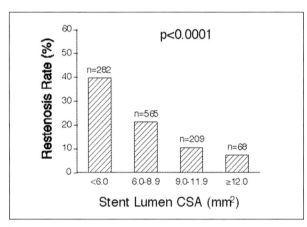

b

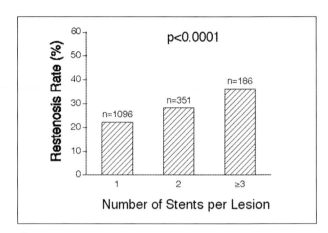

a

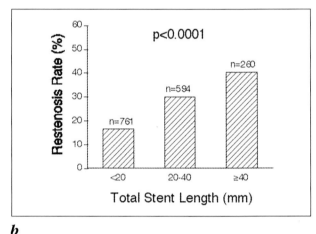

b

Figure 4.1 *(a) Effect of final minimum lumen diameter on in-stent restenosis rate (p < 0.0001). n, total number of patients at risk per category. (b) Effect of stent lumen cross-sectional area on in-stent restenosis rate (p < 0.001). n, total number of patients at risk per category.*

Figure 4.2 *(a) Effect of number of stents per lesion on in-stent restenosis rate (p < 0.0001). n, total number of patients at risk per category. (b) Effect of total stent length on in-stent restenosis (p < 0.0001). n, total number of patients at risk per category.*

restenosis rate ($p < 0.0001$). There was also a significant correlation between the total stent length and in-stent restenosis rate ($p < 0.0001$) (see *Fig. 4.2b*).

To address multiple influences, *Fig. 4.3a* compares the incidence of restenosis correlated with angiographic reference lumen diameter as affected by total stent length. There were significant differences in restenosis rates with all subgroups of total stent length for each reference lumen diameter (p for trend < 0.0001 for total stent length < 20 mm, $p < 0.0001$ for total stent length ≥ 20 mm but < 40 mm; and $p = 0.04$ for total stent length ≥ 40 mm). *Figure 4.3b*

demonstrates the incidence of restenosis compared with IVUS stent lumen cross-sectional area as affected by total stent length. There were significant differences in restenosis rates with total stent length < 20 mm, and with total stent length ≥ 20 but < 40 mm for each stent lumen cross-sectional area (p for trend < 0.0001; $p = 0.0001$, respectively). Despite a total stent length ≥ 40 mm, the restenosis rate was still acceptable (20%) when the stent lumen cross-sectional area was ≥ 9 mm². This rate was significantly lower than if the cross-sectional area was < 6 mm² (44%, $p < 0.05$) or if the cross-sectional area

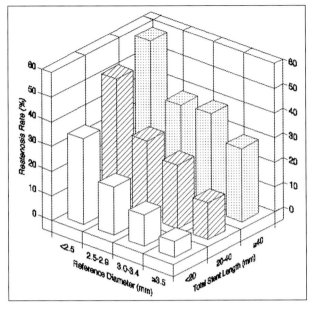

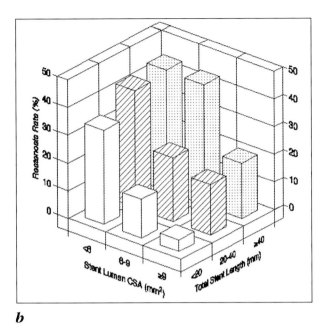

a

b

Figure 4.3 *(a) Effect of angiographic reference lumen diameter and total stent length on in-stent restenosis rate. There were significant differences in restenosis rates with all subgroups of total stent length for each reference lumen diameter (p for trend < 0.0001 for total stent length < 20 mm, p < 0.0001 for total stent length 20–40 mm, and p = 0.04 for total stent length ≥ 40 mm). (b) Effect of IVUS stent lumen cross-sectional area and total stent length on in-stent restenosis rate. There were significant differences in restenosis rates for total stent length < 20 mm or 20–40 mm for each stent lumen cross-sectional area (p for trend < 0.0001; p = 0.0001, respectively). For total stent length > 40 mm, restenosis rate (20%) with stent lumen cross-sectional area ≥ 9 mm² was significantly lower than that with cross-sectional area < 6 mm² (44%, p < 0.05) or cross-sectional area 6–9 mm² (43%, p < 0.05).*

was ≥ 6 mm² but < 9 mm² (43%, $p < 0.05$) in the long lesion subset.

COMPARISON BETWEEN IVUS AND NO-IVUS GUIDANCE

The patients who did or did not receive IVUS imaging to guide the stent implantation are separated in *Table 4.4*. The group with IVUS guidance had a significantly larger final minimum lumen diameter (3.2 ± 0.6 mm versus 3.0 ± 0.5 mm, $p < 0.0001$) and a smaller final percentage diameter stenosis (−0.3 ± 13.2% versus 4.3 ± 12.0%, $p < 0.0001$) as well as a larger acute gain (2.2 ± 0.7 mm versus 2.0 ± 0.6 mm, $p < 0.0001$) than the group without IVUS guidance. In addition, stents that were implanted with IVUS

guidance had a significantly lower in-stent restenosis rate (24% versus 29%, $p = 0.03$). There were no differences in the number of stents per lesion, total stent length, and lesion length between the two groups; however, the group without IVUS guidance had a smaller angiographic reference lumen diameter (3.0 ± 0.5 mm versus 3.1 ± 0.5 mm, $p = 0.0008$), and a higher incidence of dissection (9% versus 6%, $p = 0.03$) and type C lesions (27% vs. 22%, p=0.03) than the group with IVUS guidance.

MULTIVARIATE LOGISTIC REGRESSION ANALYSIS

As shown in *Table 4.5*, there were 13 parameters that had a univariate correlation with restenosis at the

Table 4.4

Comparison of clinical, angiographic and procedural variables between IVUS and no-IVUS guidance

	IVUS n (%)	No-IVUS n (%)	p value
Number of patients	904	245	
Number of lesions	1248	385	
Restenosis	296 (24)	113 (29)	0.03
Final MLD (mm)	3.2 ± 0.6	3.0 ± 0.5	<0.0001
Final %DS	−0.3 ± 13.2	4.3 ± 12.0	<0.0001
Acute gain (mm)	2.2 ± 0.7	2.0 ± 0.6	<0.0001
Angiographic RLD (mm)	3.1 ± 0.5	3.0 ± 0.5	0.0008
Number of stents per lesion	1.6 ± 0.9	1.5 ± 0.9	NS
Total stent length (mm)	26 ± 16	26 ± 17	NS
Lesion length (mm)	11 ± 7	11 ± 7	NS
Age, yr	58 ± 10	58 ± 9	NS
Diabetes	117 (13)	33 (14)	NS
Prior CABG	89 (10)	33 (14)	NS
Type C lesion	266 (22)	102 (27)	0.03
Dissection	69 (6)	33 (9)	0.03

CABG = coronary artery bypass graft, MLD = minimal lumen diameter, RLD = reference lumen diameter, %DS = percent diameter stenosis

Table 4.5

Predictors of in-stent restenosis by logistic regression analysis (n = 1501)

Variables	Univariate			Multivariate (r^2 = 0.1)		
	Odds ratio	95% CI	p value	Odds ratio	95% CI	p value
Total stent length	1.26/10 mm	1.17-1.34	< 0.0001	1.26/10 mm	1.17–1.35	< 0.0001
Angiographic RLD	0.32/1 mm	0.25-0.42	< 0.0001	0.47/1 mm	0.34–0.65	< 0.0001
Final MLD	0.37/1 mm	0.29-0.47	< 0.0001	0.55/1 mm	0.41–0.75	0.0001
Prior CABG	1.58	1.14-2.19	0.024	1.33	1.11–1.60	0.0024
Age	1.14/10 yr	1.02-1.29	0.025	1.17/10 yr	1.03–1.33	0.018
Diabetes	1.45	1.06-1.97	0.020	1.20	1.01–1.43	0.038
Lesion length	1.30/10 mm	1.11-1.52	0.0009			
Active smoker	0.76	0.59-0.97	0.032			
Dissection	1.94	1.27-2.93	0.0018			
PS stent	0.51	0.40-0.65	< 0.0001			
Single stent	0.64	0.51-0.80	0.0001			
Type C lesion	1.66	1.29-2.14	0.0001			
IVUS guidance	0.75	0.58-0.97	0.026			

CABG = coronary artery bypass graft, CI = confidence interval, IVUS = intravascular ultrasound, MLD = minimal lumen diameter, PS = Palmaz–Schatz, RLD = reference lumen diameter

Table 4.6

Predictors of in-stent restenosis in lesions with IVUS guidance by multivariate logistic regression analysis

Variables	Odds ratio	95% CI	p value
IVUS stent L-CSA	$0.81/1 \text{ mm}^2$	0.74–0.88	<0.0001
Total stent length	1.21/10 mm	1.11–1.33	<0.0001
Angiographic RLD	0.60/1 mm	0.40–0.89	0.012
Dissection	1.47	1.08–1.99	0.014
Age	1.19/10 yr	1.02–1.39	0.03
Prior CABG	1.27	1.00–1.60	0.046

CABG = coronary artery bypass graft, CI = confidence interval, IVUS = intravascular ultrasound, L-CSA = lumen cross-sectional area, RLD = reference lumen diameter

$P<0.05$ level: four clinical parameters (age, previous coronary artery bypass grafts, diabetes mellitus and active smoking), four procedural parameters (IVUS guidance, total stent length, single stent, and Palmaz–Schatz stent), and five angiographic parameters (final minimum lumen diameter, reference lumen diameter, lesion length, dissection, and type C lesion). These 13 variables were entered into a multivariate logistic regression model for the binomial variable of angiographic restenosis. In-stent restenosis was predicted independently by six variables (see *Table 4.5*). Of these variables, a longer total stent length, previous coronary artery bypass grafts, patient age, and diabetes mellitus increased the risk of restenosis. A larger reference lumen diameter and a larger final minimum lumen diameter decreased the risk of restenosis. The best predictors of restenosis were total stent length and angiographic reference lumen diameter. The odds ratio indicates that the predicted risk of restenosis increases 26% for every 10 mm increase in total stent length, restenosis risk decreases 53% for every 1 mm increase in reference lumen diameter and restenosis decreases 45% for every 1 mm increment in final MLD. The use of IVUS guidance did not reach statistical significance in the multivariate model.

To assess the predictors of in-stent restenosis in lesions where IVUS measurements were obtained, stent lumen cross-sectional area by IVUS was entered into the multivariate model. As shown in *Table 4.6*, IVUS stent lumen cross-sectional area and total stent length were the best predictors of in-stent restenosis. The odds ratio indicates that the predicted risk of restenosis decreased 19% for every 1 mm^2 increase in stent lumen cross-sectional area. When IVUS measurements were entered into the multivariate

model, final minimum lumen diameter by angiography was no longer an independent predictor of restenosis.

DISCUSSION

The analysis of our database suggests that multiple factors combine to influence the incidence of restenosis following stent insertion in coronary arteries. The independent predictors of restenosis by multivariate logistic regression analysis were:

(a) total stent length
(b) angiographic reference lumen diameter
(c) angiographic final minimum lumen diameter
(d) previous coronary artery bypass grafts
(e) age
(f) diabetes mellitus.

In the group of patients where IVUS observations were obtained, the stent lumen cross-sectional area by IVUS was a stronger predictor of restenosis than the angiographic parameters; in fact, final minimum lumen diameter by angiography was no longer an independent predictor. In the group of patients who had IVUS guidance, the independent predictors of restenosis were:

(a) IVUS stent lumen cross-sectional area
(b) total stent length
(c) angiographic reference lumen diameter
(d) dissection

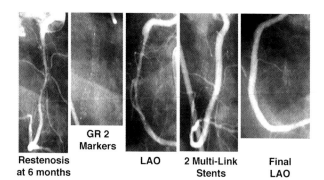

Figure 4.4 *Severe diffuse in-stent restenosis occurred in this right coronary artery six months following placement of a 40 mm long Gianturco–Roubin II stent. This was treated by placing two multi-link stents to cover the restenotic section. The patient has remained asymptomatic for 1 year.*

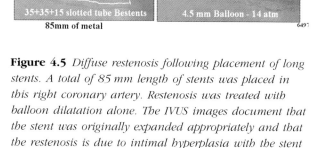

Figure 4.5 *Diffuse restenosis following placement of long stents. A total of 85 mm length of stents was placed in this right coronary artery. Restenosis was treated with balloon dilatation alone. The IVUS images document that the stent was originally expanded appropriately and that the restenosis is due to intimal hyperplasia with the stent struts.*

(e) age
(f) previous coronary artery bypass grafts.

An example of aggressive restenosis is demonstrated in *Fig. 4.4*. This 62-year-old woman initially presented with an acute myocardial infarction from an occluded right coronary artery (RCA). This was reopened successfully and a 40 mm Gianturco– Roubin II stent was placed in the RCA. Over the next few months the patient did well and denied any symptoms of angina. However, 6 months after placement of the stent, she had a sudden onset of pulmonary edema. After being stabilized in the emergency room with intravenous heparin and nitroglycerin she had cardiac catheterization, which revealed diffuse restenosis throughout the entire length of the Gianturco–Roubin stent. This was treated with repeat dilatation followed by two ACS Multilink stents (as shown in the last two panels of *Fig. 4.4*).

Another example of diffuse restenosis following deployment of long stents is provided in *Fig. 4.5*. This patient had several lesions throughout the RCA which were treated by placement of sequential BeStents covering a total length of 85 mm. Three months later the patient returned with recurrent angina, and the angiogram demonstrated diffuse in-stent restenosis. The ultrasound image demonstrates that the initial stent was adequately deployed with a 3.5 mm diameter; however, intense intimal hyperplasia has narrowed the lumen dramatically. In this case, the restenosis was treated with balloon dilatation using a 4.5 mm balloon at 14 atmospheres. An adequate cross-sectional area (9.2 mm²) and lumen diameter was documented by IVUS. The patient remained asymptomatic for 3 months but returned with recurrent angina. Follow-up by angiography demonstrated a focal restenosis isolated to the mid-RCA. This was treated by balloon dilatation alone. The patient remained asymptomatic over the next six months.

COMPARISON WITH OTHER STUDIES

Several investigators have reported clinical or angiographic predictors of in-stent restenosis. Klugherz and colleagues[18] reported that predictors of clinical events 3 years after Palmaz–Schatz stenting included diabetes mellitus, higher angina score at follow-up, smaller stent deployment balloon size, and greater number of stents implanted. Haude and colleagues[19] and Ellis and colleagues[20] reported that multiple stents were an important predictor of angiographic restenosis. Carrozza and colleagues[21] reported that diabetes mellitus, small post-procedure lumen diameter, and stenting of the left anterior descending artery were associated with higher rates of restenosis by multivariate logistic regression analysis. The numbers of patients in these studies (between 50 and 227) were smaller and the patients were more selected than in our study. Kastrati and colleagues[11] reported that the strongest predictors of in-stent restenosis after Palmaz–Schatz stent implantation in 1399 lesions were diabetes mellitus, multiple stents, and smaller final minimum lumen diameter.

THE EFFECTS OF THE NUMBER OR LENGTH OF STENTS

A frequent finding in these previous studies is that in-stent restenosis is more common with multiple stents.[19,20] Our results support this finding, but since we used a variety of stents with different lengths, we analysed total stent length as well as the number of stents per lesion. By univariate logistic regression analysis, both total stent length and the number of stents per lesion were significant variables. By multiple logistic regression analysis, total stent length was the strongest predictor of restenosis, but the number of stents per lesion was not an independent predictor. In addition, lesion length, which was only roughly related to total stent length, did not enter into the multivariate model. These results suggest that achieving an optimal result with a minimal total stent length during the procedure may reduce in-stent restenosis. This analysis of our experience has significantly influenced our current practice; owing to the recognition of the higher restenosis rate with multiple stents, we tend to dilate longer lesions and stent only those dissected areas that appear to compromise the lumen. This has been called 'spot stenting' and it is described more completely in Chapter 20.

ROLE OF ANGIOGRAPHY AND IVUS

In contrast to the initial reports of stent utilization where the risk of subacute stent thrombosis was thought to be due to the presence of a metallic prosthesis, subsequent studies have suggested that adequate stent expansion may be the most important factor to decrease the risk of complications after stent deployment.[20,22] Several studies have demonstrated that the incidence of restenosis is decreased when a larger final lumen is achieved for balloon angioplasty, directed atherectomy, or stent insertion.[20,21,23,24]. Our prospective analysis extends these observations. Both larger final minimum lumen diameter and larger reference lumen diameter are inversely correlated with restenosis. This combination is understandable because it is easier to obtain a larger stented lumen area in larger vessels. In arteries with a reference lumen diameter ≥ 3.5 mm, the incidence of angiographic restenosis was only 12%. The persistent problem is how to optimize the results for smaller arteries[20,25,26] and diffuse disease.

Although angiographic guidance has been the traditional method of assessing stent deployment, we have reported that 40% of stents with an acceptable angiographic result still require additional dilatation with a larger balloon to achieve an optimal result by IVUS.[14] Using IVUS guidance, we have also shown that high-pressure balloon inflations increase the percentage of patients who achieve adequate stent expansion from 12% to 60%.[14] With the stent deployment technique used in this large group of patients, IVUS provided critical information about the adequacy of stent deployment and reference vessel dimensions. This information was utilized for determining balloon size and whether to use a stent, and for maximizing stent expansion. The lesions with IVUS guidance had a larger final minimum lumen diameter and a lower final percentage diameter stenosis than the lesions without IVUS guidance. These results indicate that IVUS guidance may be useful for optimizing stent implantation. In addition, the restenosis rate in the lesions in which IVUS guidance was used (24%) was significantly lower than in the lesions without IVUS guidance (29%, $p = 0.03$).

Because this study was not a randomized comparison between angiography and IVUS guidance of coronary stenting, no definitive conclusions can be made from this analysis. There were some differences in angiographic characteristics between the IVUS group and the no-IVUS group, although each of these differences may have biased either group toward a different restenosis rate. Although the binomial variable of IVUS guidance was not an independent predictor of restenosis by multivariate logistic regression analysis, this does not necessarily imply that IVUS guidance does not help decrease restenosis. Because IVUS guidance was associated with a larger final minimum lumen diameter, these two variables parallel each other and therefore IVUS guidance may not appear in the model as an independent predictor of restenosis. In lesions with IVUS guidance, stent lumen cross-sectional area by IVUS was a better predictor of restenosis than the angiographic measurements. If the lumen cross-sectional area was ≥ 12 mm², the angiographic restenosis rate was only 7%. Our interpretation is that IVUS guidance is helpful in achieving an optimal result, which may in turn reduce in-stent restenosis.

STUDY LIMITATIONS

Several important limitations should be noted when assessing the results of this study. Although it was a prospective, unselected case analysis, there was no randomized protocol for the use of different stents or IVUS guidance. Although the stent types may affect in-stent restenosis, it was impossible to compare the different stent types individually because the type of stent was not randomly assigned. Angiographic follow-up was obtained in only 70% of the lesions studied during this period. However, there were only minimal differences in the baseline characteristics of those with or without angiographic follow-up, so the study group does not represent a significantly biased population.

It is important to note that in the multivariate model, $r^2 = 0.1$ which means that only 10% of the variance for restenosis is predicted by these clinical, or quantitative variables. The majority of restenosis is not accounted for in this analysis (or by other investigators' studies). One alternative explanation may be that there are biologic predictors that are not measurable at the present time.[27] Despite these limitations, this study is based on one of the largest available databases of coronary stents with angiographic follow-up. Therefore, these observations may be useful guidelines as predictors of in-stent restenosis since it is unlikely that many of these individual variables will be studied in prospective randomized trials.

CONCLUSIONS

This study has identified several factors that predispose to in-stent restenosis:

(a) total stent length
(b) angiographic reference lumen diameter
(c) angiographic final minimum lumen diameter
(d) previous coronary artery bypass grafts
(e) age
(f) diabetes mellitus.

In addition, when IVUS guidance was used, the most important inverse predictor of restenosis was stent lumen cross-sectional area. Achieving an optimal stented lumen cross-sectional area with the use of IVUS guidance and with a minimal total stent length may reduce in-stent restenosis.

REFERENCES

1. Serruys PW, de Jaegere P, Kiemeneij F et al. A comparison of balloon-expandable-stent implantation with balloon angioplasty in patients with coronary artery disease. Benestent Study Group. *N Engl J Med* 1994; **331**: 489–495.
2. Fischman DL, Leon MB, Baim DS et al. A randomized comparison of coronary-stent placement and balloon angioplasty in the treatment of coronary artery disease. Stent Restenosis Study Investigators. *N Engl J Med* 1994; **331**: 496–501.
3. Macaya C, Serruys PW, Ruygrok P et al. Continued benefit of coronary stenting versus balloon angioplasty: one-year clinical follow-up of Benestent trial. Benestent Study Group. *J Am Coll Cardiol* 1996; **27**: 255–261.
4. Kimura T, Nosaka H, Yokoi H et al. Serial angiographic follow-up after Palmaz–Schatz stent implantation: comparison with conventional balloon angioplasty. *J Am Coll Cardiol* 1993; **21**: 1557–1563.
5. Gordon PC, Gibson CM, Cohen DJ et al. Mechanisms of restenosis and redilation within coronary stents – quantitative angiographic assessment. *J Am Coll Cardiol* 1993; **21**: 1166–1174.
6. Hoffmann R, Mintz GS, Dussaillant GR et al. Patterns and mechanisms of in-stent restenosis. A serial intravascular ultrasound study. *Circulation* 1996; **94**: 1247–1254.
7. Reimers B, Moussa I, Akiyama T et al. Long-term clinical follow-up after successful repeat percutaneous intervention for stent restenosis. *J Am Coll Cardiol* 1997; **30**: 186–192.
8. Savage MP, Fischman DL, Schatz RA et al. Long-term angiographic and clinical outcome after implantation of a balloon-expandable stent in the native coronary circulation. Palmaz–Schatz Stent Study Group. *J Am Coll Cardiol* 1994; **24**: 1207–1212.
9. Laham RJ, Carrozza JP, Berger C et al. Long-term (4- to 6-year) outcome of Palmaz–Schatz stenting: paucity of late clinical stent-related problems. *J Am Coll Cardiol* 1996; **28**: 820–826.
10. Mintz GS, Popma JJ, Pichard AD et al. Intravascular ultrasound predictors of restenosis after percutaneous transcatheter coronary revascularization. *J Am Coll Cardiol* 1996; **27**: 1678–1687.
11. Kastrati A, Schomig A, Elezi S et al. Predictive factors of restenosis after coronary stent placement. *J Am Coll Cardiol* 1997; **30**: 1428–1436.
12. Hoffmann R, Mintz GS, Mehran R et al. Intravascular ultrasound predictors of angiographic restenosis in lesions treated with Palmaz–Schatz stents. *J Am Coll Cardiol* 1998; **31**: 43–49.
13. Bauters C, Hubert E, Prat A et al. Predictors of restenosis after coronary stent implantation. *J Am Coll Cardiol* 1998; **31**: 1291–1298.
14. Colombo A, Hall P, Nakamura S et al. Intracoronary

stenting without anticoagulation accomplished with intravascular ultrasound guidance. *Circulation* 1995; **91**: 1676–1688.

15. Nakamura S, Colombo A, Gaglione A et al. Intracoronary ultrasound observations during stent implantation. *Circulation* 1994; **89**: 2026–2034.

16. Theron HD, Lambert CR, Pepine CJ. Videodensitometry versus digital calipers for quantitative coronary angiography. *Am J Cardiol* 1990; **66**: 1186–1190.

17. Uehata A, Matsuguchi T, Bittl JA et al. Accuracy of electronic digital calipers compared with quantitative angiography in measuring coronary arterial diameter. *Circulation* 1993; **88**: 1724–1729.

18. Klugherz BD, DeAngelo DL, Kim BK et al. Three-year clinical follow-up after Palmaz–Schatz stenting. *J Am Coll Cardiol* 1996; **27**: 1185–1191.

19. Haude M, Erbel R, Straub U et al. Short and long term results after intracoronary stenting in human coronary arteries: monocentre experience with the balloon-expandable Palmaz–Schatz stent. *Br Heart J* 1991; **66**: 337–345.

20. Ellis SG, Savage M, Fischman D et al. Restenosis after placement of Palmaz–Schatz stents in native coronary arteries. Initial results of a multicenter experience. *Circulation* 1992; **86**: 1836–1844.

21. Carrozza J, Kuntz R, Schatz R et al. Inter-series differences in the restenosis rate of Palmaz–Schatz coronary stent placement: differences in demographics and post-procedure lumen diameter. *Cathet Cardiovasc Diagn* 1994; **31**: 173–178.

22. Moussa I, Di Mario C, Moses J et al. Coronary stenting after rotational atherectomy in calcified and complex lesions: angiographic and clinical follow-up results. *Circulation* 1997; **96**: 128–136.

23. Kuntz RE, Gibson CM, Nobuyoshi M, Baim DS. Generalized model of restenosis after conventional balloon angioplasty, stenting and directional atherectomy. *J Am Coll Cardiol* 1993; **21**: 15–25.

24. Kuntz R, Safian R, Carrozza J et al. The importance of acute luminal diameter in determining restenosis after coronary atherectomy or stenting. *Circulation* 1992; **86**: 1827–1835.

25. Dussaillant GR, Mintz GS, Pichard AD et al. Small stent size and intimal hyperplasia contribute to restenosis: a volumetric intravascular ultrasound analysis. *J Am Coll Cardiol* 1995; **26**: 720–724.

26. Sutton JM, Ellis SG, Roubin GS et al. Major clinical events after coronary stenting. The multicenter registry of acute and elective Gianturco–Roubin stent placement. The Gianturco–Roubin Intracoronary Stent Investigator Group. *Circulation* 1994; **89**: 1126–1137.

27. Amant C, Bauters C, Bodart JC et al. D allele of the angiotensin I-converting enzyme is a major risk factor for restenosis after coronary stenting. *Circulation* 1997; **96**: 56–60.

Chapter 5 Use of physiologic measurements of lesion severity to guide interventions

Carlo Di Mario

INTRODUCTION

An intracoronary Doppler catheter or guidewire can measure the velocity of blood in humans and assess any change in this velocity caused by coronary stenoses.[1] Technical improvements have made it possible to use this method during coronary interventions to determine which lesions should be treated and to determine that specific physiologic end-points of the procedure have been achieved. More recently, pressure-based indices of stenosis severity have been proposed, with the potential of overcoming some of the limitations of intracoronary Doppler.[2]

This chapter reviews the techniques of intracoronary Doppler and pressure measurements and the results of clinical studies of these techniques, and discusses their current indications in clinical practice.

EXAMINATION TECHNIQUES

INTRACORONARY DOPPLER MEASUREMENTS

The past 20 years have seen rapid changes in Doppler technology, with progressive miniaturization of the transducers and refinement of signal analysis. The large piezoelectric crystals mounted at the tip of standard 8 Fr Sones or Judkins catheters have been replaced by circular transducers attached to 3 Fr intracoronary catheters and, more recently, by miniaturized crystals at the tip of 0.46 mm (0.018-inch) and 0.36 mm (0.014-inch) guidewires.[3] Because of its small diameter, the Doppler guidewire can be passed distal to coronary stenoses without creating significant obstruction to flow. The forward directed ultra-sound beam diverges at 14° from the Doppler transducer to include a large portion of the flow velocity profile.[3] Although experienced operators can achieve a stable and optimal signal in most cases, recent in vivo experiments have shown that the measured flow velocity is 20% lower than the true maximal velocity in 40% of cases and suggested a method to help the operator in the optimal positioning of the Doppler sample volume based on the assessment of the normalized first Doppler moment.[4]

A real-time spectral analyser using on-line fast Fourier transformation provides a gray-scale spectral display.[5] The system software automatically tracks the instantaneous peak velocity and calculates on-line the average peak velocity over two consecutive beats. The Doppler guidewire can be detached from the rotary connection so that percutaneous transluminal coronary angioplasty (PTCA) balloons or other interventional devices can be advanced over it. The wire can then be reconnected to monitor the flow velocity changes during and immediately after PTCA and to repeat the flow reserve assessment after treatment.

Flow velocity measurements using the Doppler guidewire have been validated in straight tubes and canine coronary arteries by Doucette and colleagues.[3] These studies showed a linear correlation with absolute flow measured by electromagnetic flowmeters.

Coronary flow reserve

Although many Doppler indices of stenosis severity have been proposed (e.g. diastolic-to-systolic velocity ratio, proximal-to-distal ratio), coronary velocity reserve is the only Doppler-based index that has been shown to reflect lesion severity reliably. The tip of the Doppler guidewire should be advanced at least

2 cm distal to the stenosis to avoid recordings in segments of post-stenotic flow turbulence. The Doppler signal should be optimized by gentle rotation, advancement, or withdrawal until a stable flow velocity envelope is obtained. To increase the reproducibility of measurements, it is recommended to maintain a maximally vasodilated vessel, using intracoronary nitroglycerin (100–300 µg) or isosorbide dinitrate (1–3 mg). Basal velocity should be recorded after stabilization of the signal (at least 2–3 minutes after injection of nitrates or contrast) and should be followed by the injection of a maximally vasodilating dose of papaverine or adenosine to measure coronary flow reserve. An automatic detection system is available to search for the peak hyperemic velocity and to calculate and display the coronary flow reserve. Duplicate flow reserve measurements are highly recommended. Flow obstruction caused by having the guiding catheter engaged in the coronary ostium is rarely observed with the routine use of small (6–7 Fr) guiding catheters, but this should be excluded by careful monitoring of the pressure waveform during hyperemia (pressure damping).

In animal experiments, flow reserve discriminates between lesions of increasing severity.[6,7] Although the concept can be easily applied in humans,[8,9] it should be recognized that coronary flow reserve is influenced by several factors that are independent of the hydrodynamic characteristics of the stenotic lesion, such as the presence of scar tissue after myocardial infarction, myocardial hypertrophy, and impaired microvascular response. In addition, changes in heart rate, aortic pressure, pre-load and myocardial contractility, which occur frequently during coronary interventions, may affect the hyperemic pressure flow relationship or the basal flow and so modify the final measurement of flow reserve.[10]

Intracoronary papaverine has been reported to increase coronary blood flow velocity to between four and six times the resting value in patients with normal coronary arteries.[8,9] In these series, however, a highly selected patient population was studied, with the exclusion of myocardial hypertrophy, previous myocardial infarction, or any other condition known to increase baseline flow (e.g. anemia, hyperthyroidism). Recent experiments have challenged the results of Doucette and colleagues,[3] showing the absence of a fully developed parabolic profile (at the site of Doppler sampling maintained 5.2 mm beyond the sensor). Since the flow profile becomes flatter in high flow conditions, the ratio between maximal velocity and mean velocity drops below the level

observed at baseline. Consequently, the ratio between hyperemic and basal velocity is also reduced and the true velocity reserve is underestimated (Porenta, personal communication).

The group in St Louis (Morton Kern and coworkers) has established the normal values of flow reserve in a cohort of 490 patients, including patients with chest pain and angiographically normal arteries, in arteries without stenoses in patients with significant coronary artery disease, and in cardiac transplant recipients.[11] Although the average coronary flow reserve (CFR) ranged between 2.6 and 3.1 in all these groups and in the three major coronary arteries, a large standard deviation was observed, with 15% of measurements falling below the threshold of 2.0. Various groups have investigated the correlation of CFR measured with Doppler flow wires and [201]Thallium or [99]Technetium-MIBI single positron emission computed tomography (SPECT). Myocardial perfusion scintigraphy assesses relative differences of myocardial perfusion in the territory of distribution of different arteries, but despite this basic difference a good correlation between Doppler-based CFR and perfusion scintigraphy has been observed. A value of CFR below 2.0 to 1.7 can identify more than 90% of patients with abnormal scintigraphy[12–17] or positive high-dose dipyridamole echocardiography.[18] To improve the diagnostic accuracy of the test and identify false-positive flow reserve measurements (normal scintigraphy with CFR < 2.0), the measurement of flow reserve in a second artery without significant stenoses has been advocated so that the ratio between CFR in the artery under evaluation and CFR in the normal artery (relative flow reserve; RFR) can be calculated (*Fig. 5.1*). A cut-off measurement of RFR of 0.80 or 0.75 has been shown to improve the correlation with nuclide scintigraphy and predict event-free survival after deferral of coronary interventions.[19,20] A direct application of this method in the catheterization laboratory is cumbersome and not feasible in all patients since it requires the presence of a normal artery for comparison.

POST-STENOTIC PRESSURE AND RELATED INDICES

The measurement of post-stenotic pressure gradient was used as an end-point of coronary angioplasty by the pioneers of this technique.[21,22] It was soon realized that the large diameter of the balloon partially occluded the vessel and – especially after deflation – limited the accuracy of the measurements.

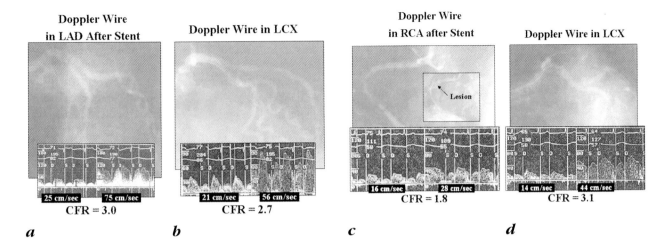

Figure 5.1 *Two examples of relative flow reserve measurement after stenting. (a) Coronary flow reserve (CFR) measured in the left anterior descending artery (LAD) after implantation of a 15 mm Palmaz–Schatz stent. Note the increase in flow velocity after adenosine from 25 cm/second to 75 cm/second; CFR = 3.0. (b) When the same wire is positioned in a normal contralateral artery, the left circumflex artery (LCX, arrowhead), similar values of CFR are obtained. Relative flow reserve can be calculated as a ratio of CFR in the LAD and LCX (1.1 in this case). (c) Despite optimal stent expansion in a lesion of the proximal right coronary artery (RCA), a persistent impairment of CFR is observed (CFR = 1.8). (d) Note that when the wire is positioned in the contralateral normal artery (left circumflex, LCX) a normal CFR of 3.1 is measured, indicating that the flow impairment is limited to the territory of distribution of the treated artery (relative flow reserve = 0.58, far below the normal value of 0.75–0.80).*

This method was abandoned until the early 1990s when intracoronary pressure guidewires became available.

Modern technology allows the manufacture of dedicated pressure guidewires with handling characteristics that are similar to those of conventional angioplasty wires. Fluid-filled guidewires transmit a very damped pressure waveform because of the small dimension of the recording channel connected with a regular electromagnetic pressure transducer.[23] More recently, a nitinol 0.36 mm (0.014-inch) fluid-filled hollow wire has been introduced; this has the advantage of a superior signal quality because of its innovative super-stiff proximal connector. With these wires, the pressure signal can be recorded using electromagnetic transducers, displayed on the standard physiologic monitoring system, and printed as part of the standard catheterization or angioplasty report (*Fig. 5.2*).

Solid-state sensor-tipped wires are also available, allowing recording with dedicated consoles of high-fidelity pressure signals. The first guidewire introduced was a 0.46 mm (0.018-inch) wire with an optical microsensor (Radi Medical, Uppsala, Sweden); this was limited by the stiffness of the shaft and the drift of the measurement in tortuous segments. The second-generation system from the same company is a 0.36 mm (0.014-inch) disconnectable flexible wire with improved handling characteristics; this system allows an easier integration during interventional procedures. The presence of a new system in advanced clinical testing confirms the revival of interest in post-stenotic pressure measurements, as a consequence of the introduction and the experimental and clinical validation of the concept of fractional flow reserve.

The technique of examination is very simple and does not require the wire manipulation and interpretation skills that are sometimes necessary during a Doppler study. After careful flushing with heparinized saline (fluid-filled) or electronic calibration (sensor-tipped), the correct calibration of the wire is tested by confirming that no mean pressure gradient is present when the pressure transducer is at the tip of the guiding catheter. In all pressure wires, the sensor is located proximal to the wire tip, at the proximal end

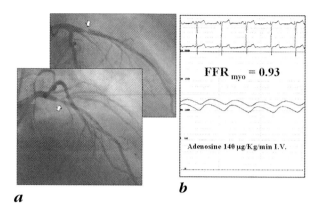

FFR$_{myo}$ = 0.93

Adenosine 140 µg/Kg/min I.V.

a *b*

Figure 5.2 *Physiologic assessment of an intermediate lesion. (a) Two angiograms showing an eccentric stenosis at the proximal edge of a 15 mm NIR stent implanted 6 months earlier. The patient was asymptomatic and bicycle stress test was negative at a maximal workload of 150 Watts. (b) Upper pressure curve (average) from the left Judkins 6 Fr guiding catheter, lower pressure curve (average) measured with a 0.36 mm (0.014-inch) Scimed Informer wire advanced distal to the stenosis. Note that a minimal pressure gradient is present during maximal hyperemia induced by a continuous intravenous infusion of adenosine. The ratio of post-stenotic pressure and driving aortic pressure is calculated as myocardial fractional flow reserve (FFR$_{myo}$) and is equal to 0.93, far above the threshold for ischemia (0.75).*

of the 2–3 cm long radiopaque platinum-covered distal segment. This permits the operator to pull back and advance the pressure sensor across the stenosis safely in order to locate its exact position.

Fractional flow reserve

Fractional flow reserve is the maximum blood flow divided by the theoretical maximum flow in the absence of the stenosis (i.e. the fraction of normal maximum flow still achievable despite the presence of the epicardial coronary stenosis). Since flow can be expressed by the ratio between driving pressure and resistance, maximum attainable flow through the myocardium equals the ratio of the perfusion pressure across the myocardium (distal coronary pressure minus central venous pressure) to the resistance during maximum vasodilatation. If no epicardial stenosis is present, the perfusion pressure across the myocardium is equal to the difference between the mean aortic pressure and the central venous pressure.

A significant coronary stenosis reduces the perfusion pressure across the myocardium by generating a pressure gradient that is maximal under conditions of maximum arteriolar vasodilatation. If the central venous pressure is negligible in comparison with the arterial driving pressure, fractional flow reserve can be calculated as the ratio between mean post-stenotic pressure and mean aortic pressure.[24] Since distal pressure is also affected by the development of collateral vessels, unlike Doppler-based coronary flow reserve, fractional flow reserve also reflects the physiologic importance of the collateral circulation in maintaining coronary flow.[25,26] The measurement of post-stenotic pressure during coronary occlusion (balloon dilatation) can be used to determine the contribution of anterograde and collateral flow to myocardial perfusion and to assess the response of collateral circulation to pharmacologic interventions. Another important difference with coronary flow reserve is that fractional flow reserve is not affected by microcirculatory changes and reflects only the severity of the lesion under assessment.

Two main features of fractional flow reserve explain why this index has largely replaced coronary flow reserve for the assessment of stenosis severity:[27]

(a) independence from hemodynamic conditions at the time of the measurement
(b) presence of well-defined cut-off criteria to distinguish between normal and abnormal response.

Experimental and clinical studies have shown that changes in heart rate, arterial blood pressure, and myocardial contractility do not affect the accuracy of fractional flow reserve. Unlike CFR, for which the wide range of normal values overlaps the results obtained in vessels with flow-limiting stenoses, fractional flow reserve has an unequivocal normal value of 1.0. There is a very high correlation between evidence of myocardial ischemia during non-invasive tests and the presence of a fractional flow reserve lower than 0.75. Large validation studies have shown that when an abnormal stress test is normalized by a successful PTCA, fractional flow reserve invariably increases to normal values.[28–31]

PHARMACOLOGIC AGENTS THAT INDUCE MAXIMUM ARTERIOLAR VASODILATATION

Widely used vasodilator agents are dipyridamole, papaverine, and adenosine. The hyperosmolar ionic and low osmolar non-ionic contrast media cannot be used because they do not produce maximum vasodilatation. Similarly, nitrates have a predominant effect on large conductance vessels and do not consistently induce a maximal flow increase. Continuous infusion of an adequate dose of dipyridamole results in maximum coronary vasodilation, but it has the disadvantage of a long duration of action.[32] The dose range of intracoronary papaverine that is needed to produce maximum coronary vasodilation has been established in humans by Wilson and White[33] at 8 mg for the right coronary artery and 12 mg for the left coronary artery.

The coronary vasodilation that occurs after intravenous or intracoronary administration of adenosine is similar in magnitude to that observed after papaverine, with the advantage that the time from intracoronary injection of adenosine to peak hyperemia, as well as the total duration of the hyperemic response, is about four times shorter.[34] Furthermore, intracoronary adenosine does not prolong the QT interval, avoids the potentially dangerous ventricular arrhythmias that occur with papaverine,[35] and does not induce significant changes in heart rate or blood pressure or cause other side effects. A continuous intravenous infusion of adenosine at 140 µg/kg per minute also induces maximum coronary vasodilation, but it requires a large infusion vein and is associated with mild hypotension and bradycardia and frequent development of flushing, chest discomfort, headache, dyspnea and first- or second-degree atrioventricular block (< 10%).[36] In view of the extremely good safety profile, the absence of side effects, and the ease of use, a bolus of intracoronary adenosine is the agent and route of administration of choice. In the left coronary artery a bolus of 24 µg is effective and well tolerated. In the right coronary artery, because of the possible development of sinus node or atrioventricular node depression, the initial dose should not exceed 12 µg. The very short duration of the maximal effect of a bolus of adenosine and the interference of the injection through the guiding catheter with the measurements that are needed to calculate fractional flow reserve explain why intravenous adenosine is more often used for pressure-based indices. A possible compromise to avoid the side effects of intravenous adenosine and still achieve a prolonged vasodilating response is the use of a continuous intracoronary infusion via the guiding catheter.

CLINICAL APPLICATIONS DURING CORONARY INTERVENTIONS

DEFERRAL OF TREATMENT FOR NON-FLOW-LIMITING STENOSES

Lesions with a diameter reduction of 40–70% in multiple angiographic projections are a dilemma for the angiographer since non-invasive tests may have not been performed before catheterization. In patients with multivessel disease, non-invasive tests are often insufficient to confirm or rule out the presence of ischemia in the territory of distribution of the artery with intermediate stenosis. If further non-invasive investigations must be performed, an immediate percutaneous treatment at the time of the diagnostic procedure is precluded,[37] the hospital stay is prolonged, and the cost of treatment and the discomfort to the patient are increased. In the PEACH study,[38] a significant cost reduction was obtained by using intracoronary Doppler to decide the treatment strategy at the time of catheterization, without the addition of 2 days of hospital stay to perform stress scintigraphy.[38] As discussed above, CFR measured with intracoronary Doppler correlates well with the results of radioisotope perfusion tests. Large clinical studies have reported the safety of deferring angioplasty on the basis of the results of flow velocity measurements or the results of the combination of CFR and pressure gradient measurements. It has been reported that 88% of 146 patients with intermediate lesions on angiography were event free if no intervention was performed because of normal flow parameters.[39–41] In the remaining patients, most of the events were not related to the stenosis assessed with intracoronary Doppler. It must be recognized, however, that while measurements of CFR in the normal range (> 2.0, ideally > 2.5) provide confidence that the lesion should not be treated, lower CFR values still raise the question of a false-positive Doppler test because of a poor vasodilatory response of the microvasculature. In some patient groups (patients with diabetes mellitus or hypertension or patients with a marked tachycardia at the time of measurement causing an increase in the basal flow), a low CFR is frequently observed in the absence of a flow-limiting stenosis. In these circumstances, a measurement of CFR in a second artery without flow-limiting stenoses can reveal the presence of diffuse impairment of the vasodilatory response so that only lesions with a flow reserve in the diseased artery of less than 75% of the flow reserve in the control normal artery will be treated. Although this strategy has been shown to be successfully applicable in the clinical setting,[20] it requires a tedious separate assessment in a normal vessel, which is by definition impossible in patients with triple–vessel disease, and it does not address two important problems: the functional significance of lesions with regional abnormalities of flow response (i.e. previous myocardial infarction), and the presence of multiple stenoses in the same artery.

The calculation of the percentage area stenosis based on the continuity equation has been shown to be applicable with the Doppler guidewire in severe stenoses and to yield good correlation with independent measurements of stenosis severity by quantitative angiography and intracoronary ultrasound.[42,43] Unfortunately, flow velocity tracings suitable for quantitative analysis are difficult to record in the stenotic segment because of misalignment of the guidewire with the stenotic jet and reduced intensity of the backscatter from blood in segments with high shear stress. Recently, there has been a revival of this technique to study moderate residual narrowings after stent implantation. There is a good correlation of Doppler-derived and intravascular ultrasound-derived calculations of percentage in-stent residual stenosis.[44]

Myocardial fractional flow reserve (FFR-myo) > 0.75 has been shown to predict a favorable long-term outcome in patients with angiographically intermediate stenoses, with 80% of patients having had no cardiac events after 18 months.[45] An interesting subgroup of patients is those with intermediate stenoses of the left main coronary artery that were left untreated. Even in this group, no cardiac events were observed if FFR-myo was normal and the lesion was left untreated.[46] A note of caution concerns culprit lesions in unstable syndromes, in which physiologically non-significant stenoses may induce sudden adverse events because of their high risk of rapid progression and thrombosis. In addition, these techniques cannot identify the 'vulnerable plaque' that may rupture spontaneously.

GUIDANCE OF CORONARY INTERVENTIONS

Percutaneous transluminal balloon angioplasty

The angiographic evaluation of the results of coronary interventions is limited by the presence of wall disruption so that the true lumen available for blood passage cannot be easily assessed. Intracoronary ultrasound gives a better definition of the presence and severity of wall disruption after angioplasty and has been instrumental in teaching us that many cases of recurrence of symptoms after PTCA are not due to restenosis but are the result of an insufficient initial lumen enlargement.[47] Intracoronary ultrasound, however, requires a separate insertion of a new catheter and is not always able to determine whether the complex neolumen created by the dilatation is sufficient to normalize vascular conductance. Intracoronary Doppler is an appealing alternative since this technique can determine the exact functional severity of the residual coronary stenosis and can be easily integrated in a standard interventional procedure. In the multicenter DEBATE I[48,49] and II[50] and DESTINI[51] studies (1600 patients in total), which tested the usefulness of intracoronary Doppler during balloon angioplasty, the Doppler guidewire could be used as the primary wire to cross the stenosis and advance the balloon or the stent in the great majority of patients.

Balloon angioplasty improves the flow velocity parameters[52–56] but an incomplete normalization is observed in most patients, often despite a good angiographic result. Hemodynamic changes during the procedure, microembolization, and transient or persistent changes in the distal microvascular BED may explain part of this discrepancy, as indicated by the late normalization in some lesions.[48,57] In other cases, however, the persistent abnormal flow response reflects persistent abnormalities in vessel conductance. The multicenter DEBATE study[49] has shown that impairment in flow reserve after PTCA is associated with a higher incidence of persistence or recurrence of angina or of a positive exercise test at 1 month and of target lesion revascularization at 6 months. The combination of an optimal angiographic result (< 35% diameter stenosis) and of a flow reserve of more than 2.5 was associated with a favorable clinical outcome at 6 months (16% incidence of major adverse cardiac events). Based on these observations, various groups are testing the hypothesis that the combination of angiographic and functional endpoints can be used to identify lesions that have a worse prognosis after PTCA alone and thus require additional treatment.[50,51,58]

The absence of cyclic flow variations (a condition that carries a risk of abrupt occlusion) and the restoration of a normal flow velocity reserve almost exclude the development of immediate complications after PTCA.[59] These findings indicate the clinical relevance of these measurements in the presence of long dissections or suboptimal PTCA results in

Baseline FFR in obtuse marginal stenosis

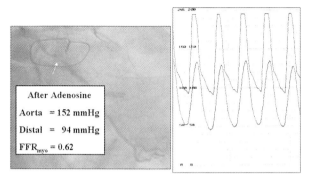

a

Assessment of Collateral Filling Pressure

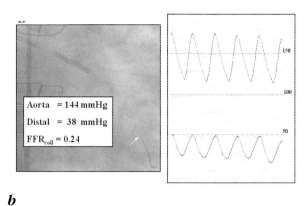

b

Post PTCA FFR=0.89 but inadequate IVUS result

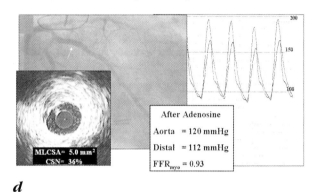

c

Final studies post stent placement

d

Figure 5.3 *(a) Pre-treatment angiogram of a severe lesion (arrow) in a large obtuse marginal branch. A distal pressure guidewire (Scimed Informer 0.36 mm (0.014 inches) detects a severe reduction in post-stenotic pressure with a calculated myocardial fractional flow reserve (FFR-myo) of 0.62. (b) During balloon occlusion the pressure in the distal vessel is generated by collateral flow and can be calculated assuming that the prolonged balloon occlusion has induced maximal distal vasodilatation. (c) IVUS images show moderate residual narrowing after percutaneous transluminal coronary angioplasty (PTCA), with a severe eccentric plaque (A) and a large dissection (B) undetected by angiography in the positions marked with arrows in the angiogram. The distal pressure during adenosine infusion, however, is markedly increased and FFR-myo is calculated as 0.89, a measurement slightly below the threshold recommended as acceptable residual FFR impairment after PTCA (0.90). (d) After stent implantation normalization of the angiogram and increased regular lumen diameter is followed by a further increase of FFR-myo. CSN is the residual cross-sectional narrowing, calculated as the ratio between plaque area and total vessel area.*

conditions that are unfavorable for stent implantation, such as long lesions or lesions in small vessels.

The stiffness of the first-generation pressure guidewires has limited their application during interventions. Initial reports, however, indicate that an almost complete normalization of FFR-myo (> 0.90) has an independent predictive value of favorable long-term outcome (*Fig. 5.3*).[60] For lesions with a good angiographic result after balloon angioplasty (residual diameter stenosis < 30%), the association of

high FFR-myo (> 0.90) predicts a low incidence of restenosis, with a need for target lesion revascularization of 11% at 6 months.[60]

ROTATIONAL AND DIRECTIONAL CORONARY ATHERECTOMY

Unlike balloon angioplasty, a flow velocity improvement is more rarely observed after rotational

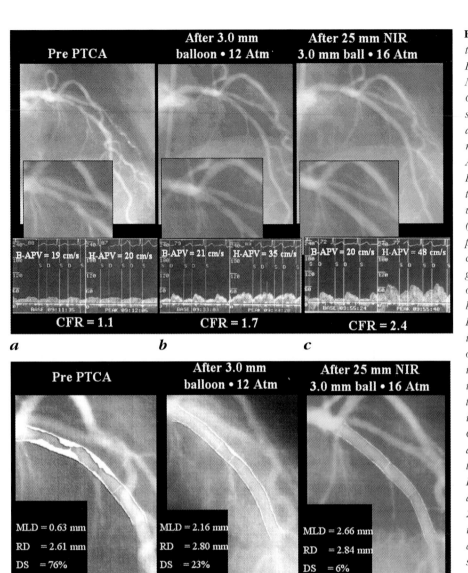

Figure 5.4 *Case example from the DESTINI-CFR trial (courtesy of Dr Dupuoy and Dr Bonan, Montreal Heart Institute, Canada). (a) Angiogram showing severe stenosis of the proximal left anterior descending artery (LAD), magnified in the smaller images. At the bottom, the corresponding Doppler measurements distal to the stenosis, showing absence of velocity increase after adenosine (CFR = 1.1). (b) After percutaneous transluminal coronary angioplasty (PTCA) a good lumen improvement is obtained, with a persistent haziness at the treated site. Because an insufficient improvement in CFR was obtained (< 2.0), a stent was implanted. (c) After stent implantation, normalization of the angiogram and further increase in CFR. (d) Corresponding quantitative angiographic measurements. Note that the lumen improvement after PTCA (e) appears acceptable, with a residual diameter stenosis of 23%. After stenting (f) further improvement in minimum lumen diameter and decrease in residual stenosis is observed. RD, reference diameter; CFR, coronary flow reserve.*

atherectomy; rather, there is a tendency to see a persistent flow impairment despite optimal angiographic results and a regular circular lumen demonstrated with ultrasound. This phenomenon may be explained by the microembolization of minute particles of plaque debris, which limits the role of intracoronary Doppler for the assessment of the results of this specific intervention.[61–63] Similarly, the higher frequency of platelet emboli created by repeated passes of the atherectomy cutter, which is responsible for the higher frequency of non-Q-wave myocardial infarction in comparison with percutaneous transluminal coronary angiography (PTCA), might account for the average lower flow reserve observed after atherectomy in comparison with PTCA. FFR-myo has potential advantages after these types of interventions but there have been no reports so far.

STENT IMPLANTATION

The chief indication of intracoronary Doppler during stent implantation is the detection of lesions with an insufficient functional recovery after balloon angioplasty, allowing the operator to limit stent deployment to the lesions that are really in need of this additional treatment. Based on the encouraging results of the DEBATE (Doppler Endpoints Balloon

Angioplasty Trial Europe) trial,[49] three independent studies[50,51,58] have randomized patients to elective stenting or a strategy of balloon angioplasty and provisional stenting according to the adequacy of the Doppler and quantitative angiographic measurements after PTCA. The differences in inclusion criteria (single lesion–single stent treatment in FROST (FRench Optimal Stent Trial)[58] and DEBATE II,[50] multivessel–multilesion deployment of multiple stents in DESTINI)[58] and in Doppler cut-off criteria (CFR > 2.0 in DESTINI (Doppler Endpoints STent INternational Investigators),[51] CFR >2.2 in FROST, CFR > 2.5 in DEBATE II), make these studies highly complementary in addressing the problem of the use of intracoronary Doppler to select the indications to stent implantation.

The largest of these studies is the DESTINI trial,[51] a randomized study carried out in 26 centers in Europe, Canada, Australia, Japan, Korea, and in 36 centers in the USA. When enrolment was complete (March 1998), 731 patients were treated and half of them were randomized to receive elective stent implantation, using slotted tubular stents in 90% of lesions (mainly Palmaz–Schatz and NIR stents). In the remaining patients randomized to guided angioplasty, all the following end-points had to be met (*Fig. 5.4*):.

(a) final residual diameter stenosis < 35%
(b) final coronary flow reserve measured with a Doppler guidewire distal to the stenosis > 2.0
(c) absence of dissections at risk of abrupt closure.

If all these criteria were not met even after additional dilatation with larger balloons or higher balloon inflation pressure, the investigators were allowed to perform coronary stent implantation. Since the goal of the study was to evaluate the impact of this strategy on the everyday patient population of a busy catheterization laboratory, the only inclusion criterion was the suitability of all the lesions under treatment for stent implantation. Exclusion criteria were the presence of chronic total occlusion, elective planned Rotablator or directional atherectomy, recent (in the previous 48 hours) myocardial infarction or previous Q-wave myocardial infarction with akinesis or dyskinesia in the territory of the artery to be treated, graft and ostial stenoses, or second restenosis.

Despite these broad inclusion criteria, multivessel treatment was actually performed in 5% of patients, treating angiographically type B2 or C lesions in 59% of cases, with an average lesion length of 12.7 ± 4.2 mm and an average reference vessel diameter of 3.07 ± 0.3 mm; these parameters were similar in the guided PTCA and stent groups. Of the 386 lesions randomized to guided PTCA, all the predetermined end-points could be achieved in 167 arteries (43%). The lesions treated with stent implantation had a larger final minimal luminal diameter (2.84 mm and 2.95 mm in the primary and conditional stenting groups versus 2.30 mm in the group treated with PTCA alone, $p < 0.00001$) and a lower final residual diameter stenosis (8.8% in the stent groups versus 26.2% in the group treated with PTCA only, $p < 0.00001$).

At the time of preparation of this manuscript, the 6-month follow-up reports of 551 patients (75%) were received and reviewed at the Core Laboratory in Milan. On an intention-to-treat analysis, the early and late cardiac events did not show significant differences in the two groups. The odds ratio (95% confidence intervals) for cumulative major adverse cardiac events of the stent group versus the optimal PTCA group was 0.97 (0.55–1.76) (*Fig. 5.5*). In particular, overall (PTCA and bypass graft operation) 6-month target lesion revascularization involving the lesions initially treated was 14.9% in the PTCA group and 14.6% in the stent group (not significant). Complete cost analysis was performed only for the US centers and showed a significantly lower catheter laboratory cost in the guided PTCA than in the stent group ($US5,848 versus $US6,269, $p < 0.05$), owing to a lower use of balloons and stents per patient.

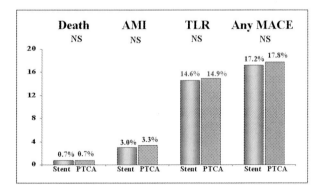

Figure 5.5 *Destini Trial Preliminary Results. Histogram reporting the cardiac events 6 months after treatment in the patients treated with elective stent implantation or guided percutaneous transluminal coronary angioplasty (PTCA). Note that similar percentages are observed for cardiac death, acute myocardial infarction (AMI), target lesion revascularization (TLR), and all major adverse cardiac events (MACE).*

The preliminary results of the DESTINI study indicate that when optimal angiographic and physiologic end-points are met after PTCA, the early and late clinical outcome is equivalent to the outcome observed after elective stent implantation. In the PTCA group, however, a minority (43%) of patients could achieve the predetermined end-points and the remaining patients ultimately received a stent. Despite the frequent need to cross over to stenting, initial cost analysis suggests that a provisional stenting strategy still has a lower cost than stenting all suitable lesions. In the most recent and the largest PTCA versus stent trial (BENESTENT II),[64] a significantly lower incidence of major cardiac events and target lesion revascularization was observed at 6 months. The conflicting result of the DESTINI trial (almost perfect equivalence of treatment outcome in both groups) can be explained by the implantation of stents in all patients not meeting predetermined angiographic and velocity criteria (57% of patients stented) and not only as bail-out (13% in BENESTENT II). A second explanation could be the inclusion of bifurcation and longer lesions (average lesion length 12.5 mm in DESTINI and 8.2 mm in BENESTENT II), which may have a smaller benefit from stenting. Despite the high expectation that pressure-based indices, unaffected by the changing hemodynamic conditions during interventions, may overcome the limitations of intracoronary Doppler and yield better prognostic long-term clinical outcome after PTCA, the unfriendly mechanical characteristics of the first-generation pressure wires have limited their application to experienced centers and precluded large multicenter trials. Based on this initial clinical experience, a measurement of FFR < 0.90 has been proposed as a cut-off result after PTCA below which stent implantation should be performed.

When the decision to implant a stent has been made prior to the intervention, the usefulness of intracoronary Doppler or pressure-based indices of stenosis severity appears more limited. Although stent implantation achieves a higher average CFR than balloon angioplasty,[65,66] optimal lumen expansion after stenting is insufficient to normalize CFR in all vessels with low CFR after balloon angioplasty.[67] The measurement of FFR or CFR detects significant differences in patients receiving slotted tubular or coil stents, reflecting an incomplete lumen expansion with this last stent design. CFR and RFR correlate with the minimal cross-sectional area measured with intracoronary ultrasound after PTCA or stent implantation. A FFR < 0.94 has been confirmed by intracoronary ultrasound to detect residual narrowings after stenting. The clinical usefulness of these findings remains questionable since the direct lumen measurement with intracoronary ultrasound gives the additional benefit of a proper selection of balloon size and pressure to obtain safe further stent enlargement.[68]

The application of the continuity equation for the evaluation of the velocity changes within the stented segment may detect segments of velocity acceleration indicating residual lumen reduction that require further stent expansion. The practical application of the technique, however, requires further refinements in transducer technology to maintain a stable high-quality signal including the centerline of flow throughout the entire stented segment.[44]

ACUTE MYOCARDIAL INFARCTION

In the presence of acute myocardial infarction, flow velocity measurements do not correlate with angiographic thrombolysis in myocardial infarction (TIMI) flow or frame count to disappearance of contrast. In particular, a very low flow velocity is observed in the majority of patients with TIMI 2 flow, and a similar low flow velocity is observed in patients with TIMI 1 flow,[69] suggesting that incomplete recanalization is responsible for the poor prognosis and limited recovery of left ventricular function in these cases.[70,71] Continuous monitoring of flow velocity with the Doppler guidewire confirms the restoration of blood flow after thrombolysis and the persistence of anterograde flow in the hours following thrombolysis.[72,73] A persistent impairment in flow is present in many patients with angiographically successful thrombolysis after acute myocardial infarction, which may improve after PTCA and stenting. An abnormal pattern of early systolic retrograde flow and prolonged diastolic flow velocity has been shown to be associated with the presence of the 'no reflow' phenomenon.[74] Recent reports have shown a correlation between recovery of left ventricular function after acute myocardial infarction and velocity-derived indices based on the diastolic velocity pattern or on the slope of the diastolic velocity–pressure relationship.[75-77]

CONCLUSION

The coronary Doppler guidewire was the first practical method of physiologic assessment of coronary stenosis severity that was applicable in the everyday practice of a busy catheterization laboratory. This invasive method correlated closely to the results of non-invasive nuclear stress tests. Despite the positive results of the large observational DEBATE study and the encouraging consistent preliminary data of more recent randomized trials, Doppler ultrasound is rarely used during coronary interventions.

The development of flexible pressure sensors and the validation of FFR-myo has the potential to allow a more widespread use of physiological indices, overcoming some of the limitations of CFR (measurement variability, dependency on hemodynamic conditions at the time of measurement,[78] inability to differentiate flow impairment caused by epicardial stenoses and that caused by microvascular disease).[79] It will be more difficult to overcome the resistance of operators who have been trained to rely purely on morphological parameters (conventional angiography much more than IVUS) to accept and learn these new techniques. A second practical barrier is created by the absence of a specific reimbursement policy for these procedures in many countries. Simple guidelines based on the large knowledge summarized here and endorsed by the Scientific Societies[80] are required to identify areas in which overwhelming data indicate the usefulness and the necessity of the application of these techniques (e.g. assessment of intermediate stenosis) and areas in which clinical research is still in progress (e.g. decision making during interventions). The boundary between research and clinical application needs a case-by-case evaluation.

REFERENCES

1. Serruys PW, Di Mario C, Kern MJ. Intracoronary Doppler. In: Topol EJ, ed. *Textbook of Interventional Cardiology*. Philadelphia: Saunders, 1994, pp 1324–1404.
2. Kern JM, de Bruyne BD, Pijls NHJ. From research to clinical practice. Current role of intracoronary physiologically based decision making in the cardiac catheterization laboratory. *J Am Coll Cardiol* 1997; **30**: 613–620.
3. Doucette JW, Douglas Corl P, Payne HP et al. Validation of a doppler guide wire for intravascular measurement of coronary artery flow velocity. *Circulation* 1992; **85**: 1899–1911.
4. Jenni R, Buchi M, Jakob M, Ritter M. Position control of intravascular Doppler guidewire: concept of tracking indicator and its clinical implications. *Cathet Cardiovasc Diagn* 1998; **44**: 28–33.
5. Di Mario C , Roelandt JRTC, Serruys PW. Limitations of the zero-crossing detector for the analysis of intracoronary

Doppler. A comparison with fast Fourier transform analysis of basal, hyperemic and transtenotic blood flow velocity in patients with coronary artery disease. *Cathet Cardiovasc Diag* 1993; **28**: 56–64.
6. Gould KL, Lipscomb K, Hamilton GW. Physiologic basis for assessing critical coronary stenosis: instantaneous flow response and regional distribution during coronary hyperemia as measures of coronary flow reserve. *Am J Cardiol* 1974; **33**: 87–94.
7. Klocke FJ. Measurements of coronary flow reserve: defining pathophysiology versus making decisions about patient care. *Circulation* 1987; **76**: 245–253.
8. Wilson RF, Marcus ML, White CW. Prediction of the physiologic significance of coronary arterial lesions by quantitative lesion geometry in patients with limited coronary artery disease. *Circulation* 1987; **75**: 723–732.
9. Harrison DG, White CW, Hiratzkam LF. The value of lesional cross-sectional area determined by quantitative coronary angiography in assessing the physiologic significance of proximal left anterior descending coronary artery stenoses. *Circulation* 1984; **69**: 111–119.
10. Klocke FJ. Cognition in the era of technology: 'seeing the shades of gray'. *J Am Coll Cardiol* 1990; **16**: 763–769.
11. Kern MJ, Bach RG, Donohue TJ. Variations in normal coronary vasodilatory reserve stratified by artery, gender, heart transplantation and coronary artery disease. *J Am Coll Cardiol* 1996; **28**: 1154–1160.
12. Donohue TJ, Miller DD, Bach RG et al. Correlation of poststenotic hyperemic coronary flow velocity and pressure with abnormal stress myocardial perfusion imaging in coronary artery disease. *Am J Cardiol* 1996; **77**: 948–954.
13. Miller DD, Donohue TJ, Younis LT et al. Correlation of pharmacological 99mTc-SestaMIBI myocardial perfusion imaging with post-stenotic coronary flow reserve in patients with angiographically intermediate artery stenoses. *Circulation* 1994; **89**: 2150–2160.
14. Tron C, Donohue TJ, Bach RG et al. Comparison of pressure-derived fractional flow reserve with poststenotic coronary flow velocity reserve for prediction of stress myocardial perfusion imaging results. *Am Heart J* 1995; **130**: 723–733.
15. Joye JD, Schulman DS, Lasorda D et al. Intracoronary Doppler guide wire versus stress single photon emission computed tomographic Thallium-201 imaging in assessment of intermediate coronary stenoses. *J Am Coll Cardiol* 1994; **24**: 940–947.
16. Deychak YA, Segal J, Reiner SR et al. Doppler guide wire flow velocity indexes measured distal to coronary stenoses associated with reversible thallium perfusion defects. *Am Heart J* 1995; **129**: 219–227.
17. Heller LI, Cates C, Popma J et al. Intracoronary Doppler assessment of moderate coronary artery disease: comparison with 201Tl imaging and coronary angiography. FACTS Study Group. *Circulation* 1997; **96**: 484–90 .
18. Danzi GB, Pirelli S, Mauri L et al. Which variable of stenosis severity best describes the significance of an isolated left anterior descending coronary artery lesion? Correlation between quantitative coronary angiography, intracoronary Doppler measurements and high dose dipyridamole echocardiography. *J Am Coll Cardiol* 1998; **31**: 526–533.
19. Stikovac MM, Kern MJ, Donohue TJ et al. Additive value of coronary flow reserve in the assessment of intermediate

coronary stenosis: comparison to myocardial stress perfusion imaging. *J Am Coll Cardiol* 1998; **31**: 404A.

20. Baumgart D, Haude M, Vetter S et al. Event-free survival following deferral of coronary interventions based on relative flow reserve derived from intracoronary Doppler measurements. *J Am Coll Cardiol* 1998; **31**: 405A.

21. Gruntzig AR, Siegenthaler WE. Non-operative dilatation of coronary artery stenosis. *N Engl J Med* 1979; **301**: 61–68.

22. Anderson HV, Leimgruber PP, Cox WR et al. Measurement of transstenotic pressure gradient during percutaneous transluminal coronary angioplasty. *Circulation* 1986; **73**: 1223–1230.

23. De Bruyne B, Pijls NH, Paulus WJ et al. Transtenotic coronary pressure gradient measurement in humans: in vitro and in vivo evaluation of a new pressure monitoring angioplasty guidewire. *J Am Coll Cardiol* 1993; **22**: 119–126.

24. Pijls NHJ, van Son JAM, Kirkeeide RL et al. Experimental basis of determining maximum coronary, myocardial, and collateral blood flow by pressure measurements for assessing functional stenosis severity before and after percutaneous transluminal coronary angioplasty. *Circulation* 1993; **87**: 1354–1367.

25. Pijls NHJ, Bech GJW, el Gamal MIH et al. Quantification of recruitable coronary collateral flow in conscious humans and its potential to predict future ischemic event. *J Am Coll Cardiol* 1995; **25**: 1522–1528.

26. Seiler C, Fleisch M, Meier B. Direct intracoronary evidence of collateral steal in humans. *Circulation* 1997; **96**: 4261–4267.

27. De Bruyne B, Baudhuin T, Melin JA et al. Coronary flow reserve calculated from pressure measurements in humans: validation with positron emission tomography. *Circulation* 1994; **89**: 1013–1022.

28. Pijls NHJ, De Bruyne B, Peels K et al. Measurement of fractional flow reserve to assess the functional severity of coronary-artery stenoses. *N Engl J Med* 1996; **334**: 1703–1708.

29. Pijls NHJ, Van Gelder B, Van der Voort P et al. Fractional flow reserve: a useful index to evaluate the influence of an epicardial coronary stenosis on myocardial blood flow. *Circulation* 1995; **92**: 3183–3193.

30. De Bruyne B, Bartunek J, Sys SU, Heyndrickx GR. Relation between myocardial fractional flow reserve calculated from coronary pressure measurements and exercise-induced myocardial ischemia. *Circulation* 1995; **92**: 39–46.

31. Bartunek J, Marwick TH, Rodrigues AC et al. Dobutamine-induced wall motion abnormalities: correlations with myocardial fractional flow reserve and quantitative coronary angiography. *J Am Coll Cardiol* 1996; **27**: 1429–1436.

32. Bookstein JJ, Higgins CB. Comparative efficacy of coronary vasodilatory methods. *Invest Radiol* 1977; **12**: 121–127.

33. Wilson RF, White CW. Intracoronary papaverine: an ideal coronary vasodilator for studies of the coronary circulation in conscious humans. *Circulation* 1986; **73**: 444–451.

34. Wilson RF, Wyche K, Christensen BV, Laxson DD. Effects of adenosine on human coronary arterial circulation. *Circulation* 1990; **82**: 1595–1606.

35. Wilson RF, White CW. Serious ventricular dysrhythmias after intracoronary papaverine. *Am J Cardiol* 1988; **62**: 1301–1305.

36. Kern MJ, Deligonul U, Aguirre F, Hilton TC. Intravenous adenosine: continuous infusion and low dose bolus administration for determination of coronary vasodilator

37. reserve in patients with and without coronary artery disease. *J Am Coll Cardiol* 1991; **18**: 718–731.

37. Hill JA. Single-stage coronary angiography and angioplasty: a new standard? *Am J Cardiol* 1995; **75**: 75–76.

38. Joye JD, Cates CU, Farah T et al. Cost analysis of intracoronary doppler determination of lesion significance: preliminary results of the PEACH study (abstract). *J Invasive Cardiol* 1995; **7**: 22A.

39. Kern MJ, Donohue TJ, Aguirre FV et al. Clinical outcome of deferring angioplasty in patients with normal translesional pressure-flow velocity measurements. *J Am Coll Cardiol* 1995; **25**: 178–187.

40. Moses JW, Shaknovich A, Kreps EM et al. Clinical follow-up of intermediate coronary lesions not hemodynamically significant by doppler flow wire criteria (abstract). *Circulation* 1994; I-227.

41. Deychak YA, Segal G, Reiner JS, Nachnani S. Doppler guidewire-derived coronary flow reserve distal to intermediate stenosis used in clinical decision making regarding interventional therapy. *Am Heart J* 1994; **128**: 178–181.

42. Di Mario C, Meneveau N, Gil R et al. Maximal blood flow velocity in severe coronary stenoses measured with a Doppler guidewire. *Am J Cardiol* 1993; **71**: 54D–61D.

43. Tahk SJ, Cho YN, Shin JH, Chooi BIW. Clinical application of Doppler guide wire and modified continuity equation method during coronary angioplasty. A validation with intracoronary ultrasound. *Eur Heart J* 1998; **19**: 276.

44. Lerman A, Higano ST, Garratt KN et al. Measuring percent area stenosis with intracoronary Doppler and the continuity equation: correlation with intracoronary ultrasound and angiography. *Circulation* 1997; I-79.

45. Bech GJW, Pijls NHJ, De Bruyne B et al. Long-term follow-up after deferral of percutaneous transluminal coronary angioplasty of intermediate stenosis, on the basis of coronary pressure measurement. *J Am Coll Cardiol* 1998; **31**: 841–847.

46. Droste HT, De Bruyne B, Bech GJW et al. Deferral of bypass surgery in equivocal left main disease based upon coronary pressure measurements. *Eur Heart J* 1997; **18**: 239.

47. Nakamura S, Mahon DJ, Maheswaran B et al. An explanation for discrepancy between angiographic and intravascular ultrasound measurements after percutaneous transluminal coronary angioplasty. *J Am Coll Cardiol* 1995; **25**: 633–639.

48. Piek JJ, Boersma E, Serruys PW, on behalf of the DEBATE Investigators Group. The immediate and long-term effect of balloon coronary angioplasty on the distal coronary flow velocity reserve. *Eur Heart J* 1998; **19**: 566.

49. Serruys PW, Di Mario C, Piek J et al. Prognostic value of intracoronary flow velocity and diameter stenosis in assessing the short and long term outcome of coronary balloon angioplasty. The DEBATE Study (Doppler End-points Balloon Angioplasty Trial Europe). *Circulation* 1997; **96**: 3369–3377.

50. Serruys PW, de Bruyne B, de Sousa JE et al, on behalf of the DEBATE II Investigators. DEBATE II: a randomized study to evaluate the need of additional stenting after guided balloon angioplasty (abstract). *Eur Heart J* 1998; **19**: 567.

51. Di Mario C, Moses J, Muramatsu T et al, on the behalf of the DESTINI-CRF Study Group. Multicenter randomized

comparison of primary stenting vs balloon angioplasty optimized by QCA and intracoronary Doppler: procedural results in 580 patients (abstract). *Eur Heart J* 1998; **19**: 567.

52. Segal J, Kern MJ, Scott NA. Alteration of phasic coronary artery flow velocity in human during percutaneous coronary angioplasty. *J Am Coll Cardiol* 1992; **20**: 276–286.

53. Ofili EO, Kern MJ, Labovitz AJ et al. Analysis of coronary blood flow velocity dynamics in angiographically normal and stenosed arteries before and after endolumen enlargement by angioplasty. *J Am Coll Cardiol* 1993; **21**: 308–316.

54. Heller LI, Silver KH, Vilegas BJ et al. Blood flow velocity in the right coronary artery: assessment before and after angioplasty. *J Am Coll Cardiol* 1994; **24**: 1012–1017.

55. Donohue TJ, Kern MJ, Aguirre FV, Ofili EO. Assessing the hemodynamic significance of coronary artery stenosis: analysis of translesional pressure–flow velocity relationship in patients. *J Am Coll Cardiol* 1993; **22**: 449–458.

56. Serruys PW, Di Mario C, Meneveau N et al. Intracoronary pressure and flow velocity from sensor tip guidewires. A new methodological comprehensive approach for the assessment of coronary hemodynamics before and after interventions. *Am J Cardiol* 1993; **71**: 41D–53D.

57. Wilson RF, Johnson MR, Marcus ML et al. The effect of coronary angioplasty on coronary blood flow reserve. *Circulation* 1988; **71**: 873–885.

58. Steg PG, on the behalf of the FROST Study Group. A multicenter randomized trial comparing systematic stenting to provisional stenting guided by angiography and coronary flow reserve: final results (abstract). *Eur Heart J* 1998; **19**: 567.

59. Sunamura M, Di Mario C, Serruys PW, on behalf of the DEBATE Study Group. Cyclic flow variations after angioplasty: a rare phenomenon predictive of immediate complications. *Am Heart J* 1996; **131**: 843–848.

60. Pijls NHJ, Bech GJW, De Bruyne B et al. Prognostic value of pressure derived coronary flow reserve to predict restenosis after regular balloon angioplasty. *Circulation* 1997; **96**: I-649.

61. Kumar K, Dorros G, Dufek C, Mathiak L. Coronary blood flow velocities during rotational atherectomy. *Cathet Cardiovasc Diagn* 1997; **41**: 152–156.

62. Bowers TR, Stewart RE, O'Neill WW et al. Effect of Rotablator atherectomy and adjunctive balloon angioplasty on coronary blood flow. *Circulation* 1997; **95**: 1157–1164.

63. Khoury AF, Aguirre FV, Bach RG et al. Influence of percutaneous transluminal coronary rotational atherectomy with adjunctive percutaneous transluminal coronary angioplasty on coronary blood flow. *Am Heart J* 1996; **131**: 631–638.

64. Serruys PW, van Hout B, Bonnier H et al, on behalf of the BENESTENT II Study Group. Effectiveness, cost and cost-effectiveness of a strategy of elective stenting compared to a strategy of balloon angioplasty allowing bailout stenting in patients with coronary artery disease. *Lancet* 1998; **352**: 673–681.

65. Verna E, Gil R, Di Mario C et al, on behalf of the DEBATE Study Group. Does coronary stenting following angioplasty improve distal coronary flow reserve? *Circulation* 1995; **92**: I-551.

66. Haude M, Baumgart D, Verna E et al. Doppler flow velocity reserve after coronary stent implantation: results of the DEBATE ancillary trial (abstract). *Eur Heart J* 1998; **19**: 567.

67. Di Mario C, Di Francesco L, De Gregorio J et al, on behalf of the DESTINI-CFR Investigators. Heterogeneity of persistent impairment of coronary flow reserve after stenting. *J Am Coll Cardiol* 1998; **31**: 404A.

68. Colombo A, Hall P, Nakamura S et al. Intracoronary stenting without anticoagulation accomplished with intravascular ultrasound guidance. *Circulation* 1995; **91**: 1676–1688.

69. Moore JA, Kern MJ, Donohue TJ et al. Disparity of TIMI grade flow and directly measured coronary flow velocity during direct angioplasty for acute myocardial infarction (abstract). *Cathet Cardiovasc Diagn* 1994; **32**: 86.

70. Karagounis L, Sorensen SG, Menlove RL et al, for the TEAM-2 Investigators. Does Thrombolysis In Myocardial Infarction (TIMI) perfusion grade 2 represent a mostly patent artery or mostly occluded artery? Enzymatic and electrocardiographic evidence from the TEAM-2 study. *J Am Coll Cardiol* 1992; **19**: 1–10.

71. Keiman NS, White HD, Ohman EM et al, for the GUSTO Investigators. Mortality within 24 hours of thrombolysis for myocardial infarction: the importance of early reperfusion. *Circulation* 1994; **90**: 2658–2665.

72. Gershony G, Cishek MB, Galloway M. Intracoronary Doppler flow to monitor the results of selective saphenous vein graft thrombolytic therapy. *Cathet Cardiovasc Diagn* 1995; **35**: 277–281.

73. Tsunoda T, Nakamura M, Wakatsuki T et al. Continuous monitoring of coronary flow velocity in acute myocardial infarction using Doppler guidewire (abstract). *Circulation* 1994; **90**: I-449.

74. Iwakura K, Ito H, Takiuchi S et al. Alteration in the coronary blood flow velocity pattern in patients with no reflow and reperfused acute myocardial infarction. *Circulation* 1996; **94**: 1261–1275.

75. Wakatsuki T, Oki T, Sakabe K et al. Relationship between temporal changes in coronary flow velocity pattern and recovery of left ventricular wall motion after successful direct angioplasty in patients with acute myocardial infarction. *J Am Coll Cardiol* 1998; **31**: 419A.

76. Takano Y, Nanto T, Ohara T et al. Quantitative relationship between coronary microvascular damage and myocardial viability assessed by Doppler guide wire. *J Am Coll Cardiol* 1998; **31**: 418A.

77. Di Mario C, Krams R, Gil R, Serruys PW. Slope of the instantaneous hyperemic diastolic coronary flow velocity–pressure relation. A new index for assessment of coronary stenoses in humans. *Circulation* 1994; **90**: 2016–2027.

78. Di Mario C, Gil R, Serruys PW. Long-term reproducibility of intracoronary Doppler measurement. *Am J Cardiol* 1995; **75**: 1177–1180.

79. Di Mario C, Gil R, de Feyter PJ et al. Utilization of translesional hemodynamics: comparison of pressure and flow methods in stenosis assessment in patients with coronary artery disease. *Cathet Cardiovasc Diagn* 1996; **38**: 189–201.

80. Di Mario C, Gorge G, Peters R et al. Clnical application and image interpretation in intracoronary ultrasound. *Eur Heart J* 1998; **19**: 207–229.

Chapter 6 Evolution in our approach to stenting

Antonio Colombo and Jonathan Tobis

INTRODUCTION

This chapter explains the evolution in our thinking and approach to coronary artery stenting based on experience and the development of newer technology between 1988 and 1998. This chapter serves not only as an introduction to our recommendations for different lesion subsets, but also provides an explanation of why our suggestions have changed over time. As George Santayana said, 'Those who cannot remember the past are condemned to repeat it.' We hope that we have learned from our experiences and continue to evolve as we attempt to improve the results of coronary artery stenting.

STENTS TO BAIL OUT COMPLICATIONS OF PERCUTANEOUS TRANSLUMINAL CORONARY ANGIOPLASTY

Coronary stents were available in Europe in 1986 but their use was reserved primarily for situations in which coronary angioplasty was complicated by a severe dissection with threatened closure of the artery, so-called 'bail-out stenting'. The application of stents was restricted because of the high incidence (24%) of subacute stent thrombosis associated with their use.[1] On the basis of preliminary data in animals, the presence of subacute stent thrombosis was believed to be due to platelet stimulation from the metallic foreign body within the bloodstream. To prevent subacute thrombosis, an aggressive regimen of anticoagulation was recommended; this included heparin and dextran infusion during the procedure, as well as a combination of aspirin and warfarin after stent placement.[2] This prolonged the patient's hospital stay since heparin had to be continued until the effect of coumadin became therapeutic. This not only increased the cost of the procedure, but also increased the possibility of signif-

icant vascular problems and bleeding, requiring blood transfusions in 8% of cases. An example of the type of extensive dissection for which stents were reserved is shown in *Fig. 6.1*. After balloon angioplasty in this patient, there was a long spiral dissection from the

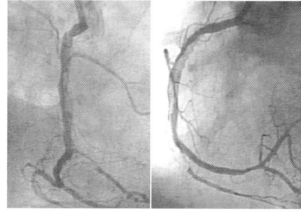

a

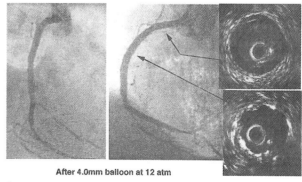

After 4.0mm balloon at 12 atm

b

Figure 6.1 *(a) Bailout use of stents. Large dissection after PTCA threatens complete occlusion. (b) Three Palmaz–Schatz stents were placed sequentially in the proximal and mid-right coronary artery. The ultrasound image (top insert) demonstrates the reference lumen size of the proximal RCA, the bottom insert shows the stent struts as bright echo reflections.*

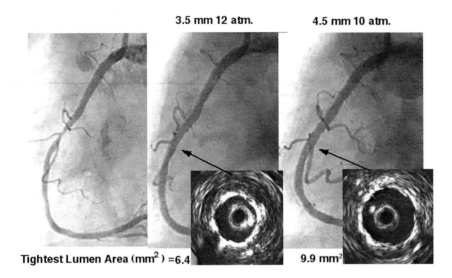

3.5 mm 12 atm.   **4.5 mm 10 atm.**

Tightest Lumen Area (mm²) = 6.4   **9.9 mm²**

Figure 6.2 *Intravascular ultrasound-guided stent implantation.*

proximal right coronary artery (RCA) to the acute margin of the vessel. This was successfully supported by the use of three sequential Palmaz–Schatz stents, which were dilated to 12 atmospheres with a 4.0 mm balloon (*Fig. 6.1b*).

INTRAVASCULAR ULTRASOUND-GUIDED STENT INSERTION: HIGHER PRESSURES AND LARGER BALLOONS

At the same time that we were gaining more experience with this conservative approach for the use of coronary artery stents, we also began investigating the effect of stent deployment with intravascular ultrasound (IVUS) imaging. This process began in October 1992 and led to the realization that, despite an adequate appearance on angiography, ultrasound images frequently revealed inadequate expansion of the stent. As shown in *Fig. 6.2*, a Palmaz–Schatz stent was placed in this mid-RCA tubular stenosis and inflated with a fairly aggressive balloon size at 3.5 mm diameter and relatively high pressure for that time period (12 atmospheres). Despite what appeared to be an angiographic success, IVUS imaging revealed that the tightest area within the stent was 6.4 mm², which was significantly smaller than the proximal or distal reference lumen areas.

Based on these observations, a larger balloon was chosen – 4.5 mm in diameter – and inflated at a moderate pressure (10 atmospheres). The resulting angiographic image showed a larger lumen but the

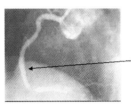
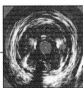

ACS MultiLink
25 mm stent
on 3.5 mm Ellipse
balloon @ 9atm   Angiographic Result   IVUS

Figure 6.3 *Incomplete stent expansion despite delivery balloon inflation to 9 atm. IVUS = intravascular ultrasound.*

ultrasound cross-sectional area dramatically improved by 50% to 9.9 mm².

Stent underexpansion occurred not only during our early experience; this phenomenon is still seen occasionally with some of the newer stents. In *Fig. 6.3*, an ACS Multilink stent has negotiated a tortuous RCA and is deployed at the recommended balloon delivery inflation pressure of 9 atmospheres. Despite a successful angiographic result, the ultrasound image showed that several of the stent struts were not apposed to the wall of the artery and remained in an underexpanded state in the middle of the lumen. The stent was re-expanded at 16 atmospheres and repeat ultrasound imaging documented appropriate strut apposition and expansion.

In other cases of deployed stents examined with ultrasound imaging, it was found that some stents

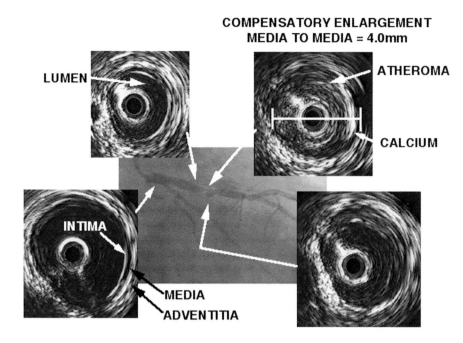

COMPENSATORY ENLARGEMENT
MEDIA TO MEDIA = 4.0mm

LUMEN

ATHEROMA

CALCIUM

INTIMA

MEDIA
ADVENTITIA

Figure 6.4 *Pre-intervention IVUS imaging reveals compensatory enlargement at the lesion site.*

had slipped off the deployment balloon or were underexpanded despite the use of what was considered to be an adequate pressure. This could occur in the presence of an excellent angiographic result, which emphasized the additional benefit of IVUS in understanding the mechanisms involved during stenting. These recurrent observations[3,4] reinforced for us the necessity of deploying stents at higher pressures to obtain full expansion and of using ultrasound to guarantee that the deployment was satisfactory and then to optimize the cross-sectional area by using an appropriately sized balloon.

PRE-INTERVENTION IVUS

In addition to using ultrasound imaging after stent deployment, we took advantage of IVUS to image the artery before any intervention. Pre-intervention imaging (*Fig. 6.4*) is very useful not only for identifying the area of stenosis but also for interrogating the rest of the vessel to determine the length of the stenosis and the diameter of the lumen proximal and distal to the lesion, and for assessing the true size of the artery as measured by the media-to-media diameter. In *Fig. 6.4*, the proximal left anterior descending artery (LAD) by ultrasound is just under 3 mm, but at the site of stenosis the media has expanded to 4 mm

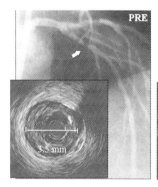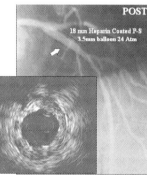

PRE

POST

18 mm Heparin Coated P-S
3.5mm balloon 24 Atm

3.5 mm

Figure 6.5 *Pre-interventional ultrasound imaging demonstrates the amount of plaque. Based on the media to media measurement, a 3.5 mm diameter balloon was chosen to post dilate the Palmaz–Schatz stent.*

to accommodate the large plaque deposition (compensatory remodeling). As described in other chapters, the use of pre-intervention ultrasound is extremely helpful in choosing the type of device, such as a Rotablator or directional atherectomy, as well as the size of the balloon and stent to be used. In *Fig. 6.5* pre-intervention IVUS imaging revealed that the diameter of the vessel, as measured from media to media, was 3.5 mm. Based on this measurement, a Palmaz–Schatz stent was hand crimped on a 3.5 mm balloon and deployed at 24 atmospheres. With this aggressive approach, a successful angio-

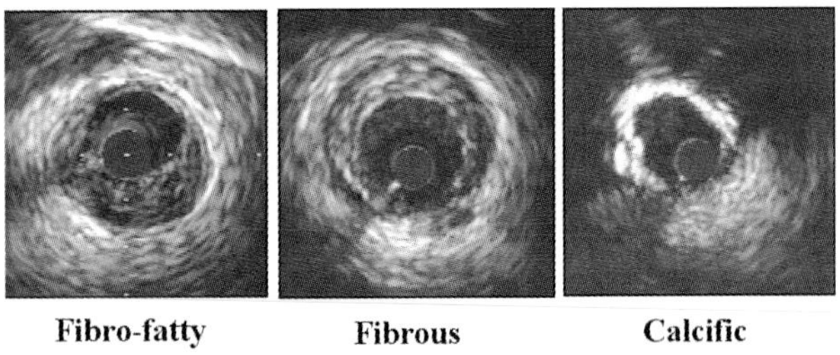

Fibro-fatty   **Fibrous**   **Calcific**

Figure 6.6 *Pre-intervention assessment of plaque composition*

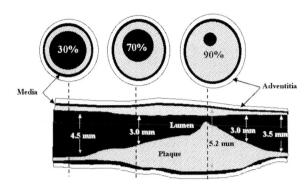

Figure 6.7 *Intravascular ultrasound for selection of stent size and length*

graphic result was obtained with significant step up and step down; however, the lumen diameter by ultrasound (at 2.8 mm) is still less than expected given the balloon size and pressure.

There are two lessons that we gained from these observations:

(a) without the use of IVUS to optimize stent expansion, the lumen area would be significantly smaller and the rate of restenosis would be higher (evidence for this is provided in Chapter 18);

(b) despite the improved results with larger balloons and higher pressures, the lumen cross-sectional area was still limited by the large amount of plaque.

This has led to our current use of atherectomy, before stenting, in a larger percentage of our patients. Pre-intervention imaging is also very useful for determining plaque composition (*Fig. 6.6*). The recognition of extensive calcification within the plaque frequently directs us to use rotational atherectomy before we attempt to dilate the lesion or place a stent. Not only does this increase the lumen size, but it also alters the mechanical characteristics of the plaque to improve the compliance so that the balloon is able to expand the stent to a larger dimension than would otherwise be possible. A list of the uses of IVUS imaging in coronary stenting is provided in *Table 6.1.*

IVUS FOR SELECTION OF STENT SIZE AND LENGTH

A schematic representation of what we have learned from pre-intervention IVUS imaging is provided in *Fig.*

Table 6.1

Uses of intravascular ultrasound imaging in coronary stenting

Pre	Post
1. Lesion severity	1. Stent expansion
2. Lesion length	2. Stent apposition
3. Amount of calcium	3. Edge dissection
4. Precise positioning	4. 'Lost' stent
5. Balloon size	5. Ostial, edge placement
	6. Side branch entrapment

6.7. This figure presents a longitudinal reconstruction of the cross-sectional ultrasound images as if they were stacked together and then cut down the long axis. This permits us to visualize not only the change in the lumen size at the stenosis relative to the reference areas, but also the fact that the outer wall of the artery expands in the process of compensatory dilatation to accommodate the increased growth in plaque.

What we have learned from this analysis is that these lesions do better if some of the plaque can be removed before stenting. In addition, a final balloon size can be chosen on the basis of the media-to-media width. This results in an improved lumen cross-sectional area without increasing the risk of proximal or distal dissections, provided that the shoulders of the balloon are inflated within the stent. In those situations where the length of the lesion is not obvious from the angiogram, IVUS imaging can be used with a continuous mechanical pull-back to determine more accurately the length of artery that needs to be stented.

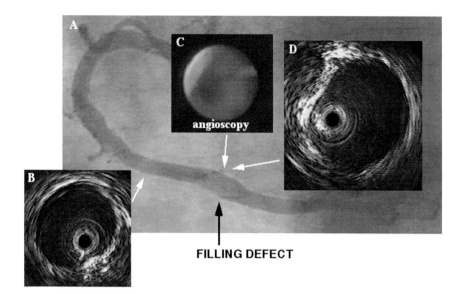

Figure 6.8 *On the cine angiograms, there appeared to be a filling defect in the distal right coronary artery. Pre-intervention imaging by IVUS and angioscopy demonstrate the absence of any intraluminal pathology. The IVUS image shows that the artery is aneurysmally dilated at the lesion site with loss of the medial layer.*

WHEN NOT TO STENT

As we continued to expand our experience with IVUS, we realized that intraluminal imaging was very useful to show us, on occasion, that a lesion did not have to be stented or even treated. The real-time cineangiogram in *Fig. 6.8* appeared to show a filling defect in the distal portion of the right coronary artery. The referring physicians were convinced that this angiographic observation corresponded to a thrombus and so the patient had angioplasty on two occasions before being referred to us. Instead of stenting this filling defect, we performed IVUS imaging. The ultrasound image of the artery proximal to the filling defect shows a large patent lumen without significant atherosclerosis (see *Fig. 6.8b*). At the level of concern (see *Fig. 6.8d*), the ultrasound image reveals that the artery is ectatic with loss of circular symmetry. In addition, the media is not visualized between 12 o'clock and 6 o'clock, which is consistent with an aneurysm of the wall of the artery caused by medial degeneration, but despite repeated passes, there was no evidence for a filling defect, thrombus, or even any atherosclerosis. This was also confirmed with angioscopy (see *Fig. 6.8c*). As a result of the information provided by these IVUS techniques, no intervention was performed. The apparent filling defect was caused by the flow of contrast into the ectatic zone.

STENTING WITH IVUS GUIDANCE AND THE ABSENCE OF COUMADIN

As our experience with the use of stents grew, we became more confident that we could obtain a consistent satisfactory angiographic result without the fear of dissection or sudden occlusion, as was common following balloon angioplasty. In addition, the use of ultrasound imaging guidance to optimize the stent lumen emboldened us to try to deploy stents without using coumadin anticoagulation. Contrary to our concerns, the subacute stent thrombosis rate plummeted despite the absence of coumadin anticoagulation because the lumen cross-sectional area was optimized by IVUS guidance of the procedure. By maintaining the patient on an antiplatelet regimen of aspirin or ticlopidine, or both, we were able to discharge patients sooner and did not sustain the high vascular complication rate associated with anticoagulation therapy. With these alterations in the procedure, the success rate was extremely gratifying despite the array of challenging cases that were treated.

This early experience with stent deployment without anticoagulation therapy using ultrasound guidance was published in 1995.[5] Our use of stents expanded dramatically, to the point where the majority of lesions were treated with stents (*Fig. 6.9*). This led, on occasion, to an excessive use of metal in an attempt to reconstruct arteries by placing multiple

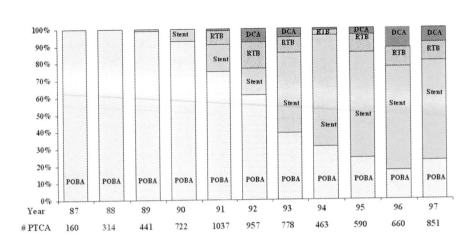

Figure 6.9 *Summary of 11 years of percutaneous transluminal coronary angioplasty (PTCA) at Centro Cuore Columbus, Milan, Italy.*

Full metal jacket

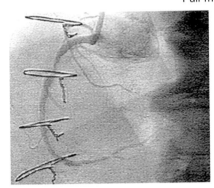

Baseline

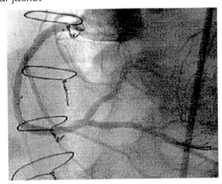

After 8.5 Palmaz–Schatz stents

Figure 6.10 *Multiple stents for long lesions. Prior to the development of long stents, multiple 15 mm long Palmaz–Schatz stents had to be placed to treat diffuse disease. Although the immediate angiographic result was often satisfactory, the restenosis rate was high.*

stents. An example of a 'full metal jacket' for an RCA is presented in *Fig. 6.10*. This arterial reconstruction was a laborious process because long stents were not available at that time. In addition, the pleasing angiographic appearance of the immediate result soon yielded to the reality of diffuse in-stent restenosis, as described below.

BARE STENTING VERSUS THE STENT DELIVERY SYSTEM

Between 1989 and 1997, there were two major differences between the way that stents were deployed in the USA versus other parts of the world. The first difference was that outside the USA there was a greater variety of stents available. The second difference was that within the USA, strict adherence to guidelines of the Food and Drug Administration

meant that the Palmaz–Schatz stent had to be deployed with the stent delivery system. The stent delivery system consisted of an outer plastic sheath, which was felt to be necessary to protect the stent from being displaced from the balloon as the stent passed through the proximal vessels prior to its deployment at the lesion site. The negative aspect of the delivery system was that it increased the profile of the stent, which inhibited access through tortuous arteries or in smaller vessels. This required the use of stiffer guidewires or the use of a second 'buddy' wire to straighten the artery and facilitate passage of the bulky delivery system. In addition, the balloon that was used to deliver the stent was not an appropriate balloon to expand the stent at high pressures. Therefore, after pre-dilating the lesion with one balloon to permit access, the stent had to be deployed with its bulky delivery system and then a second balloon had to be used to expand the stent at a higher pressure. Outside the USA, the Palmaz–Schatz stent was available as a separate entity

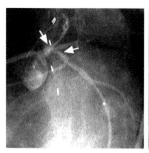
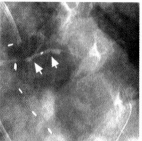
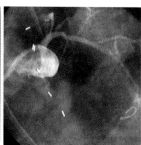

Figure 6.11 *Stent delivery system (SDS) versus bare stenting*

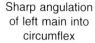

Sharp angulation of left main into circumflex

Bare stent passes through where SDS would not

Final angiogram

without the balloon or stent delivery system. This facilitated the procedure because a single balloon could be used to pre-dilate the lesion, then the Palmaz–Schatz stent could be hand crimped on to the same balloon for stent deployment. The same balloon, which was specifically chosen as a non-compliant high-pressure device, could then expand the stent without changing its position.

An example of how the bare stenting technique was useful in approaching tortuous or angulated lesions is demonstrated in *Fig. 6.11*. This proximal circumflex artery had a significant stenosis with documented ischemia in the lateral wall. There was a 90° take-off of the circumflex artery from the left main coronary artery. The Palmaz–Schatz stent delivery system would not negotiate this angle despite the use of a platinum-plus guidewire. Therefore, the stent was removed from the sheath delivery system and hand crimped on to a 3.0 mm × 20 mm NC Shadow balloon. The bare stent successfully negotiated the sharp angle and was inflated at 16 atmospheres with a satisfactory angiographic result and relief of the patient's symptoms.

A retrospective analysis was performed on 209 patients. This analysis compared the stent delivery system in 107 lesions to 150 lesions that had the bare stenting approach.[6] The measured diameter of the stent delivery system with a 3.0 mm balloon was 1.8 mm. The same stent manually mounted on an NC Bandit 3.5 mm balloon measured 1.3 mm in diameter. Significantly fewer balloons were used per lesion in the bare stent group than in the stent delivery group (1.9 ± 0.6 versus 3.8 ± 1.2, $p < 0.0001$). In addition, the procedure time in the bare stent group was significantly shorter than in the stent delivery system group (106 ± 55 minutes versus 134 ± 60 minutes, $p = 0.001$). There was no difference in the frequency of adverse events or stent displacement during the procedure.

The bare stenting technique decreased the procedure time, reduced the number of balloons used, and was as safe as the stent delivery system approach.

Another approach that we developed to improve stent delivery through tortuous arterial segments was to cut the Palmaz–Schatz stent in half at the articulation site and then mount the 7-mm-long half stent on to a low-profile balloon. By decreasing the length of the rigid segment, the stent was more easily manipulated through tortuous or small vessels or even through previously deployed stents.[7] The use of bare stenting and half stenting with Palmaz–Schatz stents had a significant impact on our ability to treat complex lesions and decreased the time of the procedure. However, the response of the medical industry to the demand for improved stent design has had an even greater impact on our ability to perform coronary stenting in complex anatomy and these earlier methods of bare stenting and use of half stents are only rarely used in current practice.

NEWER STENT DESIGNS FACILITATE TREATMENT OF COMPLEX LESIONS

In addition to the hand-crimped, bare stenting technique, stent deployment was facilitated by the proliferation of new stent designs. The increased flexibility and various length options made it easier to treat complex lesions such as stenoses in tortuous vessels or bifurcations. A brief description of our experience with many of the new stents is provided in Chapter 2. An example of the use of a second-generation stent to treat a complex lesion in a hairpin turn of a sclerotic coronary artery is shown in *Fig. 6.12*. To treat this lesion, two NIR stents were used.

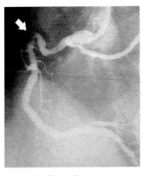
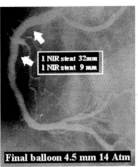
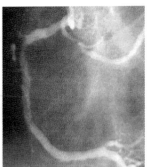

Figure 6.12 *Treatment of a tortuous vessel; MLD, minimum lumen diameter.*

	Baseline		Final Result		6 months FU	
-----------------	--------		------------		-----------	
Ref Vessel	3.99 mm		4.01 mm		3.35 mm	
MLD	1.35 mm		4.04 mm		2.05 mm	
Diam. Stenosis	66 %		0 %		39 %	

The first was 9 mm long and the second was 32 mm long. These were expanded with a 4.5 mm balloon at 14 atmospheres on the basis of the ultrasound assessment of the vessel size. The high radial strength of the NIR stent provided adequate scaffolding to support the vessel and reduce the severe tortuosity of the proximal segment without creating a pleat or hinge effect at the proximal or distal ends of the stent.

THE USE OF PHYSIOLOGIC MEASUREMENTS TO ASSESS LESION SEVERITY

One of the other techniques that has influenced the way we perform interventional procedures has been the use of physiologic assessment of lesion severity either with the Doppler flow wire or by measuring the pressure gradient across the lesion before and after hyperemia (see Chapter 5). The velocity of blood flow in the artery can be measured with the Doppler technique using a 0.36 mm (0.014-inch) wire (Flowire, Cardiometrics Inc., Mountain View, California, USA). Following successful deployment of a stent, the flow in the treated artery should be equal to that in the non-obstructed arterial system. The Doppler flow velocity is measured at baseline and then after the administration of 12–18 µg adenosine injected as a bolus through the guiding catheter. The coronary flow reserve (CFR) is defined as the average peak velocity after hyperemia divided by the baseline measurement. In *Fig. 16.13* the blood flow velocity was measured in the LAD after deploying a spiral design Palmaz–Schatz stent 30 mm in length. The baseline average peak velocity was 23 cm/second which increased to 57 cm/second after adenosine. The CFR was calculated as 2.5 in the LAD. Although this ratio is considered to be indicative of normal flow, there are conditions that diminish the CFR as a result of altered vascular tone in the distal resistance vessels secondary to hypertension, myocardial infarction, or diabetes mellitus. Therefore, the non-obstructed vessel, such as the left circumflex artery in this example, was also examined before and after infusion of adenosine. This yielded a coronary flow reserve of 2.8 (see *Fig. 6.13c*).

Although not required on a routine basis, the use of physiologic measurements to assess the severity of the lesion before treatment or the adequacy of the intervention has been very useful. This information is frequently combined with the anatomical information obtained by angiography and intravascular ultrasound. *Figure 6.14* demonstrates how the analysis of Doppler flow can be used before and after treatment to guide interventional therapy. The angiogram in *Fig. 6.14a* shows a stenosis in the proximal circumflex artery. The 0.36 mm (0.014-inch) Doppler flow wire was passed into the large obtuse marginal branch. The baseline average peak velocity was 33 cm/second which increased after adenosine infusion to only 44 cm/second, producing a coronary flow reserve of 1.3. Following balloon dilatation with a balloon of 3.0 mm diameter, the angiogram is consistent with a successful angioplasty result; however, the CFR has not increased and is still 1.2 (see *Fig. 6.14b*). A stent was then deployed at 10 atmospheres on a 3.5 mm balloon. Despite 10 atmospheres of pressure there is still some indentation in the distal aspect of the balloon (insert) and the angiogram does not show complete efface-ment of the lesion (see *Fig. 6.14c*). The corresponding coronary flow reserve is still below normal at 1.6. The balloon was then inflated to 16 atmospheres, which

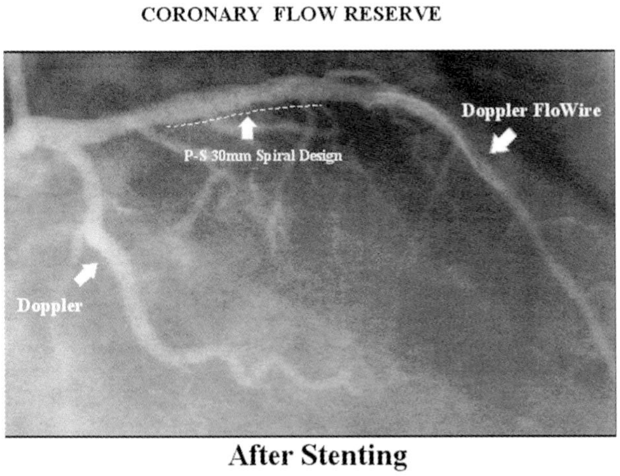

CORONARY FLOW RESERVE

a

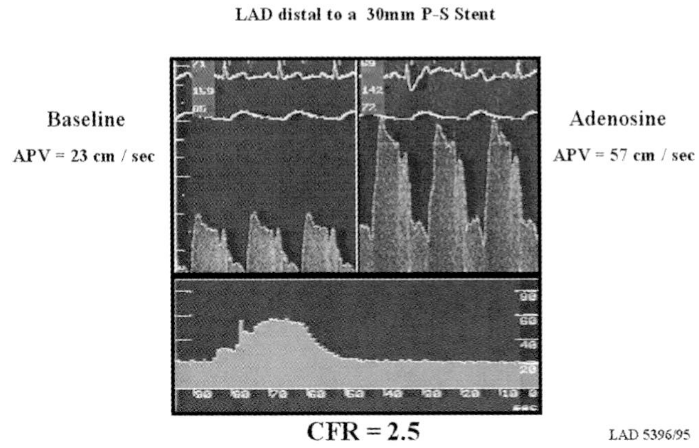

b

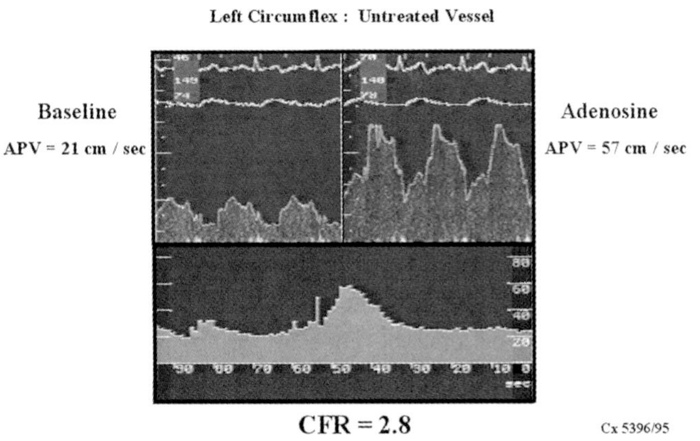

c

Figure 6.13 *Intracoronary Doppler after stenting. CFR, coronary flow reserve; LAD, left anterior descending artery; APV, average peak velocity.*

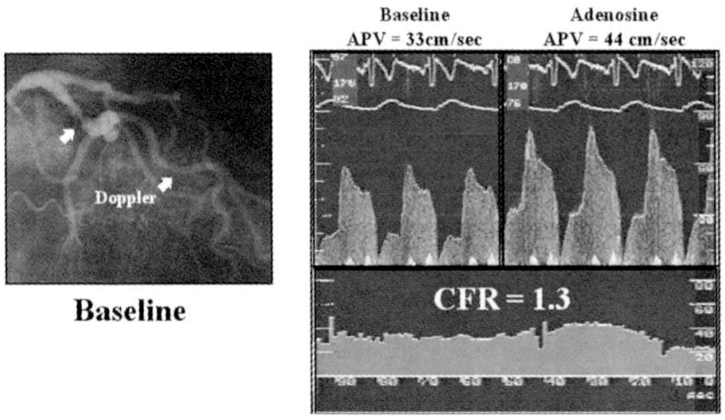

a

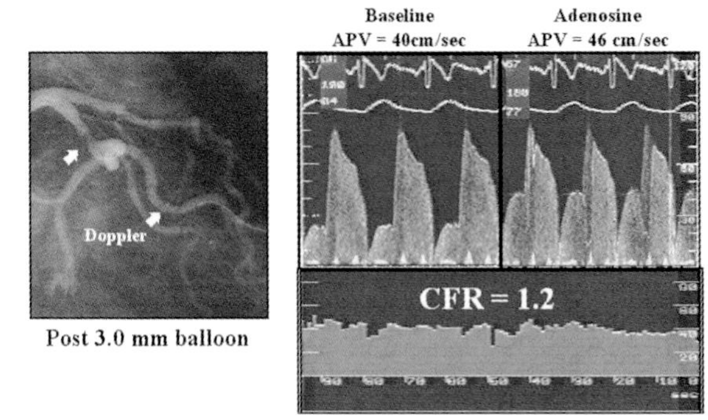

b

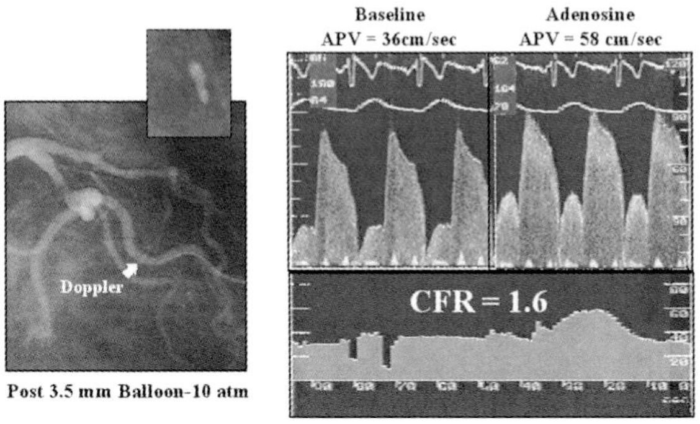

c

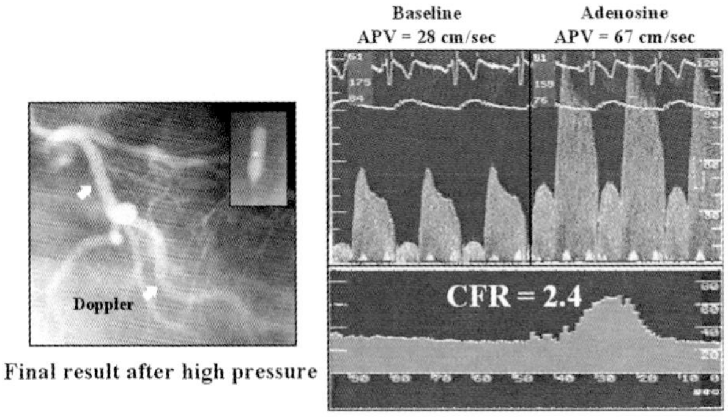

d

Figure 6.14 *(a) Doppler flow before treatment; (b) Doppler flow after pre-dilatation; (c) Doppler flow after stenting at 10 atm; (d) Doppler flow after stenting at 16 atm. CFR, coronary flow reserve; APV, average peak velocity.*

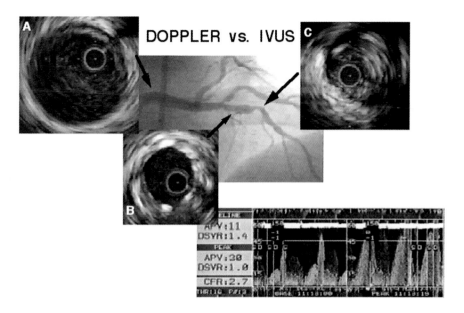

Figure 6.15 *Assessment of an intermediate lesion. Although the IVUS study (c) shows a small lumen (1.4 × 1.2 mm in diameter) surrounded by a large atheroma, the Doppler flow analysis revealed a normal coronary flow reserve (CFR). The threshold for diagnosing a severe stenosis is higher for physiologic measurements than it is by IVUS cross-sectional imaging.*

produced an angiographic appearance of complete expansion of the stenosis. In addition, the CFR improved to 2.4 as the average peak velocity reached 67 cm/second following adenosine infusion.

The threshold for a normal CFR response is somewhat different from the 'occulo-stenotic reflex' that occurs when viewing either an angiogram or an IVUS anatomic image. The angiogram in *Fig. 6.15* was obtained 5 years after the placement of a Palmaz–Schatz stent in the LAD distal to the first septal perforator. There is a significant step up and step down with a relative stenosis distal to the stent. By IVUS the distal narrowing also appears to be significant as the plaque encroaches near the ultrasound catheter. The lumen measured 1.4 mm in diameter. However, this appeared to be adequate to maintain blood flow, both at rest and following hyperemia induced by adenosine, as shown in the Doppler flow wire insert where the coronary flow reserve was calculated as 2.7. Since the stent had been present for 5 years without any symptoms, it was decided not to treat the stenosis distal to the stent on the basis of the physiologic assessment and lack of symptoms.

DEBULKING THE PLAQUE BEFORE STENTING

As described in Chapter 1, our excitement with coronary artery stenting evolved from the results of

a study of using IVUS to optimize the effects of rotational atherectomy and directional atherectomy. The concept at the time of that project (the autumn of 1992) was that restenosis might be reduced if we could decrease the plaque burden prior to balloon dilatation. The method of accomplishing this was to measure the plaque cross-sectional area by IVUS and attempt to remove the plaque with either rotational or directional atherectomy until the lumen was > 50% of the vessel cross-sectional area defined as the boundary of the media. Not only was this process laborious, but the preliminary results revealed that the restenosis rate was highest in the group of arteries that were most aggressively treated, the exact antithesis to our original hypothesis. The only cases that had markedly reduced restenosis rates were those lesions that were treated aggressively by debulking the plaque mass with an iterative process of IVUS-guided atherectomy followed by coronary artery stenting. The results of this study encouraged us to use stents more frequently.

Despite our early enthusiasm for the beneficial results of using stents compared to balloon dilatation alone, we realized that the process was still limited by a restenosis rate of 20–40% depending on the lesion subset. We then reviewed the concept that by removing some of the plaque, the restenosis rate might be reduced further. Although we were using rotational atherectomy throughout our experience with stenting, this was usually limited to calcified arteries or diffuse disease. The use of directional

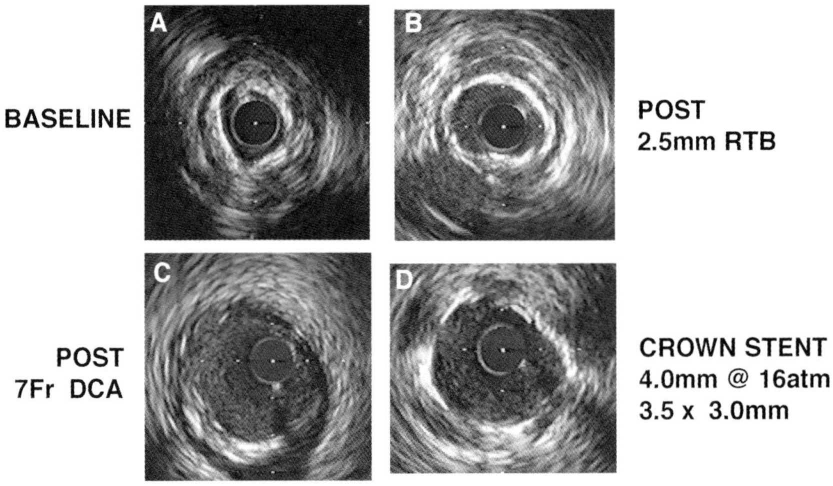

Figure 6.16 *Debulking prior to stenting. IVUS guided rotational atherectomy, directional atherectomy, and stenting.*

atherectomy had suffered significantly because of the less than impressive results of the CAVEAT Trial.[8] In 1997 we returned to the idea of trying to remove a significant amount of plaque so that the lumen cross-sectional area would be more than 50% of the vessel area before deploying the stent. This iterative process is demonstrated in *Fig. 6.16*. Using IVUS imaging before the intervention, the tissue characteristics reveal significant calcification at the lumen–plaque interface (see *Fig. 6.16a*). Therefore, progressive rotational atherectomy burrs were used from a 1.5 mm up to a 2.5 mm burr (see *Fig. 6.16b*). Although this resulted in the lumen being slightly larger than 2 mm in diameter, the vessel size measured at the media was less than 4 mm. Based on this IVUS observation, directional atherectomy was performed with a 7 Fr catheter, which removed a significant amount of plaque (see *Fig. 6.16c*). At this cross-section, the lumen measured 7.3 mm² and the area bounded by the media measured 15 mm², giving a lumen-to-vessel ratio of 0.49. After removing the bulk of this plaque, a Crown stent was deployed on a 4 mm balloon at 16 atmospheres. The final dimensions of the lumen were 3.0 mm × 3.5 mm (8.1 mm²). In our experience with lesions that have such a large plaque burden, the attainment of a large lumen would not be possible without initially debulking the plaque. In addition, our early data from debulking plaques before stenting suggest that the restenosis rate is significantly reduced[9] (see Chapter 19).

'PROVISIONAL STENTING' – BALLOON ANGIOPLASTY WITH STENTING AS A BACK-UP

The STRESS[10] and BENESTENT[11] trials demonstrated that stents reduce restenosis by one-third compared to balloon angioplasty. Faced with these results, many operators, including ourselves, elected to place stents in the majority (75%) of lesions. In general, the results with stenting were predictable and successfully relieved symptoms. However, the STRESS and BENESTENT studies were limited to short lesions (< 15 mm) and large arteries (> 3.0 mm). As we applied stents to more complex settings and diffuse disease, we were faced with the recurrent problem of restenosis. In an attempt to decrease restenosis yet diminish the cost associated with stenting, the concept of 'provisional stenting' has been developed.

The basic principle of this technique is that angioplasty alone will be tried first and a stent will be used only if the results are unsatisfactory as assessed by angiography, ultrasound, or physiologic parameters such as Doppler flow wire or fractional flow reserve. The concept of provisional stenting is a testimony to the fact that the results achieved with balloon angioplasty have improved because of the advent of stenting. Since stents are available to provide back-up, a larger balloon size can be chosen to optimize the results of dilatation. Higher pressures can be used during the initial dilatation and, if a dissection occurs, the artery can be satisfactorily treated by the deployment of a stent.

A clinical example of 'provisional stenting' using IVUS-guided angioplasty is demonstrated in *Fig. 6.17*. The baseline angiogram demonstrates a diffusely involved mid-section of the LAD. The lesion was 30 mm long and involved both the first and second

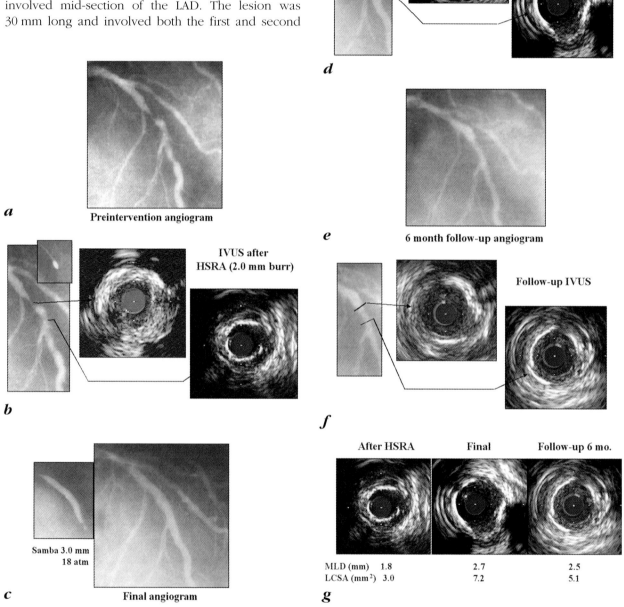

a **Preintervention angiogram**

IVUS after HSRA (2.0 mm burr)

b

Samba 3.0 mm 18 atm

c **Final angiogram**

Final IVUS CSA = 7.2mm²

d

e **6 month follow-up angiogram**

Follow-up IVUS

f

	After HSRA	Final	Follow-up 6 mo.
MLD (mm)	1.8	2.7	2.5
LCSA (mm²)	3.0	7.2	5.1

g

Figure 6.17 *Provisional stenting: IVUS-guided angioplasty. Sequential steps when trying to obtain a 'stent like result' during coronary angioplasty without having to place a stent. (a) Baseline coronary angiogram. (b) IVUS after rotational atherectomy with a 2.0 mm burr. (c) Aggressive balloon dilatation using the measurements from the IVUS study. (d) Assessment of lumen diameter by angiography as well as IVUS. If lumen cross-sectional area is greater than 5.5 mm², then the procedure is terminated without the use of a stent. (e) Follow-up angiogram at six months shows minimal lumen loss. (f) IVUS exam obtained at the six-month follow-up study. (g) Comparison of IVUS exams at the same cross-section following initial rotational atherectomy, after the final balloon dilatation, and at the six-month follow-up study.*

septal perforating branches. This was initially treated with a 1.5 mm and then a 2.0 mm rotational atherectomy burr. The IVUS images, after rotational atherectomy, are shown in *Fig. 6.17b*. The lumen measures < 2 mm in the proximal portion and exactly 2.0 mm in the calcified distal half. This was then dilated with a 3.0 mm Samba balloon at 18 atmospheres; the final angiogram is shown in *Fig. 6.17c*. Following rotational atherectomy and balloon dilatation the final examination demonstrates an adequate lumen cross-sectional area of 7.2 mm² (*Fig. 6.17d*). On the basis of these ultrasound measurements, a decision was made not to place a stent in this artery. The follow-up angiogram obtained 6 months after the procedure demonstrates patency of the vessel with minimal restenosis. The angiographic results are confirmed by the follow-up IVUS study (see *Fig. 6.17f*). These sequential changes in the ultrasound images after initial rotational atherectomy, final balloon dilatation and the follow-up are summarized in *Fig. 6.17g*.

As outlined more fully in Chapter 20, if an initial lumen cross-sectional area > 5.5 mm² is obtained following balloon dilatation, then we feel comfortable leaving the result without placing a stent. Using this combined approach, the restenosis rate appears very favorable and the aggressive form of diffuse in-stent restenosis is avoided. In this technique of 'provisional stenting', stents are reserved only for those situations where there is a large dissection that compromises the lumen or where the lumen cross-sectional area does not meet our minimum criteria.

Abizaid and Pichard and co-workers at the Washington Hospital Center developed a practical algorithm for optimizing balloon angioplasty with stent rescue.[12] In their technique, IVUS imaging is performed before the intervention. A balloon is chosen whose diameter is equal to the media-to-media distance at the lesion site. The balloon is inflated to > 10 atmospheres (mean 13.5 ± 3.3 atmospheres). By angiography this corresponds to a balloon-to-artery ratio of 1.16. The end-points are a lumen area > 75% of the average reference areas by ultrasound and the absence of any lumen-compromising dissections observed either by angiography or ultrasound. In 243 lesions, 148 (61%) did not achieve this result and had stents deployed at the lesion site. In the 95 lesions treated with angioplasty alone, the final lumen area was 6.0 ± 2.0 mm², which corresponded to a cross-sectional percentage stenosis of 44%. In this group of patients treated with angioplasty alone, there were no abrupt vessel closures and the 6-month target lesion revascularization rate was 17%. This would qualify as a 'stent-like' angioplasty result.

Based on our experience, we believe the lesions that are preferable for balloon dilatation alone are discrete lesions that are < 10 mm in length in relatively large vessels (> 3 mm in diameter) that respond well at a low inflation pressure. These are the types of lesions that were included in the BENES-TENT[11] and STRESS[10] studies. PTCA works well alone in at least 50% of these lesions. If a successful result is not achieved, then a stent can always be used with confidence. On the other hand, more complex lesions would do better by having a stent placed as primary therapy. These include lesions at the aorto-ostial junction, large ulcerated plaques, severely calcified lesions, restenotic lesions, chronic total occlusions, and saphenous vein graft lesions.

'SPOT STENTING' – BALLOON ANGIOPLASTY WITH SELECTIVE STENTING USING IVUS OR PHYSIOLOGIC GUIDANCE

In patients who have long lesions or diffuse disease, the use of long stents has facilitated our ability to obtain a satisfactory angiographic result. Unfortunately, despite the initial apparent success, the restenosis rate with multiple stents or long stent lengths is disappointingly high (see Chapter 4). In response to the high restenosis rate associated with long stent lengths, the concept of 'spot stenting' has been developed. With 'spot stenting' balloon dilatation is performed initially throughout the long diseased segment. If the result, based on angiography, ultrasound, or physiologic assessment of flow, is satisfactory, then the artery is left alone and no stent is placed. However, if these parameters uncover segments within the artery that are inadequately dilated, then a stent is placed only in those residual stenotic zones with the intention of using as short a stent as possible. Our criterion for a successful balloon dilatation is a lumen cross-sectional area ≥ 5.5 mm² or, for small vessels, a lumen that is > 50% of the vessel cross-sectional area (measured at the external elastic membrane) (*Table 6.2*). In addition, dissections are left unstented if they do not compromise flow and subtend an area less than the true lumen.

An example of IVUS 'spot stenting' is provided in *Fig. 6.18*. The baseline angiogram shows diffuse disease in the proximal and mid-portions of the RCA. By quantitative coronary angiography, the minimum

Pre-intervention angiogram

IVUS

QCA

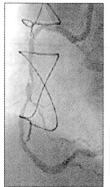

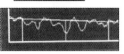

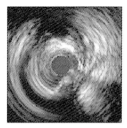

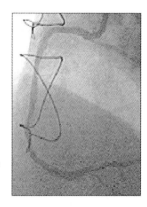

Media to media: 4.1 mm

Balloon size: 3.75 mm

Ref.: 2.67 mm
MLD: 0.98 mm
Lesion length: 49.2 mm

a

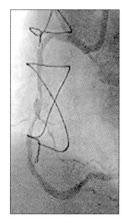

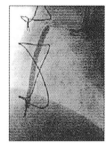

Balloon angioplasty

D: 3.75 mm
L: 40 mm
P: 14 atm

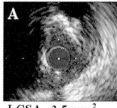

After balloon angioplasty

Pre-intervention

b

IVUS after balloon angioplasty

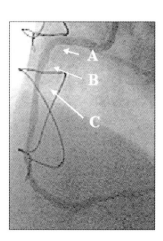

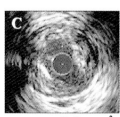

LCSA 3.5 mm^2

LCSA 5.6 mm^2

Dissection

LCSA 7.3 mm^2

c

Figure 6.18 *IVUS-guided SPOT stenting. (a) Pre-intervention angiogram reveals diffuse disease in this right coronary artery. Although the lumen reference by QCA measures 2.67 mm, the media to media measurement by IVUS is 4.1 mm. (b) Based on the ultrasound measurement, a 3.75 mm balloon was chosen to dilate the long lesion. (c) The IVUS exam after balloon angioplasty demonstrates that the proximal RCA has an insufficient lumen cross-sectional area. (d) Based on this IVUS analysis, a relatively short 16 mm stent was placed only in the proximal portion of the artery. (e) The final angiogram and ultrasound studies demonstrate a satisfactory lumen with a cross-sectional area greater than 5.5 mm². Based on the IVUS results, only a short stent was used to treat this extensive lesion.*

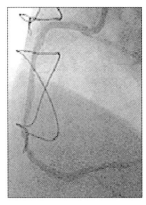

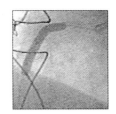

Stent: DART 16 mm

Post dilatation
D: 4.0 mm
L: 20 mm
P: 10 atm

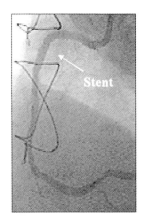

After balloon angioplasty

After spot stenting

d

IVUS after final procedure

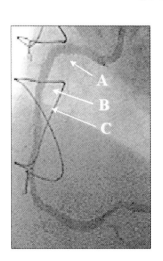

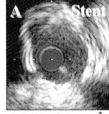

LCSA 8.1 mm^2

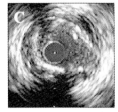

LCSA   6.6 mm^2

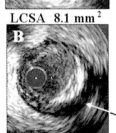

LCSA 10.2 mm^2

Dissection

e

Table 6.2
What is 'optimal' IVUS criteria that defines a successful stent result?

We have used different criteria over time:
  The optimal stented lumen minimum CSA should be:
1. ≥ 60% of proximal and distal vessel (EEM) CSA, or
2. ≥ 90% of distal lumen CSA.
BUT: we can attain this criteria in only 66% of cases.
THEREFORE, we now use this method:
1. Choose a balloon 0.5 mm < the vessel (EEM) diameter at lesion site or average reference diameter. Strive for the optimal criteria, but:
2. Minimally acceptable criteria: lumen CSA ≥ 5.5 mm² and lumen ≥ 50% of vessel (EEM) at lesion site.
3. Use as short a stent as possible.
4. Although we strive for the optimal criteria, the acute and long term results appear adequate using the minimally acceptable threshold, especially with long lesions.

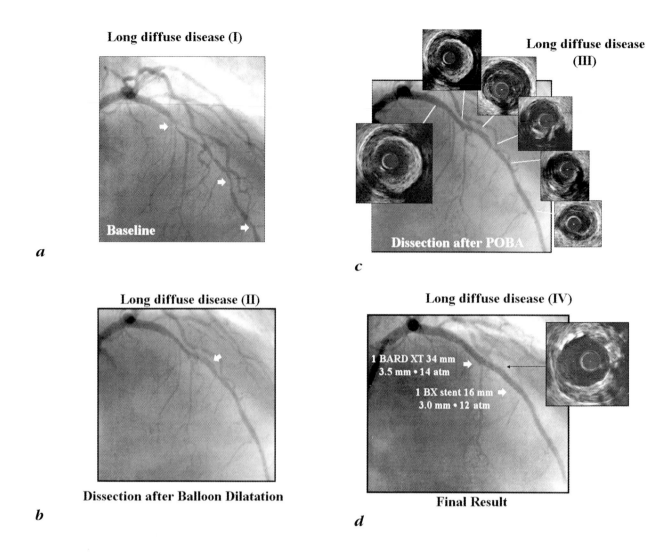

Figure 6.19 *The use of IVUS to assess coronary dissections. (a) Baseline angiogram reveals diffuse disease in the mid and distal left anterior descending artery. (b) Following balloon dilatation, there is evidence for dissection by angiography. (c) The ultrasound exam helps to identify the extent of the dissection and where the lumen may be compromised. (d) Based on the ultrasound and angiographic appearance, several stents were used to provide a scaffold for this artery.*

lumen diameter was 1 mm and the reference was 2.7 mm in diameter, with a total lesion length of 49 mm. However, by IVUS imaging, the media-to-media diameter measured 4.1 mm. Therefore, a 3.75 mm diameter balloon was chosen to perform the initial dilatation, which is a much larger device than would have been chosen based on angiography. The 40 mm balloon was inflated at 14 atmospheres (see *Fig. 6.18b*). The angioplasty result appeared to be successful by angiographic criteria. The results of IVUS imaging are shown in *Fig. 6.18c*. IVUS imaging demonstrated that the lumen cross-sectional area in

Panel A was inadequate at 3.5 mm². Based on this observation, a 16 mm DART stent was placed in the proximal portion of the artery just at the initial bend. The stent was deployed on a 4 mm diameter balloon at 10 atmospheres (see *Fig. 6.18d*). The size of this balloon also was chosen based on the IVUS measurements. The subsequent ultrasound study (see *Fig. 6.18e*) showed that an adequate cross-sectional area was obtained in the stented zone at 8.1 mm² (Panel A) as well as the non-stented zone at 10.2 mm² (Panel B), and even more distal to the stent at site C, which measured 6.6 mm². The presence of the dissection behind the plaque in Panel B is not an indication for placing a stent since the plaque did not compromise the lumen.

This technique of 'spot stenting' may be useful for small vessels (< 2.5 mm), long lesions (> 20 mm in length) and diffuse disease.[13] A more complete description of our experience with 'spot stenting' is presented in Chapter 20.

DO ALL DISSECTIONS NEED TO BE STENTED?

Our thinking with respect to dissections has also evolved. Especially when treating diffuse disease, a successful balloon dilatation is often associated with a dissection. However, not every dissection is occlusive or needs to be treated with a coronary artery stent.[14,15] If possible, dissections should be assessed with both the anatomic parameter of IVUS cross-sectional imaging and physiologic measures such as pressure gradients or coronary flow reserve following hyperemia.

Even when we try to avoid using stents or, at least, limit the length of artery that is stented, it is important to know when long stents should be used to cover severe dissections. In *Fig. 6.19a*, we attempted to treat the diffuse disease in the mid- and distal LAD with balloon dilatation alone. However, dilatation with a 40 mm long balloon resulted in a type C dissection (see *Fig. 6.19b*). Although the lumen did not appear compromised, by ultrasound examination this dissection extended further than appreciated by angiography and the disrupted plaque fell into the lumen (see *Fig. 6.19c*). This dissection was treated with a 34 mm long Bard XT stent and a 16 mm long BX stent. Although the risk of restenosis may be over 40% owing to the length of these stents, it is imperative that arterial patency is maintained.

CONCLUSION

This chapter has attempted to summarize the changes in our thinking and our approach to coronary artery stenting. The procedures will continue to evolve as more refinements are developed and our knowledge about coronary artery stenting increases. It is our hope that the reader will have a greater appreciation of our decision-making process by understanding the evolution of our concepts of coronary artery stenting over the past decade.

REFERENCES

1. Serruys PW, Strauss BH, Beatt KJ et al. Angiographic follow-up after placement of a self-expanding coronary-artery stent. *N Engl J Med* 1991; **324**: 13–17.
2. Schatz RA, Baim DS, Leon M et al. Clinical experience with the Palmaz–Schatz coronary stent. Initial results of a multicenter study. *Circulation* 1991; **83**: 148–161.
3. Nakamura S, Colombo A, Gaglione A et al. Intracoronary ultrasound observations during stent implantation. *Circulation* 1994; **89**: 2026–2034.
4. Goldberg SL, Colombo A, Nakamura S et al. Benefit of intracoronary ultrasound in the deployment of Palmaz–Schatz stents. *J Am Coll Cardiol* 1994; **24**: 996–1003.
5. Colombo A, Hall P, Nakamura S et al. Intracoronary stenting without anticoagulation accomplished with intravascular ultrasound guidance. *Circulation* 1995; **91**: 1676–1688.
6. Kasaoka S, Son R, Eslami M et al. Comparison of the sheath delivery system versus bare stenting for coronary stent implantation. *Cathet Cardiovasc Diagn* 1998; **43**: 386–394; discussion 395–396.
7. Colombo A, Hall P, Thomas J et al. Initial experience with the disarticulated (one-half) Palmaz–Schatz stent: a technical report. *Cathet Cardiovasc Diagn* 1992; **25**: 304–308.
8. Topol EJ, Leya F, Pinkerton CA et al. A comparison of directional atherectomy with coronary angioplasty in patients with coronary artery disease. The CAVEAT Study Group. *N Engl J Med* 1993; **329**: 221–227.
9. Moussa I, Moses J, Di Mario C et al. Stenting after optimal lesion debulking (SOLD) registry. Angiographic and clinical outcome. *Circulation* 1998; **98**: 1604–1609.
10. Fischman DL, Leon MB, Baim DS et al. A randomized comparison of coronary-stent placement and balloon angioplasty in the treatment of coronary artery disease. Stent Restenosis Study Investigators. *N Engl J Med* 1994; **331**: 496–501.
11. Serruys PW, de Jaegere P, Kiemeneij F et al. A comparison of balloon-expandable-stent implantation with balloon angioplasty in patients with coronary artery disease. Benestent Study Group. *N Engl J Med* 1994; **331**: 489–495.
12. Abizaid A, Mehran R, Pichard AD et al. Results of high pressure ultrasound-guided 'over-sized' balloon PTCA to achieve 'stent-like' results. *J Am Coll Cardiol* 1997; **29 (suppl A)**: 280A.
13. Moussa I, De Gregorio J, Di Mario C et al. The use of intravascular ultrasound and spot stenting for the treatment of long lesions and small vessels. *J Invas Cardiol* 1999; **11**: 36–42.
14. Kobayashi N, De Gregorio J, Adamian M et al. Dissections post coronary stenting: is it worth extending your stent length to cover all dissections (abstract)? *J Am Coll Cardiol* 1999; **33**: 58A.
15. Reimers B, Spedicato L, Sacca S et al. Residual dissections after coronary stenting not covered by additional stents. *J Am Coll Cardiol* 1999; **33 (suppl A)**: 27A.

Chapter 7 Saphenous vein grafts

Antonio Colombo and Jonathan Tobis

When approaching the patient with coronary artery graft disease, the first question the interventionalist must confront is whether to do an intervention at all or to refer the patient for another bypass operation. Since the incidence of complications with treating bypass grafts is higher than with native disease,[1] it is important to be selective in deciding which grafts should be treated with percutaneous therapy. Repeat surgery may be preferable if:

(a) the left internal mammary artery was not used in the first operation;
(b) there are multiple degenerated grafts;
(c) the grafts are more than 7 years old; or
(d) there is an occluded major graft that cannot be reopened for technical reasons.

Repeat surgery also has more complications than the first operation, with several studies reporting a perioperative infarction rate of 2–8% and an operative mortality that is between two and four times higher than that of the original surgery.[2]

The use of balloon angioplasty alone has not been very successful for treating graft stenosis. Although the primary success rate is reported as being between 80 and 92%, there is a major event rate between 2 and 12% and the restenosis rate is reported as varying between 39 and 58% (*Table 7.1*).[3,4] In the CAVEAT II study,[5] atherectomy of saphenous vein grafts was not significantly better than balloon angioplasty alone (*Table 7.2*). Although the primary success rate with directional coronary atherectomy was higher than with percutaneous transluminal coronary angioplasty (PTCA) (89% versus 79%, $p < 0.05$), the complications of acute closure, embolization, and myocardial infarction (MI) were also higher. Ellis and colleagues,[6] reporting on 103 patients who were treated for saphenous vein graft disease, found that the event-free survival from death, MI, or repeat vascularization was only 28% in 33 months of follow-up. Their analysis demonstrated not only that the treated saphenous vein graft was frequently the site of repeat procedures, but also that the untreated saphenous vein grafts with lesions less than 50% at baseline often progressed and required further treatment.

Results with transluminal extraction catheter (TEC) atherectomy have also been less than satisfactory. Patients with a large thrombus load can be treated successfully with TEC atherectomy, but the reported mortality and restenosis rates are high (*Table 7.3*). Braden and colleagues[7] reported a 95% procedural

Table 7.1

Balloon angioplasty without stenting in vein graft stenosis

	Year	Pts	Success	Events	Restenosis
Douglas	1986	235	92%	8%	–
Cote	1987	101	85%	2%	39%
Platko	1989	101	92%	5%	61%
Plokker	1991	454	90%	2%	–
Douglas	1991	599	90%	7%	58%
Holmes	1994	156	79%	12%	51%

Table 7.2

Atherectomy (DCA) failed to show a superior effect compared to balloon dilatation (BA) (CAVEAT II)

	DCA	BA	
Lesions	149	156	
Lesion length (mm)	10.9	11	
Success	89%	79%	$p < 0.05$
Acute closure	4.7%	2.6%	
Embolization	13.4%	5.1%	
MI (Q + non-Q)	17.4%	11.5%	
Death	2%	1.9%	
Angio restenosis	45%	50%	

Table 7.3

Transluminal extraction catheter atherectomy in saphenous vein grafting

US TEC Multicenter Registry

Lesions	538
Mortality	3.2%
Emergency CABG	0.7%
Major complicafions	4.3%

William Beaumont Hospital

Lesions	158
Procedural success	84%
Distal embolization	11%
Abrupt closure	5%
Clinical restenosis	42%
Angio restenosis	83%

Table 7.5

Late clinical outcome with saphenous vein graft stenting. Washington Hospital experience 1996

	6 m (n=1261)	12 m (n=1040)
No event	65%	57%
Death	8.4%	10.2%
CABG	5.3%	6.4%
PTCA	20%	24%
PTCA on the lesion	5.2%	5.8%

mellitus (odds ratio (OR) 1.9), unstable angina (OR 1.5), ostial location (OR 3.1), or low left ventricular ejection fraction (OR 28.3) (*Table 7.6*).

NON-DEGENERATED GRAFTS

The use of coronary stents to treat saphenous vein graft lesions increases the likelihood of long-term survival over balloon angioplasty alone. In the multicenter prospective randomized trial of 220 patients

success rate when combining TEC atherectomy with stenting in 53 vein grafts that were over 9 years old. Distal embolization occurred in 2% and hospital death occurred in 3% of the patients. However, after 13 months of follow-up, the rate of target lesion revascularization was 11%, the rate of MI was 9%, and death occurred in 11% of the patients. At least one major event occurred in 28% of the 49 patients. The Washington Hospital Center group has reported on their large experience of treating saphenous vein graft disease. They had a 97% procedural success rate in 1898 lesions that were treated in 1379 patients (*Table 7.4*). In hospital, death occurred in only 0.9% of this population; however, MI developed in 17%. The late clinical outcome shown in *Table 7.5* is less optimistic. Death occurred in 8.4% at 6 months and in 10.2% at 12 months. Clearly, this is a high-risk subgroup of patients. The likelihood of a late clinical event was predicted by the presence of diabetes

Table 7.6

Predictors of a late clinical event. Washington Hospital experience 1996

	p	*Odds ratio*
Diabetes mellitus	0.0001	1.9
Unstable angina	0.001	1.5
Ostial lesion	0.0001	3.1
LV EF	0.0002	28.3

Table 7.4

Washington Hospital experience

1379 pts with 1898 saphenous vein graft lesions

Unstable angina	78%	Degeneration	31%
Graft age (mths)	93±50	Proced. success	97%
Diabetes mellitus	46%	Death	0.9%
Ostial location	2300	MI	17.1%
Thrombus	16%		

Multivariate predictors of failure:Thrombus odds ratio 2.6, *p* = 0.04

Table 7.7

The SAVED Trial. Stent vs PTCA in vein grafts non-ostial lesions, max 2 stents, mean graft age 10 years

	Stent	*PTCA*	*p*
Clinical success	95%	75%	<0.0001
MACE 9 m	27%	42%	<0.05
Restenosis	37%	46%	=0.24

treated with PTCA versus Palmaz–Schatz coronary stents in vein grafts (the SAVED trial),[8] stenting achieved a superior minimum lumen diameter, a higher procedural success, and a lower incidence of repeat bypass surgery. The incidence of restenosis was not statistically different (46% with angioplasty and 37% with stents, p = 0.24), but the incidence of event-free survival at 9 months was 58% for angioplasty and 73% for stenting (p = 0.03) (*Table 7.7*).

In contrast to PTCA, the result of placing a stent in a non-degenerated vein graft does not appear to be influenced by the graft age: acute and long-term results are similar for vein grafts less than or greater than 4 years of age. However, the 2-year event-free survival after vein graft stenting is only 55%, which is similar to the results of angioplasty alone. This attrition in late outcome is due to increasing mortality, recurrent ischemia, and the unfavorable clinical characteristics of many patients with old bypass grafts.

A straightforward example of treating saphenous vein graft disease is shown in *Fig. 7.1*. Although there appears to be a relatively short stenosis in the midsection of the graft, there is also a more proximal 50% narrowing. Rather than just treating the distal stenosis, a 32 mm NIR stent was placed across both lesions (see *Fig. 7.1b*). The 6-month follow-up demonstrated that the vein graft was widely patent with excellent flow into the left anterior descending artery (LAD).

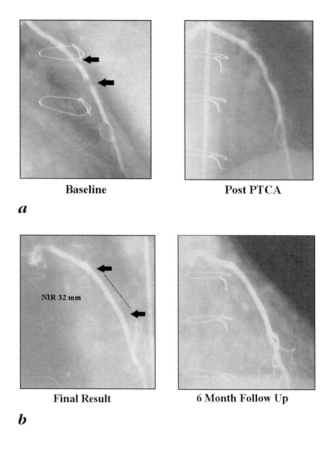

Figure 7.1 *Use of a long NIR stent to treat two lesions in a saphenous vein graft. There was no evidence for restenosis at the six-month follow-up angiogram.*

DEGENERATED GRAFTS

The ideal intervention for degenerated vein grafts is unknown. Some operators recommend TEC atherectomy followed by stent implantation to achieve definitive lumen enlargement, with decreased restenosis compared to balloon dilatation alone.[7] Other authors have recommended a strategy of initial TEC atherectomy followed by 1–2 months of oral warfarin with a staged stent implantation. Compared to the immediate placement of a stent, this deferred stent strategy resulted in less distal embolization (10.7% versus 22.7%) and fewer in-hospital ischemic complications (0% versus 11.4%), but silent total occlusion occurred in 15% of cases. Some authors have reported good results using urokinase infusion into the graft to facilitate the results of stenting. In one report, procedural success was achieved in 93%, with stent thrombosis in 7%, Q-wave myocardial infarction in 3%, and serious vascular injury in 17%.[9]

Because the incidence of distal embolization is high with stent insertion in old vein grafts, the use of other devices has been proposed to debulk the clot and friable tissue within the graft. One device to remove thrombus is the Angiojet, which uses a high-speed saline flush to create a Venturi effect to break up thrombus and then remove it by vacuum.[10]

An example of the Angiojet used in a saphenous vein graft is provided in *Fig. 7.2*. This 60-year-old man with diabetes mellitus developed sudden onset of chest pain with ischemic ECG changes 1 month after five-vessel coronary artery bypass surgery. The initial creatine phosphokinase level was elevated at 250 mg%. The baseline angiogram shows two saphenous vein grafts that emanate from a common ostium. The vein graft to the diagonal artery was patent but the saphenous graft to the obtuse marginal artery was completely occluded after the first centimeter.

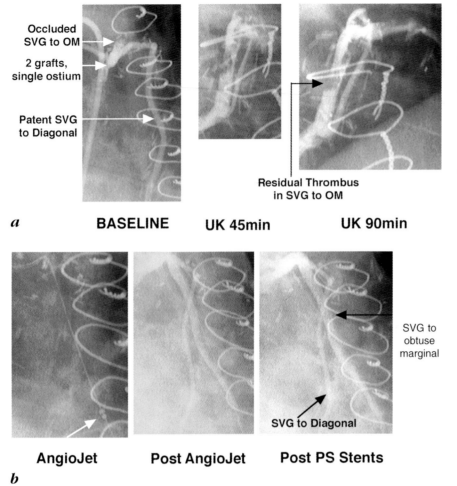

Occluded
SVG to OM

2 grafts,
single ostium

Patent SVG
to Diagonal

Residual Thrombus
in SVG to OM

a   **BASELINE**   **UK 45min**   **UK 90min**

SVG to
obtuse
marginal

SVG to Diagonal

AngioJet   **Post AngioJet**   **Post PS Stents**

b

Figure 7.2 *This saphenous vein graft thrombosed one month after coronary artery bypass surgery. It did not respond to urokinase infusion (a). An Angio jet thrombectomy device was used to remove the clot. This was followed by placement of three Palmaz–Schatz stents into the proximal portion of the vein graft.*

Urokinase was infused through the guiding catheter with some improvement in blood flow, but the angiogram in *Fig. 7.2a* shows a large residual thrombus burden after 90 minutes of urokinase infusion at 4000 units/minute. The Angiojet device was passed over an extra support guidewire and was manipulated to the distal portion of the vein graft (see *Fig. 7.2b*, Panel 1). The Angiojet was turned on for intervals of 45 seconds for a total of five passes. The last pass was performed in the proximal portion of the vein graft after removal of the guidewire. This facilitated lateral motion of the Angiojet to try to pick up more of the clot. The angiogram following the use of the Angiojet is shown in Panel 2 of *Fig. 7.2b*, and no residual thrombus is evident. Three Palmaz stents were placed in the proximal portion of the vein graft (see *Fig. 7.2b*, Panel 3). In this case there was no evidence of distal embolization, either before or after use of the Angiojet.

Another device that is being investigated is called the Exciser. This uses a recessed reverse Archimedes screw, which cuts and extracts thrombus and soft tissue without significant distal embolization. Clinical trials are just beginning with this device. A separate device (Percusurge) has been developed to decrease distal embolization. This device consists of a guidewire that has an inflatable balloon at its tip. The wire can be passed through the vein graft and then the balloon is inflated during the use of any of the thrombectomy devices to prevent embolization of material beyond the graft into the native coronary bed. With this device, stents could be placed in the vein graft and then a final passage of the thrombectomy device could be performed before releasing the distal balloon. Multicenter evaluation of this device is already under way in Europe.[11] Another approach to treating degenerated vein grafts is to use a plastic-covered stent to isolate the lumen from the wall of

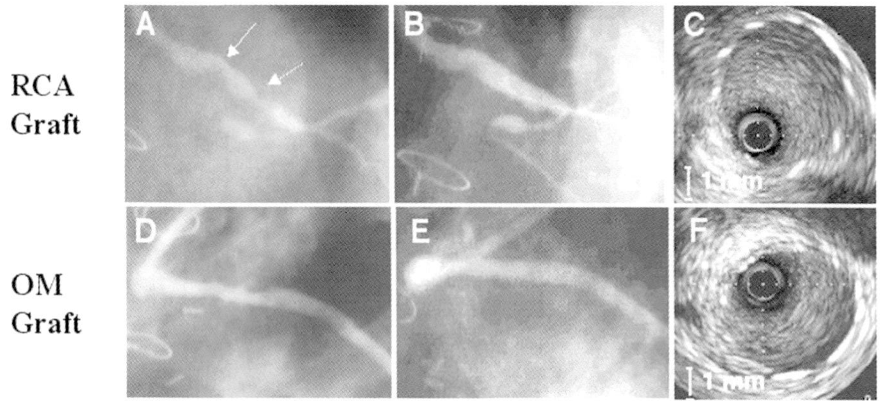

RCA
Graft

OM
Graft

Figure 7.3 *The use of a Wallstent to treat diffuse disease in saphenous vein grafts.*

the vein.[12] Since there are no side branches in a vein graft, there is no need for the stent to be porous. It is hoped that these long plastic-covered stents could decrease the possibility of dislodging friable material within the stent. They may also decrease the restenosis rate by inhibiting the influx of intimal cells.

Among the various stents currently available, the Wallstent is a very useful device for treating saphenous vein graft stenoses. Since the disease process in vein grafts tends to be diffuse and the conduits are long, the self-expanding Wallstent is ideal for this application. Wallstents come in variable lengths and diameters that are appropriate for vein grafts. An example of a diffusely diseased vein graft to a distal right coronary artery is shown in *Fig. 7.3*; Panel A is before insertion of the stent and Panel B is after. The ultrasound image shown in Panel C reveals a widely patent lumen of 5 mm diameter. A second Wallstent was then placed into a vein graft to the obtuse marginal system. The baseline angiogram is shown in Panel D and the angiogram after stent insertion is shown in Panel E. The ultrasound image of the second Wallstent (Panel F) demonstrates the typical symmetrical expansion achieved with this device.

OUR CURRENT APPROACH TO TREATMENT OF SAPHENOUS VEIN GRAFT DISEASE

Our current approach to the treatment of saphenous vein graft disease is to pre-dilate and stent if the lesion is relatively short. If a large thrombus burden is present, we try to remove it with the Angiojet. We

also use abciximab when there is a large thrombus burden or if the vein grafts are more than 7 years old. The treatment of long lesions in vein grafts with long stents is complicated by a 35% incidence of restenosis. In an attempt to lower this restenosis rate, polymer-covered stents such as polytetrafluoroethylene (PTFE) are being developed. It is hoped that the use of PTFE-covered stents may decrease the incidence of restenosis, but the results with this newly developed device are still early. As of May 1998, 32 PTFE-covered stents had been placed in 31 patients at Centro Cuore Columbus. The lesion characteristics included placement of the PTFE stents in 24 de novo lesions (*Table 7.8*). The lesions were located in a saphenous vein graft in 19 cases and in a native coronary artery in 13 cases. An ostial location accounted for 25% of the indications for placing a PTFE-covered stent. Twenty-one of the lesions were

Table 7.8

Initial experience with PTFE-covered stents – lesion characteristics

	Total 32 lesions			
De novo	24 (75%)		Lesion type	
SVG	19 (59%)		A	8
Native artery	13 (41%)		B1	8
LAD	6		B2	3
RCA	6		C	21
OM	1		Indication (/lesion)	
Ostium	8 (25%)		Rupture	3
			Aneurysm	5
			Stenosis	24

type C. The indications for placing the PTFE-covered stent included an arterial rupture in three cases and an aneurysm of the artery in five cases. There was one death associated with placement of a PTFE-covered stent, which was placed urgently into an artery that had ruptured during balloon inflation. The PTFE-covered stent was placed in an attempt to stop the arterial bleeding. This patient was sent to bypass surgery but suffered a significant myocardial infarction during the angioplasty and died subsequently. From a technical standpoint, the stents are relatively easy to place, although the stent is stiffer than single layered stents. The procedure success rate without a major adverse cardiac event was 97%.

The rationale for using a plastic-covered stent is that the circumferential layer of plastic may inhibit the growth of intimal cells and thus prevent restenosis. This device would be appropriate for arterial segments that do not have branching vessels, such as vein grafts. An example of the PTFE-covered stent is shown in Chapter 2, *Fig. 2.49*. In this configuration, the PTFE is sandwiched between two slotted tubular stents. The entire system is low profile and can fit in a 6 Fr guiding catheter. The following provides a guideline for deploying the PTFE-covered stent:

(a) the lesion is pre-dilated with a long balloon 2.0 mm or 2.5 mm in diameter at a pressure sufficient to obtain full balloon expansion;
(b) the stent is deployed without oversizing the balloon at a pressure not to exceed 12 atmospheres; this is done to avoid any trauma to the pliable vein graft with consequent distal embolization. It is important to keep the balloon inflated for at least 1 minute to allow full stent expansion;
(c) intravascular ultrasound (IVUS) imaging is performed to confirm that adequate apposition and lumen size are obtained. The stent is redilated only if the stent lumen is smaller than the distal reference segment of the graft.

This approach differs somewhat from our usual concept of trying to achieve the maximal possible stent lumen. The reasoning behind this approach is the need to reduce the risk of distal embolization which, we believe, occurs when more aggressive stent dilatation is performed inside a vein graft. Even with a covered stent, thrombus or friable tissue can be expressed longitudinally behind the stent, like toothpaste from a tube, and embolize downstream.

A clinical example of a PTFE-covered stent that was placed in a vein graft is shown in *Fig. 7.4*. The

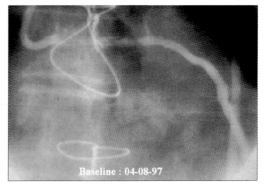

Complex (ulcerated) plaque post SVG PTCA

a

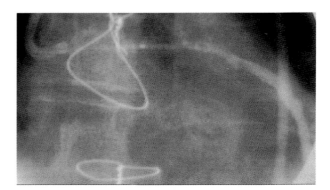

JOMED 16 mm PTFE covered Stent in place

b

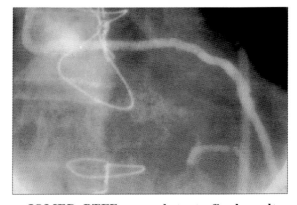

JOMED PTFE covered stent : final result

c

Figure 7.4

baseline angiogram demonstrates a complex ulcerated plaque in the proximal portion of the vein graft extending to the aorto-ostial junction. This was pre-dilated with a 3 mm balloon and then a JOMED

Baseline

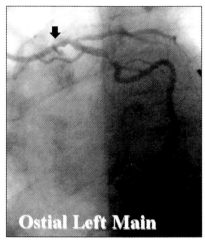

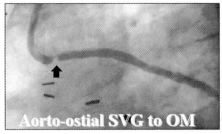

IABP support

a

Final Result

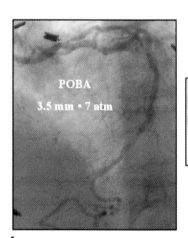

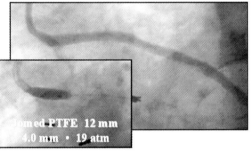

b

Figure 7.5 *Treatment of a stenosis at the aorto-ostial junction in a saphenous vein graft to an obtuse marginal artery. This was a high-risk patient with poor left ventricular function. He was pretreated with placement of an intra-aortic balloon pump. A 12 mm long JoMed PTFE covered stent was used to treat the vein graft. The native left coronary system was also treated with balloon angioplasty.*

16 mm long PTFE-covered stent was placed in the lesion (see *Fig. 7.4b*). The stent was inflated at 12 atmospheres with a 3 mm balloon, and the final results are demonstrated in *Fig. 7.4c*.

A second example of the use of a PTFE-covered stent for treatment of saphenous vein graft disease is provided in *Fig. 7.5*. This high-risk patient had poor left ventricular function associated with an aorto-ostial stenosis in the saphenous vein graft to an obtuse marginal artery, as well as native coronary artery disease involving the ostium of the left main coronary artery. The saphenous vein graft was treated first by placing a 12 mm long JOMED PTFE-covered stent on a 4 mm balloon that was expanded to 19

atmospheres. During this procedure, the patient was supported prophylactically with an intra-aortic balloon pump. The left main artery was treated with balloon dilatation alone using a 3.5 mm balloon expanded at 7 atmospheres.

ARTERIAL CONDUIT GRAFTS

In addition to dealing with saphenous vein grafts, the interventionalist occasionally has to respond to problems in free-standing autologous arterial grafts. The case shown in *Fig. 7.6* describes a complication

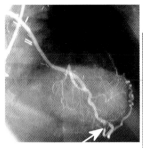

**Lesion in Distal LAD
Collaterals to OM**

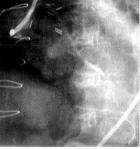

**Dissection and
Closure of RIMA**

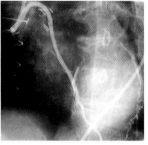

**After 5
Multilink Stents**

Figure 7.6 *Reconstruction of a dissected right internal mammary artery graft*

that may occur when working with these transplanted arteries. The patient had a 10-year-old right internal mammary artery (RIMA) graft that was detached from its origin and reinserted from the ascending aorta into the mid-LAD. Although the body of the graft appeared angiographically intact, a severe lesion had developed in the distal LAD, which compromised collateral blood flow to the lateral wall. There was evidence of ischemia on a thallium study. We were able to pass a guidewire and a 2.0 mm balloon easily through the arterial graft into the distal LAD and successfully dilated the stenosis. Immediately after balloon dilatation, there was markedly reduced flow in the bypass graft. It was not immediately apparent whether this was a dissection, spasm, or 'no reflow' phenomenon since there was no obvious guidewire or guide catheter trauma to the graft. However, the poor flow did not respond to intracoronary nitrates or verapamil. We concluded that this had to be due to an extensive dissection throughout the RIMA graft. An intra-aortic balloon pump was inserted and abciximab was started. This complication was successfully treated by the placement of five sequential Multilink stents expanded with a 3.0 mm balloon.

Treatment of lesions within the left internal mammary artery (LIMA) or distal to its anastomosis can be difficult, owing to tortuosity of the vessel and its propensity for spasm. An example of this is demonstrated in *Fig. 7.7*, where there is a tight stenosis in the body of the LIMA prior to the anastomosis with an obtuse marginal artery. Pre-imaging the stenosis with IVUS demonstrated that the media-to-media boundary was slightly less than 4 mm.

Therefore a 3.5 mm balloon was used to dilate the lesion at 6 atmospheres (see *Fig. 7.7b*). A flexible 15 mm long DivYsio stent was placed in the LIMA, and the 3.5 mm balloon was dilated to 20 atmospheres; the final result is shown in *Fig. 7.7c*. The ultrasound examination revealed a symmetrical lumen of 3.4 mm in diameter.

MILAN RESULTS WITH SAPHENOUS VEIN GRAFT LESIONS

The results of our experience with stenting saphenous vein grafts are provided in *Tables 7.9, 7.10,*

Table 7.9
Coronary stenting in saphenous vein grafts

	n (%)
No. of patients	71
No. of lesions	93
No. of stents/lesion	1.4 ± 0.9
Total stent length (mm)	26 ± 15
Age, yr	63 ± 8
Male	57 (90%)
EF	53 ± 14%
Angiographic success	88 (99%)
Angiographic F/U	52 (68%)
IVUS used	53 (60%)

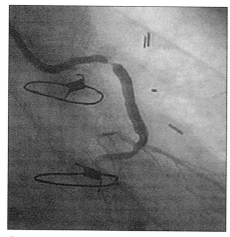

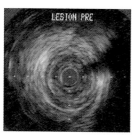

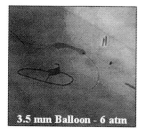

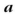

Baseline

a

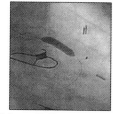

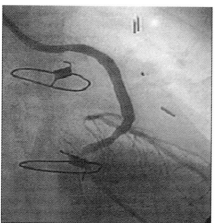

3.5 mm Balloon - 6 atm

b

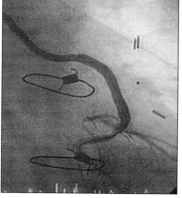

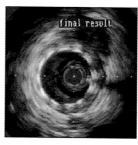

3.5 mm Balloon - 20 atm

c

Final Result

Figure 7.7 *Implantation of a DivYsio stent in the body of a left internal mammary artery graft to an obtuse marginal artery. The LIMA (left internal mammary artery) measured almost 4.0 mm on the preintervention IVUS exam. A 3.5 mm balloon was used to pre-dilate the lesion and then expand the stent at 20 atmospheres.*

7.11 and *7.12.* In 93 vein grafts, the mean total stent length was 26 ± 15 mm, which represents our preference for using long stents in these diffusely diseased grafts (see *Table 7.9*). Stent deployment was successful in 99% of the cases. The variety of stents that were used is shown in *Table 7.10*. The high use of the Palmaz–Schatz stent was due to the initial availability of this stent in our early experience. Our

Table 7.10

Coronary stenting in saphenous vein grafts

Type of stents	n	(%)
Palmaz–Schatz	33	(36%)
Wallstent	24	(26%)
JOMED PTFE	15	(16%)
NIR	7	(8%)
BeStent	3	(3%)
Cook GR I	2	(2%)
IRIS	2	(2%)
PURA	2	(2%)
AVE	1	(1%)
TENSUM	1	(1%)
DivYsio	1	(1%)
Paragon	1	(1%)

Table 7.11

Coronary Stenting in saphenous vein grafts. Angiographic measurements

	Pre	Final	F/U
Ref. diam. (mm)	3.3 ± 0.7	3.5 ± 0.7	3.4 ± 0.6
MLD (mm)	1.1 ± 0.6	3.4 ± 0.6	2.1 ± 1.5
Percentage diameter stenosis	67 ± 16	0.4 ± 12	41 ± 40
Lesion length (mm)	13 ± 8		

IVUS measurements	
Prox. ref. L-CSA (mm²)	10.9 ± 5.2
Stented L-CSA (mm²)	8.8 ± 3.4
Distal ref. L-CSA (mm²)	9.6 ± 4.6

Table 7.12

Early or late outcome after coronary stenting in saphenous vein grafts

	n	(%)
No. of patients	71	
No. of lesions	93	
Procedure		
MI	4	(7%)
CABG	1	(1%)
Death	0	
Stent thrombosis		
Acute	0	
Subacute	1	(2%)
Out-of-hospital		
MI	2	(4%)
CABG	1	(2%)
Death	9	(17%)
Angiographic F/U	52	(68%)
Angiographic restenosis	18	(36%)

SUMMARY

In summary, the only role of balloon angioplasty for treating saphenous vein graft lesions is in the treatment of distal anastomotic stenoses. For treating focal lesions with a vein graft, the best approach is to place a stent. The necessity for debulking depends on the amount of thrombus present. The use of abciximab significantly improves the acute results; however, the long-term outcome is related not only to successful treatment of the target lesion, but also to disease progression in the untreated portion in all the grafts. Studies are currently in progress to assess the benefits of angiographic treatment of non-critical areas located in vein grafts. Technical developments in stent design have made vein graft intervention safer. Although still experimental, PTFE-covered stents are being evaluated for treatment of disease at the aorto-ostial junction or for long lesions within degenerated grafts. Radioactive beta-emitting stents may also have a role in treating these diffusely involved vein grafts. In addition, the development of oral 2B3A platelet inhibitors may have significant benefit in preventing thrombotic events after the stent is placed.

current preference would be to use a more flexible and longer stent, such as the Wallstent, the NIR, or the PTFE-covered stent. The angiographic and IVUS measurements are provided in *Table 7.11*. The clinical outcome in our patient population is shown in *Table 7.12*. There were no immediate deaths related to the procedure but, in follow-up, death occurred in 17% of patients. This is a high incidence of mortality but is similar to the Washington Hospital Center experience. Of the 52 lesions that had angiographic follow-up, restenosis was evident in 18 (36%).

REFERENCES

1. Mehran R, Lansky A, Hong MK et al. Percutaneous revascularization of patients with prior coronary bypass surgery: saphenous vein graft or native coronary stenting? *J Am Coll Cardiol* 1999; **33**: 51A.

2. Borst C, Grundeman PF. Minimally invasive coronary artery bypass grafting: an experimental perspective. *Circulation* 1999; **99**: 1400–1403.

3. Meester BJ, Samson M, Suryapranata H et al. Long-term follow-up after attempted angioplasty of saphenous vein grafts: the Thoraxcenter experience 1981–1988. *Eur Heart J* 1991; **12**: 648–653.

4. Morrison DA, Crowley ST, Veerakul G et al. Percutaneous transluminal angioplasty of saphenous vein grafts for medically refractory unstable angina. *J Am Coll Cardiol* 1994; **23**: 1066–1070.

5. Holmes DR Jr, Topol EJ, Califf RM et al. A multicenter, randomized trial of coronary angioplasty versus directional atherectomy for patients with saphenous vein bypass graft lesions. CAVEAT-II Investigators. *Circulation.*1995; **91**: 1966–1974.

6. Ellis SG, Brener SJ, DeLuca S et al. Late myocardial ischemic events after saphenous vein graft intervention – importance of initially 'nonsignificant' vein graft lesions. *Am J Cardiol* 1997; **79**: 1460–1464.

7. Braden GA, Xenopoulos NP, Young T et al. Transluminal extraction catheter atherectomy followed by immediate stenting in treatment of saphenous vein grafts. *J Am Coll Cardiol* 1997; **30**: 657–663.

8. Savage MP, Douglas JS Jr, Fischman DL et al. Stent placement compared with balloon angioplasty for obstructed coronary bypass grafts. Saphenous Vein De Novo Trial Investigators. *N Engl J Med* 1997; **337**: 740–747.

9. Denardo SJ, Morris NB, Rocha-Singh KJ et al. Safety and efficacy of extended urokinase infusion plus stent deployment for treatment of obstructed, older saphenous vein grafts. *Am J Cardiol* 1995; **76**: 776–780.

10. Hamburger JN, Serruys PW. Treatment of thrombus containing lesions in diseased native coronary arteries and saphenous vein bypass grafts using the AngioJet Rapid Thrombectomy System. *Herz* 1997; **22**: 318–321.

11. Grube E, Webb J. The SAFE study: multicenter evaluation of a protection catheter system for distal embolization in coronary venous bypass grafts (abstract). *J Am Coll Cardiol* 1999; **33**: 37A.

12. Moussa I, Inglese L, Di Mario C et al. Immediate and short-term results of the implantation of PTFE covered stents in saphenous vein grafts (abstract). *Eur Heart J* 1998; **19**: P2822.

Chapter 8 Long lesions in arteries with diffuse disease

Antonio Colombo and Jonathan Tobis

Perhaps with the exception of bifurcation lesions, there are few other conditions that are more difficult to treat than long lesions in arteries with diffuse disease. When only the 15 mm long Palmaz–Schatz stent and the 20 mm long Gianturco–Roubin I stent were available, patients with diffuse disease had to be treated with multiple stents. These were difficult to deliver and it was hard to know the exact placement of the serial stents. Technical alterations in stent flexibility, profile, and length have significantly improved our ability to treat patients with diffuse disease. Unfortunately, the restenosis rate is still quite high in patients with long lesions. This is probably due to a combination of increased restenosis with longer stented length[1] and greater plaque burden,[2,3] as well as to the fact that long lesions taper distally and result in a smaller minimum lumen diameter (MLD). Our approach to treating long lesions has changed over the past few years. This chapter reviews our experience and describes several ways that we have tried to treat these challenging lesions.

The definition of a long lesion is not clearly stipulated. We have segregated the length of stented artery into three groups: ≤ 20 mm, > 20 but ≤ 35 mm, or > 35 mm in length. Between April 1993 and March 1997, we treated 2313 lesions in 1706 patients with intracoronary stents. As shown in *Table 8.1*, there were 607 lesions between 20 mm and 35 mm, and 433 lesions > 35 mm in length. A significant proportion (23%) of the patients with the longest lesions had chronic total occlusions. The distribution of the arteries treated and the type of stents used are described in *Table 8.2*. The Palmaz–Schatz stent was used more commonly in the shorter stenoses whereas the newer, longer stents tended to be used in lesions > 20 mm. As shown in *Table 8.3*, a higher number of stents per lesion was used with longer lesions (this number had more significance when stents were only

Table 8.1

Stenting long lesions. Clinical background

	Stented segment ≤ 20 mm	*Stented segment $> 20 \leq 35$*	*Stented segment > 35 mm*	*p*
Lesions	1273	607	433	
Prior MI (%)	52	54	65	0.01
Prior CABG (%)	10	10	10	NS
Elective stent (%)	69	64	53	0.01
Restenotic lesion (%)	7	6	2	0.01
CTO	4	12	23	0.01

Table 8.2

Stenting long lesions. Arteries and stents

	Stented segment ≤ 20 mm	*Stented segment $> 20 \leq 35$*	*Stented segment > 35 mm*	*p*
Lesions	1273	607	433	
LAD (%)	47	53	47	NS
RCA (%)	25	27	35	0.01
LCX (%)	22	17	14	0.01
Type of stent (%)				
Palmaz–Schatz	59	41	22	0.01
Combinations	1	9	28	0.01
Wallstent	1	4	14	0.01
Gianturco–Roubin	8	2	13	0.01
NIR	10	17	6	0.01
AVE	6	6	6	NS
Wiktor	5	4	3	NS
ACS Multilink	4	2	2	NS
Crown	1	4	1	0.01
Cordis	2	2	1	NS

Table 8.3

Stenting long lesions. Results

	Stented segment ≤ 20 mm	Stented segment > 20 ≤ 35	Stented segment > 35 mm	p
Lesions	1273	607	433	
Stents per lesion	1.0	1.6	2.6	0.01
Stent length (mm)	15.0 ± 3.3	29.2 ± 3.8	53.5 ± 18.5	<0.0001
Final balloon (mm)	3.5 ± 0.5	3.6 ± 0.5	3.6 ± 0.5	0.01
CABG (%)	1.5	1.8	2.5	NS
Death (%)	0.1	0.9	0.3	0.05
Subacute thrombosis (%)	0.9	1.7	2.7	0.05

Table 8.4

Stenting long lesions. Angiographic results

	Stented segment ≤ 20 mm	Stented segment > 20 ≤ 35	Stented segment > 35 mm	p
Lesions	1273	607	433	
Angio F-Up (%)	68	70	74	
Reference (mm)	3.06 ± 0.5	3.02 ± 0.5	3.01 ± 0.6	ns
MLD pre (mm)	0.99 ± 0.5	0.84 ± 0.5	0.70 ± 0.6	0.01
Stenosis post (%)	0.9 ± 13	0.2 ± 13	4 ± 14	0.01
Les. length (mm)	9.1 ± 5.2	12.3 ± 6.9	14.8 ± 9.9	0.01
Acute gain (mm)	2.11 ± 0.67	2.29 ± 0.66	2.29 ± 0.74	0.01
Late loss (mm)	0.94 + 0.84	1.12 + 0.97	1.39 + 0.91	0.01
Loss index	0.44 + 1.09	0.51 ± 0.48	0.62 + 0.74	0.05

available in 15 mm and 20 mm lengths). A more meaningful number in its effect on restenosis is the mean stent length, which is also provided in *Table 8.3*. The mean stent length increased among the three groups from 15 mm to 29 mm, with 54 mm for the longest group. There was a high rate of success with the first two groups but a slightly lower rate of procedural success (92%) in lesions that were longer than 35 mm. In this third subgroup, the incidence of bypass surgery was higher, although this did not reach statistical significance. The incidence of subacute thrombosis was also higher in the group with stented segments > 35 mm (2.7%; $p < 0.05$). Although the overall death rate was low, it was slightly higher in the group with lesions between 20 and 35 mm ($p < 0.05$).

The angiographic analysis showed that there was no significant difference in the proximal reference lumen size for any of the three groups although the MLD was slightly smaller in the group with the longest lesions (*Table 8.4*). The lesion length was statistically different in the three groups. Although the mean lesion length for the third group was 14.8 ± 9.9 mm, these patients had more diffuse disease and therefore received longer stents even though the primary lesion was not as long as the stented segment. A second reason that the stented length could be significantly longer than the lesion length is dissection. This inconsistency is created by the artificial definition of lesion length, which is measured from the shoulders of an assumed normal segment of the artery; with diffuse disease, there often is no

normal segment. Although the acute gain was similar in all three groups, the late lumen loss was greater in the patients who received longer stents with an increase in loss index from 0.44 to 0.62. The intravascular ultrasound findings paralleled the angiographic results in that the stented lumen minimum cross-sectional area was significantly smaller, at 6.82 mm², for the patients who received stents longer than 35 mm (*Table 8.5*).

The restenosis rates for the 1633 patients who had angiographic follow-up at 6 months is shown in *Fig. 8.1*. The restenosis rate was 19% for stents < 20 mm,

Table 8.5

Stenting long lesions. IVUS results

	Stented segment ≤20 mm	Stented segment >20 ≤35	Stented segment >35 mm	p
Lesions	1273	607	433	
Prox. ref. CSA (mm²)	8.99	9.19	9.21	NS
Stent CSA	7.85	7.58	6.82	<0.01

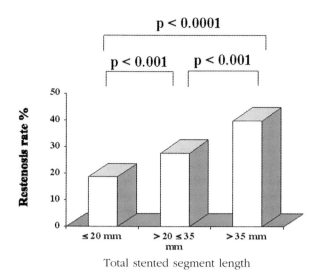

Figure 8.1 *Restenosis after stenting long lesions*

28% for stents 20–35 mm, and 40% for lesions with stent segments > 35 mm in length (p < 0.0001). Lesions in which there was restenosis (n = 409) are compared to the group of lesions without restenosis (n = 1224) in *Table 8.6*. By multivariate analysis, the three significant predictors of restensosis were longer stent length, smaller reference lumen diameter, and smaller final percent stenosis. It is interesting to note that although the final minimum lumen diameter was significantly different between the two groups (3.2 ± 0.6 mm versus 2.9 ± 0.5 mm), this was not independently predictive of restenosis and did not enter into the multiple logistic regression model.

CLINICAL EXAMPLES

PALMAZ–SCHATZ STENTS

An example of how long lesions were treated during our early experience is shown in *Fig. 8.2*. This lesion in the proximal to mid-left anterior descending artery (LAD) measured 32 mm in length and contained three sharp bends. Since long stents were not available at this time, a total of six Palmaz–Schatz half stents were inserted sequentially. The half stents were prepared by cutting a 15 mm Palmaz–Schatz stent at the articulation, then hand crimping the stent to a balloon.[4] Although laborious, the process can be performed expeditiously and the shorter length and bare stenting technique improved the trackability during passage of the stent (see Chapter 6 for more on bare stenting). The stented segment was dilated to 12 atmospheres with a 4.0 mm balloon, with an excellent angiographic result (see *Fig. 8.2b*). Interrogation with intravascular ultrasound (IVUS), however, demonstrated a section that was unsupported by stent struts with a cross-sectional area of only 6.5 mm² (Panel C). Repeat dilatation was performed at 16 atmospheres and resulted in an enlarged lumen area of 9.9 mm² (see *Fig. 8.2c*), which is impressive considering the diffuse nature of the lesion at baseline.

STENTING LONG LESIONS WITH A SINGLE STENT

Another example of a long lesion in the proximal LAD is shown in *Fig. 8.3*. This stenosis was first treated with rotational atherectomy using a 1.5 mm burr followed by pre-dilatation with a balloon of

Table 8.6
Stenting long lesions. Angiographic follow-up

	No restenosis *n = 1224*	*Restenosis* *n = 409*	*Univ*	*Mult*
Stent length (mm)	24.1 ± 14.9	30.8 ± 19.1	< 0.001	< 0.001
Refer. diameter (mm)	3.12 ± 0.52	2.84 ± 0.51	< 0.001	< 0.001
Final % stenosis	0 ± 13	3 ± 14	< 0.01	< 0.01
Multiple stenting (%)	30	41	< 0.001	NS
Final MLD (mm)	3.17 ± 0.56	2.89 ± 0.52	< 0.001	NS
Lesion length (mm)	10.7 ± 7.0	12.1 ± 7.5	< 0.01	NS

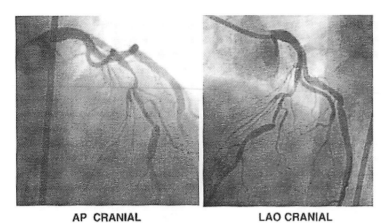

AP CRANIAL   LAO CRANIAL

Lesion Length = 32 mm

a

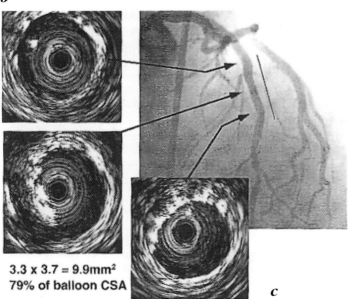

4.0 mm 12 atm

2.7 x 3.2 = 6.5 mm²
51% of balloon CSA

b

3.3 x 3.7 = 9.9mm²
79% of balloon CSA

c

Figure 8.2 *Treatment of diffuse disease with the Palmaz–Schatz stent. (a) A 32 mm long tortuous lesion in the proximal and mid-left anterior ascending coronary artery. (b) The stenosis was treated by cutting three Palmaz–Schatz stents in half. The six short stents were then placed sequentially throughout the length of the stenosis. The shorter length of the cut stent facilitated passage through the tortuous segments. (c) To optimize the cross-sectional area as documented by IVUS imaging, repeat balloon inflation was performed at 16 atmospheres with a 4.0 mm balloon.*

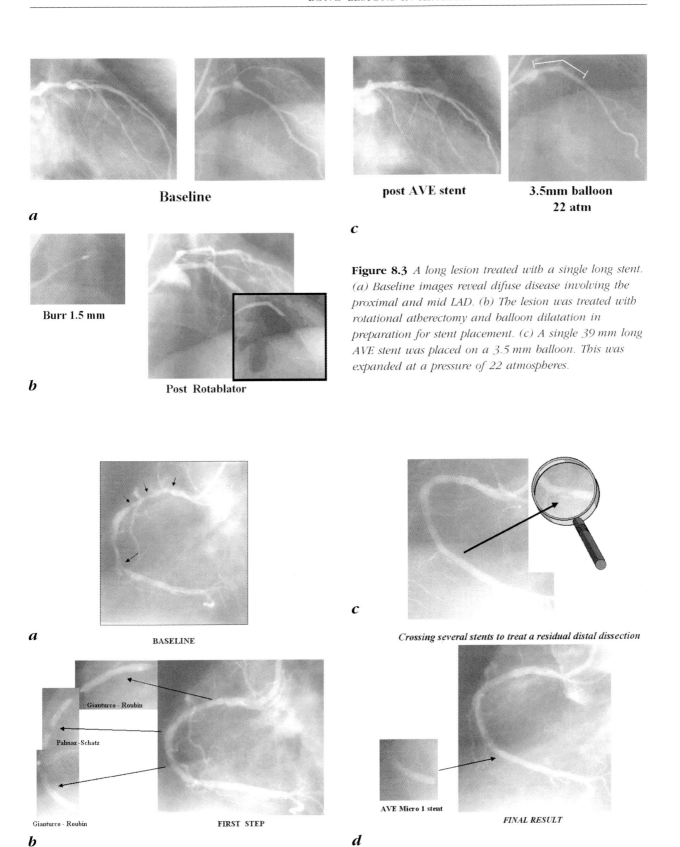

Figure 8.3 *A long lesion treated with a single long stent. (a) Baseline images reveal difuse disease involving the proximal and mid LAD. (b) The lesion was treated with rotational atherectomy and balloon dilatation in preparation for stent placement. (c) A single 39 mm long AVE stent was placed on a 3.5 mm balloon. This was expanded at a pressure of 22 atmospheres.*

Figure 8.4 *Multiple stents for diffuse disease. (a) Baseline angiogram reveals diffuse sequential stenoses throughout the proximal and mid-right coronary artery. (b) A combination of Gianturco–Roubin I and Palmaz–Schatz stents was used. (c) A dissection that was inadequately supported by the GR I stent. (d) This was treated by placing a single AVE Micro1 stent inside the GR 1 stent.*

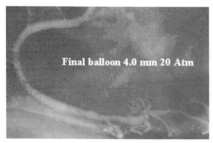

A   **Baseline**

Ref Vessel	3.06 mm
MLD	0.64 mm
Diam. Stenosis	79 %

B   **After 35mm beStent**

Ref Vessel	2.99 mm
MLD	3.46 mm
Diam. Stenosis	- 16 %

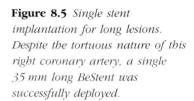

Figure 8.5 *Single stent implantation for long lesions. Despite the tortuous nature of this right coronary artery, a single 35 mm long BeStent was successfully deployed.*

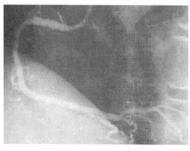

C   **4 months Follow-Up**

Ref Vessel	3.11 mm
MLD	2.00 mm
Diam. Stenosis	36 %

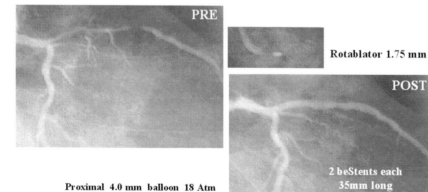

Figure 8.6 *Treatment of long calcified lesions. This diffusely diseased and calcified proximal LAD was treated with rotational atherectomy followed by the placement of two BeStents.*

3.5 mm diameter and 40 mm length. A 39 mm long AVE stent was inserted and then post-dilated at 22 atmospheres. The subselective final angiographic result shows a smooth, large lumen throughout the stented segment. The comparison of these first two cases dramatizes the technologic changes that have occurred in coronary stenting.

STENTING LONG LESIONS WITH STENT COMBINATIONS

A right coronary artery (RCA) with more extensive disease is demonstrated in *Fig. 8.4*. After pre-dilatation, this artery was treated with a combination of stents using a Gianturco–Roubin I stent in the proximal and

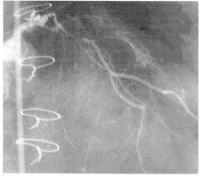

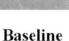

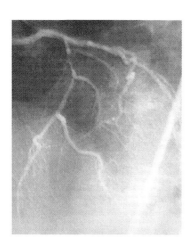

Baseline

a

Figure 8.7 *Treatment of long diffuse disease with a 32 mm long NIR 7 cell stent.*

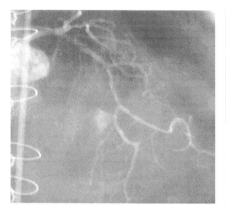

Following PTCA

b

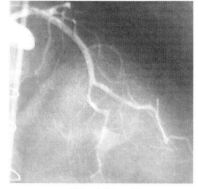

Stent deployment

Stent 15 atm dilatation

c

Final Result

distal segments and a Palmaz–Schatz stent for the mid-section (see *Fig. 8.4b*). Following post-deployment balloon inflation, there was a dissection in the distal Gianturco–Roubin I stent (see *Fig. 8.4c*). This was treated by passing a flexible AVE stent through the proximal and mid-stents to buttress the wall in the dissected zone. At the present time, there are lower-profile, longer stents that could be used instead of those used initially, but this and other examples will demonstrate how the treatment of diffuse disease has evolved over the past few years as the technology has changed.

Figure 8.5 (Panel A) shows an RCA with a severe stenosis in the proximal portion and a more moderate stenosis in the mid-section. This was treated with one long 35 mm BeStent. The stent was expanded after deployment with a 4 mm diameter balloon at 20 atmospheres with a final MLD of 3.46 mm (*Fig. 8.5*, Panel B). Figure 8.5 (Panel C) shows the result at 4

months: there is significant intimal hyperplasia in the proximal portion of the artery; however, the MLD is still acceptable at 2.0 mm or 36% diameter stenosis.

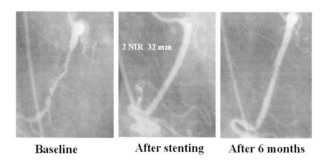

Baseline   After stenting   After 6 months

Figure 8.8 *Six months follow-up after treatment for diffuse disease.*

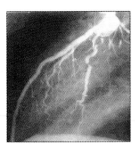
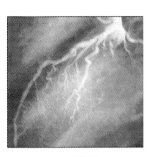

Figure 8.9 *The NIR stent for long lesions.*

Baseline	Final Result	1 year F-Up
Ref Vessel 2.11 mm	Ref Vessel 2.65 mm	Ref Vessel 2.66 mm
MLD 0.70 mm	MLD 2.82 mm	MLD 1.19 mm
Diam. Stenosis 67 %	Diam. Stenosis - 7 %	Diam. Stenosis 55 %

ROTATIONAL ATHERECTOMY AS AN ADJUNCT FOR TREATING LONG LESIONS

The treatment of a long calcified lesion is shown in *Fig. 8.6*. This extensive disease in the proximal and mid-LAD was initially treated with rotational atherectomy with progressively larger burrs. This was followed by placement of two BeStents, each 35 mm in length. The proximal portion of the artery was dilated with a 4 mm balloon at 18 atmospheres and, owing to tapering, the distal stent was dilated with a 3.5 mm balloon at 24 atmospheres. The size of the balloon was chosen on the basis of the ultrasound image, which demonstrated that proximally the media-to-media vessel diameter was 4 mm. Rotational atherectomy is extremely useful in obtaining an optimal result when treating patients with diffuse disease. By removing some of the plaque burden and changing the compliance of calcified lesions, the stent can be expanded more completely with a greater final MLD.[5,6]

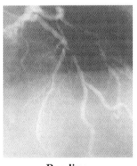
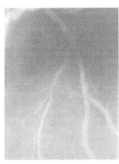
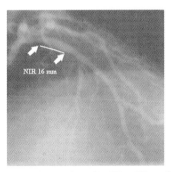

Baseline	Post PTCA	6 months Follow-Up Final Result

a

c

Figure 8.10 *Peri-stent restensosis following deployment of a 32 mm long NIR stent.*

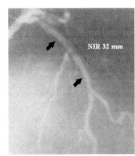
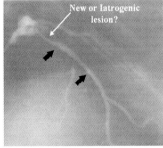

Final Result	6 months F-Up

b

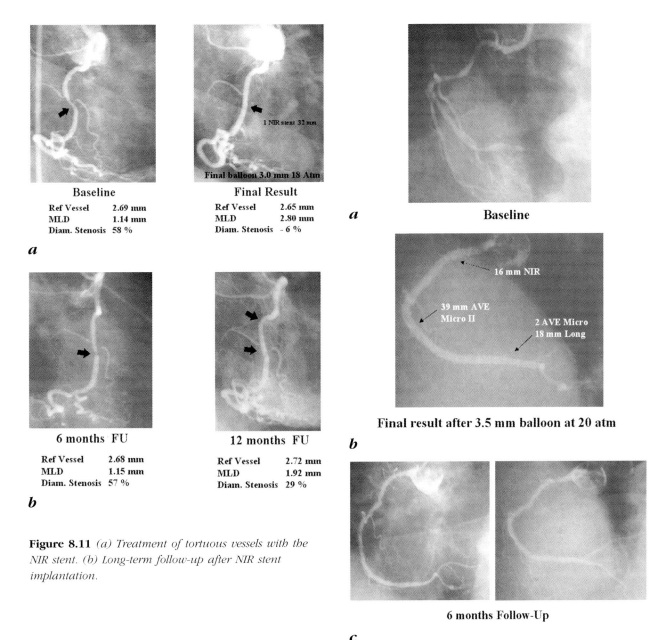

Baseline

Ref Vessel	2.69 mm
MLD	1.14 mm
Diam. Stenosis	58 %

a

Final Result

Ref Vessel	2.65 mm
MLD	2.80 mm
Diam. Stenosis	- 6 %

6 months FU

Ref Vessel	2.68 mm
MLD	1.15 mm
Diam. Stenosis	57 %

b

12 months FU

Ref Vessel	2.72 mm
MLD	1.92 mm
Diam. Stenosis	29 %

Figure 8.11 *(a) Treatment of tortuous vessels with the NIR stent. (b) Long-term follow-up after NIR stent implantation.*

a   **Baseline**

b   **Final result after 3.5 mm balloon at 20 atm**

c   **6 months Follow-Up**

Figure 8.12 *Vessel reconstruction. (a) Baseline angiogram of a diffusely diseased right coronary artery. (b) 'Full metal jacket'. The use of multiple stents to cover over 70 mm length of diseased artery. (c) Surprisingly, the six-month follow-up angiogram does not reveal any significant restenosis.*

THE NIR STENT FOR LONG LESIONS

Another long, diffusely diseased artery is demonstrated in *Fig. 8.7a.* Following balloon dilatation at 10 atmospheres with a 3.0 mm balloon, the LAD lumen is improved but has several areas of dissection (see *Fig. 8.7b*). A 32 mm long, seven-cell NIR stent was deployed in the proximal to mid-LAD and post-dilated at 15 atmospheres with a 3.0 mm × 20 mm balloon. The final result shows a widely patent lumen with smooth borders in this previously diffusely diseased vessel (see *Fig. 8.7c*).

Another example of the use of the 32 mm NIR stent is shown in *Fig. 8.8.* In this diffusely narrowed RCA,

two NIR 32 mm long stents were placed in tandem throughout the length of the proximal and mid-RCA. In this instance, not only is the immediate result significantly improved, but at 6 months there is only minimal narrowing in a short segment of the RCA.

A third example of use of the NIR stent for long lesions is shown in *Fig. 8.9.* The mid- to distal section of this diffusely diseased LAD was treated with three NIR stents, each 32 mm long, and was post-inflated with a 3.0 mm balloon at 20 atmospheres, with an excellent immediate result. In addition, the 1-year follow-up demonstrated continued patency and acceptable lumen size despite the diffuse nature of the disease and the distal position of the stent.

FOLLOW-UP STUDIES: RESTENOSIS

Although the use of longer stents to treat diffuse disease has improved the initial success rate, restenosis remains a major concern. This is demonstrated in *Fig. 8.10* where there is a long irregular lesion in the proximal to mid-LAD. A 32 mm long NIR stent was placed overlapping the large first septal perforator. This was expanded with a 3.5 mm balloon. On the 6-month follow-up angiogram (see *Fig. 8.10b*), there is some mild intimal encroachment in the distal portion of the stent but there is no hemodynamically significant in-stent restenosis; however, proximal to the stent, there is an area of severe tubular narrowing that was not present at the time of the initial study. Whether this rapid progression of luminal narrowing is due to intimal hyperplasia from the presence of the stent or trauma during insertion or whether it represents progression of atherosclerosis is unknown. This narrowing was treated by balloon dilatation and placement of a 16 mm long NIR stent, with the final result shown in *Fig. 8.10c.* Currently, we would approach the initial lesion by using a shorter stent, probably a 15 mm AVE stent. Even though this may not completely cover the distal aspect of the lesion, the balloon dilatation would be adequate and the predicted restenosis rate would be lessened by using a shorter stent.

A variation of the possible alternatives that can occur during follow-up is demonstrated in *Fig. 8.11.* This RCA was a moderately tortuous vessel with a concentric stenosis in the mid-portion. This was treated with one NIR stent, 32 mm in length, which was expanded with a 3.0 mm balloon at 18 atmospheres. The final result was successful with an MLD of 2.8 mm, which was larger than the reference vessel segment, giving a diameter stenosis of –6%. The 6- and 12-month follow-up angiograms are shown in *Fig. 8.11b.* At 6 months there was angiographic evidence of restenosis at the site of the original lesion, with an MLD of 1.15 mm and

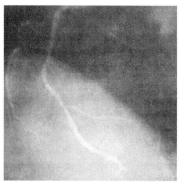

a **Baseline**

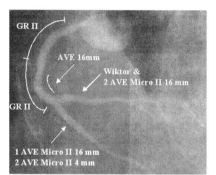

b **Following vessel reconstruction**

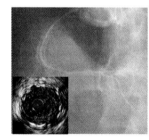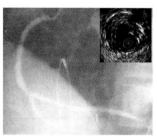

6 months Follow-Up   **Following 2.0mm Excimer Laser + 2.5mm RTB**

c

Figure 8.13 *Vessel reconstruction with development of diffuse in-stent restenosis. (a) Baseline angiogram. (b) Placement of multiple variety of intracoronary stents. (c) Angiogram follow-up at six months reveals diffuse in-stent restenosis. This was treated with an aggressive attempt to remove the neointimal hyperplasia with an excimer laser and a 2.5 mm rotablator burr.*

diameter stenosis of 57%. Despite this quantitative coronary angiography (QCA) result, no intervention was performed because the patient was asymptomatic and had a negative stress test. Six months after the follow-up angiogram and 12 months after the original angioplasty, the lumen was patent and the MLD was enlarged at 1.92 mm, which represents only a 29% diameter stenosis. This finding is consistent with the serial angiographic studies from Kimura who showed that in-stent luminal narrowing may regress over time. This case also exemplifies how our approach to stenting has evolved. We now look back on this case and recognize that we would approach this lesion differently today: we would choose a shorter, more flexible stent. However, the patient did well clinically with the device that was available at the time.

VESSEL RECONSTRUCTION

The treatment of long, diffuse disease frequently requires the placement of multiple stents to reconstruct the artery. This is especially true when treating the RCA, which is primarily a long conduit that provides blood to the posterolateral and inferior walls of the left ventricle. An example of this is demonstrated in *Fig. 8.12*, which shows an RCA with diffuse disease throughout the proximal and mid-sections as well as occlusion of the bifurcation into the posterolateral and posterior descending arteries. The occlusions were reopened and multiple stents were placed in the main body of the RCA. The stents deployed were two 18 mm AVE II Microstents to the distal RCA, one

39 mm AVE II Microstent to the mid-RCA, and one 16 mm NIR stent in the proximal RCA. These were dilated with a 3.5 mm balloon at 20 atmospheres. Despite the use of multiple stents and a long treated segment length, the 6-month angiographic follow-up was quite acceptable, with adequate flow provided to the inferior and posterolateral walls (see *Fig. 8.12c*).

COMPLETE VESSEL RECONSTRUCTION MAY NOT BE APPROPRIATE

Although reconstruction of the RCA in the previous case was successful, *Fig. 8.13* reveals an example in which vessel reconstruction resulted in extensive intimal hyperplasia and diffuse restenosis. In *Fig. 8.13a* there is moderately diffuse narrowing in the body of the RCA, as well as significant disease at the bifurcation of the posterior lateral and posterior descending branches. The vessel was reconstructed with the use of multiple stents. A Wiktor stent was placed in the distal RCA and dilated at 4 mm to 10 atmospheres (see *Fig. 8.13b*). In addition, two AVE Microstents, each 16 mm in length, were placed beyond the Wiktor stent in the distal RCA and dilated with a 3 mm balloon at 12 atmospheres. The proximal portion of the posterior descending artery was treated with one AVE II Microstent, 16 mm in length, and two

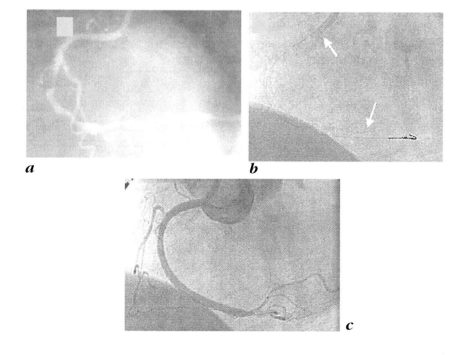

a   *b*

c

Figure 8.14 *Wallstent for diffuse disease. (a) Baseline angiogram. (b) Wallstent inserted. (c) Final angiogram.*

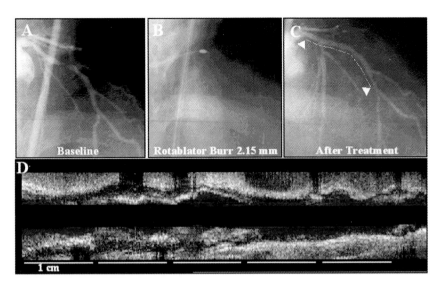

Figure 8.15 *Treatment of a long lesion. (a) Baseline angiogram and IVUS study revealed diffuse calcium which was treated with rotational atherectomy. (b) Software within the ultrasound machine can perform an automated analysis of lumen dimensions.*

a

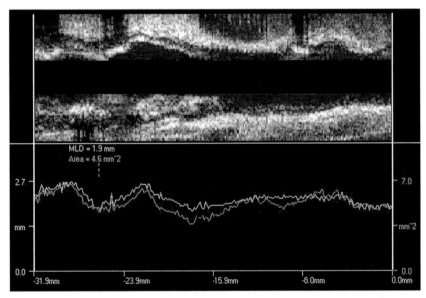

b

AVE II Microstents, each 4 mm. These were also dilated to 18 atmospheres with a 4 mm balloon. The proximal and mid-section of the RCA was treated with two 20 mm long Gianturco–Roubin II stents and dilated with a 4 mm balloon. After the insertion of the Gianturco–Roubin II stent, at the angle of the acute margin, the lumen was unsatisfactory, so an additional 16 mm long AVE stent was placed within the Gianturco–Roubin II stent and dilated with a 4 mm balloon at 18 atmospheres. Following this extensive use of metal and multiple balloon dilatations, the angiographic result was acceptable (see *Fig. 8.13b*).

Despite this pleasing angiographic result, the patient developed recurrence of symptoms and the angiogram 6 months after the procedure revealed an atretic vessel owing to severe intimal hyperplasia throughout the treated artery. The IVUS study showed that the stent struts were expanded appropriately during the initial deployment (the stent diameter measured close to 4 mm).

This is an important point, because one of the common reasons for restenosis is inadequate initial deployment. This is especially likely to occur if the first deployment was not confirmed with IVUS.

The second use of the IVUS study is to assess the amount of intimal tissue that is present after an

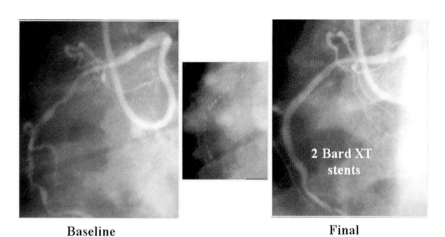

Baseline   Final

Figure 8.16 *A new modular stent for diffuse disease in tortuous vessels.*

attempt to treat the restenosis, whether by balloon alone or after debulking with a laser or Rotablator. In an attempt to remove some of the intimal hyperplasia, the vessel in *Fig. 8.13c* was treated with an excimer laser using a 1.7 mm and a 2.0 mm laser catheter, followed by rotational atherectomy using a 2.5 mm burr and final balloon dilatation using a 3.5 mm diameter balloon. The patient developed no reflow phenomenon associated with this aggressive debulking. Flow was re-established with the use of intracoronary nitroglycerin and verapamil, but the patient sustained a non-Q-wave myocardial infarction. The patient has since been followed up for 2 years and has had no recurrence of angina.

THE WALLSTENT FOR DIFFUSE DISEASE

Instead of placing multiple individual stents, an alternative for diffuse disease is to place a long flexible

stent, such as the Wallstent. This is especially useful for the RCA or saphenous vein grafts, in which the artery functions as a large conduit before any significant side branches.[8] The diffuse disease shown in *Fig. 8.14a* was pre-dilated and treated with deployment of a single Wallstent, 60 mm long by 6 mm in diameter. The radiopacity of the stent is shown in *Fig. 8.14b*. The flexible self-expanding nature of the stent provides a large lumen throughout the length of this curved and severely diseased artery (see *Fig. 8.14c*). There may be some difficulty during deployment of Wallstents in placing the stent in the precise position. The interventionalist needs to make sure that there is no movement of the stent and that the chosen length is appropriate. Sometimes this can be facilitated by using mechanical pull-back during IVUS imaging to measure the length of the lesion. Despite the practicality of treating a long lesion with a single very long stent the angiographic and clinical follow-up has been so poor that we completely abandoned this approach.

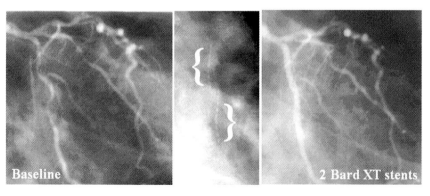

radiopaque
stent markers

Figure 8.17 *A new modular stent for tortuous vessels.*

Baseline

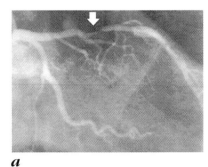

a

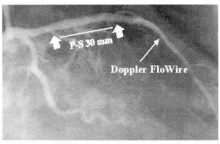

**After P-S 30mm Stent
Spiral Design**

Figure 8.18 *Coronary flow reserve assessment after stenting with the Doppler flow wire.*

Baseline APV = 27 cm/sec	Adenosine APV = 77 cm/sec

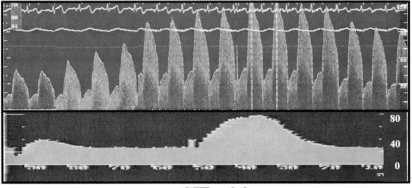

CFR = 2.9

b

LONGITUDINAL RECONSTRUCTION BY IVUS

The use of a longitudinal reconstruction from a mechanical pull-back during IVUS imaging is shown in *Fig. 8.15*. The baseline angiogram (see *Fig. 8.15a*) shows diffuse disease in the LAD diagonal system. After passage of several rotational atherectomy burrs incrementally up to 2.15 mm, the angiogram showed an adequate lumen with spasm at the distal end (see *Fig. 8.15c*). To assess the vessel dimensions as well as the length of artery that needed to be stented, IVUS imaging was performed with a mechanical pull-back device. The individual cross-sectional images are stored in computer memory and then realigned according to the internal orientation of the ultrasound catheter drive shaft that is pulled back within the guiding sheath. The images are then displayed as a longitudinal view of the artery lumen and vessel wall (see *Fig. 8.15d*). If the images are taken from a distal to a proximal bifurcation, these bifurcations can be easily identified on the longitudinal view and the distance between the bifurcations can be determined. In addition, the operator can scroll through the database images and quantitative measurements of MLD and lumen area are provided automatically with the use of automated edge detection software (see *Fig. 8.15b*). During the longitudinal pull-back of the IVUS catheter, there can be artefacts associated with the reconstruction process, especially since the ultrasound images take a curved artery and portray it as a straight tube. The operator must be sure to over-read the automated edge detection algorithm results to ensure its accuracy.

TREATING TORTUOUS ANGLES WITH NEW TECHNOLOGY

Advances in stent technology are critical for treatment of complex tortuous vessels and diffuse disease. The RCA shown in *Fig. 8.16* had an unusual take-off

Pre treatment

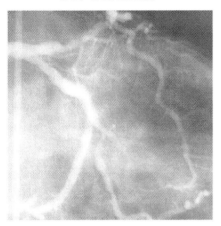

After treatment

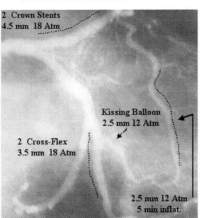

2 Crown Stents
4.5 mm 18 Atm

Kissing Balloon
2.5 mm 12 Atm

2 Cross-Flex
3.5 mm 18 Atm

2.5 mm 12 Atm
5 min inflat.

Figure 8.19 *The combination of using multiple stents as well as balloon angioplasty to treat diffuse multivessel disease.*

which could only be cannulated with a left Amplatz 2 guiding catheter. However, this provided an unfavorable entrance and a sharp angle into the artery. In addition, there was diffuse disease in the proximal and mid-portions of the vessel. This was approached with a newer stent design from Bard called the 'XT' stent, which has the beneficial property of a radiopaque marker along one side of the stent. This facilitates placement of the stent and subsequent positioning of the balloon for accurate expansion. This stent has very favorable characteristics in flexibility as well as hoop strength. It permits us to enter arteries in tortuous segments that would be difficult with most of the older types of stents. Another example of the Bard 'XT' stent is shown in *Fig. 8.17*. This circumflex artery has a long segment of diffuse narrowing with moderate tortuosity. Two 'XT' stents have been placed and the radiopaque outline of the stents can be seen in the middle panel.

THE PHYSIOLOGIC SIGNIFICANCE AFTER STENTING LONG LESIONS CAN BE ASSESSED BY DOPPLER FLOW

Figure 8.18 shows a moderately long lesion in the mid-LAD, which was treated with a 30 mm long Palmaz–Schatz spiral stent. The severity of this lesion was tested at baseline by assessing the coronary flow reserve using a Doppler flow wire. The baseline average peak velocity was 21 cm/second; increased to 42 cm/second after infusion of adenosine for a

coronary flow reserve of 2.0. After placement of the stent, the coronary flow reserve increased to 2.9 (see *Fig. 8.18b*). The physiologic measure of flow is another means of assessing the functional significance of stenosis or the adequacy of its treatment (see Chapter 5). This may be a useful method of assessing your results, especially when dealing with diffuse disease.

AN ALTERNATIVE APPROACH TO MULTIVESSEL DIFFUSE DISEASE – A COMBINATION OF STENTS AND BALLOON DILATATION

Multiple lesions with diffuse disease can be treated at the same sitting with acceptable angiographic results, as demonstrated in *Fig. 8.19*. In this case, a combination of stents as well as balloon angioplasty alone was used to treat long lesions involving bifurcations in the LAD and circumflex arteries. Two Crown stents were placed in the proximal and mid-LAD and were dilated with a 4.5 mm balloon to 18 atmospheres. The distal LAD was treated with balloon dilatation alone using a 2.5 mm balloon at 12 atmospheres for a prolonged inflation of 5 minutes. Two Crossflex stents were placed in the large obtuse marginal branch and dilated with a 3.5 mm balloon at 18 atmospheres. The branch vessel from this obtuse marginal was treated simultaneously with a 2.5 mm balloon inflated at 12 atmospheres to preserve the side branch during expansion of the stented main branch. This case demonstrates a combination of

Before procedure

Angiography

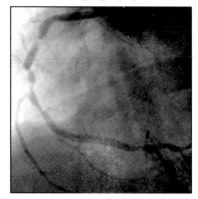

QCA

Ref.: 2.59 mm
MLD: 0.66 mm
Lesion length: 41.3 mm

a

Figure 8.20 *IVUS guided 'spot stenting'. (a) Baseline angiogram and quantitative coronary angiography (QCA). (b) Angiogram and intravascular ultrasound images after balloon angioplasty. (c) Final angiogram and IVUS images after placement of a single 16 mm long stent based on the IVUS results.*

IVUS findings after balloon angioplasty

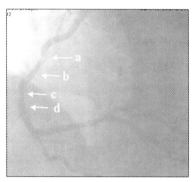

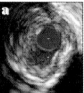

LCSA= 3.2 mm²

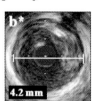

LCSA= 8.8 mm²

VOYAGER- C : 3.0 mm 20 mm 8 atm

b* : Media to media = 4.2 mm

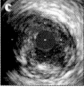

LCSA= 2.9 mm²

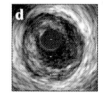

LCSA= 5.2 mm²

b

final result

angiography

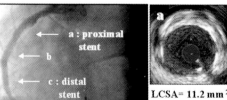

a : proximal stent

b

c : distal stent

IVUS finding

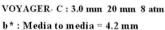

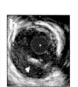

LCSA= 11.2 mm²

DART stent 16 mm

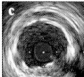

LCSA= 9.8 mm²
(➤ : flap)

LCSA= 9.9 mm²

DART stent 16mm

post dilatation

VOYAGER- C : 4.0 mm 20 mm 8 atm

c

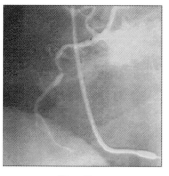

Baseline

a

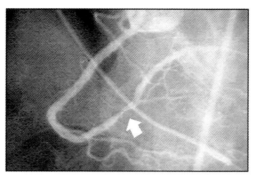

Distal lesion in the RCA after
reopening proximal total occlusion

Figure 8.21 *Complications of treating diffuse disease. (a) Baseline angiogram shows diffusely diseased and tortuous right coronary artery. The distal RCA is a chronic total occlusion. (b) Following high-pressure inflation to 15 atmospheres of a 3 mm balloon, there is rupture of the artery just before the bifurcation with the posterior descending branch. (c) Treatment of the acute rupture with a vein covered Palmaz–Schatz stent. (d) Final angiogram.*

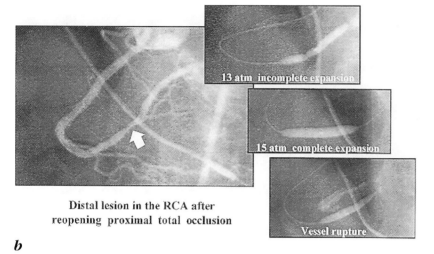

13 atm incomplete expansion

15 atm complete expansion

Vessel rupture

Distal lesion in the RCA after
reopening proximal total occlusion

b

10F

Advancement of a second PTCA system
while sealing with the first one

c

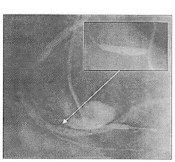

Deployment of P-S stent covered
with a vein

d

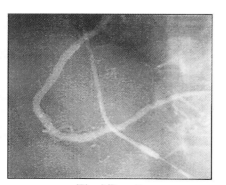

Final Result
The rupture is sealed

techniques: balloon angioplasty alone may be used when the vessels are smaller than 3 mm, whereas the larger branches with diffuse disease are supported with stents.

This type of approach has evolved into the concept of 'spot stenting', which is discussed more completely in Chapter 20. Owing to the high restenosis rate associated with longer stent length, in the 'spot stenting' technique an attempt is made to limit the total length of stents used. Stenoses in long lesions or diffuse disease are initially treated with balloon dilatation. The artery is then interrogated with IVUS, or physiologic assessment such as fractional flow reserve with a pressure wire or both. If there are focal areas where the lumen is compromised, then these segments are stented rather than placing one or several long stents throughout the dilated zone. In an attempt to reduce the restenosis rate associated with long lesions, we have abandoned the earlier recommendations that stents must be deployed without leaving an unstented segment between stents.

'SPOT STENTING' FOR DIFFUSE DISEASE

An example of IVUS-guided stenting using the 'spot stenting' approach is demonstrated in *Fig. 8.20*. The baseline angiogram shows moderately diffuse disease in the proximal and mid-section of the RCA as well as in the distal RCA just proximal and just distal to the bifurcation with the posterior descending artery. The QCA measurements (see *Fig. 8.20a*) demonstrate several areas of significant stenosis. The total lesion length in the proximal and mid-portion of the artery measured 41 mm, with a mean reference lumen diameter of 2.6 mm. Based on our experience with IVUS imaging, we suspected that this reference lumen size by QCA underestimated the true size of the artery. Therefore, balloon angioplasty was performed using a 20 mm long Voyager 3.0 mm diameter balloon inflated at 8 atmospheres. IVUS imaging obtained after balloon dilatation is shown in *Fig. 8.20b*. As distinct from the measurement of the lumen size by QCA, IVUS revealed that the media-to-media diameter was significantly larger, at 4.2 mm. Moreover, the results of balloon dilatation were unacceptable at segments A and C, but were adequate at segment B and D, with a lumen cross-sectional area of 8.8 mm² and 5.2 mm², respectively. Based on the ultrasound results, two DART stents were placed, each 16 mm long, at the proximal section A and the mid-section C (see *Fig. 8.20c*). For post-dilatation, a 20 mm long Voyager balloon was chosen; this was 4.0 mm in diameter. The size of this balloon was chosen based on the ultrasound measurement of media-to-media dimensions. This was inflated at 8 atmospheres which achieved a lumen cross-sectional area between 9.8 mm² and 11.2 mm². In addition, the ultrasound images revealed a flap of torn plaque in section B. In the past, we would have recommended stenting this flap. At the current time, however, we believe that this type of

tear is stable, especially when there is a stent proximal and distal. In addition, there is no evidence by either angiography or ultrasound that the flap is threatening to collapse into the lumen and occlude the vessel. The benefit of this approach is that less metal is used and the shorter total stent length decreases the risk of restenosis.

COMPLICATIONS OF TREATING DIFFUSE DISEASE

As demonstrated in the previous figures, our ability to treat long lesions and diffuse disease has improved dramatically over the past few years. It is not unreasonable to expect, however, that treatment of diffuse disease will also be associated with a higher incidence of complications. Several of these potential complications are described in Chapter 15, such as long dissections, no reflow phenomenon, distal embolization, and side branch closure. The case presented in *Fig. 8.21* demonstrates another severe complication that may occur while treating diffuse disease, namely, arterial rupture. This 65-year-old woman presented with stable angina and a type C lesion in her RCA. As shown in *Fig. 8.21a*, the RCA was diffusely involved with a tortuous proximal section followed by occlusion of the distal portion of the artery. The occlusion was recanalized and the artery was dilated with a balloon 20 mm long and 3 mm in diameter. Rotational atherectomy was not used. The proximal and mid-RCA were supported with two Palmaz–Schatz 204 stents. The distal lesion, just before the bifurcation with a large posterior lateral branch, did not expand completely at 13 atmospheres. The 3 mm diameter balloon was then expanded to 15 atmospheres, which resulted in perforation of the artery and extravasation of contrast (see *Fig. 8.21b*). To prevent severe hemopericardium and hemodynamic collapse, the balloon was reinflated to seal the vessel rupture, and a second angioplasty system was inserted via the left femoral artery using a 10 Fr guiding catheter. A 15 mm long segment of the basilic vein was extracted and was sewn on to a Palmaz–Schatz stent 15 mm in length. This was advanced through the second guiding catheter system to the level of the obstruction (see *Fig. 8.21c*). The first balloon was then deflated and removed and the vein-covered stent was deployed at the site of arterial rupture (see *Fig. 8.21d*). The vein-covered stent was expanded with a 3.5 mm balloon at 14 atmospheres. The final angiogram (see *Fig. 8.21d*) demonstrates good blood flow without evidence of residual extravasation of contrast into the pericardium.

This procedure was performed several years ago and we recognize now that there were several ways that we could have avoided this potentially catastrophic complication. In our current practice, if a balloon does not fully expand the lesion at 12 atmospheres, instead of using higher pressures, we remove the balloon and perform rotational atherectomy. In addition, given the presence of such diffuse disease, it would probably have been more effective to try to debulk some of the plaque by performing rotational atherectomy at the beginning of the case. At the present time, it is also easier to deal with ruptured arteries by using a PTFE-covered stent rather than hand crafting a vein-covered stent system.

REFERENCES

1. Kobayashi N, De Gregorio J, Kobayashi Y et al. Effect of varying stent length on outcome in the treatment of long lesions with subanalysis of small and large reference vessels. *Circulation* 1998; **98**: 1486.

2. Moussa I, Di Mario C, Moses J et al. The impact of preintervention plaque area as determined by intravascular ultrasound on luminal renarrowing following coronary stenting. *Circulation* 1996; **94**: 1528.

3. Hoffman R, Mintz GS, Mehran R et al. Intravascular ultrasound predictors of angiographic restenosis in lesions treated with Palmaz–Schatz stents. *J Am Coll Cardiol* 1998; **31**: 43–49.

4. Colombo A, Hall P, Thomas J et al. Initial experience with the disarticulated (one-half) Palmaz–Schatz stent: a technical report. *Cathet Cardiovasc Diagn* 1992; **25**: 304–308.

5. Moussa I, Di Mario C, Moses J et al. Coronary stenting after rotational atherectomy in calcified and complex lesions. Angiographic and clinical follow-up results. *Circulation* 1997; **96**: 128–136.

6. Hoffmann R, Mintz GS, Kent KM et al. Comparative early and nine-month results of rotational atherectomy, stents, and the combination of both for calcified lesions in large coronary arteries. *Am J Cardiol* 1998; **81**: 552–557.

7. Kimura T, Yokoi H, Nakagawa Y et al. Three-year follow-up after implantation of metallic coronary artery stents. *N Engl J Med* 1996; **334**: 561–566.

8. Itoh A, Hall P, Maiello L et al. Implantation of the peripheral Wallstent for diffuse lesions in coronary arteries and vein grafts. *Cathet Cardiovac Diagn* 1996; **37**: 322–330.

Chapter 9 Lesions in small vessels

Antonio Colombo and Jonathan Tobis

One of the more frustrating subsets of lesions that confronts the interventionalist is the approach to severe disease in small vessels. Vessels between 2 mm and 3 mm in diameter are more likely to dissect during balloon dilatation and are associated with a higher incidence of restenosis, even after stent placement.[1] Pre-intervention intravascular ultrasound (IVUS) imaging may be exceedingly helpful in this situation because IVUS may reveal a discrepancy between the angiographic dimensions of the lumen and the vessel size as measured by the media-to-media diameter. By knowing the vessel size from IVUS examination, the operator can optimize the stent placement by using appropriate debulking methods and by using a balloon diameter that approximates the media-to-media diameter. Since coronary artery disease is frequently a diffuse process, even precise measurements as performed with quantitative coronary angiography may frequently be misleading and underestimate the true size of the vessel. This chapter discusses our approach to the treatment of small-vessel disease and demonstrates that, with IVUS-guided pre-intervention studies, small-vessel stenting can be performed with a high success rate, comparable to that with stenting larger vessels.

For this analysis, small vessels were defined as those having reference lumen artery measurements of less than 3 mm. From April 1993 to September 1997, 834 lesions were identified as emanating from vessels < 3 mm in diameter, and these were compared to 929 lesions that were treated in vessels that were ≥ 3 mm in diameter at the reference segment. There was no difference between the vessel distribution in these two groups (*Table 9.1*). The majority of the lesions treated were in the left anterior descending artery (LAD). Approximately 80% of the lesions were located in the proximal or mid-portion of the artery (*Table 9.2*). There was also no difference in these two groups in the classification of the lesions and 75% of these lesions were class B1 or B2 and 20% were type

Table 9.1

Stenting small vessels. Lesion characteristics (I)

	< 3 mm	≥ 3 mm	p
Lesions	834	929	
Vessel distribution			NS
LAD	472 (56.6%)	388 (41.8%)	
Cx	168 (20.1%)	157 (16.9%)	
RCA	167 (20.0%)	337 (36.3%)	
LM	3 (0.4%)	20 (2.2%)	
SVG	24 (2.9%)	27 (2.9%)	

Table 9.2

Stenting small vessels. Lesion characteristics (II)

	< 3 mm	≥ 3 mm	p
Lesions	834	929	
Lesion location			NS
Ostium	50 (6%)	72 (7.8%)	
Proximal	300 (40.0%)	428 (40.0%)	
Mid	367 (44.0%)	360 (38.8%)	
Distal	117 (14.0%)	69 (7.4%)	

Table 9.3

Stenting small vessels. Lesion characteristics (III)

	< 3 mm	≥ 3 mm	p
Lesions	834	929	
Type of lesion			NS
A	47 (5.6%)	58 (6.2%)	
B1	268 (32.1%)	308 (33.2%)	
B2	357 (42.8%)	380 (40.9%)	
C	162 (19.4%)	183 (19.7%)	

Table 9.4

Stenting small vessels

	< 3 mm	≥ 3 mm	p
Lesions	834	929	
Age (yrs)	57 ± 10	59 ± 9	< 0.001
Refer. diameter (mm)	2.6 ± 0.3	3.4 ± 0.4	< 0.001
Percentage stenosis pre	69 ± 19	69 ± 17	NS
Lesion length (mm)	10 ± 6.7	10.8 ± 7.2	< 0.04
Final inflat. press (atm)	15.9 ± 3.3	16.3 ± 3.1	< 0.04
Balloon/artery ratio	1.3 ± 0.2	1.1 ± 0.1	< 0.001

Table 9.5

Stenting small vessels. Stent distribution

Type of stent	< 3 mm	≥ 3 mm
Palmaz–Schatz	417 (50.0%)	615 (66.3%)
Cook	95 (11.4%)	46 (5.0%)
Combinations	79 (9.5%)	56 (6.0%)
NIR	58 (7.0%)	60 (6.5%)
AVE	47 (5.6%)	22 (2.4%)
Wiktor	46 (5.5%)	49 (5.3%)
Walistent	37 (4.4%)	39 (4.2%)
Cordis	25 (3%)	14 (1.5%)
InStent	17 (2.0%)	7 (0.8%)
Crown	7 (0.8%)	10 (1.1%)
Angiostent	3 (0.4%)	1 (0.1%)
ACS	3 (0.4%)	7 (0.8%)
ACT I	0 (0.0%)	2 (0.2%)

Table 9.6

Stenting small vessels. Incidence of complications

	< 3 mm	≥ 3 mm	p
Lesions	834	929	
Success rate (%)	95.6	95.4	NS
Stent thrombosis			
Acute	4 (0.5%)	4 (0.4%)	NS
Subacute	11 (1.3%)	13 (1.4%)	NS
Major complications			
Non-Q MI	71 (7%)	48 (4%)	0.02
Q MI	29 (3%)	21 (2%)	NS
CABG	17 (2%)	13 (1%)	NS
Death	1 (0.1%)	3 (0.3%)	NS

C (*Table 9.3*). The major differences between these two groups are outlined in *Table 9.4*. The mean reference lumen diameter by angiography was 2.6 ± 0.3 mm in the small vessel group and 3.4 ± 0.4 mm in the larger vessel group (*p* < 0.001). The lesion length and final inflation pressure was slightly higher in the larger vessel group. It is of note that the balloon-to-artery ratio was significantly higher in the small vessel group (1.3) than in the larger vessel group (1.1).

The distribution of the stents is shown in *Table 9.5*. The vast majority of these procedures were performed with the Palmaz–Schatz stent since that represented the primary stent used for the first few years of our experience. At the present time we are more likely to use more dedicated stents (NIR 5 cells, BeStent mini, BioDivysio SV) for truly small vessels as documented by IVUS. Despite the presumption that treating small vessels is associated with a higher complication rate and greater difficulty, the success rate was similar in vessels < 3 mm to those vessels that were larger (*Table 9.6*). In addition, there was no difference in the incidence of stent thrombosis, whether acute or subacute; the total incidence was 1.8% in both groups. Although the incidence of non-Q-wave myocardial infarction (MI) was slightly higher with small vessels (7% versus 4%; *p* = 0.02), the incidence of other major complications, such as Q-wave MI, the need for emergency bypass surgery, or death, was similar in both groups.

An example of an angiographic result after stenting a small vessel is shown in *Fig. 9.1*. This symptomatic patient had a subtotal stenosis of the first diagonal artery. Although the artery appears to be < 2 mm in diameter, a successful result was achieved by dilating the vessel with a 2.5 mm balloon and placing a five-cell NIR stent, 19 mm long, in this branch vessel. The stent was then expanded at 20 atmospheres. Another example of treating a small branch vessel is shown in *Fig. 9.2*. In this case, a small diagonal branch that was subtotally occluded was treated initially with rotational atherectomy, using a 1.5 mm burr. In this case also, a NIR five-cell stent was placed, and the final result is shown in Panel C of *Fig. 9.2b*. The left anterior oblique view, although foreshortened, demonstrates wide patency, especially at the bifurcation with the LAD after the stent in the diagonal branch has been expanded.

We have been successful in treating this difficult lesion subset owing largely to the use of pre-intervention IVUS imaging. For patients entered into our

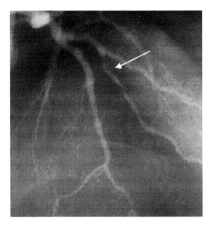
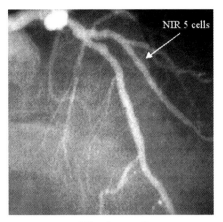

Baseline

Final result

Figure 9.1 *A small diagonal artery treated with a five cell NIR stent.*

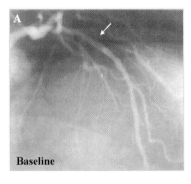

a

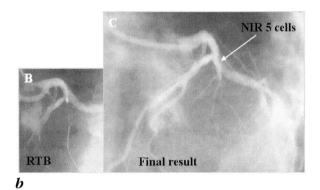

b

Figure 9.2 *A subtotal occlusion of a diagonal artery treated with rotational atherectomy and placement of a five cell NIR stent.*

database, if we use the angiographic reference lumen diameter as the measure of the size of the artery, *Fig. 9.3* reveals that we would underestimate the true vessel dimension by 28%. In the 834 vessels that were considered to be < 3 mm by angiography, the mean angiographic reference diameter lumen was 2.6 ± 0.3 mm. However, in the same arteries the ultrasound measurement of the reference minimum vessel diameter was 3.6 ± 0.5 mm ($p < 0.001$).

This discrepancy between angiography and ultrasound imaging is demonstrated visually in *Fig. 9.4*. The angiogram shows the results of quantitative coronary angiography (QCA) measurement of a posterior descending artery branch with a severe stenosis. The proximal reference was measured as 2.3 mm and the distal reference was 2.7 mm, giving an average reference of 2.5 mm. However, by IVUS, the media-to-media diameter was 3.5 mm both

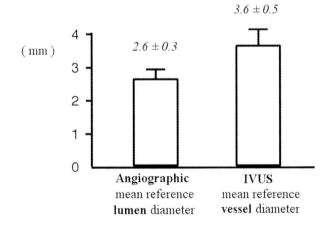

Figure 9.3 *Comparison of reference diameters by angiography and IVUS in small vessels. By angiography, the reference is measured from the lumen diameter, and by IVUS, the reference is measured at the media of the vessel.*

Proximal ref.   Lesion site   Distal ref.

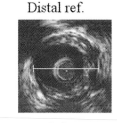

MVD   3.5 mm   3.4 mm   3.5 mm

(MVD = minimum vessel diameter)

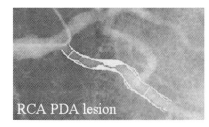

Figure 9.4 *Discrepancy of vessel size between quantitative coronary angiography (QCA) measurements of lumen diameter and IVUS image measurements of the media to media diameter. RCA, right coronary artery PDA, posterior descending artery.*

RCA PDA lesion

QCA measurement (*CMS system*)

Proximal reference	2.3 mm
Interpolated reference	2.5 mm
Distal reference	2.7 mm

QCA   # IVUS

Figure 9.5 *Stenting small vessels. Difference in definition of artery size. QCA, quantitative coronary angiography; IVUS, intravascular ultrasound; B/A, balloon-to-artery; CSA, cross-sectional area.*

Plaque   **2.6 ± 0.3 mm**   **3.7 ± 0.5 mm**

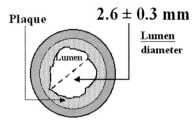   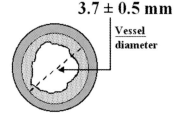

Lumen diameter   **Vessel diameter**

B / A ratio = 1.3 ± 0.2   **B / A ratio = 0.9 ± 0.1**

Vessel CSA = 11.3 ± 3.0 mm²

proximally and distally. Based on this observation, the decision was made to debulk the lesion with rotational atherectomy. We used a larger burr (2.0 mm) and a larger balloon (3.25 mm) than would be chosen if the decision were based on angiographic guidance. In addition, a stent was placed with greater expansion than would be deemed appropriate on the basis of the angiographic measurement alone. This discrepancy is shown schematically in Fig. 9.5 where the distinction is drawn between the QCA measurement of the lumen diameter being taken as the artery size and the IVUS measurement of the media-to-media diameter. The question is: What is the proper determinant of the

artery size that should drive our decisions for balloon size and the use of other interventional devices? We believe that by using the vessel size determined by IVUS as the media-to-media diameter, one can safely obtain a final stented lumen area that is larger than would be achieved by using angiographic criteria, either visually estimated or with QCA measurements. With respect to lumen measurements, it should be emphasized that, before balloon dilatation, the lumen measurements by QCA and IVUS are similar whereas, after balloon inflation, a dissection will cause a disassociation between the measurements of these two imaging techniques.[2]

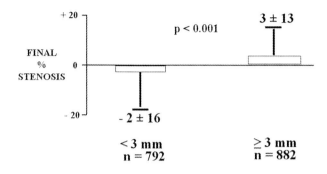

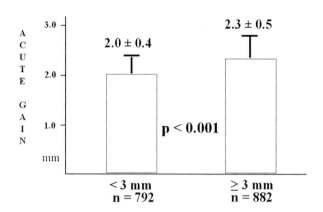

Figure 9.6 *Difference in final percent stenosis achieved when stenting arteries greater than or less than 3 mm.*

Figure 9.8 *Difference in acute gain achieved when stenting arteries greater than or less than 3 mm.*

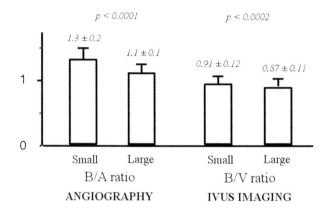

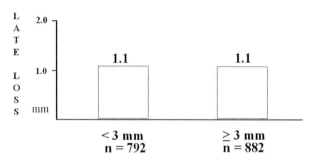

Figure 9.7 *Comparison of balloon/artery (B/A) ratio by angiography and balloon/vessel (B/V) ratio by IVUS.*

Figure 9.9 *Late lumen loss achieved when stenting arteries greater than or less than 3 mm.*

Using the guidelines described above, the results that were obtained in the 1674 lesions from our patients are demonstrated in *Figs 9.6–9.13*. The final percentage diameter stenosis is shown in *Fig. 9.6*. For vessels < 3 mm by angiography, our final diameter stenosis was –2 ± 16%, which was significantly larger than the percentage diameter stenosis in larger vessels (3 ± 13%; p < 0.001) (i.e. there was a 5 percentage points greater 'step-up' in the smaller arteries). The method of obtaining this larger final percentage diameter stenosis is presented in *Fig. 9.7*. Based on angiography, the balloon-to-artery ratio in small vessels was 1.3 ± 0.2, whereas it was only 1.1 ± 0.1 in larger vessels (p < 0.0001). However, when using IVUS imaging to guide the balloon-to-vessel ratio, the difference was much closer, the ratios in both groups averaging 0.9.

These results indicate that a larger balloon-to-artery ratio is required when using angiographic guidance; however, by ultrasound guidance, there really is no difference in the balloon-to-vessel ratio in the small or larger vessels. In other words, the apparent oversizing of the balloon by angiographic evaluation in small arteries reflects the underassessment of the vessel size by angiography. The evaluation of vessel size by IVUS permits more accurate selection of the final balloon diameter. However, since these vessels are smaller, the acute gain is still less in the small vessels (2.0 ± 0.4 mm versus 2.3 ± 0.5 mm) (see *Fig. 9.8*).

The 6-month follow-up angiographic results are demonstrated in *Figs 9.9, 9.10* and *9.11*. Angiographic follow-up was obtained in approximately 70% of the lesions. The late lumen loss was

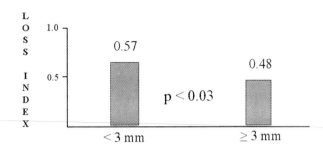

Figure 9.10 *Loss index achieved when stenting arteries greater than or less than 3 mm.*

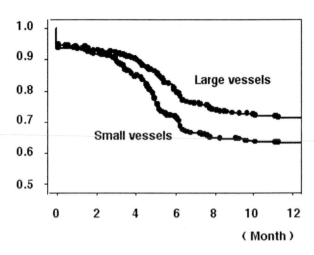

Figure 9.12 *Kaplan–Meier event-free survival curves for combined end-points of major adverse clinical events (MACE).*

similar in both groups at 1.1 mm (see *Fig. 9.9*). Loss index reflects the percentage of acute gain that is lost at follow-up; it is calculated as:

$$\text{loss index} = \frac{\text{post-procedure minimum lumen diameter} - \text{follow-up minimum lumen diameter}}{\text{acute gain}}$$

Since the late loss is similar in both groups, but the acute gain is less in smaller arteries, the loss index was higher in small vessels than in the vessels that were ≥ 3 mm (0.57 versus 0.48; $p < 0.03$) (see *Fig. 9.10*). In other words, for a given acute gain, late loss was greater in small vessels. This corresponded to a follow-up percentage diameter stenosis of 35 ± 30% in the small vessel group and 28 ± 28% in the larger vessel group ($p < 0.001$). The 6-month restenosis rate (defined as a binomial function ≥ 50% diameter narrowing on angiography) was significantly higher in the small vessel group, at 32%, than in the vessels ≥ 3 mm, in which it was 20% ($p < 0.001$) (see *Fig. 9.11*).

The predictors of restenosis are shown in *Table*

9.7. Of 21 clinical, angiographic, and ultrasound variables for 834 lesions in vessels < 3 mm by angiographic assessment, the univariate predictors of restenosis were stent lumen cross-sectional area, the reference diameter (angiographic artery size), the final minimum lumen diameter, and the patient's age. When these variables were placed in a multiple logistic regression model, the only variables that were independent predictors of restenosis were the stent lumen cross-sectional area measured by IVUS and the artery size as measured by the angiographic reference diameters. For every 1 mm² increase in stented lumen area, the chance of restenosis decreased by 23%. For every 1 mm increase in reference lumen diameter (artery size), the chance of restenosis decreased by 60%.

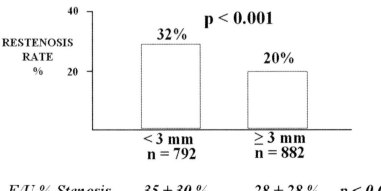

F/U % Stenosis   *35 ± 30 %*   *28 ± 28 %* *p < 0.001*

Figure 9.11 *Restenosis rate and percent diameter stenosis at follow-up when stenting arteries greater than or less than 3 mm.*

Table 9.7
Multiple logistic regression analysis stenting small vessels

	Univariate			Multivariate		
n = 834	Odds ratio	CI	p value	Odds ratio	CI	p value
IVUS stent CSA	0.72/mm²	0.63–0.81	< 0.0001	0.77/mm²	0.67–0.88	< 0.001
Angio ref. diam.	0.21/mm	0.1–035	< 0.0001	0.40/mm	0.19–0.82	< 0.05
Angio final MLD	0.47/mm	0.34–0.66	< 0.0001			
Age	1.17/10 yr	1.01–1.35	< 0.05			

The influence of small vessel size on increasing the chance for restenosis is reflected in the Kaplan–Meyer event-free survival curves with a combined end-point of death, MI, coronary bypass surgery, or target lesion revascularization during the first 12 months of stenting (*Fig. 9.12*). Patients with small vessels had a significantly higher rate of clinical events (37%) than patients with large vessels (29%) ($p = 0.007$).

Our conclusion from this analysis is that angiographic small vessels, with a reference diameter < 3 mm, have a high primary success rate with coronary artery stenting that is comparable to the results when stenting larger vessels. By using IVUS we can obtain a more accurate assessment of the vessel size, which permits us to use debulking devices or larger balloons to optimize the stent placement. When combined with antiplatelet therapy, this leads to a stent thrombosis rate in small vessels that is not different from that seen in stented larger vessels. Unfortunately, the restenosis rate is still higher after stenting smaller vessels than larger vessels. However, the angiographic restenosis rate of 32% is not so high that it should dissuade us from attempting coronary artery stenting in these vessels, especially since target lesion revascularization is significantly less than this value. These results can be achieved by performing stent dilatation with balloons that are appropriately sized to the media-to-media diameter as assessed by IVUS imaging, even though they appear to be oversized by angiography assessment. This corresponds to a balloon-to-artery ratio of 1.3 when using angiographic analysis, but a balloon-to-vessel ratio that is slightly less than 1 when using ultrasound guidance. The fact that the loss index is higher for the small vessel group is of concern and raises the question of whether greater stretching or barotrauma to the vessel, or other factors, are responsible for the higher loss index. Our attempt to address this problem has resulted in the concept of 'spot stenting,' which is discussed in depth in Chapter 20.

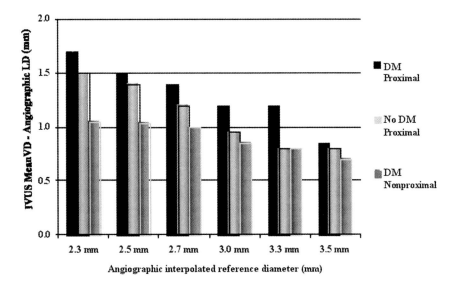

Figure 9.13 *Differences in measurement of reference diameter by angiography or IVUS as a function of artery size. The measured difference is greater in smaller vessels and is most pronounced in patients with diabetes. VD, vessel diameter; LD, lumen diameter; DM, diabetes mellitus.*

The severity of disagreement between the IVUS measurement of vessel diameter and the angiographic measurement of the lumen diameter is not the same for all artery sizes:[3] the difference between IVUS and angiographic measurements is significantly greater in smaller vessels than in larger vessels (*Fig. 9.13*). The graph in *Fig. 9.13* plots the difference between the IVUS and angiographic measurements on the vertical axis compared with the reference artery size varying between 2.3 and 3.5 mm in diameter. In addition, the graph provides information on patients with or without diabetes mellitus. The effect of whether a proximal coronary segment is involved also modulates the difference between IVUS and angiographic measurements. The largest difference between IVUS and angiographic measurements is found in patients with diabetes mellitus in whom the reference diameter of the vessel in question is 2.3 mm and whose disease is in a proximal coronary segment (mean difference of 1.7 mm). The lowest difference between the IVUS and angiographic measurements is found in non-diabetics in whom reference diameter of the vessel in question is 3.5 mm and whose disease is not in a proximal coronary segment (mean difference of 0.7 mm). This analysis emphasizes how the use of IVUS may be especially useful in arteries that appear to be small by angiography, especially in proximal or mid-locations where one might expect a larger artery. In this situation, it is more common for the angiogram to be misleading in the interpretation of the reference lumen diameter because of the presence of diffuse disease, as is commonly found in those with diabetes mellitus.

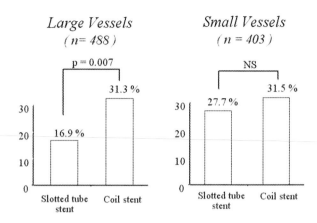

Figure 9.14 *Restenosis rates for large or small vessels as a function of different stent structures.*

was no significant difference between the restenosis rates for the slotted tubular stents and the coiled stents. In addition, the restenosis rate for the coiled stents was no worse in small vessels than in larger vessels. This last observation was analysed (*Fig. 9.15*) and the results from 713 lesions treated with slotted tubular stents were compared to the results from 178 lesions treated with coiled stents. With the slotted stents, there was a significant difference in the restenosis rate between large vessels and small vessels, yet with the coil stents, there was no significant difference on the basis of the size of the vessel. These restenosis rates for the slotted stents appear to

EFFECT ON RESTENOSIS FROM DIFFERENT KINDS OF STENTS

Another important issue is whether the type of stent used in smaller vessels impacts the restenosis rate. A subset analysis of the restenosis rate for different types of stents in 488 large vessels was compared to the results in 403 small vessels (< 3 mm in diameter). When the data were segregated according to the type of stent used (i.e. slotted tubular stents or coiled stents), there was a significant difference in the restenosis rate in large vessels, but not in the smaller vessels (*Fig. 9.14*). For vessels ≥ 3 mm in diameter, the restenosis rate for slotted tubular stents was 17%, but it was 31% for the coiled stent ($p = 0.007$). It is interesting to note that, in the smaller vessels, there

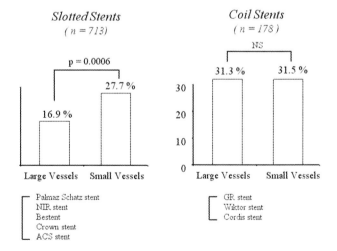

Figure 9.15 *Restenosis rate for different stent structures as a function of vessel size.*

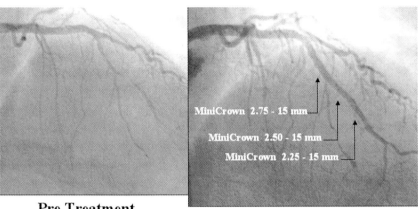

Pre Treatment
3 months after AMI

After Treatment

Figure 9.16 *The use of stents specifically made for treating smaller vessels. AMI, acute myocardial infarction.*

be consistent with the concept that the higher the final minimum lumen diameter is, the lower the restenosis rate will be. It is not clear why the restenosis rate is the same for large and small vessels with the coil stents.

SOME QUESTIONS ABOUT RESTENOSIS IN SMALLER ARTERIES

The incidence of restenosis was significantly higher following stenting in small vessels than in large vessels. This finding is in accordance with previous studies evaluating restenosis rates after standard percutaneous transluminal coronary angioplasty and atherectomy,[4,5] but it has not been consistently confirmed after coronary stenting.[6–8] In our experience, the absolute luminal reduction caused by intimal proliferation appears to be similar in small and large vessels. The bigger post-procedural lumen obtained in large vessels than in smaller vessels is the most important explanation for the lower restenosis rate seen after stenting large vessels. Serial IVUS studies after stenting have confirmed that the restenotic process is entirely due to intimal proliferation[9,10] and that chronic vessel recoil, which is the main mechanism of restenosis after other coronary interventions,[11] is prevented by the mechanical scaffolding of the stent.

It remains to be clarified why stenting elicits a relative higher proliferative response in small vessels as reflected by the higher loss index. Possible explanations include:

(a) greater vessel trauma induced by a more aggressive stent expansion strategy (higher balloon-to-vessel ratio);

(b) higher chronic wall stress imparted to a vessel with a smaller diameter and a large amount of plaque; or

(c) coronary arteries have a similar absolute amount of intimal hyperplasia in response to injury, and small arteries have less room for this scar tissue.

Attempts to limit vessel trauma in small vessels are likely to produce a smaller stent cross-sectional area, which may have a negative effect on the incidence of stent thrombosis and restenosis. Another possible explanation for the relatively higher proliferative response in small vessels is the higher metal density when a stent designed to be implanted in large vessels is used in vessels with diameters < 3.0 mm. Stents specifically designed to achieve an optimal radial force at a smaller diameter and with a lower metal-to-vessel surface ratio at these diameters have been recently introduced (NIR seven-cell and five-cell stents, Mini-Crown stents, BeStent) and these theoretically have the potential to improve long-term results. Further studies will test this hypothesis.

An example of using one of these newer stents to treat small vessels is provided in *Fig. 9.16*. This 65-year-old woman with diet-controlled diabetes mellitus suffered an anterior wall MI 3 months before admission. At the time of the angiogram she had recurrent angina. The LAD was diffusely diseased and atretic after the MI; however, it was felt that there was still some viable peri-infarction myocardium that was causing her angina. The artery was pre-treated with a 2.5 mm balloon, and then three mini-Crown stents, each 15 mm long, were placed in the distal LAD. The mini-Crown sizes were chosen to taper from 2.75 mm in the proximal segment to 2.25 mm in the distal zone. The total stent length was 45 mm. The proximal stent was inflated with a 2.75 mm balloon at 14 atmospheres. The result is shown in the right panel of *Fig. 9.16.*.

SUMMARY

(1) Small vessel stenting is associated with short-term results that are similar to stenting larger vessels.

(2) The incidence of stent thrombosis is no higher in small vessels than it is in larger vessels.

(3) These improved results for small vessels are obtained by using a significantly higher angiographic balloon-to-artery ratio (of 1.3 by QCA) for the final stent dilatation in small vessels than in larger vessels. The balloon-to-vessel ratio by IVUS measurement can be chosen safely at 0.9 in both large and small arteries.

(4) Stenting of small vessels is associated with a higher restenosis rate than stenting of larger vessels (32% versus 20%).

(5) The loss index in small vessel is higher than that in larger vessels.

(6) Achieving a larger final cross-sectional area within the stent is the major independent variable associated with a lower restenosis rate, both in large and small vessels.

(7) Slotted tubular stents perform better in large vessels than coil stents do.

(8) Both types of stents appear to have similar rates of restenosis when implanted in small vessels.

REFERENCES

1. Akiyama T, Moussa I, Reimers B et al. Angiographic and clinical outcome following coronary stenting of small vessels: a comparison with coronary stenting of large vessels. *J Am Coll Cardiol* 1998; **32**: 1610–1618.

2. Ozaki Y, Violaris AG, Kobayashi T et al. Comparison of coronary luminal quantification obtained from intracoronary ultrasound and both geometric and videodensitometric quantitative angiography before and after balloon angioplasty and directional atherectomy. *Circulation* 1997; **96**: 491–499.

3. Moussa I, Moses J, De Gregorio J et al. The discrepancy between quantitative coronary angiography and intravascular ultrasound in determining true vessel size: a homogeneous or a selective phenomena? *J Am Coll Cardiol* 1999; **33 (suppl A)**: 76A.

4. Hirshfeld JW Jr, Schwartz JS, Jugo R et al. Restenosis after coronary angioplasty: a multivariate statistical model to relate lesion and procedure variables to restenosis. The M-HEART Investigators. *J Am Coll Cardiol* 1991; **18**: 647–656.

5. Kuntz RE, Safian RD, Carrozza JP et al. The importance of acute luminal diameter in determining restenosis after coronary atherectomy or stenting. *Circulation* 1992; **86**: 1827–1835.

6. Strauss BH, Serruys PW, de Scheerder IK et al. Relative risk analysis of angiographic predictors of restenosis within the coronary Wallstent. *Circulation* 1991; **84**: 1636–1643.

7. Ellis SG, Savage M, Fischman D et al. Restenosis after placement of Palmaz–Schatz stents in native coronary arteries. Initial results of a multicenter experience. *Circulation* 1992; **86**: 1836–1844.

8. de Jaegere P, Serruys PW, Bertrand M et al. Angiographic predictors of recurrence of restenosis after Wiktor stent implantation in native coronary arteries. *Am J Cardiol* 1993; **72**: 165–170.

9. Hoffmann R, Mintz GS, Dussaillant GR et al. Patterns and mechanisms of in-stent restenosis. A serial intravascular ultrasound study. *Circulation* 1996; **94**: 1247–1254.

10. Mudra H, Regar E, Klauss V et al. Serial follow-up after optimized ultrasound-guided deployment of Palmaz–Schatz stents. In-stent neointimal proliferation without significant reference segment response. *Circulation* 1997; **95**: 363–370.

11. Mintz GS, Popma JJ, Pichard AD et al. Arterial remodeling after coronary angioplasty: a serial intravascular ultrasound study. *Circulation* 1996; **94**: 35–43.

Chapter 10 Bifurcation lesions

Bernhard Reimers, Antonio Colombo and Jonathan Tobis

Stenoses at a bifurcation remain one of the most technically challenging lesion subsets to treat by coronary angioplasty. Angioplasty operators quickly realized that dilating lesions that span a branch vessel was associated with the risk of closure of the side branch.[1-7] Dilating the side branch, in turn, frequently resulted in compression of the major artery. This was due to plaque redistribution, or 'plaque shift' across the carina of the bifurcation. Plaque shift can occur with stents as well as with balloon dilatation alone, as demonstrated conceptually in *Fig. 10.1*. In an attempt to diminish the effect of plaque shift, the technique of 'kissing balloons' was developed, whereby two guidewires were used to cannulate each branch vessel and two balloons were inflated simultaneously.[3] Despite these attempts, the results with balloon dilatation of bifurcation lesions still had a high incidence of complications, suboptimal results, and restenosis.[5-8] The results of balloon dilatation alone in this trifurcation lesion has resulted in suboptimal expansion (*Fig. 10.2*). This ultrasound image reveals that the plaque has been fractured with lumen diameters of only

1.9 mm × 2.8 mm or a lumen cross-sectional area of 3.8 mm². This unsatisfactory treatment of the bifurcation lesion with angioplasty was corrected by placing

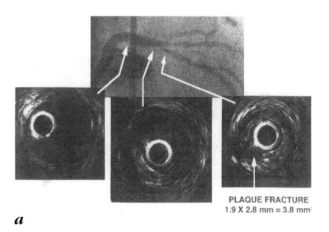

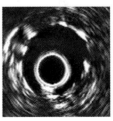

PLAQUE FRACTURE
1.9 X 2.8 mm = 3.8 mm²

a

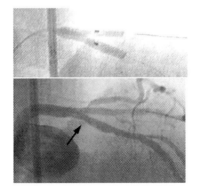

POST STENT
2.6 X 3.0 = 6.2mm²

b

Figure 10.2 *Balloon dilatation of a trifurcation lesion. (a) Following balloon dilatation with a 3.0 mm balloon, there is still significant residual stenosis. The ultrasound image reveals a fractured plaque with a total lumen cross-sectional area of 3.8 mm². (b) The lower branch was treated with a Palmaz–Schatz stent. Simultaneous balloons were inflated in the lower and middle branches.*

Mechanism of Side-branch Compromise after Stenting

Transverse Plaque Redistribution

Axial Plaque Redistribution

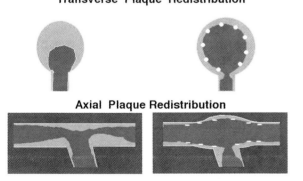

Figure 10.1 *Transverse and axial plaque redistribution following balloon dilatation or stent insertion as a cause of sidebranch compromise.*

a stent into the lower branch (*Fig. 10.2b*). The lower and middle branches were treated with 'kissing balloons'. The subsequent ultrasound of the stent at the bifurcation confirmed an improved diameter of 2.6 mm × 3.0 mm or a cross-sectional area of 6.2 mm².

Treatment of bifurcations with directional atherectomy (without stenting) has been shown to improve the immediate procedural outcome compared to balloon dilatation alone, but the incidence of restenosis remains high.[9,10] The use of coronary stents has improved the treatment of bifurcation lesions, but it is technically challenging and there is still a high incidence of compromising the branch vessel.[4,11,12] The incidence of procedural complications when stenting bifurcations, especially if both the main branch and the side branch are stented, has been reported as being up to 9%.[13] Increased operator experience and recent technical developments have improved the success rate to 98% when stenting bifurcations. There are only limited data, based on single-center experiences, on the incidence of restenosis after stenting bifurcations. The available results report an incidence of restenosis up to 36%, indicating that bifurcation stenting carries a higher risk of restenosis than stenting non-bifurcation lesions.[14,15] The unique characteristics of some of the newer stents facilitate our ability to treat bifurcation lesions. In addition, the concept of debulking has been effective in diminishing plaque redistribution at the bifurcation. This chapter reviews several of the approaches we have tried to treat this challenging anatomic variant of coronary angioplasty.

TYPES OF BIFURCATIONS

Coronary bifurcations are reported as being at high risk of developing atherosclerotic plaque, owing to turbulent flow and increased shear stress.[1,2] Lesions situated at a bifurcation account for up to 16% of coronary angioplasty procedures.[3] A true bifurcation lesion is characterized by the presence of a significant (≥ 50% diameter) stenosis involving both a main vessel and a side branch. For practical reasons, we consider a bifurcation lesion to be a stenosis that is located in the major branch close to the origin of a side branch where the treatment of the main branch may compromise the side branch. A classification of bifurcation lesions with regard to the threat of side branch occlusion during coronary angioplasty has been proposed by Koller and Safian[3] and recently modified for

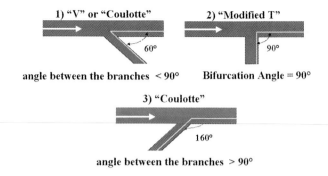

Figure 10.3 *The approach to treating bifurcation lesion depends in part on the angle of incidence of the branch vessel.*

coronary stenting by Aliabadi and colleagues.[4] These authors identified side branches at risk of occlusion when plaque is present at its origin or when the disease in the major branch is very close to the ostium of the side branch with possible plaque shift at the time of the major branch being dilated or stented.

Not all bifurcations are anatomically equivalent. The angle at which the branch vessel takes off from the main artery and the size of the branch vessel frequently dictate our approach to treatment. Our choice of treatment is determined by the angle of the bifurcation (*Fig. 10.3*) depending on whether it is less than 90°, approximately 90°, or retroflexed and greater than 90° to the antegrade approach. In general, if the branches are large enough, we prefer to debulk the bifurcation with the use of a Rotablator, stepping up to large size burrs, or we use directional atherectomy to remove a larger amount of plaque. If the angle at the bifurcation is not too sharp, then we would also recommend using directional atherectomy in the branch vessel to diminish the chance of plaque shifting. Although we have performed rotational atherectomy when both branches are calcified, the need to use multiple burrs makes this a laborious process; therefore our current practice is to use the Rotablator only in the main branch of a bifurcation. If both branches are greater than 3 mm in diameter and both branches have been debulked, our preference is to place a stent in both the main branch and the side branch vessel. If the side branch is less than 3.0 mm in diameter, we tend to stent only the main branch and use a balloon through the stent to dilate the ostium of the side branch.

The ability to perform the different techniques of bifurcation stenting that are discussed in this chapter is intimately connected to the type of stent that is

Table 10.1
Strategic approaches to bifurcational lesions: treatment of the side branch

Side branch	< 2.0 mm	≥ 2.0 mm < 3.0 mm	> 3.5 mm
Threatened side branch occlusion	Wire protection	Wire protection Pre-dilate before stenting the main branch	Wire protection Pre-dilate and/or debulk Plan to stent both branches
Non-threatened side branch	No wire protection	No wire protection	No wire protection
Side branch significantly compromised after main branch balloon dilatation	Only if clinically indicated wire and pre-dilate before stenting the main branch	Wire and pre-dilate If > 2.5 mm consider stenting both branches	Wire and pre-dilate Plan to stent both branches
Side branch significantly compromised after main branch stenting	Only if clinically indicated wire and dilate	If flow impaired or closed, try to wire and dilate If > 2.5 mm consider stenting bail-out through struts	Stent both branches

available. In addition, since larger devices or two simultaneous stents are often used, we recommend using larger guiding catheters, such as 9 Fr or 10 Fr guides, when treating bifurcation lesions. The approach to bifurcation stenting requires significant forethought in the technique and equipment to be used. This is clearly one of the areas in stenting where the technique may change significantly over the next few years as more experience is gained and newer stents and technology become available. At the present time, our recommendation is to use meshwork stents for greater support, such as the Multilink by ACS or the NIR seven-cell stent. Among coil stents we have had good success with the Crossflex LC (Cordis) and the Wiktor stent. The flexibility of the AVE stent, especially the GFX model, has facilitated our ability to stent side branches after the stent is deployed in the main branch.

GENERAL CONSIDERATIONS WHEN APPROACHING THE TREATMENT OF BIFURCATION LESIONS

An attempt should be made to preserve any side branch > 2.0 mm in diameter, and therefore the first step when treating a bifurcation is to decide:

(a) Does the side branch need wire protection?
(b) Does the side branch need balloon dilatation?
(c) Does the side branch need a stent?
(d) Does the lesion need debulking?

The following represents our approach to this decision-making process, which is outlined in *Table 10.1*.

DOES THE SIDE BRANCH NEED WIRE PROTECTION?

Side branch protection entails positioning a second wire into the daughter branch before starting the treatment of the main branch. The decision to protect the side branch depends on the risk of closure while treating the main branch and on the size of the side branch. In the experience of Aliabadi and colleagues,[4] only 4% of side branches ≥ 1 mm with a non-threatened morphology occluded after stenting the major branch, whereas 67% of threatened side branches occluded. Thus, non-threatened side branches should not be wired. Small size branches (< 2.0 mm) can be left unprotected at the beginning of the procedure and then salvaged only in case of compromise after dilatation of the main branch. Side branches ≥ 2.0 mm that are at risk of closure should be protected. If there is any doubt, we prefer to protect a side branch rather than have to respond quickly to its closure without a wire already in place.

DOES THE SIDE BRANCH NEED BALLOON DILATATION?

Operationally, there is a significant difference between elective side branch treatment with balloon dilatation followed by conditional stenting and bail-out treatment of a side branch that is compromised following dilatation of the main branch. Side branches ≥ 2.5 mm in diameter with ostial disease or at risk of plaque shift should be treated with elective balloon dilatation with or without a 'kissing balloon' simultaneously in the main branch. This may prevent side branch occlusion after stent placement in the major branch and may facilitate rewiring the side branch through the struts of the main branch stent if necessary. Dilatation of the side branch should be performed without using oversized balloons to prevent dissections, which will commit the operator to stenting the side branch.

DOES THE SIDE BRANCH NEED A STENT?

Complete bifurcation stenting with elective stent implantation of both the main branch and the side branch should be performed only if the side branch is ≥ 3.0 mm in diameter. If the side branch is < 3.0 mm, stenting both branches should be avoided because the incidence of restenosis is higher than in single stent implantation in the main artery followed by side branch dilatation. As described in more detail under Clinical Results, a retrospective evaluation of bifurcations treated between 1996 and 1997 revealed that the restenosis rate in 90 lesions treated with double stents was 39%, compared to 28% in 92 lesions treated with a single stent and side branch dilatation. If the side branch occludes, dissects, or has impaired flow during the dilatation procedure, then our threshold for stenting lowers significantly. Bail-out stenting of the occluding side branch appears reasonable if its diameter is ≥ 2.5 mm. When both branches have been treated with directional atherectomy, both branches should receive a stent.

DO WE NEED TO DEBULK THE BIFURCATION LESION?

In an attempt to optimize the minimum lumen diameter and the minimum lumen area, directional atherectomy has been applied in the treatment of bifurcations with improvement in short-term results.[7,8,16,17] The large plaque burden of a bifurcation can be reduced by directional atherectomy to a residual plaque area less than 50%. Atherectomy before stenting enhances stent expansion, reduces plaque shift, and maximizes the lumen.[17] In a recent experience of 90 consecutive cases of directional atherectomy

followed by stenting, a remarkably low target lesion revascularization rate of 7.9% was achieved.[18] Unfortunately, the current directional atherectomy catheters are not user-friendly and this limits their applicability to large vessels with favorable anatomy. In the presence of calcium, the use of rotational atherectomy may be necessary to remove some of the plaque, thereby changing its compliance and permitting better stent expansion.[19]

GUIDING CATHETERS AND WIRES

The guiding catheter and wires must be chosen according to a planned approach. New 6 Fr guiding catheters with large inner lumens combined with very low-profile dilatation balloons and a fixed wire system may allow 'kissing' inflations. The gain from the small access site with the use of a 6 Fr guiding catheter is negated by the increased friction and the reduced visualization. If the bifurcational intervention requires 'kissing balloon' inflations, an 8 Fr guiding catheter should be used to allow comfortable balloon and wire handling to guarantee reasonable contrast injections. When positioning two stents simultaneously (i.e. for the 'modified T technique'; see later) the newer, big lumen 8 Fr catheter is wide enough to accommodate two pre-mounted stents with low-profile shafts. For debulking procedures using directional atherectomy, adequate catheter sizes (10 Fr) are needed.

For most bifurcational lesions, any regular percutaneous transluminal coronary angioplasty wire and support wire can be used. For procedures with directional atherectomy, the use of two nitinol wires should be used to prevent accidental cutting of the wire. We have also performed directional atherectomy with two Platinum Plus 0.36 mm (0.014-inch) wires (Sci-Med, Boston Scientific Inc., Minneapolis, Minnesota, USA) without entrapping the second wire. Specific steerable or hydrophilic-coated wires or balloons with fixed wires are also useful to cross previously implanted stents or to cross stent struts into side branches.

STENTING BIFURCATION LESIONS

The following discussion presents different techniques of stent implantation for bifurcations that have been performed in our laboratory.[20–23] A

Table 10.2

Stenting bifurcations: a summary of techniques

Technique	Angle of origin of side branch	Advantages	Disadvantages	Suitable stents
Stent the main branch and dilate side branch through struts	20°–120°	Less complex and less expensive compared to double stenting Lower complication rate and lower incidence of restenosis compared to double stenting	Sometimes difficult to wire side branch and/or to cross struts with balloon Lesion coverage only of the main branch Often suboptimal result in case of disease at origin of side branch	Slotted tube: all, preferably with struts which allow creation of a wide side lumen Coil stents: all, often easier side branch access compared to slotted tube but higher risk of stent distortion and less scaffolding
'Culottes' stent technique	30°–90°	Optimal lesion coverage in the main branch and the side branch Second stent implantation only if necessary	Access to both branches not always maintained (possibly difficult to re-wire) Possible difficulty in crossing struts with second stent	Pre-mounted, low-profile: Slotted tube with wide expandable struts or ring design: ACS Duet, mini Crown, Crossflex lasercut, AVE GFX Coil stents easier but less scaffolding: Crossflex, Wiktor
'Modified T stent' technique	Close to 90°	Access to main branch always maintained	Only for close to 90° bifurcations Possible imperfect lesion coverage at ostium of side branch	Preferably premounted: For side branch: AVE GFX or ACS Duet For main branch: any slotted tube
'V stent' technique	≤75°	Access to both branches always maintained Safe and quick method for two large branches	Creation of a metallic neo-carina not in contact with the vessel wall	All slotted tube or ring design stents
'Y stent' technique	30°–75°	Access to main branch always maintained	Complex technique Possible gaps in lesion coverage Need for 3 stents	For branches: AVE GFX, ACS Duet Proximal stent: visible: NIR Royal, ACS Duet
Creating a proximal funnel	30°–75°	Creates wide 'inflow' into the bifurcation Avoids stenting of side branches especially if small sized Ideal in presence of disease only proximal to the bifurcation	Lesion coverage only of the main branch Often need for a second, distal stent	Visible slotted tube: NIR Royal, ACS Duet

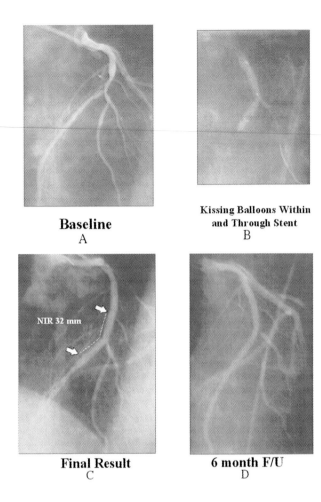

Baseline
A

Kissing Balloons Within and Through Stent
B

NIR 32 mm

Final Result
C

6 month F/U
D

Figure 10.4 *Use of a single stent in the main branch with balloon dilatation through the middle of the stent into the diagonal sidebranch.*

summary of these different approaches is provided in *Table 10.2*.

TECHNIQUE 1: PLACING A SINGLE STENT IN THE MAIN ARTERY AND DILATING THE BRANCH THROUGH THE STENT

The simplest approach to bifurcation lesions is to use one stent to cover the lesion in the major branch with the side of the stent covering the ostium of the side branch. After deploying and post-dilating the stent in the main branch of the artery, the side branch is cannulated with a second guidewire. The ostium of the side branch is then dilated with a separate balloon. To prevent plaque shift we prefer to use

rotational atherectomy or directional atherectomy in the main artery (as described above) and also use simultaneous inflations of the balloon in the main branch and side branch (i.e. the 'kissing balloon' technique). This approach is demonstrated in *Fig. 10.4* where a moderately long stenosis of the left anterior descending artery (LAD) straddles a large diagonal branch. In this case, a 32 mm NIR stent was placed in the LAD across the ostium of the diagonal branch and the diagonal branch was dilated with a 2.5 mm balloon while the LAD was simultaneously dilated with a 3.5 mm balloon (*Fig. 10.4b*). Although there was significant narrowing at the ostium of the diagonal branch at the 6-month follow-up (*Fig. 10.4d*), the patient was asymptomatic and had no evidence of ischemia. If ischemia had been documented, we would have redilated the diagonal artery or both branches if necessary with simultaneous inflations.

Usually the long-term patency rate is excellent when a side branch is even modestly patent after stenting the major branch.[11,12] It is not yet clear whether wiring the side branch is easier after low-pressure stent implantation, which may cause less plaque shift, or after high-pressure stent implantation, which provides wider expanded struts. In our institution, the stent is implanted initially in the main artery at medium or high pressure. A variety of wires may be used to cross stent struts. The wire should be shaped to approximately 90°. After the tip is engaged within the struts at the origin of the side branch, a slight backward movement with careful steering allows it to cross into the side branch. If this is not successful, the tip should be reshaped with a wider curve (> 90°). Newly developed short transition wires with prolapsing tips can be helpful because they can be easily advanced through the proximal part of the stent and then withdrawn in the manner described above. Hydrophilic-coated wires have less friction to cross the struts but the risk of dissecting the side branch is increased. If the stent cannot be crossed with a guidewire alone, a 1.5 mm over-the-wire balloon or an open-end catheter can be advanced close to the origin of the side branch to increase the support of the wire to cross the struts. This technique is especially useful for a reverse (> 90°) angle of origin of a side branch.

After crossing the stent with a wire, a balloon needs to be advanced into the side branch. This may be easy depending on the type of stent, but sometimes the use of a new, unexpanded, low-diameter, low-profile balloon is necessary. Over-the-wire balloons with higher pushability than monorail

Bifurcation Lesion
Dilatation through a single stent Technique (I)

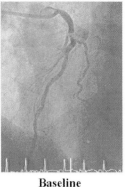

a   Baseline

Bifurcation Lesion
Dilatation through a single stent Technique (III)

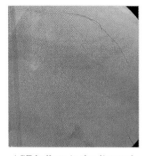 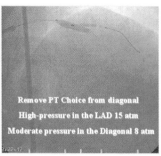

Remove PT Choice from diagonal
High-pressure in the LAD 15 atm
Moderate pressure in the Diagonal 8 atm

ACE balloon in the diagonal   **Kissing inflation**
along the Choice PT wire

c

Bifurcation Lesion
Dilatation through a single stent Technique (II)

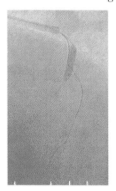 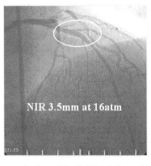

NIR 3.5mm at 16atm

Stent deployed in LAD while guidewire
(Choice PT) is in diagonal branch

b

Bifurcation Lesion
Dilatation through a single stent Technique (IV)

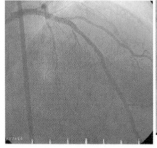 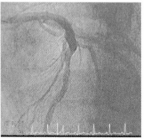

Final Result

d

Figure 10.5 *Single stent treatment of a bifurcation lesion. (a) Baseline angiogram. (b) A polymer coated guide wire was left in the diagonal branch during stent deployment at low pressures, into the LAD. This was done to help maintain patency of the diagonal as well as provide a road map for balloon dilatation after stent expansion. (c) An ACE balloon was passed along the guide wire into the diagonal branch. The guide wire was then removed and simultaneous inflations in the diagonal and the stented LAD were performed. (d) Final angiographic result.*

balloons should be used. Repeated, quick forward and backward movement of the balloon ('dottering') may help the balloon pass through the stent struts. The guiding catheter position may need to be adjusted, but patience usually leads to success. The balloon should not be advanced completely into the side branch because this increases the risk of balloon entrapment after inflation. The inflation pressure should also be kept well under the rated burst pressure because balloon rupture within a stent can also lead to balloon entrapment.

An alternative to this approach is demonstrated in *Fig. 10.5*. For this stenosis in the LAD, a NIR stent was deployed with a 3.5 mm balloon and expanded

at 16 atmospheres after deployment. To protect the diagonal branch, a Choice PT (polymer tip) guidewire was passed into the diagonal artery before balloon dilatation of the LAD. The guidewire was purposely left in the diagonal branch during stent expansion in the LAD because of concern for plaque shift (*Fig. 10.5b*). The NIR stent was then deployed in the LAD at low pressure (6 atmospheres) with the expectation that we would be able to remove the hydrophilic guidewire underneath this type of stent from the side branch. Following the low-pressure stent deployment, the ostium of the diagonal was indeed compromised. As shown in *Fig. 10.5c*, the Choice PT wire was used as a guide to pass a

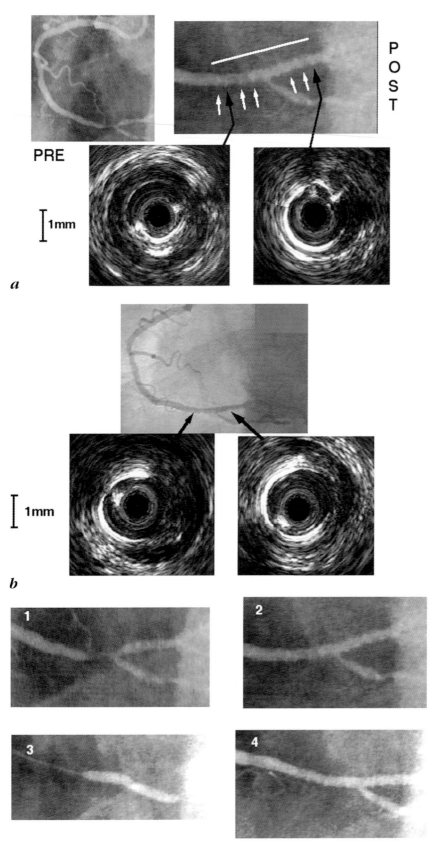

a

b

c

Figure 10.6 *A coiled stent to treat a bifurcation lesion. (a) Baseline angiogram demonstrates severe stenosis just proximal to the bifurcation of the posterior descending and posterolateral branches. A Gianturco–Roubin 1 stent was placed into the distal RCA across the ostium of the PDA. The ultrasound images reveal the scimitar shape struts of this stent. (b) Based on the ultrasound cross-sectional area, the stent was redilated at higher pressures. (c) Because of plaque shift into the ostium of the PDA branch (panel 2) a balloon was placed through this stent and the ostium of the PDA was dilated. The final angiographic result is shown in (c) Panel 4.*

balloon on a wire across the lumen and the struts of the NIR stent into the diagonal branch. The lubricious polymer-tipped guidewire was easily removed from behind the stent. Simultaneous inflations in the stent and the ostium to the diagonal artery were then performed with the use of high pressures (15 atmospheres) in the LAD balloon and only moderate pressures (8 atmospheres) in the diagonal branch (*Fig. 10.5c*). The final result is shown in *Fig. 10.5d*. The use of a balloon on a fixed wire has the advantage of using a balloon with low profile to preserve optimal pushability, yet this method is quick since only one device needs to be inserted. When a fixed wire balloon is used, the operator should be very careful because of the increased risk of side branch dissection. The final balloon chosen for side branch inflations should be adequately sized but not oversized, since side branch ruptures, especially of diagonal branches, might occur. Final simultaneous balloon inflations in the stented main branch and in the side branch should be performed because stent deformation after side branch dilatation might have occurred.

The simplest and most predictable way of performing side branch dilatation through a stent is to use a coil stent or a ring design stent. The three coil stents most frequently used are: the Wiktor stent (Medtronic Inc., Minneapolis, Minnesota, USA), the Crossflex stent (Cordis, J & J Inc., Warren, New Jersey, USA), and the Gianturco–Roubin II stent (Cook Inc., Bloomington, Indiana, USA). Although these stents do not provide the same scaffolding support as the slotted tubular stents, they permit easier access to the side branch. We tend to use one of these stents when there is more than one branch originating from the bifurcation, when the plaque burden is not very large, or when the bifurcation involves a bend or a sharp curve. An example of the use of a coil stent for a simple bifurcation is shown in *Fig. 10.6*. This stenosis, just proximal to the bifurcation of the posterior descending artery (PDA) and the distal right coronary artery (RCA), was treated with a Gianturco–Roubin I coiled stent. The ultrasound images (*Fig. 10.6a*) show the scimitar-like echo reflections from the stent coils, which do not completely surround the circumference of the plaque–lumen interface. The stent struts can be seen indenting the wall of the artery in the post-deployment angiogram (white arrows). Based on the ultrasound measurements of lumen cross-sectional area, the stent was redilated at 11 atmospheres with a 3.0 mm balloon (*Fig. 10.6b*). Although these inflations enlarged the lumen of the RCA, the bifurcation at the ostium of the PDA was

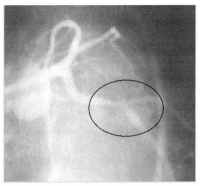

a   **Baseline**

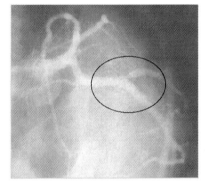

b   **Post Stenting Main Branch**

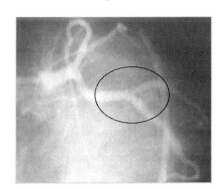

b   **Final Post Kissing Dilatation**

Figure 10.7 *Example of stent implantation in the main branch and balloon dilatation of the side branch through the struts. (a) A lesion in the mid-left circumflex artery involving the origin of an obtuse marginal branch. A Wiktor stent was deployed in the circumflex artery covering the ostium of the marginal branch (b). A wire was then passed into the marginal branch. (c) The result after 'kissing balloon' inflation of the circumflex artery and the marginal branch. Simultaneous inflation was performed to prevent stent distortion during side branch dilatation.*

Table 10.3
Side lumen creation and stent distortion during simulated side branch dilatation

Balloon diameter	AVE GFX	BeStent	Crown	ACS Multilink	NIR*
Mean side lumen diameter (mm)					
2.5 mm	2.7	2.7	2.3	2.5	2.0
3.0 mm	3.1	2.9	2.5	3.0	2.0
3.5 mm	3.6	3.0	3.0	3.5	2.2
4.0 mm	4.1	3.8†	3.7	3.7	3.6†
Distal diameter stenosis (%)					
2.5 mm	17	18	16	28	4
3.0 mm	25	42	25	38	36
3.5 mm	25	43	31	48	46
4.0 mm	50	64	38	55	58

*: Cell number not specified. †: strut rupture. From Ormiston et al.[30] with permission.

compromised (*Fig. 10.6c,* Panel 2). The stent was recrossed through its side with a guidewire and the same balloon was used to dilate the PDA without using simultaneous balloon inflations (*Fig. 10.6c,* Panel 3). In this case there was no plaque shift or compromise of the main branch after dilating through the stent into the side branch (*Fig. 10.6c,* Panel 4).

Another example of using a coil stent for a simple bifurcation approach is shown in *Fig. 10.7.* In this case no atherectomy was performed before placing a Wiktor stent in the main branch of the circumflex artery. After deployment there is apparent compromise of the large obtuse marginal branch (see *Fig. 10.7b*). However, the openings of the coil stent are amenable to the passage of a second guidewire down the obtuse marginal branch to dilate the side branch simultaneously ('kissing dilatations') without having to use an extremely low-profile balloon such as the ACE. A potential problem when using a coil stent without a longitudinal spine is the risk of stent deformation during initial stent crossing or during balloon withdrawal. A reasonable compromise between optimal support and easy recrossing ability is the use of a ring design stent such as the GFX II stent (AVE Inc., Santa Rosa, California, USA) or the new slotted tubular design with larger struts, such as the Crossflex LC (Cordis, J & J Inc., Warren, New Jersey, USA), the ACS Multilink Duet (Guidant Inc., Santa Clara, California, USA), or the Mini Crown stent (Cordis, J & J Inc., Warren, New Jersey, USA). The diameter through the sides of five stent designs

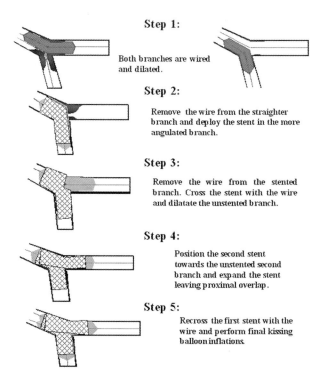

Step 1:
Both branches are wired and dilated.

Step 2:
Remove the wire from the straighter branch and deploy the stent in the more angulated branch.

Step 3:
Remove the wire from the stented branch. Cross the stent with the wire and dilatate the unstented branch.

Step 4:
Position the second stent towards the unstented second branch and expand the stent leaving proximal overlap.

Step 5:
Recross the first stent with the wire and perform final kissing balloon inflations.

Figure 10.8 *The 'culottes' technique for bifurcation stenting.*

expanded at four different balloon sizes is provided in *Table 10.3.*

TECHNIQUE 2: STENTING BOTH BRANCHES – THE 'CULOTTES' METHOD

If the side branch is compromised despite balloon dilatation, an alternative is to stent the side branch as well. The 'kissing' stent technique was first described by Chevalier and colleagues[23] and, in our view, it is the most elegant method for stenting both branches of a bifurcation (*Fig. 10.8*). We call this the 'through the stent' technique or the 'culottes' method, using an analogy from the world of fashion. In this approach, both branches are wired and each branch is pre-dilated sequentially (*Fig. 10.8*, Panel 1). The guidewire from the straighter branch is removed and a coil stent or flexible open design meshwork stent (e.g. the Multilink stent or the Crossflex stent) is passed down the more angulated branch (see *Fig. 10.8*, Panel 2). If an important dissection or occlusion is present in one branch, this branch should be stented first, since wire removal might be risky. After successful deployment, the guidewire from the angulated branch is removed and the same wire and balloon (if the size is appropriate) are used to enter the other branch. In some cases, a new low-profile, uninflated balloon may be necessary. The unstented ostium is then dilated with the balloon halfway back into the proximal portion of the stent to dilate the entrance into the unstented branch (*Fig. 10.8*, Panel 3). A second stent is then advanced and placed across the ostium with overlap in the proximal portion of the stent (*Fig. 10.8*, Panel 4). After deployment, a second balloon and guidewire are reinserted down the original stent and simultaneous dilatations of both stents and the proximal portion of the artery are performed (*Fig. 10.8*, Panel 5).

With this technique, the vessel proximal to the bifurcation is covered by two overlapping stents and each branch is covered by a single stent. This technique is particularly suitable for bifurcation angles between 30° and 90° but it can also be performed for reverse angles (> 90°). This technique can also be used when the initial plan was to stent only one vessel but the second branch becomes compromised and requires a stent too. When utilizing this technique, the operator does not need to overlap the proximal stents equally. One of the two stents can be asymmetrically advanced into one branch as long as the bifurcation is covered. Drawbacks of this approach are the possible difficulties of rewiring and redilatation (in steps 3 and 5) and of crossing the second stent through the struts of the first stent (step 4). However, these difficulties occur less frequently with the new low-profile pre-mounted

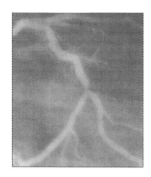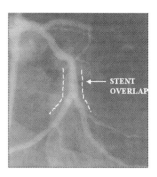

Atherectomy of both branches + NIR Medinol Scimed stents (inserted across each other)

Figure 10.9 *'Culottes' technique for bifurcation stenting. This circumflex-obtuse marginal stenosis was treated with directional atherectomy into each branch vessel. A NIR stent was then deployed in the circumflex artery. A second NIR stent was then passed through the side of the first stent into the obtuse marginal branch.*

stents with large expandable strut areas. Initially, coil stents were used for this technique; however, new slotted tube or ring design stents such as the ACS Duet, the Crossflex LaserCut and the AVE GFX are ideal for this approach and provide excellent scaffolding of the entire bifurcation. Using these stent designs, large side lumens can be created and the smoother strut edges decrease the chance of balloon rupture.

An example of the 'through the stent' or 'culottes' technique is demonstrated in *Fig. 10.9*. This circumflex artery bends posteriorly so that the obtuse marginal bifurcation is close to 90°. Because of the large amount of plaque burden proximal to the ostium of both branches, directional atherectomy was performed down each branch sequentially. After deploying a NIR stent in the circumflex artery across the ostium of the obtuse marginal branch, a second wire and balloon were directed through the side of the NIR stent into the obtuse marginal artery. A second NIR stent was then placed through the first one into the proximal portion of the obtuse marginal artery, with the proximal half of the stent overlapping the original stent in the circumflex artery. The NIR stent used in this instance has a larger opening in the middle segment to facilitate stenting bifurcations. This is called a 'NIR side' stent. Another variety of large-cell aperture to permit passage into a bifurcation branch is produced by Jomed (Sweden) (*Fig. 2.47*).

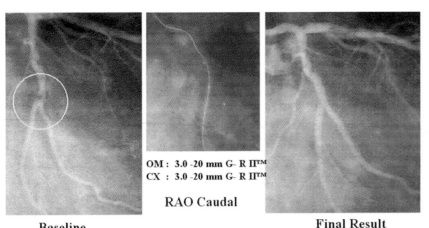

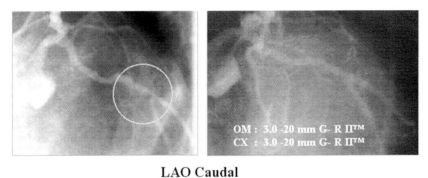

Figure 10.10 *The 'culottes' technique for bifurcation stenting using two coiled stents.*

An example of the use of two coil stents with the 'culottes' technique for stenting a bifurcation lesion is demonstrated in *Fig. 10.10*. In this instance the bifurcation lesion of the large obtuse marginal and circumflex artery was treated by sequentially placing a 3 mm × 20 mm long Gianturco–Roubin II stent down the obtuse marginal branch and then placing a second stent through the first one into the main branch of the circumflex artery. The final dilatation was performed with two balloons inflated simultaneously in both branches to prevent plaque shifting.

An example of newer stent technology to treat bifurcational lesions is provided in *Fig. 10.11*. The baseline angiogram reveals a significant stenosis in the proximal LAD that extends into a large diagonal branch as well as the mid-LAD. This was initially treated with progressive Rotablator burr sizes from 1.5 mm to 2.0 mm. The lesion was pre-dilated with simultaneous balloon inflations into both branches.

An 18 mm long Crossflex laser cut stent was then passed into the diagonal branch over a balance middle-weight wire. The diagonal branch was stented first because it had more of an angle to negotiate. The stent was placed so that the proximal third was still within the LAD. It was deployed at 16 atmospheres. The wire in the diagonal branch was withdrawn and repositioned into the LAD. A second Crossflex laser cut stent, 18 mm long, was then passed on a 3.5 mm balloon. This was positioned into the LAD and one-half to two-thirds of the stent was kept proximal to the bifurcation. After the stent in the LAD had been deployed, a 3.0 mm balloon (over a second wire) was passed into the stent in the diagonal branch. The 3.5 mm balloon was repositioned into the LAD stent. Both stents were inflated simultaneously at 12 atmospheres. The radiographic outline of the stents without contrast is shown in *Fig. 10.11b*. Proximal to the bifurcation, the two stents

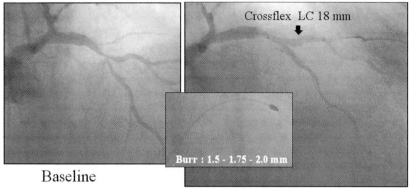

Baseline

Crossflex LC 18 mm

Burr : 1.5 - 1.75 - 2.0 mm

First stent deployment

a

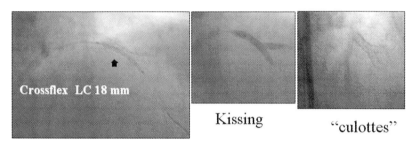

Crossflex LC 18 mm

Kissing

"culottes"

Second stent deployment

b

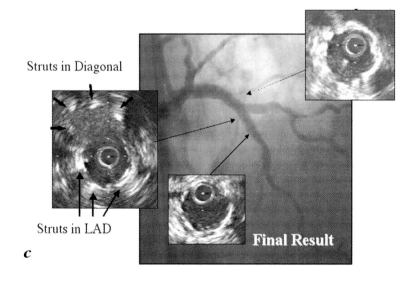

Struts in Diagonal

Struts in LAD

Final Result

c

Figure 10.11 *Example of the 'culottes' technique using an open meshwork design Crossflex LC stent. (a) The left panel shows a lesion at a bifurcation of the LAD with a diagonal branch. Rotational atherectomy with a 1.5 mm, 1.75 mm, and a 2.0 mm burr was performed due to the presence of calcium on angiography. Both branches were wired and predilated. An 18 mm Crossflex laser cut stent was positioned from the LAD into the diagonal branch. (b) After expansion of the stent in the diagonal branch, the wire was withdrawn and advanced across the struts of the stent into the LAD. The side struts of the stent were dilated permitting passage of a second 18 mm Crossflex LC stent to pass through the side of the first stent into the LAD with proximal overlap of both stents (left panel). After stent deployment, the diagonal branch was crossed again with a second wire and simultaneous balloon inflations were performed (middle panel). The right panel shows the expanded stents without contrast injection. (c) The final result demonstrated by angiography and IVUS imaging. Note the stented lumen of the diagonal branch visible on the left ultrasound image. On the right ultrasound image, the proximal two overlapping stents have more prominent echoes than the single stent on the ultrasound image in the middle panel.*

are superimposed, with each 'leg' of the culottes extending into the respective branch. The final angiographic result is shown in *Fig. 10.11c*. The ultrasound study documents that the bifurcation is widely patent and the stent struts are well apposed in both the LAD and diagonal arteries. There is no evidence of plaque shift.

TECHNIQUE 3: 'KISSING' STENTS OR THE 'V' METHOD

Another variation on the technique of using two stents to treat a bifurcation lesion is to place the two stents parallel to each other, such that a new metal carina is made more proximal to the bifurcation where the two

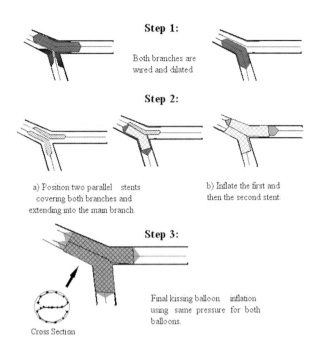

Step 1:

Both branches are wired and dilated

Step 2:

a) Position two parallel stents covering both branches and extending into the main branch.

b) Inflate the first and then the second stent.

Step 3:

Final kissing balloon inflation using same pressure for both balloons.

Cross Section

Figure 10.12 *The 'V' technique for bifurcation stenting.*

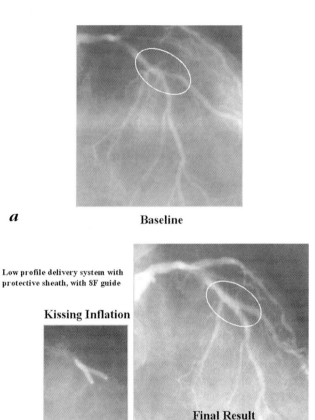

a

Baseline

Low profile delivery system with protective sheath, with 8F guide

Kissing Inflation

Final Result

b

Figure 10.13 *Use of the mini-Crown stent for a LAD-diagonal bifurcation with the 'V' technique.*

stents press against each other. This 'kissing' stents technique is suitable for bifurcations of two large side branches with a large diameter of the vessel proximal to the bifurcation. This technique is best suited for branches that originate with a narrow angle (<70°). This technique is called the 'V' technique (*Fig. 10.12*). In using this technique it is important to start with a large guiding catheter and to pre-dilate both branches.

Step 1: An extra support guidewire is passed down each branch of the bifurcation. Both branches are pre-dilated.

Step 2: Each stent is loaded on a separate balloon and advanced to the lesion. The stents are positioned simultaneously but each stent is dilated and deployed separately to avoid forward displacement of either delivery balloon.

Step 3: Following this initial sequential stent deployment, the final inflation is performed simultaneously in a 'kissing' technique using the same pressure in each balloon.

It is preferable to deliver the stents with a high-pressure balloon that can also be used for the final inflation without having to exchange balloons. One of the problems with this technique is that the proximal

stent struts may puncture the opposing balloon; however, the new generation of meshwork stents and the AVE GFX are less likely to cause balloon puncture.

An example of this 'V' technique is demonstrated in *Fig. 10.13*. At this bifurcation of the LAD and diagonal branch, the take-off of the side branch is approximately 60°. A guidewire was passed into both the LAD and the diagonal branches and both arteries were pre-dilated. Two mini-Crown stents were then advanced using their low-profile delivery system and protective sheath. The stents were placed alongside each other in the proximal portion, with half of each stent extending into its respective branch. The stents were then deployed separately but the final inflations were performed simultaneously (*Fig. 10.13b*).

Another example of the 'V' technique is shown in *Fig. 10.14*. Here, intravascular ultrasound (IVUS) clearly demonstrates a double barrel from the two opposing stents in the segment of the artery proximal to the bifurcation. This bifurcation of the obtuse

9 mm NIR Stent X 2

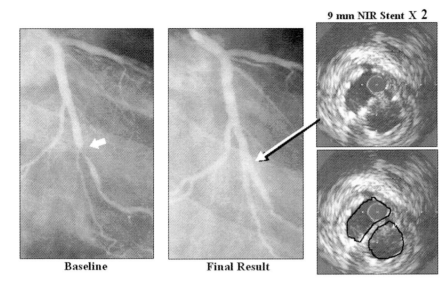

Baseline   Final Result

Figure 10.14 *Bifurcation stenting with the 'V' technique using two 9 mm-long NIR stents.*

marginal and circumflex arteries was treated with two 9 mm NIR stents.

In our early experience with ultrasound imaging of coronary artery stents, we were initially concerned that leaving stent struts unapposed in the artery lumen would predispose to subacute stent thrombosis. However, in our experience of 'V stenting' bifurcation lesions as well as of placing the stent across a side branch, there does not appear to be an increased incidence of subacute stent thrombosis. We believe the conditions that predispose to subacute stent thrombosis (see Chapter 3), are inadequate expansion of the artery as well as poor flow. The presence of a metal carina in the middle of the artery, if it is well expanded, does not appear to predispose to subacute thrombosis. An additional example of the 'double-barrel' stents in the proximal segment of an RCA–PDA bifurcation is shown in *Fig. 10.15*. This was treated with two short 9 mm NIR stents placed simultaneously side by side.

The most appropriate stents for the 'V' technique are two slotted tube stents of equal design with good radial strength to preserve the best configuration of the original carina. This technique is relatively safe to perform since access to both branches is always maintained. Lesion coverage is also complete. However, compared to the 'culottes' technique, the 'V' technique has more limited applications: it is best suited for very large branches with a narrow angle of origin. Rapid performance and easy execution are the major advantages of the 'V' technique. As a minimum, a large lumen 8 Fr guiding catheter is needed for this technique. The use of IVUS to

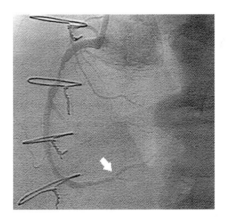

Baseline

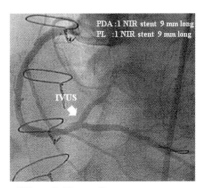
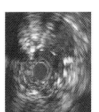
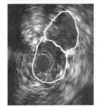

PDA : 1 NIR stent 9 mm long
PL : 1 NIR stent 9 mm long

IVUS

Final Result

Figure 10.15 *Bifurcation stenting with the 'V' technique using two 9 mm-long NIR stents. PDA, posterior descending artery; PL, postero-lateral artery.*

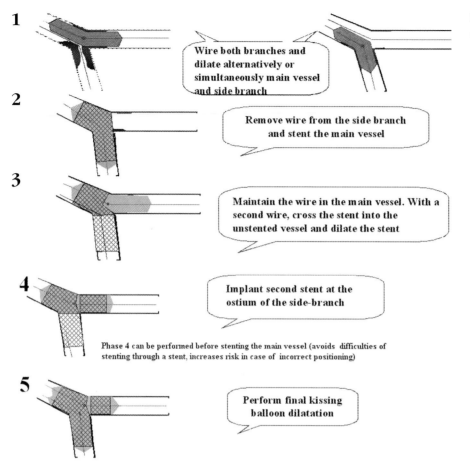

1

Wire both branches and dilate alternatively or simultaneously main vessel and side branch

2

Remove wire from the side branch and stent the main vessel

3

Maintain the wire in the main vessel. With a second wire, cross the stent into the unstented vessel and dilate the stent

4

Implant second stent at the ostium of the side-branch

Phase 4 can be performed before stenting the main vessel (avoids difficulties of stenting through a stent, increases risk in case of incorrect positioning)

5

Perform final kissing balloon dilatation

Figure 10.16 *'T' stenting for bifurcation lesions.*

document expansion of both stents is recommended. Alternative 'V' techniques have been described in which only the ostium of the two branches is stented without creating a new carina.[26,27] In one technique, the articulation of a Palmaz–Schatz stent was bent and the two half-stents were mounted on two balloons and advanced on two wires until the articulation reached the carina of the bifurcation.

TECHNIQUE 4: 'T' STENTING – THROUGH THE STENT SIDE

A variation of the 'through the stent' technique has been termed 'T' stenting. A guidewire is placed down both branches and each branch is dilated alternatively or simultaneously (*Fig. 10.16*, Panel 1). The wire from the side branch is then removed and a stent is placed in the main vessel across the ostium of the side branch (*Fig. 10.16*, Panel 2). With the guidewire remaining in the main vessel, a second wire recrosses the stent into the unstented side branch vessel. A balloon is then passed and dilates through the side of the stent into the ostium of the side branch (*Fig. 10.16*, Panel 3). A second stent (usually shorter than the first) is then passed through this side opening into the ostium of the side branch (*Fig. 10.16*, Panel 4). Final simultaneous inflations into both branches are then performed to diminish plaque shift or damage to either of the stents *Fig. 10.16*, Panel 5). The difference between this approach and the 'through the stent culottes' technique is that in this method there is no overlapping of the stents in the proximal portion of the artery. We tend to reserve this method only for those instances where the first stent in the main artery compromises the ostium of the branch. It is a bailout method to use when the initial plan for only one stent results in narrowing of the side branch.

TECHNIQUE 5: THE MODIFIED 'T' TECHNIQUE

For the treatment of 90° bifurcations, a true 'T' shape deployment of stents has been tried. Because this technique developed later it has been called the 'modified T' technique (*Fig. 10.17*).[22,25]

Step 1: Both branches are wired and pre-dilated.

Step 2: Two stents are then advanced sequentially to the side branch and then into the main branch, with the stent of the main branch straddling the side branch. Once again, in order to perform this technique, a larger 8 Fr guiding catheter is necessary.

Step 3: The stent in the side branch is then deployed first with an attempt to have 1 mm of the proximal portion of the stent sticking out into the main branch so that the ostium is completely covered. The stent should be deployed on a high-pressure balloon to optimize the lumen area without having to recross with a separate balloon. While the stent in the side branch is being deployed, the stent in the main branch should be left undeployed but straddling the ostium to the side branch. If the stent in the main branch is not left in this position, it may be difficult to reposition it once the stent in the side branch is deployed, owing to extension of the stent struts from the ostium of the side branch back into the main lumen.

Step 4: The balloon and guidewire in the side branch are removed after the side branch stent has been fully dilated. The stent in the main branch of the bifurcation is then deployed and inflated at high pressure.

Step 5: If necessary, you can rewire the side branch for a final simultaneous balloon dilatation.

In order to approach these 90° angulations, a stent such as the AVE GFX or Crossflex is preferred for the branch vessel. In addition, the smooth, round edges of these stents minimize the risk of balloon rupture. The second stent for the main branch can be any slotted tube stent but preferably one with a large space between struts to facilitate rewiring and dilatation of the side branch.

Disadvantages of this procedure are that it is limited to bifurcations that are close to 90°; furthermore, if the stent in the side branch is implanted too distally, an uncovered gap might remain at the ostium of the side branch.

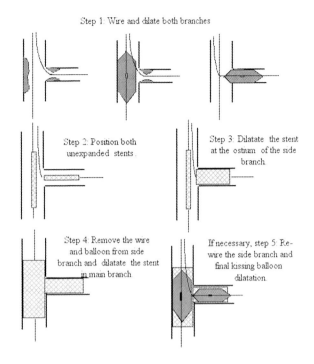

Figure 10.17 *The 'modified T' technique.*

An example of this 'modified T' stenting technique is shown in *Fig. 10.18*. In this instance the bifurcation consists of the left main artery with significant extension of the stenosis into the circumflex artery and the proximal LAD. Both branches were pre-dilated and then a 12 mm AVE GFX stent was placed into the ostium of the circumflex artery and a second stent (an 18 mm AVE GFX stent) was positioned in the LAD. As the insert shows, the stent in the circumflex was deployed on a 3.5 mm balloon at 12 atmospheres while the second stent was left undeployed but in position in the distal left main and the LAD. After the circumflex stent had been deployed, the balloon and wire were removed and then the stent in the left main artery and the LAD was deployed at 12 atmospheres with a 3.5 × 20 mm balloon.

Figure 10.19 provides an example of an approach to treating a complex bifurcation lesion in the LAD and diagonal artery using two new stent technologies. The baseline angiograms reveal that there is an extensive amount of plaque proximal to the bifurcation and that the take-off of the diagonal artery is approximately 90°. Both branches were wired and pre-dilated. Next, an AVE GFX stent, 12 mm long × 3.0 mm wide, was advanced into the diagonal branch

RAO   **LAO**

Pre

LM LAD: AVE GFx
3.5 mm 12 atm

Post

LAO Caudal

Circ: AVE GFx
3.5 mm 12 atm

Figure 10.18 *'Modified T' technique for treating a left main bifurcation lesion. The LAD and circumflex arteries were both dilated. The 18 mm long AVE GFX stent was placed into the ostium of the circumflex artery and the second 18 mm long AVE GFX stent was positioned in the proximal LAD. The stent in the circumflex was deployed at 12 atmospheres while the second stent was left undeployed covering the distal left main and LAD. The circumflex balloon and wire were then removed and the stent in the left main and LAD was deployed at 12 atmospheres.*

Simultaneous Insertion, Successive Deployment

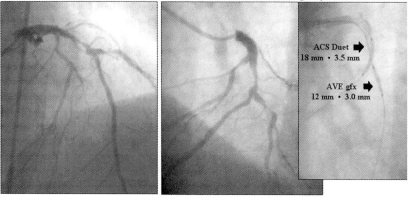

ACS Duet
18 mm · 3.5 mm

AVE gfx
12 mm · 3.0 mm

BASELINE

a

Figure 10.19 *Example of the 'modified T' technique. (a) The presence of diffuse disease in the LAD and the diagonal branch is noted in the baseline images. After wiring and predilatation of both branches, a 12 mm AVE GFX stent was positioned in the diagonal branch. A second stent (ACS Duet, 18 mm) was positioned in the LAD to cover the ostium of the diagonal branch (right panel). The stent in the diagonal artery was first inflated, then balloon and the wire were removed. The stent in the LAD was then deployed. Another stent was implanted in the proximal LAD to treat the proximal disease. (b) The final result and a radiograph without contrast of the expanded stents are shown.*

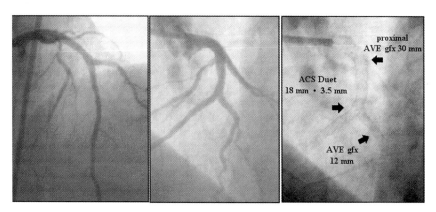

proximal
AVE gfx 30 mm

ACS Duet
18 mm · 3.5 mm

AVE gfx
12 mm

b   **Final Result**

with the proximal end of the stent positioned at the ostium. An 18 mm ACS Duet stent was then passed over a second guidewire into the LAD and positioned so that it straddled the bifurcation with the diagonal branch (*Fig. 10.19a*, inset). The diagonal artery stent was inflated at 14 atmospheres and the balloon and guidewire in the diagonal branch were then removed. The ACS Duet stent had been kept in place in the LAD during inflation of the diagonal stent. The LAD stent was now inflated to 16 atmospheres with a 3.5 mm balloon. The proximal disease in the LAD was then treated with another AVE GFX stent (30 mm long). The final result is provided in *Fig. 10.19b*.

TECHNIQUE 6: THE 'Y' TECHNIQUE

Another option for treating bifurcation lesions has been termed the 'Y' technique.[28] The technique can be summarized in three steps (*Fig. 10.20*).

Step 1: Each branch of the bifurcation is wired and pre-dilated.
Step 2: Two short stents are deployed sequentially and then inflated simultaneously at the ostium of both branches. The balloons are removed and the guidewires are left in place.
Step 3: A third stent is then hand crimped on the proximal half of two balloons, and the balloons are threaded over the guidewires such that the distal end of each balloon enters the ostium of its branch. The proximal stent is then deployed by inflating both balloons simultaneously, which also prevents plaque from shifting at the bifurcation.

This is a complicated procedure and requires that the two guidewires should not coil around each other. This is achieved by using a special catheter with two lumens to position the guidewires so that they are not crossed as they pass through the guiding catheter and down the respective branches of the coronary artery (Ultrafuse-X by SciMed or the Multifunctional probe by Schneider).

The advantage of the 'Y' technique is that wire access to both branches is always maintained. The lesion coverage, however, is less complete than with the 'culottes' method or the 'V' method. An alternative to using two balloons simultaneously inside the third stent is to mount the third stent on only one balloon, deploy it proximally after removing the second wire, and add the second balloon subsequently and then inflate both branches with 'kissing' balloon expansion.

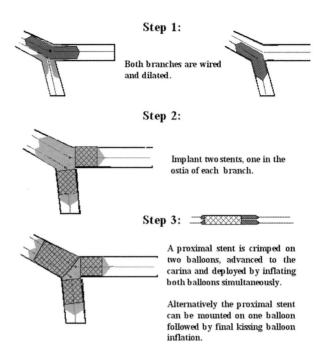

Step 1:

Both branches are wired and dilated.

Step 2:

Implant two stents, one in the ostia of each branch.

Step 3:

A proximal stent is crimped on two balloons, advanced to the carina and deployed by inflating both balloons simultaneously.

Alternatively the proximal stent can be mounted on one balloon followed by final kissing balloon inflation.

Figure 10.20 *The 'Y' or three-stent technique*

A clinical example of this 'Y' technique for bifurcation stenting is shown in *Fig. 10.21*. Baseline images reveal a severe stenosis just proximal to and extending into the LAD and diagonal branches. Both arteries were treated with directional atherectomy and then the diagonal branch was stented with a 15 mm long Crown stent using a 4 mm balloon at 6 atmospheres. A second 15 mm long Crown stent was then passed into the LAD, also using a 4 mm balloon and deployed at 14 atmospheres. A third Crown stent was then placed in the LAD proximal to the bifurcation (*Fig. 10.21c*).

Figure 10.22 provides an example of severe disease involving the ostium of the LAD and extending into the bifurcation of a large diagonal branch. This case occurred early on in our experience when only the Palmaz–Schatz stent was available. Two Palmaz–Schatz stents were implanted in the LAD diagonal bifurcation after pre-dilating both branches (see *Fig. 10.22b*). A third Palmaz– Schatz stent was then hand crimped on to two balloons which were threaded over the two guidewires. The third stent was deployed proximal to the bifurcation and then all three stents were expanded with a final simultaneous balloon dilatation. The final result (*Fig. 10.22c* shows wide patency from the ostium of the LAD into the ostia of the bifurcation.

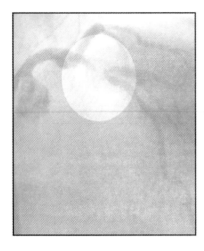
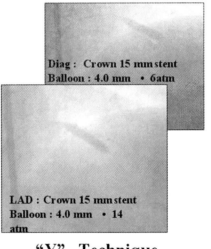

a **Baseline**

Figure 10.21 *The 'Y' technique for bifurcation stenting. (a) Baseline images demonstrate a severe stenosis in the proximal LAD extending into a large diagonal branch. (b) Both arteries were treated with directional atherectomy. Each branch was then dilated and stented sequentially. (c) A third Crown stent was then placed in the LAD proximal to the bifurcation.*

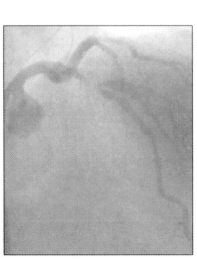
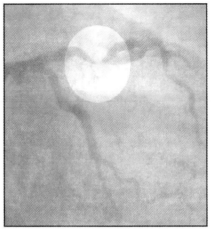

Diag : Crown 15 mm stent
Balloon : 4.0 mm • 6atm

LAD : Crown 15 mm stent
Balloon : 4.0 mm • 14 atm

b **"Y" Technique**

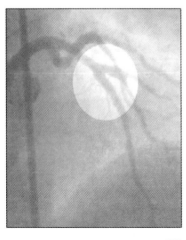
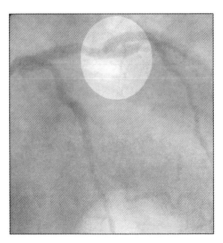

c **Final Result**

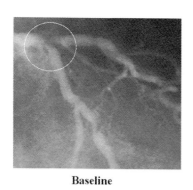

Baseline

Debulking with Rotational Atherectomy

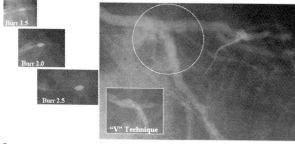

a

b   Final Result

Figure 10.26 *Left main bifurcation stenting. Progressive rotational atherectomy burr sizes up to 2.5 mm, through a 10 French guiding catheter, were used to diminish the bulk of plaque. Two AVE GFX stents were then placed using the 'V' technique.*

diagonal branch. An ACS Multilink stent was placed into the LAD. After deployment, the diagonal artery was re-entered with an ACE balloon and then a high-pressure inflation of the LAD stent was performed with a Titan 4 mm diameter balloon at 18 atmospheres. Simultaneous inflations were then performed at the bifurcation. A 9 mm short, low-compliance Titan balloon was chosen so that the proximal portion of the LAD would not be overstretched when the two balloons were simultaneously inflated.

In *Fig. 10.28* the bifurcation of the circumflex artery and the obtuse marginal artery was treated with directional atherectomy sequentially down both branches (*Fig. 10.28b*). A NIR seven-cell stent was placed in the larger obtuse marginal branch, and then the smaller circumflex was dilated through the side of the NIR stent with a 2.5 mm ACE balloon. Simultaneous inflations were performed, and the final result is demonstrated in *Fig. 10.28c*. The use of atherectomy before stent deployment has a dramatic effect in preventing plaque shift or compromise to the ostium of either branch at the bifurcation.

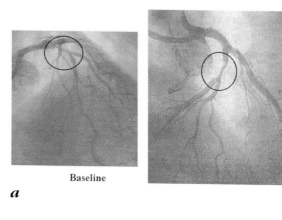

Baseline

a

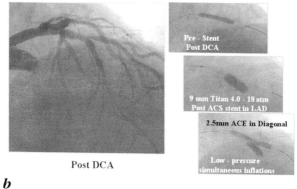

Post DCA

b

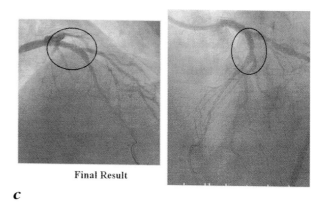

Final Result

c

Figure 10.27 *Directional atherectomy to debulk a bifurcation lesion prior to stenting.*

CLINICAL RESULTS

Our results in 182 cases of bifurcation lesions are presented in *Tables 10.4–10.13*. The lesions are separated into two groups; the first group is called the 'kissing stent' group (n = 90) – patients in whom both branches received a stent, and the second group is

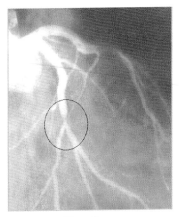

Baseline

a

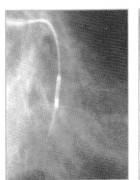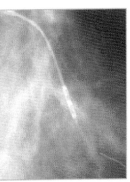

DCA in Circumflex   DCA in Obtuse Marginal

b

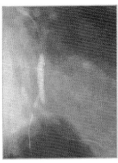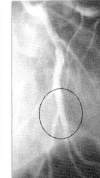

Kissing Inflation
3.5mm NIR 7 cell in OM
2.5mm ACE in Circ   **Final Result**

c

Figure 10.28 *Directional atherectomy to debulk a bifurcation lesion prior to stenting. OM, obtuse marginal.*

called the 'side branch inflation' group (n = 92) – patients in whom only the main branch was stented and the side branch received balloon inflation. The patient characteristics for these two groups are presented in *Table 10.4*. Patients who received stents in both branches tended to have more disease, as manifested by the group having a greater prevalence of diabetes mellitus, previous bypass surgery, and multivessel involvement. The angiographic characteristics for the two groups are listed in *Table 10.5*. The majority of these cases were performed electively, and a total occlusion existed at the bifurcation in approximately 9% of cases. Larger artery bifurcations (such

Table 10.4
Bifurcation lesions. Patient characteristics

	Kissing stent n = 90	Side branch inflation n = 92	p
Age (years)	58 ± 11	58 ± 10	NS
Male (%)	93	93	NS
Diabetes (%)	23	12	<0.05
Previous CABG (%)	18	2	<0.01
Unstable angina (%)	29	28	NS
Multivessel disease (%)	80	60	< 0.01

Table 10.5
Bifurcation lesions. Angiographic characteristics

	Kissing stent n = 90	Side branch inflation n = 92	p
Indication for stenting			NS
Elective (%)	82	86	
Acute (%)	8	8	
Total occlusion (%)	10	7	
Bifurcation site			< 0.01
LAD–LCX (%)	24	8	
LAD–Diag (%)	31	60	
LCX–OM (%)	29	22	
RCA–RCA (%)	16	11	
DCA prior to stenting (%)	14	10	NS
RTB prior to stenting (%)	17	13	NS

Table 10.6

Bifurcation lesions. Type of stent

	Kissing stent n = 90	Side branch inflation n = 92	p
Palmaz–Schatz	17	25	NS
AVE Micro	22	11	NS
NIR	19	21	NS
Gianturco–Roubin	14	45	NS
Multilink	8	9	NS
Other stents	12	18	NS
Combination of stents	8	1	NS

Table 10.7

Bifurcation lesions. Procedural characteristics

	Kissing stent n = 90	Side branch inflation n = 92	p
Multiple stents (%)	26	22	NS
Length of stents (mm)	22 ± 17	25 ± 13	NS
Balloon size (mm)	3.34 ± 0.37	3.44 ± 0.40	NS
Final B/A ratio	1.20 ± 0.20	1.17 ± 0.18	NS
Max pressure (atm)	14.6 ± 3.5	16.0 ± 4.0	<0.05

B/A, balloon to artery ratio.

Table 10.8

Bifurcation lesions. Procedural outcomes and clinical events

	Kissing stent n = 90	Side branch inflation n = 92	p
Procedural success (%)	94	95	NS
Angiographic success (%)	99	96	NS
Procedural MI (%)	4.4	0	<0.05
Procedural CABG (%)	2.2	1.1	NS
Procedural death (%)	2.2	1.1	NS
Acute thrombosis (%)	1.1	0	NS
Subacute thrombosis (%)	3.3	2.2	NS

Table 10.9

Bifurcation lesions. Quantitative angiographic results (I)

	Kissing stent n = 90	Side branch inflation n = 92	p
	Main vessel		
Before the procedure			
Refer vessel diam (mm)	2.83 ± 0.50	2.99 ± 0.44	<0.05
MLD (mm)	0.79 ± 0.49	0.86 ± 0.44	NS
Percentage stenosis	72 ± 16	71 ± 14	NS
Lesion length (mm)	9.4 ± 6.2	11.3 ± 7.6	NS
After stenting			
Refer vessel diam (mm)	2.99 ± 0.44	3.11 ± 0.45	NS
MLD (mm)	2.84 ± 0.59	2.92 ± 0.59	NS
Percentage stenosis	5 ± 15	7 ± 12	NS

as LAD–circumflex bifurcations) were more likely to be treated with 'kissing stents' whereas LAD–diagonal bifurcations were more often approached with a single stent and dilatation through the side branch. Directional coronary atherectomy was performed before stenting in 13% of patients and rotational atherectomy was performed in 15% of cases.

The variety of stents that were deployed for each group is shown in *Table 10.6*. The procedural characteristics, including the length of the stents, balloon size, balloon-to-vessel ratio, and maximum pressure are shown in *Table 10.7*. There was no difference in the length of the stents or the balloon-to-artery ratio, but the maximum pressure used was slightly higher for the side branch inflation group. The procedural outcomes and clinical events listed in *Table 10.8* demonstrate a high initial success rate (95%), although the incidence of procedural myocardial infarction (2.2%) and subacute thrombosis (2.7%) is higher than in non-bifurcational lesions.

The quantitative angiographic results before and after stenting are shown in *Table 10.9* and angiographic follow-up is shown in *Table 10.10*. These data show that a large final minimum lumen diameter (2.8 mm) is obtained on average from both groups in this difficult anatomic setting but that the late loss index (0.59) is high compared to non-bifurcational lesions. The loss index is worse for the kissing stent group (0.65 versus 0.52) than when a single stent was used. The 6-month restenosis rate for the 128 patients who had follow-up angiography is shown in *Tables 10.11* and *10.12*. The total restenosis rate for the

Table 10.10

Bifurcation lesions. Quantitative angiographic results (II)

	Kissing stent n = 90	Side branch inflation n = 92	p
Angio follow-up (%)	81	73	NS
At follow-up			
Refer vessel diam (mm)	2.83 ± 0.55	2.90 ± 0.47	NS
MLD (mm)	1.57 ± 0.95	1.90 ± 0.96	0.05
Percentage stenosis	46 ± 27	36 ± 28	0.05
Acute gain (mm)	2.08 ± 0.64	2.05 ± 0.63	NS
Late loss (mm)	1.25 ± 0.91	0.97 ± 0.81	NS
Loss index	0.65 ± 0.55	0.52 ± 0.47	NS

Table 10.11

Bifurcation lesions. Restenosis rate (I)

	Kissing stent	Side branch inflation	p
Total	39.3 (26/66)	27.4 (17/62)	NS
Bifurcation site (%)			
LAD–LCX	33.3 (5/15)	40.0 (2/5)	NS
LAD–Diagonal	27.3 (6/22)	25.6 (10/39)	NS
LCX–GM	47.4 (9/19)	27.3 (3/11)	NS
RCA–RCA	60.0 (6/10)	28.6 (2/7)	NS

Table 10.12

Bifurcation lesions. Restenosis rate (II)

	Kissing stent	Side branch inflation	p
Slotted tube stent (%)	31.4 (11/35)	20.9 (9/43)	NS
DCA prior to stent (%)	16.7 (2/12)	16.7 (1/6)	NS
RTB prior to stent (%)	38.5 (5/13)	22.2 (2/9)	NS
IVUS used (%)	38.7 (12/31)	29.3 (12/41)	NS
DCA + slot, tub. stenting	10.0 (1/10)	0 (0/4)	NS

Table 10.13

Bifurcation lesions. Final IVUS results

	Kissing stent n = 40	Side branch inflation n = 56	p
Proximal reference			
LD (mm)	3.10 ± 0.63	3.31 ± 0.60	NS
LCSA (mm²)	9.13 ± 3.17	10.35 ± 3.65	NS
Stented segment			
MLD (mm)	2.61 ± 0.37	2.71 ± 0.50	NS
MLCSA (mm²)	6.24 ± 1.62	6.89 ± 2.29	NS
Distal Reference			
LD (mm)	2.66 ± 0.35	2.68 ± 0.46	NS
LCSA (mm²)	6.31 ± 1.81	6.48 ± 2.18	NS

LD = lumen diameter; LCSA lumen cross sectional area; MLD = minimal lumen diameter; MLCSA= minimal lumen cross sectional area

'kissing' stent technique was 39.3%; it was 27.4% when the side branch inflation technique was used (not significant). Given the small number of patients in each group there was no statistically significant difference in restenosis whether the 'kissing' stent or side branch inflation technique was used. The location of the bifurcation also did not appear to influence restenosis either. It is of note that there was a trend towards a lower restenosis rate (17%) when directional atherectomy was used before stenting.

The higher rate of restenosis for bifurcation lesions can be understood more clearly by the IVUS results (*Table 10.13*). In the 96 patients studied with ultrasound following stent insertion, the minimum lumen cross-sectional area was 6.2 mm² for the kissing stent group and 6.9 mm² for the side branch inflation groups. This is smaller than our average result for non-bifurcational lesions and is consistent with the

fact that the bifurcation often extends into smaller vessels, which have an inherent higher restenosis rate. Based on these results, we currently try to perform atherectomy more frequently for bifurcation lesions and stent both branches only when the diameter of the side branch is > 3.0 mm.

CHOICE OF STENT FOR BIFURCATION LESIONS

A list of some of the advantages and disadvantages of different types of stents when treating bifurcation lesions is provided in *Tables 10.14* and *10.15*. The benefit of using coil stents for bifurcation lesions is primarily that their placement is technically less

Table 10.14

Coil stents for bifurcation lesions

Advantages	Disadvantages
Technically less demanding Second stent inserted only if necessary Crossing with the wire and balloon dilatation through the stent facilitated	Possible plaque prolapse through stent struts Coil stents without axial support may be damaged during recrossing and balloon dilatation

Table 10.15

Mesh stents for bifurcation lesions

	Advantages	Disadvantages
T stenting	• Technically less demanding • Suitable for treatment of large side branches • Second stent inserted only if needed	• Positioning second stent cumbersome (gaps at the ostium or protrusion of the side branch stent into the main vessel possible) • Access to side branch lost while stenting main vessel (occasionally rewiring and ballooning side branch difficult)
Kissing stent	• More complete lesion coverage • Access to both vessels always maintained • Suitable for treatment of two large arteries (left main stenting)	• Technically very demanding • Even with the best technique gaps among stents possible (three-stent technique) • Metallic neo-carina in the middle of main vessel, not in contact with the vessel wall (two-stent technique)

demanding. Because the coils are more easily separated by balloon dilation, it is easier to recross the stent through its side into the branch vessel. An initial attempt to use only one stent in the main branch and dilating through the side branch can be tried; if that is unsuccessful then a second stent can be inserted with one of the 'through the stent' techniques. The disadvantages of the coil stents is that, owing to the wider separation and lower coverage of the plaque, there may be prolapse of plaque tissue through the stent struts. In addition, in association with the lower axial support, the stents can be damaged through recrossing and balloon dilatation.

Table 10.15 lists the advantages and disadvantages for the newer meshwork stents. Compared to the less flexible slotted tubular design stents, the meshwork stents are technically less demanding and yet provide more complete lesion coverage than the coil stents. These characteristics make the meshwork stents more suitable for treatment of two large branches, such as in left main stenting. The disadvantage of these stents, however, is that they are more difficult to cross into the side branch than the coil stents are. If access is lost to the side branch while the main vessel is being stented, it may be difficult to rewire and dilate the side branch. Some of the newer stents, such as the Crossflex laser cut stent, appear to have excellent support and still permit easy access for a second stent to pass through the side into the bifurcation.

COMPLICATIONS OF BIFURCATION STENTING

The primary difficulty with stenting bifurcation lesions is the technical challenge of delivering the

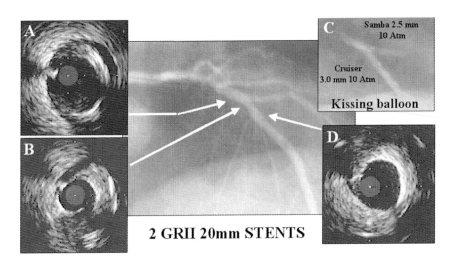

Figure 10.29 *Stent deformation after side branch dilatation.*

stent to the proper position. When only the Palmaz–Schatz slotted tubular design stent was available, the incidence of failure to deliver the stent to the appropriate position was more common than with the low-profile flexible coil and meshwork stents that are currently available. Other complications include stent jail of the side branch vessel with inability to recross the initially deployed stent, side branch compression, deformation of the stent, and malposition of the stent. These problems are more easily recognized by IVUS than by angiography, as demonstrated in the following examples. In *Fig. 10.29*, the angiographic result is shown after stent deployment in the LAD and the diagonal branch with the 'kissing stent culottes' technique. The angiographic appearance is excellent, with wide patency to both branches. However the ultrasound image at the bifurcation (*Fig. 10.29*, Panel B) shows a compromised lumen compared to the proximal and distal stented portions of the artery. Two coiled stents (Gianturco-Roubin II stents) were used, and these provided less than adequate support. On the basis of this ultrasound observation, the two balloons were repositioned and reinflated simultaneously at higher pressures until an adequate lumen throughout the LAD was obtained.

When stenting bifurcation lesions, it is possible to traumatize one or both stents owing to repeated passage of balloons through the stents. *Figure 10.30a* shows a bifurcation of the left main artery that appears widely patent on angiography after stent deployment. However, the ultrasound image reveals compression of the stent in the circumflex artery despite simultaneous inflations in both main branches. Based on the ultrasound information, the

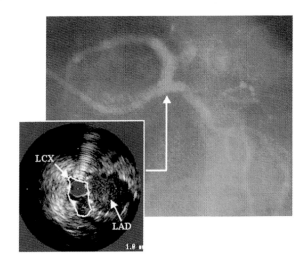

a

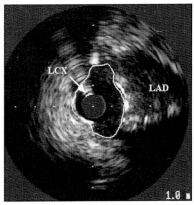

b **After Repeat Dilatation**

Figure 10.30 *IVUS evaluation of a compressed stent in a bifurcation. LCX, left circumflex.*

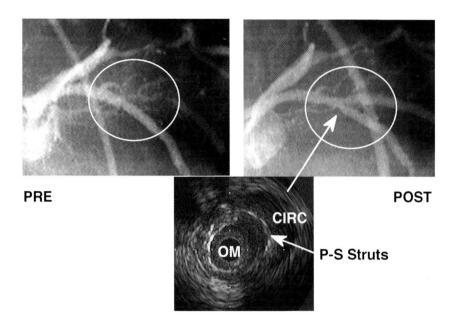

Figure 10.31 *'Stent Jail'. Stenting across a bifurcation inhibiting access to the side branch. P–S, Palmaz–Schatz.*

stent was redilated with simultaneous inflations. The subsequent ultrasound study demonstrates a significantly increased cross-sectional area into the circumflex artery (*Fig. 10.30b*). As we have stated elsewhere in this book, the more complicated the stenting technique or lesion substrate, the more important it is to check your results with IVUS imaging because problems that are not appreciated by angiography are often discovered.

Another complication that may occur when stenting near a bifurcation is stent obstruction of the side branch, which has been graciously called 'stent jail'. Although it is frequently possible with the newer stents to pass a wire and balloon or an ACE balloon across a stent into the side branch, this is not always successful. A case of 'stent jail' is shown in *Fig. 10.31*, where the ultrasound image taken in the obtuse marginal artery reveals that stent struts extend into the main branch of the circumflex. In this instance, a second guidewire had not been left in the circumflex artery and, after deployment of the stent into the obtuse marginal branch, a balloon over a wire or an ACE balloon could not be passed alongside the deployed stent to help expand the circumflex artery.

THREE-DIMENSIONAL IVUS IMAGING OF BIFURCATION LESIONS

On occasion a three-dimensional reconstruction of the IVUS images obtained on pull-back may be helpful for understanding the anatomy immediately surrounding a bifurcation. A three-dimensional reconstruction of ultrasound images is provided in *Fig. 10.32*. The bifurcation of this circumflex artery and obtuse marginal branch was treated with two Gianturco–Roubin II stents, each 20 mm long. The 'culottes' method of passing one stent through the other was used. IVUS imaging was obtained in each branch; the reconstruction of the pull-back from the circumflex artery is shown in *Fig. 10.32b* (left panel) and the pull-back through the obtuse marginal branch is shown in *Fig. 10.32b* (right panel). IVUS images can be presented in a variety of ways, including the standard cross-sectional images (*Fig. 10.32c*, Panel A), the three-dimensional projection (*Fig. 10.32c*, Panel C) and the longitudinal projection (*Fig. 10.32c*, Panel D), where the bifurcation of the circumflex and obtuse marginal is more clearly defined.

BIFURCATION STENTS

Several companies have tried to approach the problem of adequate support during bifurcational stenting by developing stents that have larger stent struts that can be placed at the bifurcation, such as the NIR side (SciMed), the Jostent B (Jomed International AB, Drottninggatan, Sweden) and the Devon side-arm stent (Devon Medical, Hamburg, Germany). This permits passage of a balloon, or even a second stent, through the first stent into the side branch while

Gianturco Roubin II

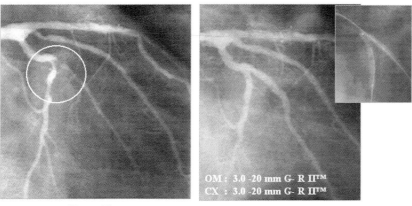

Baseline   **Final Result**

a

Figure 10.32 *The use of intravascular ultrasound with three-dimensional reconstruction and longitudinal reconstruction to identify the ostium of the side branches. OM, obtuse marginal; CX, circumflex.*

3-D Reconstruction

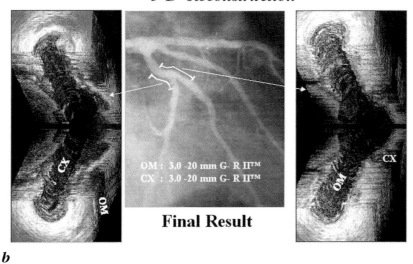

Final Result

b

3-D Reconstruction

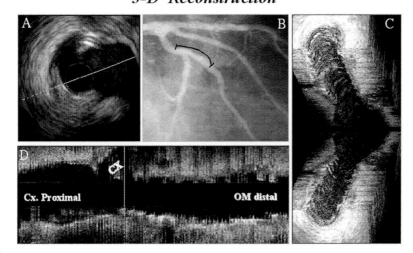

c

maintaining greater support and integrity to the main vessel. Some examples of these side branch stents are shown in *Figs 2.46, 2.47* and *2.48*. Bard Inc. (Billerico, Massachusetts, USA) has been experimenting with a bifurcational stent that has a larger proximal segment with two separate legs in the distal half of the stent (*Fig. 2.55*). This stent comes pre-mounted on two balloons with the balloons extending into the individual legs; the two balloons sit side by side within the proximal portion of the stent. Each monorail balloon is fed over a guidewire with the attempt to pass each leg of the stent into the separate branch of the bifurcation. The more proximal half of the stent then covers the area of the main vessel proximal to the bifurcation. Preliminary experience with this stent has been variable in terms of the ability to pass the bifurcating stent simultaneously over both wires without getting them crossed.

PHARMACOLOGICAL THERAPY

When dealing with a bifurcation lesion, it must be kept in mind that the increased trauma created by the dilatation of two branches and the shear stress induced by the new angle formed by the single or double stent may create a more thrombogenic environment. Therefore it is important to pay attention to the use of antiplatelet therapy. If possible, ticlopidine should be started 3 days before the procedure, and the use of abciximab should be quite liberal. We use abciximab, especially if debulking is performed before bifurcational stenting. The routine use of abciximab during bifurcational stenting may improve patency of the side branch following maneuvers which could compromise the lumen and flow. Recent data from the EPISTENT trial support this approach.[31]

CONCLUSION

In summary, bifurcation lesions remains a technically challenging subset for interventional cardiologists to stent. When possible, debulking the plaque with rotational atherectomy (if it is calcified) or directional atherectomy should be used. Owing to the high rate of restenosis, we prefer to stent the main branch and use simultaneous balloon inflations into both branches for the final expansion. Stenting both branches is recommended only when the side branch is larger than 3.0 mm. Abciximab is often helpful in this setting because the treatment of bifurcations either starts out or becomes complicated. Significant forethought as to the approach and equipment that will be necessary will go a long way in helping to attain a successful result.

REFERENCES

1. Pinkerton CA, Slack JD. Complex coronary angioplasty: a technique for dilatation of bifurcation stenosis. *Angiology* 1985; **34**: 543–548.
2. Renkin J, Wijns W, Hanet C et al. Angioplasty of coronary bifurcation stenoses. *Cathet Cardiovasc Diagn* 1991; **22**: 167–173.
3. Koller P, Safian RD. Bifurcation stenosis. In: Freed M, Grines C, Safian RD, eds. *The New Manual of Interventional Cardiology*. Birmingham, MI: Physicians Press, 1996, 233–243.
4. Aliabadi D, Tilli FV, Bowers TR et al. Incidence and angiographic predictors of side branch occlusion following high-pressure intracoronary stenting. *Am J Cardiol* 1997; **80**: 994–997.
5. Meier B, Grüntzig AR, King SB III et al. Risk of side branch occlusion during coronary angioplasty. *Am J Cardiol* 1984; **53**: 10–14.
6. Arora RR, Raymond RE, Dimas AP et al. Side branch occlusion during coronary angioplasty: incidence, angiographic characteristics and outcome. *Cathet Cardiovasc Diagn* 1989; **18**: 210–212.
7. Mathias DW, Mooney JF, Lange HW et al. Frequency of success and complications of coronary angioplasty of a stenosis at the ostium of a branch vessel. *Am J Cardiol* 1991; **67**: 491–495.
8. Weinstein JS, Baim DS, Sipperly ME et al. Salvage of branch vessels during bifurcation lesion angioplasty: acute and long term follow up. *Cathet Cardiovasc Diagn* 1991; **22**: 1–6.
9. Adelman AG, Cohen EA, Kimball BP et al. A comparison of directional atherectomy with balloon angioplasty for lesions of the left anterior descending artery. *N Engl J Med* 1993; **329**: 228–233.
10. Boehrer JD, Ellis SG, Pieper K et al. Directional atherectomy versus balloon angioplasty for coronary ostial and nonostial left anterior descending artery lesions: results from a randomized multicenter trial. *J Am Coll Cardiol* 1995; **25**: 1380–1386.
11. Fischman DL, Savage MP, Leon MB et al. Fate of lesion-related side branches after coronary artery stenting. *J Am Coll Cardiol* 1993; **22**: 1641–1646.
12. Pan M, Medina A, Suarez de Lezo J et al. Follow-up patency of side branches covered by intracoronary Palmaz–Schatz stent. *Am Heart J* 1995; **129**: 436–440.
13. Colombo A, Maiello L, Itoh A. Coronary stenting of bifurcation lesions: immediate and follow-up results (abstract). *J Am Coll Cardiol* 1996; **27**: 277A.
14. Lefèfre T, Louvard Y, Morice MC et al. Should we stent a

bifurcation lesion? A single center experience (abstract). *Eur Heart J* 1997; **18**: 26.

15. Kobayashi Y, Colombo A, Reimers B, Di Mario C. Coronary stenting in bifurcational lesions: immediate and follow up results (abstract). *Circulation* 1997; **96 (suppl)**: I-693.

16. Spokojny AM, Sanborn TA. The bifurcation lesion. In: Ellis SG, Holmes DR Jr, eds. *Strategic Approaches in Coronary Intervention.* Baltimore: Williams and Wilkins, 1996: 286–291.

17. Di Mario C, De Gregorio J, Kobayashi Y, Colombo A. Atherectomy for ostial LAD stenosis: a cut above. *Cathet Cardiovasc Diagn* 1998; **43**: 101–104.

18. Moussa I, Moses J, Di Mario C et al. The stenting after optimal lesion debulking registry 'SOLD': angiographic and clinical outcome. *Circulation* 1998; **98**: 1604–1609.

19. Moussa I, Di Mario C, Moses J et al. Coronary stenting after rotationl atherectomy in calcified and complex lesions: Angiopgraphic and clinical follow-up results. *Circulation* 1997; **96**: 128–136.

20. Di Mario C, Colombo A. Trousers-stents: how to choose the right size and shape? *Cathet Cardiovasc Diagn* 1997; **41**: 197–199.

21. Colombo A, Gaglione A, Nakamura S, Finci L. 'Kissing' stents for bifurcational coronary lesions. *Cathet Cardiovasc Diagn* 1993; **30**: 327–330.

22. Nakamura S, Hall P, Maiello L, Colombo A. Technique for Palmaz–Schatz stent deployment in lesions with a large side branch. *Cathet Cardiovasc Diagn* 1995; **34**: 353–361.

23. Kobayashi Y, Colombo A, Akiyama T et al. Modified 'T' stenting: a technique for kissing stents in bifurcational coronary lesions. *Cathet Cardiovasc Diagn* 1998; **43**: 323–326.

24. Chevalier B, Glatt B, Royer T. Kissing stenting in bifurcation lesions (abstract). *Eur Heart J* 1996; **17**: 218.

25. Carrie D, Karouny E, Chouairi S, Puel J. 'T'-shaped stent placement: a technique for the treatment of dissected bifurcation lesions. *Cathet Cardiovasc Diagn* 1996; **37**: 311–313.

26. Schampaert E, Fort S, Adelman AG, Schwartz L. The V-stent: a novel technique for coronary bifurcation stenting. *Cathet Cardiovasc Diagn* 1996; **39**: 320–326.

27. Khoja A, Özbek C, Bay W, Heisel A. Trouser-like stenting: a new technique for bifurcation lesions. *Cathet Cardiovasc Diagn* 1997; **41**: 192–196.

28. Baim DS. Is bifurcation stenting the answer? *Cathet Cardiovasc Diagn* 1996; **37**: 314–316.

29. Pomerantz RM, Ling FS. Distortion of Palmaz–Schatz geometry following side-branch balloon dilatation through the stent in a rabbit model. *Cathet Cardiovasc Diagn* 1997; **40**: 422–426.

30. Ormiston JA, Webster MWI, Ruygrok PN et al. Stent distortion during simulated side-branch dilatation (abstract). *J Am Coll Cardiol* 1998; **37**: 18A.

31. The EPISTENT Investigators. Randomised placebo-controlled and balloon-angioplasty-controlled trial to assess safety of coronary stenting with use of platelet glycoprotein-IIb/IIIa blockade. *Lancet* 1998; **352**: 87–92.

Chapter 11 Ostial lesions

Antonio Colombo and Jonathan Tobis

The treatment of aorto-ostial coronary artery lesions has always been a paradox in interventional cardiology. What appears to be the easiest target to reach in the coronary artery tree frequently turns out to be a technical challenge that can turn all too quickly into a nightmare. The treatment of aorto-ostial lesions by conventional balloon angioplasty and other devices, such as laser or directional atherectomy, has been limited to a low success rate and high incidence of restenosis.[1-4] Coronary stenting is an attractive alternative for this subset of lesions because it provides the necessary scaffolding to support the artery in this very resistant position. Because these lesions are at the entrance to the coronary artery, they are more difficult to evaluate, since the diagnostic or guiding catheter frequently protrudes beyond the lesion so that the catheter can intubate and fill the artery with contrast. Although the guiding catheter may occlude blood flow to the artery, this problem can be alleviated by using a guiding catheter with side holes. Passing a guidewire through the stenosis into the distal vessel is usually not technically difficult in these cases. However, preparing the lesion for a stent with balloon dilatation may be a significant challenge because these lesions tend to have a high incidence of calcification. Even without apparent calcification, these lesions tend to be very resistant because the balloon has to stretch against the longitudinal direction of the aortic wall.

To address these issues of calcification and lesion resistance, we frequently use rotational atherectomy or directional atherectomy to debulk the plaque and prepare the entrance for the stent. Stent implantation in the aorto-ostial location is technically challenging because of difficulties in seating the guiding catheter, obtaining adequate images to enhance stent placement, ensuring proper stent position to cover the entire lesion adequately, and preventing stent migration or embolization. The next difficulty in deploying the stent is to determine the exact position where the stent is to lie. If the stent is placed in too far, it misses the ostium and the tightest portion of the stenosis. On the other hand, if the stent is placed too proximally, it extends into the aorta and may be subject to trauma from the guiding catheter, which could collapse the stent and prevent passage of a balloon or other therapy to treat the rest of the vessel, as well as potentially compromising the lumen and subjecting the patient to a higher incidence of subacute stent thrombosis or restenosis. We have found that precise placement of a stent can be facilitated by using a stent that is clearly visible, such as the Palmaz biliary stent. Moreover, the use of intravascular ultrasound (IVUS) guidance is critical for optimum deployment and correct positioning during ostial lesion stenting. We perform IVUS imaging before any intervention if possible, or certainly after the lesion is prepared with rotational or directional atherectomy. The ultrasound images are used to determine the media-to-media diameter of the vessel, which in turn allows us to choose the correct stent and balloon size. In addition, contrast can be injected under fluoroscopy during ultrasound imaging to correlate the exact ostium of the artery with the angiographic appearance in the view that is going to be used to place the stent. The ultrasound distinction between the aorta and the ostium of the artery is very obvious and is not obscured by the superimposed projection of the sinus of Valsalva and the ostium of the artery, as occurs with X-ray imaging. After the stent is placed and expanded to high pressure, the artery and stent are again interrogated with IVUS to confirm that the stent struts extend right up to the ostium or perhaps 1 mm beyond this into the aorta. If the ostium appears to be compromised or if the stent is not within 1 mm of the true ostium, then a second stent should be placed.

Another concern when stenting ostial lesions is the higher restenosis rate that is expected on the basis of historical reports of treating these lesions. From our assessment of the predictors of restenosis (see Chapter 4), we believe that the best approach for decreasing restenosis in ostial lesions is to maximize the lumen cross-sectional area. This is obtained by debulking the lesion with rotational atherectomy or directional atherectomy and using a stent that has very high radial strength, such as the Palmaz biliary stent. This stent is hand crimped on to a large high-pressure balloon, which does not have to be a very low-profile device since it may bind better to a bulkier balloon (e.g. the Chubby or Orion balloon). Furthermore, the stent should be expanded with an optimally sized balloon as determined by IVUS measurements of the media-to-media diameter. Polymer-covered stents, such as the JoMed poly-

tetrafluoroethylene (PTFE)-covered stent (*Fig. 2.49*) may also reduce restenosis for ostial lesions.

Some examples of treating aorto-ostial lesions are presented in *Figs 11.1, 11.2* and *11.3*. *Figure 11.1* demonstrates a right coronary artery (RCA) in which

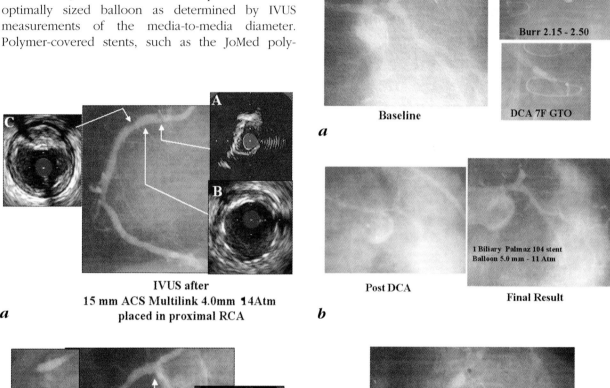

**IVUS after
15 mm ACS Multilink 4.0mm 14Atm
placed in proximal RCA**

a

**After Palmaz 104 4.5 mm
Chubby 14 Atm**

b

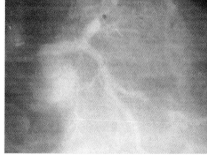

Baseline   Burr 2.15 - 2.50   **DCA 7F GTO**

a

Post DCA   1 Biliary Palmaz 104 stent Balloon 5.0 mm - 11 Atm   **Final Result**

b

5 months Follow-Up

c

Figure 11.1 *IVUS guidance for a right coronary artery aorto-ostial stenosis. (a) IVUS imaging helped to clarify the presence of a residual stenosis after deployment of a MultiLink stent to treat a proximal stenosis. (b) Angiogram and IVUS study after deployment of a second stent to treat the ostial lesion.*

Figure 11.2 *Aorto-ostial left main stenosis. (a) This severe left main disease was treated with progressive rotational atherectomy followed by debulking with directional atherectomy. (b) A Palmaz biliary stent was deployed on a 5 mm diameter balloon. (c) The five month follow-up angiogram reveals no evidence of restenosis.*

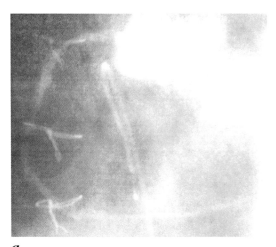

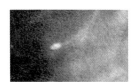

Figure 11.3 *(a) Severe diffuse disease throughout the length of the right coronary artery. This was treated with rotational atherectomy and placement of multiple stents. (b) Angiogram 4 months later reveals restenosis isolated to the ostium of the RCA This was treated by placement of a Palmaz 204 stent.*

a

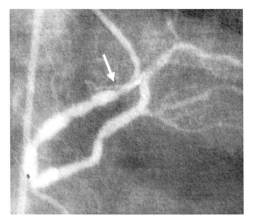

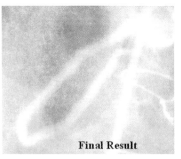

Final Result

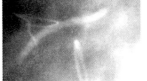

Ostial Restenosis

b

40 x 4.0mm balloon at 16 atm

a stent was deployed for a proximal stenosis. Following placement of a 15 mm long ACS Multilink stent expanded to 14 atmospheres with a 4.0 mm balloon, there is an irregular linear density at the interface of the guiding catheter and the coronary artery. The linear density is not very long, which makes it difficult to assess the severity. The IVUS image (*Fig. 11.1*, Panel A) at the ostium shows that the lumen is oblong in shape with intense calcification that diminishes penetration of the ultrasound into the plaque so that no more than 0.5 mm of the surrounding artery wall is visualized. The lumen at the aorto-ostial inlet measures only 1.5 mm × 2.0 mm (*Fig. 11.1*, Panel A). The proximal portion of the RCA covered by the stent is adequately expanded, with a lumen by IVUS of 4.0 mm × 3.5 mm (*Fig. 11.1*, Panel B). Distal to the stent, there is some lumen narrow-

ing but the eccentric lumen is adequate at 3.5 mm × 2.3 mm (*Fig. 11.1*, Panel C); 5 mm distal to the stent, the artery is quite large and measures 5.0 × 4.0 mm in diameter (media to media). Based on this ultrasound evaluation, a Palmaz 104 biliary stent was placed on a 4.5 mm Chubby balloon and deployed at 14 atmospheres at the ostium of the RCA. The final angiogram (*Fig. 11.1b*) shows a patent ostium, and the ultrasound study demonstrates that the lumen at the ostium is 3.5 mm × 3.0 mm. During the IVUS examination, it is important to withdraw the guiding catheter back into the aorta so that the IVUS catheter can document adequate coverage right at the aorto-ostial junction.

The clinical example shown in *Fig. 11.2* demonstrates severe aorto-ostial disease involving the left main coronary artery in a patient who has had bypass surgery. There was a patent graft to the left anterior descending artery (LAD) but the graft to the obtuse marginal system was occluded. This lesion was addressed by using rotational atherectomy with sequentially larger burrs reaching a maximum of 2.5 mm in diameter. A 10 Fr guiding catheter was necessary to use this large burr size. In addition, the bulk of the plaque was removed by using directional atherectomy with a 7 Fr GTO cutter. Following the atherectomy, a Palmaz biliary 104 stent was placed on a 5 mm balloon and deployed at 11 atmospheres (*Fig. 11.2b*). The follow-up angiogram at 5 months (*Fig. 11.2c*) is remarkable for the lack of intimal hyperplasia and the minimal amount of late lumen loss.

The next patient (*Fig. 11.3*) developed aorto-ostial stenosis as a complication of restenosis. The RCA was initially diffusely diseased (see *Fig. 11.3a*). This was treated with rotational atherectomy using progressively larger sized burrs from 1.25 mm to 1.5 mm, and then finally a 2.0 mm burr. The entire artery was treated with long stents, which included four Crown stents, each 32 mm long. In addition, the proximal portion of the artery was treated with a 15 mm Palmaz–Schatz stent. The patient returned 4 months later with recurrent symptoms, and angiography revealed restenosis in the distal and proximal portion of the artery (*Fig. 11.3b*). The distal section was treated with balloon dilatation followed by placement of a 39 mm long AVE stent. This was inflated with a 4 mm balloon at 16 atmospheres. The new stenosis at the aorto-ostial junction was treated with a 20 mm long Palmaz 204 stent, which was inflated with a 4.5 mm balloon at 18 atmospheres. The rest of the artery was also dilated with a 40 mm × 4.0 mm balloon at 16 atmospheres, with a final angiographic result shown in *Fig. 11.3b*.

A REVIEW OF OUR CASES WITH AORTO-OSTIAL DISEASE

There were 187 patients treated between March 1993 and May 1998 who had coronary ostial disease. Of these cases, there were 89 lesions that were at the aorto-ostial junction. In addition, there were 191 coronary ostial lesions that were not at the aortic ostium (i.e. they were at the ostial LAD, ostial circumflex artery, large diagonal or other branches). A comparison of the patient characteristics for these two classes of ostial lesions is shown in *Table 11.1*. The risk factors and previous history are typical for our patient population except that the incidence of multivessel disease (78%) is higher, which implies

Table 11.1

Patient characteristics of ostial lesions

187 patients *n (%)*	*Aorto-ostial* *67 pts.*	*Ostial (non-aortic)* *120 pts.*	*p value*
Age (yrs)	62 ± 10	59 ± 11	NS
Male	41 (77)	90 (89)	0.052
Risk factors			
Hypercholesterolemia	42 (63)	69 (58)	NS
Tobacco (active + former)	34 (51)	63 (53)	NS
Family history	26 (39)	49 (41)	NS
Diabetes	4 (6)	15 (13)	u.s.
Hypertension	29 (43)	56 (47)	NS
Previous MI	35 (52)	53 (44)	NS
Unstable angina	21 (32)	39 (33)	NS
Prior coronary bypass	27 (40)	16 (13)	< 0.0001
Multivessel disease	51 (78)	68 (57)	< 0.005

Table 11.2

Vessel distribution (total 280 lesions)

Aorto-ostial: 89 lesions	n	%	Ostial (non-aortic): 191 lesions	n	%
RCA	47	53	LAD	85	30
LM	25	28	Diag.	35	13
SVG	17	19	Cx	29	10
			OM	27	10
			Ramus	6	2
			RCA-PD	5	2
			IMA	2	1
			RCA-PL	1	0
			Cx-PD	1	0

Table 11.3

Type of stent used

Stent type	Aorto-ostial n (%)	Ostial (non-aortic) n (%)
Palmaz–Schatz	37 (42)	53 (28)
NIR	17 (19)	40 (21)
PURA	9 (10)	11 (6)
Combination	8 (9)	8 (4)
JOMED PTFE	8 (9)	0
BeStent	3 (3)	2 (1)
Radio BX	2 (2)	1 (1)
AVE	1 (1)	32 (17)
ACS	1 (1)	8 (4)
DART	1 (1)	4 (2)
Wiktor	1 (1)	2 (1)
Radio PS	1 (1)	1 (1)
Crossflex	0	7 (4)
Cook	0	6 (3)
CROWN	0	4 (2)
INFLOW	0	4 (2)
BX	0	3 (2)
Cordis	0	2 (1)
CF II	0	1 (1)

Table 11.4

Quantitative angiographic measurements

	Baseline	Post-procedure	Follow-up
Aorto-ostial			
MLD (mm)	1.16 ± 0.68	3.65 ± 0.66	2.18 ± 1.37
Percentage DS	66 ± 20	0 ± 11	39 ± 33
Ostial (non-aortic)			
MLD (mm)	0.89 ± 0.60	3.01 ± 0.65	1.99 ± 1.06
Percentage DS	70 ± 20	4 ± 15	35 ± a31

Table 11.2. The majority (53%) of the aorto-ostial lesions occurred in the RCA, but 28% of the lesions were present in the left main artery. The type of stent used to treat these lesions is shown in *Table 11.3.* The high use of Palmaz stents or Palmaz–Schatz stents reflects not only their availability in our early experience but also the fact that they have excellent radial support, which is appropriate for this set of highly resistant ostial lesions.

The quantitative angiographic measurements presented in *Table 11.4* demonstrate that a large final minimum lumen diameter (MLD) was obtained using the method of IVUS-guided optimization and debulking. IVUS imaging was used to guide the stenting process in 60% of cases. Since ostial lesions occur in the largest portion of the artery, there is a greater potential to obtain a large lumen after an intervention. On the other hand, the aorta ostium frequently

Table 11.5

Procedural complications and clinical events aorto-ostial + ostial (non-aortic) lesions

Patients	Pro-cedural	In-hospital	Early (< 2 months)	Late (> 2 months)
Subacute stent thrombosis.	na	2	0	NA
Vascular comp.	5	1	0	0
MI non-Q-wave	5	2	0	0
Q-wave	2	1	0	1
Repeat PTCA	0	2	1	38
CABG	3	0	1	3
Death	0	1	2	8

Clinical follow-up duration 6 months.

that these patients had more diffuse disease. All of these 280 lesions were treated with coronary stents. Most of these procedures were performed electively, although 10% of the lesions had been previously treated and had restenosis following balloon angioplasty. The vessel distribution is demonstrated in has a lot of calcium, which limits the results obtained with balloon dilatation alone. The average MLD at follow-up (2.18 mm) is also larger than the MLD of most stented lesions on angiographic follow-up.

The procedural complications and clinical events are outlined in *Table 11.5*. Two patients developed acute or subacute stent thrombosis. Repeat percutaneous transluminal coronary angioplasty (PTCA) for restenosis was performed in 39 lesions, and four patients had elective coronary artery bypass surgery between 2 and 12 months after the procedure. The target lesion revascularization rate was 15%. There were two Q-wave myocardial infarctions but no deaths occurred during the procedure. One death occurred in hospital and 10 patients died between 2 and 12 months after this procedure (giving a 6% 1-year mortality).

The incidence of restenosis is shown in *Table 11.6*. The mean duration of angiographic follow-up was 4.9 ± 1.6 months. With an angiographic follow-up rate of 55%, the incidence of restenosis was 40% for aorto-ostial lesions using the dichotomous definition of > 50% diameter stenosis. In these 51 lesions, the frequency of target lesion revascularization was 32%. Although this restenosis rate of 40% appears high, it is significantly better than previously reported treatments of aorto-ostial disease with PTCA alone, in which restenosis ranged between 60% and 71%.[5] Recently, Noboyoshi and colleagues reported a series of 40 RCA aorto-ostial lesions treated with stents. Their angiographic restenosis rate was greater than 60%. One of the reasons for the difference in restenosis rates may be our liberal use of atherectomy for debulking the plaque within aorto-ostial lesions.

SAPHENOUS VEIN GRAFT AORTO-OSTIAL LESIONS

Catheter-based coronary interventions for aorto-ostial lesions in saphenous vein grafts have been a challenge in terms of technique and long-term outcome.[6,7] Stenoses involving the ostium of saphenous vein grafts have some similarities with coronary aorto-ostial disease. These lesions are frequently difficult to cannulate with the guiding catheter and therefore are hard to image adequately. The aorto-ostial location makes it difficult to position the stent precisely and difficult to document that the placement of the stent is performed correctly. An example of an aorto-ostial saphenous vein graft stenosis is shown in *Fig. 11.4*. The baseline angiogram showed a tight lesion in the proximal

Table 11.6

Ostial lesions: incidence of restenosis (total 153 lesions with angiographic follow-up)

	n	*Restenosis*	*TLR*
Aorto-ostial: 51 lesions			
RCA	31	40%	40%
LM	11	25%	17%
SVG	9	56%	40%
Overall	40%	32%	
Ostial (non-aortic) 102 lesions			
LAD	54	17%	17%
DIAG	15	0%	0%
Cx	14	50%	44%
OM	15	27%	20%
Ramus	2	100%	100%
RCA-PD	2	0%	0%
Overall	26%	24%	

Angiographic F/U rate = 55%
Angiographic F/U duration = 4.9 ± 1.6 months
TLR, target lesion vascularization

portion of the graft, which extended to the entrance at the aorta (arrow *a*). In addition, there was disease in the distal portion of the graft and at the anastomosis of the vein graft and the native coronary artery (arrow *b*). The distal lesion was treated with a 15 mm Omega stent and dilated with a 3.5 mm × 30 mm Calypso balloon at 12 atmospheres. The proximal lesion was treated with a 19 mm PTFE-covered stent (see Chapter 2). This was expanded to 4 mm with a 20 mm Calypso balloon at 14 atmospheres. PTFE-covered stents are useful in vein grafts because there are no bifurcating branches that could be occluded by the covered stent. In addition, it is hoped that the lack of contact between the intima and the inner lumen of the stent diminishes the chance of restenosis, which is especially high at aorto-ostial junctions. The final angiographic result is shown in *Fig. 11.4b*, which now demonstrates excellent flow throughout the length of the stent and into the body of the native coronary artery. In addition, the stent lumen cross-sectional area by IVUS is well expanded, with an 11.0 mm² lumen proximally (*Fig. 11.4b*, Panel A) and 7.5 mm² at the anastomotic site (*Fig. 11.4b*, Panel B).

The ostial stenosis in the vein graft shown in *Fig. 11.5a* documents how difficult it can be to show the exact position of the aorto-ostial junction, owing to interference from the guiding catheter. As shown in

baseline

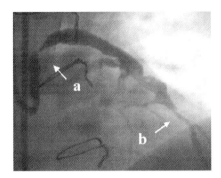

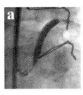

during procedure

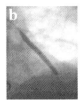

PTFE 19 mm

CALYPSO
4.0 mm
20 mm
14 atm

OMEGA 15mm

CALYPSO
3.5 mm
30 mm
12 atm

Figure 11.4 *Aorto-ostial stenosis involving a saphenous vein graft. (a) The baseline angiogram demonstrates the stenosis in the proximal and distal segments of the graft extending into the anastomosis with the native coronary artery. (b) Angiogram and IVUS study following treatment of the proximal vein graft with a PTFE covered stent. LCSA, lumen cross sectional area.*

a

Final Angiogram

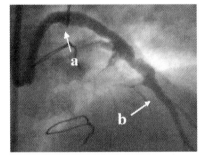

IVUS Results

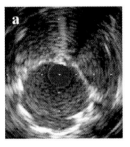

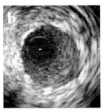

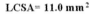

LCSA= 7.5 mm²

LCSA= 11.0 mm²

b

Fig. 11.5b, by withdrawing the guiding catheter and using multiple injections of contrast, a 27 mm JOMED PTFE-covered stent was positioned at the aorto-ostial junction of the vein graft. This was deployed on a 5 mm diameter balloon at 20 atmospheres, with the final angiographic result shown in *Fig. 11.5b.* In addition, the IVUS images in the vein graft, as well as in the PTFE-covered stent, are documented in *Fig. 11.5c.* By removing the guiding catheter out of the vein graft ostium, the IVUS pull-back study showed that there was no residual obstruction at the aorto-ostial junction.

(a) coronary stenting of aorto-ostial lesions in native coronary arteries and bypass vein grafts can be performed safely with a high rate of success;

(b) no episodes of acute stent thrombosis occurred in this series of patients;

(c) the restenosis and target lesion revascularization rates are low compared to results obtained with other interventional strategies for ostial lesions; to reduce the incidence of restenosis even further, we are currently testing the hypothesis that the use of PTFE-covered stents may inhibit the protrusion of intimal hyperplasia into the stented zone.

SUMMARY

We draw the following conclusions from this analysis of our experience:

OSTIAL LAD OR CIRCUMFLEX LESIONS

Although stenoses of the initial portion of the LAD or circumflex arteries are referred to as ostial lesions,

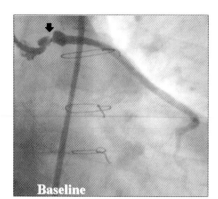

a

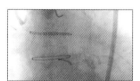

Jomed PTFE stent 27 mm
5.0 mm • 20 atm

b

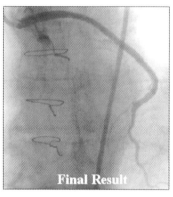

c

Figure 11.5 *An aorto-ostial saphenous vein graft lesion treated with a PTFE covered stent.*

aorto-ostial lesion. These ostial lesions are similar to the aorto-ostial stenoses in that precise placement of the stent may be difficult. The other major difference between these two sets of lesions is that the LAD or circumflex ostial lesion frequently involves the bifurcation, either because the disease extends into the bifurcation (although this may not be apparent by angiography) or because placement of the stent too proximally may entrap the other vessel. In addition, retrograde dissection may cause complications at the bifurcation and involve the branch vessel. One similarity in treating the ostial LAD or circumflex lesions compared with aorta-ostial lesions is that we have found both sets of lesions respond better to debulking with directional atherectomy, or rotational atherectomy if the arteries are calcified.[8] The patient characteristics are shown in *Table 11.1* and the vessel distribution is provided in *Table 11.2.* The overall restenosis rate for 102 non-aortocoronary ostial lesions with angiographic follow-up was 26% (*Table 11.6*). Most of these restenosis lesions were treated by repeat dilatation with a target lesion revascularization of 24%. Descriptive examples of our approach to the treatment of ostial circumflex and LAD lesions are provided in *Figs 11.6–11.10.* In addition, the treatment of ostial lesions is also covered in Chapter 10 on bifurcations because the stenosis frequently involves the bifurcation directly or else the bifurcation has to be treated, due to complications that occur when attempting to stent an ostial LAD or circumflex artery.

Our preferred method for treatment of an ostial LAD lesion is demonstrated in *Fig. 11.6.* Pre-intervention imaging with IVUS is very useful for identifying the extent of the disease and whether it extends back into the bifurcation. IVUS is used also to determine the media-to-media vessel size. The baseline angiogram in *Fig. 11.6* shows a severe stenosis in the ostium of the LAD with a large eccentric plaque on IVUS. There is a 90° arc of calcification in the mid-portion of the plaque between 3 o'clock and 6 o'clock. This was treated with directional atherectomy using a 7 Fr GTO device. Fifteen atherectomy cuts were performed. The repeat ultrasound study showed that the plaque area had been reduced to 48% of the vessel cross-sectional area. Since our criterion for successful directional coronary atherectomy is a plaque area of less than 50%, we proceeded to place a 16 mm long NIR stent which was expanded with a 3.5 mm balloon at 24 atmospheres. Both angiographic and IVUS images demonstrated a large lumen without compromise to the left main artery or the ostium of the circumflex artery.

these differ somewhat from the true aorto-ostial lesions described above. The obvious difference is that the take-off of these vessels is not from the aorta itself, so that the ostial LAD or circumflex lesion usually does not have the same resistance as a true

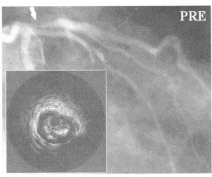
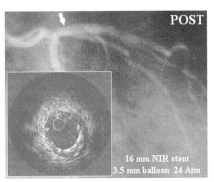
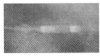

15 cuts DVI GTO 7 Fr

Figure 11.6 *Treatment of a coronary ostial lesion. The disease process frequently extends back into the bifurcation and is more successfully treated with removal of plaque. In this LAD ostial lesion, directional atherectomy was performed prior to placement of a 16 mm long NIR stent.*

Figure 11.7 provides another example of a very tight ostial stenosis of the LAD treated with directional atherectomy, with 24 cuts. A 15 mm long Palmaz–Schatz stent was inserted and inflated at 24 atmospheres with a 4.0 mm balloon. The final angiogram in the left anterior oblique caudal projection shows that not only is the LAD widely patent, but there has also been no compromise to the left main artery or the bifurcation with the circumflex artery. Without debulking these plaques, we observed a higher incidence of plaque shifting and compromise of the branch vessel.

An example of treating a severely diseased ostial LAD lesion without debulking is provided in *Fig. 11.8*. In this case, directional atherectomy was not performed. The lesion was pre-dilated and a Palmaz–Schatz 154 spiral articulated stent was placed at 20 atmospheres using a 4 mm balloon. The final angiogram demonstrated an excellent lumen diameter, which was confirmed by IVUS. This showed an MLD of 3.4 mm and a cross-sectional area of 10.1 mm² (*Fig. 11.8*). Plaque shifting was less likely to occur in this case because the origin of the LAD from the bifurcation had a 90° angle.

The previous case showed that sometimes it is possible to get by with simple balloon dilatation and stent insertion, even for ostial lesions. However, in *Fig. 11.9* treatment of the ostial circumflex lesion resulted in compromise to the distal left main artery and the proximal circumflex artery. The lesion was initially treated with rotational atherectomy with sequentially increasing burr sizes from 1.5 mm to 2.15 mm. Following balloon dilatation of the circumflex lesion, there was evidence of plaque shift into the

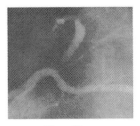
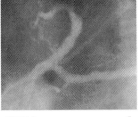
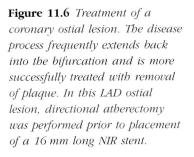

Baseline　　　**DCA** (7 Fr 24 cuts) **and
P-S 15 mm** (4.0 mm - 24 Atm)

Figure 11.7 *Treatment of an LAD ostial stenosis with directional atherectomy prior to stenting. DCA, directional coronary atherectomy; P–S, Palmaz–Schatz.*

distal left main. Therefore, directional atherectomy was performed using a 7 Fr cutter to debulk the plaque in the left main artery, as well as in the proximal circumflex artery. The distal left main artery and proximal circumflex artery were then treated with balloon dilatation alone using a 3.5 mm balloon inflated at 9 atmospheres. The patient returned 6 months later with stable angina. Restenosis was present with a 74% diameter narrowing, which was treated successfully with balloon dilatation without the use of a stent.

The case example in *Fig. 11.10* provides a dramatic example of how IVUS may be critical in the treatment of ostial lesions. The angiogram in *Fig. 11.10a* revealed an eccentric stenosis at the ostium of the LAD; this stenosis was not dramatic by angiography. However, the IVUS examination showed that

Preintervention angiogram

RAO view   Spider view

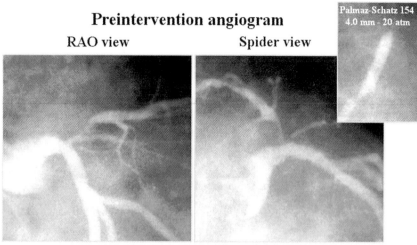

Ostial LAD lesion

Post-stenting

Angiogram   IVUS

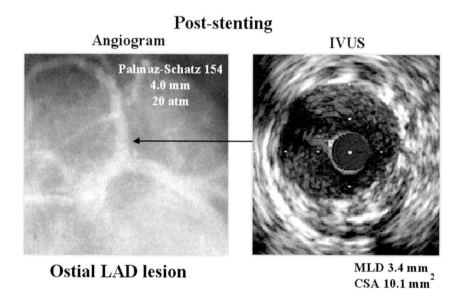

Ostial LAD lesion

MLD 3.4 mm
CSA 10.1 mm^2

Figure 11.8 *An ostial LAD lesion treated without debulking atherectomy. The 90 degree takeoff of this LAD decreases the risk of plaque shifting.*

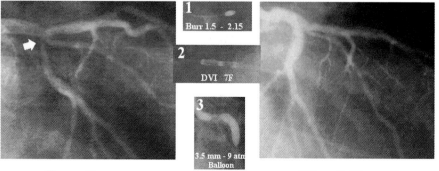

Baseline   **Final Result**

Figure 11.9 *An ostial circumflex lesion initially treated with rotational atherectomy and balloon dilatation. This resulted in plaque shifting to the distal left main artery. Directional atherectomy was performed followed by balloon dilatation without placement of a stent.*

Ostial LAD lesion

Circ Bifurcation

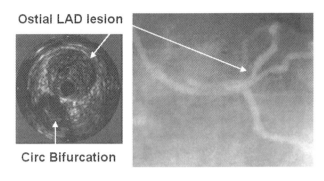

a **Baseline**

Figure 11.10 *IVUS guidance during coronary stenting for ostial lesions. (a) Preintervention IVUS imaging documented the presence of severe stenosis in the ostial LAD despite an adequate appearing angiogram. (b) After what appeared to be a successful stent deployment by angiography, IVUS imaging demonstrated that there was no stent in the ostial LAD. The stent had slipped off the balloon and was dislodged without adequate dilatation in the body in the left main coronary artery. (c) Following balloon expansion of the stent in the left main artery and placement of a half Palmaz–Schatz stent in the ostium of the LAD.*

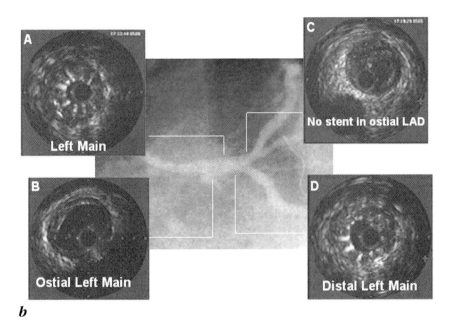

b

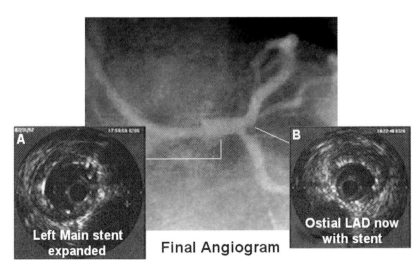

c

there was extensive eccentric plaque surrounding the ultrasound catheter and extending up to the bifurcation with the circumflex artery. In addition, the take-off of the LAD was tortuous, which could make placement of a stent more difficult. A Palmaz–Schatz stent was hand crimped on to a balloon and placed in the ostium of the LAD under fluoroscopic guidance. An acceptable angiographic result was obtained (*Fig. 11.10b*). IVUS was then performed to confirm that the stent had been placed precisely at the ostium without obstructing the circumflex artery. The ultrasound images shown in *Fig. 11.10b* provided a surprise for us. The reflections from the metallic stent struts were seen in the distal left main artery (*Fig. 11.10b*, Panel A) and no stent struts were seen at the ostium of the LAD. In addition, the stent struts were only mildly expanded in the distal left main and were not expanded at all in the mid left main. This indicates that the stent had slipped off the balloon and migrated to the more proximal left main artery instead of being positioned correctly in the ostium of the LAD. To correct this problem, a 4.0 mm balloon was placed across the stent and expanded in the left main coronary artery to secure the migrated stent. In addition, a second Palmaz–Schatz stent was cut in half and a half-stent was placed into the ostium of the LAD and expanded with a 3.0 mm balloon (*Fig. 11.10c*, Panel B). These experiences with stent migration or inadequate placement of a stent at critical junctions reinforce our belief that IVUS imaging is essential when treating ostial stenoses.

REFERENCES

1. Eigler NL, Weinstock B, Douglas JS Jr et al. Excimer laser coronary angioplasty of aorto-ostial stenoses. Results of the excimer laser coronary angioplasty (ELCA) registry in the first 200 patients. *Circulation* 1993; **88**: 2049–2057.
2. Kerwin PM, McKeever LS, Marek JC et al. Directional atherectomy of aorto-ostial stenoses. *Cathet Cardiovasc Diagn* 1993; **Suppl 1**: 17–25.
3. Koller PT, Freed M, Grines CL, O'Neill WW. Success, complications, and restenosis following rotational and transluminal extraction atherectomy of ostial stenoses. *Cathet Cardiovasc Diagn* 1994; **31**: 255–260.
4. Kereiakes DJ. Percutaneous transcatheter therapy of aorto-ostial stenoses. *Cathet Cardiovasc Diagn* 1996; **38**: 292–300.
5. Tan KH, Sulke N, Taub N, Sowton E. Percutaneous transluminal coronary angioplasty of aorta ostial, non-aorta ostial, and branch ostial stenoses: acute and long-term outcome. *Eur Heart J* 1995; **16**: 631–639.
6. Abdel-Meguid AE, Whitlow PL, Simpfendorfer C et al. Percutaneous revascularization of ostial saphenous vein graft stenoses. *J Am Coll Cardiol* 1995; **26**: 955–960.
7. Rocha-Singh K, Morris N, Wong SC et al. Coronary stenting for treatment of ostial stenoses of native coronary arteries or aortocoronary saphenous venous grafts. *Am J Cardiol* 1995; **75**: 26–29.
8. Kobayashi N, Vaghetti M, Kobayashi Y et al. Coronary stenting of ostial lesions: results are different between arteries. *Circulation* 1998; **98**: 1491.

Chapter 12 **Left main artery disease**

Antonio Colombo and Jonathan Tobis

Treatment of an unprotected left main coronary artery with non-stent catheter-based coronary interventions carries an unacceptable immediate and long-term risk.[1,2] On the other hand, stenting an unprotected left main coronary artery may decrease some of these risks, but it has several unique characteristics and risks that need to be clearly understood before attempting to stent this unusual lesion subset. Obviously the risk is increased if the circumflex artery or the left anterior descending artery (LAD) is not bypassed, (i.e. if the lesion is an unprotected left main artery lesion). In addition, there are significant differences between placing a stent at the aorto-ostial junction, in the body of the left main trunk, or at the bifurcation of the LAD and circumflex artery. In some respects, stenting the left main artery appears to be technically easier because it is in the most proximal portion of the vessel and therefore readily accessible. Although this may be the case for balloon dilatation alone, when stenting a stenosis in the left main artery it is more critical to have exact placement of the stent, and this can be a problem for less radiopaque stents. Based on our experience over the past 7 years in stenting left main coronary arteries, we suggest the following recommendations for interventionalists who attempt this procedure.

GENERAL CONSIDERATIONS IN STENTING THE LEFT MAIN CORONARY ARTERY

These general considerations are summarized in *Table 12.1*.

(a) We like to use 9 Fr or 10 Fr guiding catheters when treating left main coronary arteries for several reasons. The larger guiding catheter permits the use of debulking devices, such as large rotational atherectomy burrs or directional atherectomy catheters. In addition, if stenting the bifurcation becomes necessary, the larger guiding catheters accept two balloon catheters with stents of any type for simultaneous placement with excellent angiographic visualization during contrast injections.

(b) Because hemodynamic compromise and catastrophes can occur rapidly when ischemia or occlusion of the left main artery occurs, we prophylactically place an intra-aortic balloon pump before attempting this procedure in most patients. This stabilizes the patient hemodynamically and permits a more methodical approach to the lesion, with adequate debulking to maximize the results.

(c) By intravascular ultrasound (IVUS), the left main coronary artery frequently has a media-to-media diameter of 5 mm despite the narrowed appearance on angiography. Compared to the rest of the artery, cross-sectional area of plaque is much

Table 12.1
Guidelines for stenting the left main coronary artery

1) Use a 10 French guiding catheter
2) Use an intra-aortic balloon pump prior to the procedure
3) Debulk the majority of the lesions
4) The Palmaz 104 stent is useful for ostial lesions or in the body of the left main, NIR and Multilink stents also provide adequate radial strength. Use the AVE GFX for more complicated cases that involve the LAD/circumflex bifurcation.
5) Be prepared to stent the left anterior descending/ circumflex bifurcation even if it does not appear to be involved on the baseline angiogram.

larger. Since the risk of restenosis is critical when stenting the left main coronary artery, we prefer to debulk the lesion, which not only facilitates deployment of the stent but also, we believe, lowers the restenosis rate by half.

(d) Choose a stent that provides strong radial support, such as the biliary Palmaz 10-4 stent or the newer generation meshwork stents such as the NIR nine-cell stent or the Multilink stent for vessels ≤ 4 mm. If the bifurcation of the LAD and circumflex artery is involved, then a more flexible stent, such as the AVE GFX, is preferable.

(e) Even though an angiogram shows a stenosis isolated to the body of the left main coronary artery, there may be involvement of the bifurcation that is not appreciated until IVUS is performed. In addition to assessing the bifurcation, IVUS provides accurate sizing of the left main artery and visualizes the amount of plaque that may need to be removed. This information is important in planning the approach to the lesion, but the operator must also be prepared for the unexpected. After pre-dilating the left main artery, there may be a dissection, which may extend into the bifurcation and require that stents be placed in both branches to stabilize the anatomy.

RESULTS

A summary of our results in 62 patients treated for stenoses of the left main coronary artery is presented in *Tables 12.2–12.5*. There were 28 patients with protected left main lesions and 34 patients with unprotected left main stenoses. The majority of these cases were treated electively and in only 10% was a stent placed in the left main artery because of a retrograde dissection or acute closure that occurred while treating a more distal lesion. There was a 92% procedural success rate; three patients (5%) required emergency bypass surgery and two patients had an unsuccessful stent deployment (*Table 12.3*). Atherectomy devices were used in half the cases; balloon dilatation and stent placement alone were used in the other half. A variety of stents were used to treat this cohort of patients; the majority were of the Palmaz–Schatz design (*Table 12.4*). The quantitative coronary angiography results are shown in *Table 12.5*. Compared with lesions in other portions of the coronary arteries, the baseline minimum lumen

Table 12.2

Left main coronary artery stenting

Patient characteristics		Stent indications	
Patients	62	Elective	53 (85%)
Unprotected LM	34 pts	Dissection	6 (8%)
Protected LM	28 pts	Suboptimal PTCA	2 (3%)
Age	64 ± 10 years	Acute closure	1 (2%)
Males	80%		
Mean LVEF	54 ± 13%		

LM, left main; LVEF, left ventricular ejection fraction

Table 12.3

Left main coronary artery stenting. Results

Results	
No. of patients	62
Lesion success	57 (92%)
Unsuccessful stent deployment	2 pt
Emergency CABG	3 pt
B/V	1.1 ± 0.2
Final balloon size (mm)	40 ± 05
Final pressure (mmHg)	16.2 ± 3.6

B/V, balloon to vessel ratio

Table 12.4

Left main coronary artery stenting. Methods

Adjunctive device		Stent design	
IVUS	30 pts (48%)	Palmaz–Schatz	21
DCA	11 pts (18%)	NIR	13
Rotablator	19 pts (31%)	AVE Micro	7
		ACS Multilink	5
		PURA	4
		Crown	2
		Combination	3

diameter (MLD) (1.3 ± 0.8 mm) was larger, as was the post-stent MLD (3.7 ± 0.7 mm). At follow-up, the MLD was 2.7 ± 1.0 mm or (27% ± 25% diameter stenosis). Clinical follow-up was obtained in all patients at a mean of 20 months.

There were five deaths. Two of the deaths were caused by closure of the left main artery within 3

Table 12.5

Left main coronary artery stenting. Angiographic data

	Pie	Final	Follow-up
Reference diameter (mm)	3.7 ± 0.7	3.8 ± 0.6	3.7 ± 0.5
MLD (mm)	1.3 ± 0.8	3.7 ± 0.6	2.7 ± 1.1
Percentage stenosis	64.5 ± 18.0	2.2 ± 9.2	26.9 ± 25.2
Lesion length (mm)	7.2 ± 4.7		
Percentage of angio. F/U			50 (31/62)
Restenosis rate (%)			16 (5/31)

Table 12.6

Left main coronary artery stenting. Follow-up results

Clinical follow-up in all patients	
Deaths	5 patients
≤ 2 months	3 patients
> 2 months	2 patients
Angiographic follow-up in 31 patients (50%)	
Restenosis (> 50%)	5 lesions (16%)
Repeat PTCA	2 patients

months of the procedure. One patient died of carcinoma and another died of a non-cardiac cause. The last patient's death had an uncertain etiology. Two of the three patients who died within 3 months of the procedure did not have IVUS imaging performed, so it is unclear whether there was a technical factor that predisposed to subacute stent thrombosis and was not appreciated with angiography at the time of the procedure (these cases were done early in our experience).

There was no difference in left ventricular function in the patients who survived (ejection fraction = 53%) versus those who died (ejection fraction = 51%). Angiographic follow-up was obtained in 50% of the patients and restenosis defined as > 50% diameter narrowing occurred in five lesions, giving a restenosis rate of 16%. Two of these patients were treated with repeat balloon dilatation and none of the patients required bypass surgery during the period of follow-up.

These results are in concordance with recent data reported by Park and colleagues.[3] In this series, 74 patients with significant left main artery stenosis underwent elective stent implantation with (n = 24) or without (n = 50) prior debulking with directional atherectomy. The overall angiographic restenosis rate was 16.7% and repeat revascularization was necessary in 12.2%. The need for repeat revascularization was significantly lower in patients who underwent debulking before stent implantation (0/25 versus 9/49; $p = 0.02$).

CLINICAL EXAMPLES

This patient in *Fig. 12.1* had diffuse atherosclerosis of the remaining LAD and obtuse marginal arteries. The

Figure 12.1 *Elective stenting for protected left main coronary artery disease.*

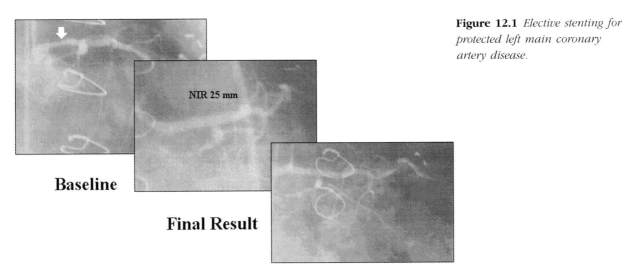

Baseline

Final Result

Follow - Up

First lesion: Left Main

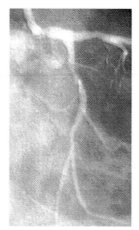

BASELINE RAO

a

Second lesion :LCx

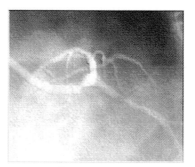

BASELINE LAO

Figure 12.2 *Unprotected left main coronary disease treated with several Palmaz–Schatz stents. LCX, left circumflex; LAO, left anterior oblique; RAO, right anterior oblique.*

Early Experience with Palmaz-Schatz Stents

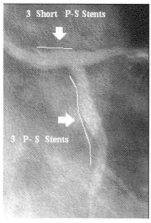

FINAL RESULT RAO

b

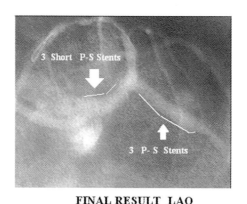

FINAL RESULT LAO

left main artery had a long tubular segment of stenosis. This was treated with pre-dilatation followed by placement of a 25 mm NIR stent into the left main artery across the entrance to the circumflex artery and into the proximal LAD. Because there are patent bypass grafts in this setting, stenting a protected left main artery carries significantly less risk than in the next example.

In *Fig. 12.2* there is a severe stenosis in the proximal portion of the left main artery in a patient who has not undergone bypass surgery. This challenging

case was attempted early in our experience before the newer flexible meshwork stents were available. To obtain adequate radial support and still have the flexibility to follow the curve into the circumflex artery, the decision was made to use three Palmaz–Schatz stents in the circumflex artery and three Palmaz–Schatz half-stents in the left main artery. To obtain a half-stent, the standard coronary Palmaz–Schatz stent was cut at the articulation and hand crimped on to a balloon. The three half-stents were positioned sequentially in the body of the left

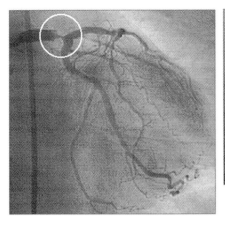
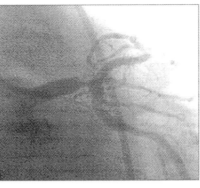

Baseline

a

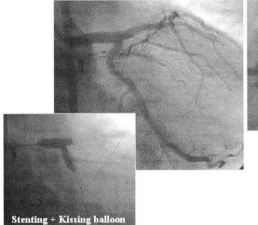
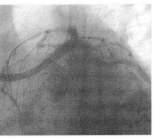

Final Result

Stenting + Kissing balloon

b

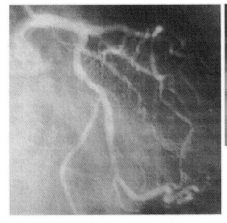
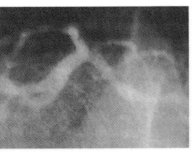

6 months Follow - Up

c

Figure 12.3 *Severe distal left main disease treated with directional atherectomy. (a) Baseline coronary angiograms. (b) Following atherectomy, an ACS MultiLink stent was placed in the left main artery extending into the LAD. Simultaneous inflations were performed into the bifurcation vessels. (c) Angiograms obtained in follow-up at six months.*

main artery. This provided strong radial support without the inconvenience of the articulation through which tissue could prolapse. In addition, the shorter length improved the trackability around tortuous segments. With the availability of newer stent designs, this method is no longer necessary.

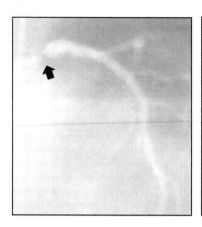

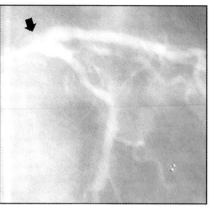

a **Baseline**

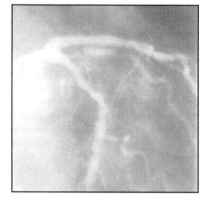

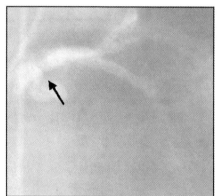

b **After predilatation**   **After AVE gfx stent**

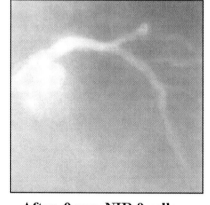

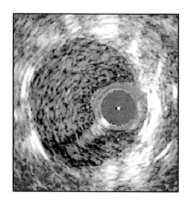

After 9 mm NIR 9 cells   **Final IVUS**

c

Figure 12.4 *Treatment of ostial left main disease without atherectomy resulting in tissue prolapse through an AVE GFX stent.*

DEBULKING FOR OPTIMIZATION OF LUMEN DIAMETER (AMIGO TRIAL)

As described more fully in Chapter 19, we believe that large arteries have a lower restenosis rate if a significant amount of plaque is removed before a stent is deployed.[4] This concept of debulking before stenting is being tested in a randomized trial, the Atherectomy and Multi Improve Gain (AMIGO) trial. An example of this approach as applied to left main coronary artery disease is demonstrated in *Fig. 12.3.*

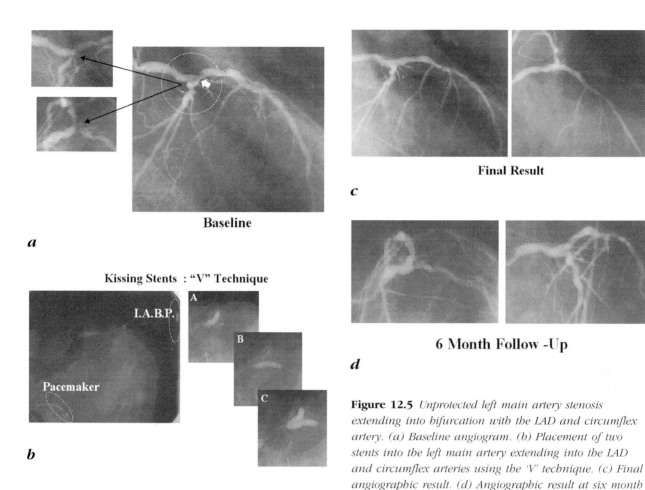

Baseline

a

Kissing Stents : "V" Technique

I.A.B.P.

Pacemaker

A
B
C

b

Final Result

c

6 Month Follow -Up

d

Figure 12.5 *Unprotected left main artery stenosis extending into bifurcation with the LAD and circumflex artery. (a) Baseline angiogram. (b) Placement of two stents into the left main artery extending into the LAD and circumflex arteries using the 'V' technique. (c) Final angiographic result. (d) Angiographic result at six month follow-up study. IABP, Intra-aortic balloon pump.*

This critical stenosis in the distal left main artery was first treated by debulking the plaque with directional atherectomy. Following removal of tissue with directional coronary atherectomy (DCA), an ACS Multilink stent was placed in the left main artery across the ostium of the circumflex artery into the LAD. The left main artery stent and the ostium of the circumflex artery were dilated simultaneously with two 3.5 mm balloons at 7 atmospheres (*Fig. 12.3b*). A lower pressure was used because the bulk of plaque had been removed and the combined balloon size was large. The angiogram at the 6-month follow-up demonstrates a widely patent left main and bifurcation system (*Fig. 12.3c*). This type of result has encouraged us to perform directional atherectomy more frequently in the setting of left main artery disease.

One of the problems of not debulking is the possibility of tissue prolapse when the stents are dilated to a large size to increase the diameter of the left main coronary artery. This is demonstrated in *Fig. 12.4*,

where a tight stenosis of a short left main artery with involvement of the ostium to both the circumflex artery and the LAD was treated with an AVE GFX stent. Following placement of the AVE stent, the angiogram shows a band-like lucency in the proximal portion of the left main artery (see *Fig. 12.4b*). This was interpreted as being consistent with tissue prolapse. Therefore, a second stent was placed through the AVE stent. In this case a 9 mm NIR nine-cell stent was placed, and this provided adequate wall coverage to force the tissue out of the lumen. The final angiogram and ultrasound image demonstrate wide patency of this 4 mm lumen (*Fig. 12.4c*).

The unprotected left main artery bifurcation lesion demonstrated in *Fig. 12.5* represents what can be accomplished with the principles outlined above. This patient had a long left main artery with severe stenosis before the entrance into the bifurcation of the circumflex artery and the LAD, which are both involved. *Figure 12.5b* demonstrates that an intra-aortic balloon pump and pacemaker have been put

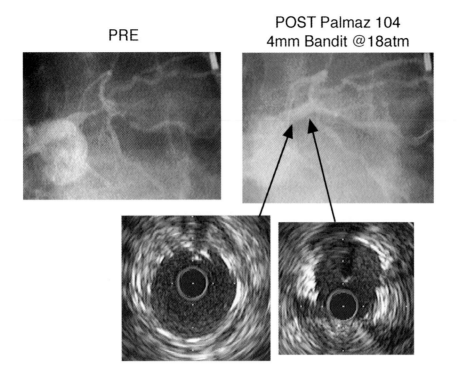

PRE

POST Palmaz 104
4mm Bandit @18atm

Figure 12.6 *IVUS guidance during left main stenting helps to identify inadequate expansion of the stent in the distal left main artery.*

in prophylactically. The inserts reveal that a guidewire was passed down each branch. The LAD and the circumflex artery were pre-dilated sequentially and then simultaneously with a 3.5 mm Tacker balloon. An AVE stent was passed over each guidewire and was deployed sequentially. The stents were then expanded with simultaneous balloon inflation using the 'V' technique (see Chapter 10). Not only was the final result acceptable, but the angiogram at 6-month follow-up also demonstrated wide patency of the distal left main artery and the bifurcation into the major branches (*Fig. 12.5d*).

In the case in *Fig. 12.6*, the patient had unusual coronary anatomy. The left main artery is severely narrowed in the mid- to distal segment, which then enters into a confluence from which four vessels emanate like spokes in a wheel. Since each of these vessels was comparatively small and had a sharp angle relative to the left main artery, we elected not to perform DCA or rotational atherectomy. After placing an intra-aortic balloon pump, the left main artery was pre-dilated with a 4.0 mm Bandit balloon. A Palmaz 104 stent was then hand crimped on to the same balloon and deployed in the left main artery at 18 atmospheres. Despite a satisfactory angiographic result, the ultrasound images show that the distal section was asymmetric and underexpanded. Repeat

dilatation increased the lumen diameter to 3.5 mm × 3.8 mm. Stenoses in two of the branch vessels were then dilated with a 2.5 mm balloon but were not stented.

A useful way of approaching bifurcation left main artery disease is the modified 'T' stent (see Chapter 10). The 71-year-old patient represented in *Fig. 12.7*, had severe distal left main disease that extended into the ostium of both the LAD and the circumflex artery. He had bypass surgery 9 years ago but the graft to the LAD was not adequate owing to sequential lesions in the LAD. Guidewires were placed in both the LAD and the circumflex artery and simultaneous inflations were performed with a 3.5 mm balloon at 5 atmospheres in the LAD and 10 atmospheres in the circumflex artery. The proximal end of the balloons extended back into the distal left main artery. A 16 mm Puro Vario stent pre-mounted on a 3.5 mm balloon was positioned at the ostium of the LAD (*Fig. 12.7*, Panel C). A second 16 mm Puro Vario stent pre-mounted on a 3.5 mm balloon was advanced into the circumflex artery until the center of the stent was positioned near the origin of the LAD and extended into the left main artery. The stent within the ostium of the LAD was then deployed with minimal protrusion into the left main artery (*Fig. 12.7*, Panel C) while the stent in the circumflex artery was held in

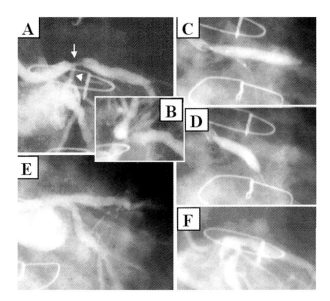

Figure 12.7 *Modified T stenting technique for left main disease. Panels A. and B: baseline coronary angiogram reveals severe stenosis of distal left main and ostial LAD and circumflex arteries. Panel C: deployment of a stent in the proximal LAD while a second stent was kept in the left main-circumflex artery in an undeployed state. Panel D: after removal of the balloon in the LAD, the stent in the circumflex artery was deployed. Panel E: Final angiographic result. Panel F: follow-up angiographic result at five months.*

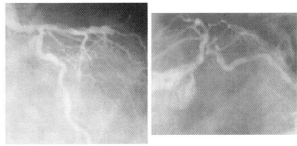

Baseline

a

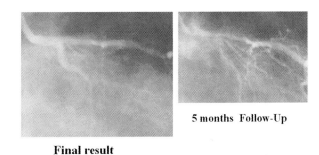

Bifurcation stenting

b

5 months Follow-Up

Final result

c

Figure 12.8 *Diffuse restenosis after stenting left main coronary artery disease.*

place to prevent dislodgement. The balloon and guidewire in the LAD were removed after expanding the stent to 18 atmospheres. The stent in the proximal circumflex artery extending into the mid left main artery was then deployed at 16 atmospheres (*Fig. 12.7*, Panel D). The final result is shown in *Fig. 12.7*, Panel E and the 5-month follow-up result is shown in *Fig. 12.7*, Panel F. There is some narrowing in the proximal portion of the circumflex artery, but the left main artery and the LAD are widely patent and the patient was asymptomatic.

Figure 12.8 provides an example of a patient who did not have a successful long-term result with this approach to stenting left main coronary artery disease. The baseline angiogram shows diffuse disease involving the distal left main artery as well as the ostium of the LAD and the circumflex artery. Directional atherectomy was performed in the left main artery and the circumflex artery. The LAD was treated with balloon dilatation alone using a 3.0 mm balloon inflated at 8 atmospheres. A 12 mm GFX stent was placed into the circumflex and inflated at

11 atmospheres on a 3.5 mm balloon. The left main artery was treated with an 18 mm long AVE GFX stent deployed on a 3.5 mm balloon at 12 atmospheres. The immediate result shown in *Fig. 12.8c* revealed a smooth luminal surface in the left main artery, the proximal LAD, and circumflex artery. However, on angiographic follow-up at 5 months, there was diffuse in-stent restenosis involving the distal left main artery as well as the proximal LAD and the circumflex artery. Owing to this poor long-term result with diffuse aggressive restenosis, it was elected to send this patient to bypass surgery. As mentioned earlier, the danger of stenting left main coronary

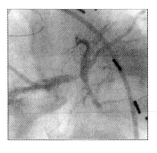
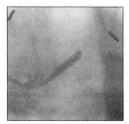
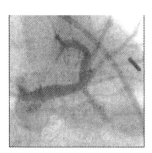

Figure 12.9 *Stenting left main coronary artery disease without debulking atherectomy. The 90 degree angulation of the LAD and circumflex arteries decreases the likelihood of plaque shifting.*

pre-intervention

Stent: Dart 16 mm

Post dilatation Maxxum 4.0 mm 9 mm 17 atm

post intervention

artery disease is that, if restenosis occurs, it could be associated with abrupt closure of the proximal vessels and so present as sudden death.

LEFT MAIN STENTING WITHOUT ATHERECTOMY

An alternative to the approach of debulking left main coronary arteries is shown in *Fig. 12.9*. The pre-intervention angiogram shows distal left main artery disease but the bifurcation of the LAD and the circumflex artery is at a 90° angle. This would make directional atherectomy or rotational atherectomy a higher-risk procedure. In addition, it is less likely for plaque shift to obstruct the proximal LAD or the circumflex artery when their take-off is at 90° to the left main artery. Therefore, the left main artery was pre-dilated and then a 16 mm long Dart stent was placed on a 4.0 mm Maxxum balloon. This was inflated at 17 atmospheres with a satisfactory post-intervention result. The patient has remained asymptomatic for two years following this procedure.

PHYSIOLOGIC ASSESSMENT OF LEFT MAIN ARTERY DISEASE

One of the most difficult questions to address when a moderate stenosis is seen in the left main coronary artery is when is it appropriate to treat and when is it better to leave such a lesion alone.[5] The patient

Significant Left Main Stenosis?

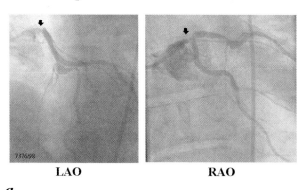

LAO   RAO

a

Figure 12.10 *The use of physiologic testing to determine the functional significance of a moderate left main coronary artery stenosis.*

Fractional Flow Reserve for Intermediate Lesion Scimed Informer 0.014" • Proximal LAD

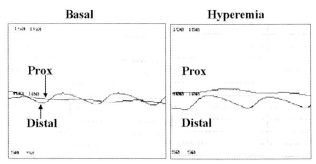

Fractional Flow Reserve = 0.92

b

whose angiogram is shown in *Fig. 12.10a* was a 56-year-old man with a normal ejection fraction and significant disease in the RCA. There is moderate stenosis of the distal left main coronary artery seen best in the left anterior oblique cranial projection. To determine the functional significance of this lesion,[6] an assessment of fractional flow reserve was performed using a SciMed 0.36 mm (0.014-inch) guidewire to measure pressure in the LAD distal to the left main artery stenosis. There was no significant pressure gradient distal to the lesion at rest (*Fig. 12.10b*). Following hyperemia induced with 18 μg adenosine administered through the guiding catheter, there was a slight drop in pressure distal to the lesion. However, the ratio of mean distal pressure to proximal pressure was still 0.92. Although this type of assessment does not tell us whether the plaque is vulnerable to sudden rupture, the fractional flow demonstrates that the lesion was not hemodynamically significant at that time. We elected to leave this left main artery stenosis alone and treat the patient with medical therapy including an HMG reductase inhibitor to lower his lipid levels. The RCA was treated with placement of a stent during the same procedure.

CONCLUSIONS

This experience of stenting the left main coronary artery suggests that treatment of this lesion subset is feasible in selected patients. Availability of the new generation of stents has permitted an expansion of the indications for treating left main artery stenoses. Our initial results with debulking the artery with rotational atherectomy or directional atherectomy suggest that restenosis can be significantly impeded with this approach. Clearly this remains a high-risk patient subset that should only be treated in this way by experienced operators, but if the treatment is performed correctly the results can be extremely gratifying.

REFERENCES

1. Ellis SG, Tamai H, Nobuyoshi M et al. Contemporary percutaneous treatment of unprotected left main coronary stenoses: initial results from a multicenter registry analysis 1994–1996. *Circulation* 1997; **96**: 3867–3872.
2. Kosuga K, Tamai H, Ueda K et al. Initial and long-term results of angioplasty in unprotected left main coronary artery. *Am J Cardiol* 1999; **83**: 32–37.
3. Park SJ, Park SW, Lee CW et al. Long-term outcome of unprotected left main coronary stenting in patients with normal left ventricular function: is debulking atherectomy prior to stenting beneficial? *J Am Coll Cardiol* 1999; **33**: 15A.
4. Moussa I, Moses J, Di Mario C et al. Stenting after optimal lesion debulking (SOLD) registry. Angiographic and clinical outcome. *Circulation* 1998; **98**: 1604–1609.
5. Wilson RF. Assessing the severity of coronary artery stenoses. *N Engl J Med* 1996; **334**: 1735–1737.
6. Pijls NHJ, De Bruyne B, Peels K et al. Measurement of fractional flow reserve to assess the functional severity of coronary artery stenoses. *N Engl J Med* 1996; **334**: 1703–1708.

Chapter 13 Chronic total occlusions

Bernhard Reimers

Percutaneous transluminal coronary angioplasty of total occlusions comprises 10–20% of all coronary angioplasty procedures.[1,2] Despite rapid evolution in technical equipment, the primary success rate for treating total occlusions remains lower, and the incidence of restenosis higher, than that for treating non-occluded lesions. The treatment of chronic total occlusions needs to be discussed separately from that of stenotic lesions because there are different indications, different technical approaches, and different outcomes. This chapter describes some general aspects of chronic total occlusions before concentrating on a practical description of the recanalization techniques performed in our patients.

DEFINITION

A total coronary occlusion is defined as a vessel stenosis with lumen compromise resulting in:

(a) complete interruption of anterograde flow thrombolysis in myocardial infarction ((TIMI) 0); or

(b) functional occlusions (99%) with delayed, faint, distal opacification (TIMI 1 or 2).

The presence of anterograde flow in functional occlusions is due to the presence of intraluminal microchannels or dilated vasa vasorum.[3,4] According to the time of occurrence, a total coronary occlusion can be considered acute or chronic. Acute occlusions are angiographically diagnosed in the setting of an acute myocardial infarction (MI). Chronic total occlusions are more difficult to define because it is frequently impossible to date the moment of occlusion. The American College of Cardiology's definition of a chronic occlusion as one older than 3 months is useful in cases of a datable MI or if there is previous angiographic documentation.[5] It does not help in cases of undatable occlusions, which are present, in our experience, in one-third of cases.[6,7] In our institution, the age of chronic total occlusion is determined as the time interval from the first angiogram demonstrating the occlusion. When no angiogram is available, a history of MI or prolonged chest pain with electrocardiographic changes in the distribution of the occluded artery is used to date the occlusion. In the absence of clinical events, the occlusion is classified as of undetermined age. Unfortunately, the heterogeneity of coronary occlusions (whether anatomic or functional and whether acute, chronic, or of uncertain age) and the lack of generally accepted definitions makes it difficult to interpret the literature and predisposes to limited reproducibility between various studies.

RATIONALE FOR OPENING CHRONIC OCCLUSIONS

Chronic total occlusions are by definition complex lesions. Angioplasty of a total occlusion is generally a more time-consuming and more expensive procedure than an intervention on a stenotic lesion. Therefore, the decision to attempt a recanalization procedure needs an individualized risk–benefit and cost–benefit analysis. Therapeutic alternatives such as medical therapy or surgical revascularization must be discussed. The main rationale for opening a chronic total occlusion is to provide adequate revascularization of viable myocardium. An occlusion may not necessarily result in a transmural infarction because of the presence of collateral vessels at the time of the closure.[8] Viable myocardium may be present after non-Q-wave infarctions. Evidence for muscle viability includes:

(a) residual resting or exercise angina in the absence of other significant coronary lesions;
(b) inducibility of left ventricular wall motion;
(c) reversibility of perfusion defects; and
(d) metabolism–perfusion mismatch.

Well-developed collateral flow to viable myocardium may be sufficient for myocardial demands at rest but may behave as a 90% stenosis during exercise.[9] Anterograde revascularization could relieve symptoms of exercise-induced ischemia. Vessel occlusion may also result in hibernating myocardium, and restoration of blood flow may result in improved ventricular function.[10]

The clinical objectives in opening chronically occluded arteries are:

(a) reduction of symptoms;
(b) reduction of silent ischemia;
(c) improvement of left ventricular function;
(d) limitation of remodeling and a decrease in the need for bypass surgery.[11–15]

These objectives, however, are met with variable success.[3] Prior studies have shown that the need for surgery can be reduced,[15,16] while left ventricular function is only modestly improved[13,17,18] after reopening a chronic total occlusion. In one study, two-thirds of successfully treated patients were free from angina at 4 years.[19] Another series of patients had an event-free survival of 86% after 5 years following successful recanalization, compared with 76% ($p < 0.01$) among unsuccessful cases.[20] Another group, however, has reported the incidence of MI and death to be similar whether or not the chronic occlusion was reopened.[21]

Another theoretic rationale for opening an occluded vessel is that the presence of a reopened artery might provide collaterals to other vascular territories with stenotic lesions. If the other stenotic vessel were to close, an MI could be prevented by the availability of the collaterals from the recanalized artery. There are several anecdotal case examples of this phenomenon.

A further indication to reopen a chronic total occlusion is a planned treatment of other stenotic coronary arteries in order to achieve a more complete revascularization. By opening the occluded vessel initially, the risk of the procedure may be reduced by providing reverse collaterals for the stenotic vessel. In case of failure to open the occlusion, an alternative treatment such as bypass surgery might be more appropriate.

PROCEDURAL SUCCESS

The success rates of recanalization of chronic total occlusions varies from 50% to 80% in published series and is dependent on several variables, such as the estimated age of occlusion, the angiographic type of occlusion (tapered or abrupt), the presence of bridging collaterals or side branches originating at the point of occlusion, and length of the occlusion.[2,9,23–25] Several recanalization devices have been proposed with improved primary success,[26–36] but the best published primary success rates still remain below the success rate for stenotic lesions.[2,23] Variables that predict the success of a recanalization procedure are:[2]

(a) more recent occlusions;
(b) the presence of anterograde flow (i.e. functional occlusion);
(c) tapered morphology;
(d) the absence of bridging collaterals;
(e) the absence of side branches at the occlusion site;
(f) shorter occluded segment; and
(g) absence of multivessel disease.[2]

The main reason for procedural failure is the inability to advance the guidewire into the distal lumen in 75% of cases.[2] Less frequent causes of failure are the inability to advance a dilatation balloon or other device through the occluded segment after successfully crossing it with a wire, or the inability to dilate the lesion. Acute reocclusion after dilatation has been a cause of procedural failure but currently may be obviated by the use of stents. The distinction between success defined as the ability to cross the occlusion (passage of any device into the distal lumen) and a procedural success with ≤ 50% residual stenosis and TIMI flow ≥ 2 is important for correct interpretation of the literature.

The long-term outcome of treating occlusive lesions is also inferior to that of non-occlusive lesions. Before the availability of coronary stents, the restenosis rates after reopening a chronic total occlusion were reported to be between 33% and 65%, and there was a high incidence of reocclusion.[37–39] The mean restenosis rate in nine studies using balloon angioplasty after reopening total occlusions was 53% as calculated by Puma and colleagues.[2] The introduction of coronary stenting dramatically reduced the restenosis rate when treating total occlusions, with an incidence in more recent studies of between 27% and 31%.[40–45] A randomized study comparing stent implantation with balloon angioplasty in chronic total occlusions showed an angiographic restenosis of 31.6% in the stent group and 73.7% in the balloon group.[45]

PROCEDURAL COMPLICATIONS

The initial concept that it was impossible to make a previously occluded artery worse during an attempt at recanalization has been shown to be incorrect. The incidence of complications might be lower than that encountered when treating stenotic lesions but all major complications, such as MI, arrhythmias and death, have been described. Serious complications include arterial wall dissection at the occlusion site and vessel perforation, with consequences varying from local contrast staining to tamponade and the need for urgent surgery. In the presence of perivessel contrast staining or larger vessel perforation with pericardial staining, the immediate use of protamine sulphate to reverse heparin is essential. The availability of covered stents may be critical for this setting. Rarer complications include dissections that extend proximally, compromise of proximal side branches, compromise of collateral flow by dissection and distal embolization causing MI.

In addition, some studies have reported acute reocclusion with sudden death and slow flow or no flow in the reopened vessel, with eventual thrombosis causing infarction or thrombotic occlusion of proximal branches.[46,47] The occurrence of slow or no flow has been observed in our experience after reopening vessels that lead into an akinetic or dyskinetic territory.

Figure 13.1 provides an example of slow flow that occurred after reopening an occluded left anterior descending artery (LAD). The LAD territory had sustained a large MI 3 years earlier. The occluded segment was treated with directional atherectomy and stent implantation. After 12 hours, stent thrombosis occurred despite infusion of abciximab, with reocclusion of the LAD (*Fig. 13.1c*). In addition, a stented intermediate branch became occluded, probably due to retrograde extension of the thrombus leading to re-infarction with significant cardiac enzyme rise.

Table 13.1 shows the procedural success rate and the incidence of complications in our series of 322 treated total occlusions. The attempt to cross the occlusion was successful in 73%, with a procedural success rate (TIMI 3 flow) in 62%. Although the

Table 13.1

Results of 322 consecutive total coronary occlusions attempted at Milan between January 1996 and July 1997

	Lesions	%
Crossing success	227	73
Coated, floppy wire success	103	45
Stiff wire success	60	26
Combined wire success*	64	29
Contralateral injection	105	33
Procedure time (minutes)†	97 ± 51	
Fluoroscopy time (minutes)	34 ± 22	
Further treatment in 227 crossed lesions		
Stent implantation	179	79
Rotational atherectomy	27	12
Directional atherectomy	23	10
Complications		
Death	1	0.3
Urgent coronary artery bypass grafts	3	1
Q-wave MI	2	0.6
Non-Q-wave MI	10	3
Cardiac tamponade	1	0.3
Local contrast staining	35	11
Angiographic success with TIMI 3 flow at end of procedure	200	62
Angiographic follow-up obtained	134	67
≥ 50% diameter restenosis	40	30

* More than one wire required for progression through the occlusion
† Patient stay in the catheterization laboratory

complication rate is small, the attempt to treat a chronic total occlusion is not without risk, and an accurate risk–benefit analysis before the procedure is indispensable. The frequent requirement of a high contrast load and extensive X-ray exposure during complex recanalization procedures should also be considered in this analysis. Angiographic restenosis was present in 30% of the patients who returned for a follow-up exam.

OCCLUSION HISTOLOGY

Total coronary occlusions are usually characterized by two histologic components.[48] The first is a lumen-

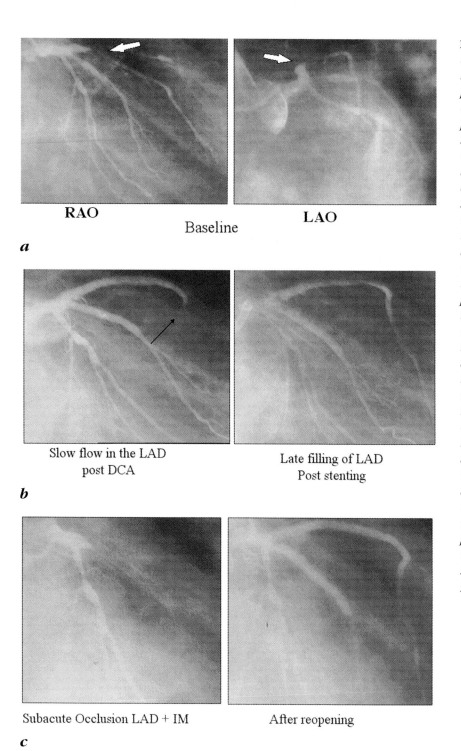

RAO

LAO

Baseline

a

Slow flow in the LAD
post DCA

Late filling of LAD
Post stenting

b

Subacute Occlusion LAD + IM

After reopening

c

Figure 13.1 *(a) Baseline coronary angiograms in the right anterior oblique projection (left panel) and the left anterior oblique caudal projection (right panel). This 72-year-old man had severe diffuse disease. The LAD was occluded following an anterior wall infarction 3 years earlier. The diagonal branch was subtotally occluded and there were significant stenoses in both the intermediate and circumflex arteries. (b) The LAD was reopened with a guidewire and then directional atherectomy was performed. Despite insertion of two Crossflex stents (4.0 mm × 15 mm) expanded at 13 atmospheres, there was slow flow, as demonstrated by the late filling of the distal LAD (right panel). The intermediate artery was also treated with insertion of two Crossflex stents (3.0 mm × 15 mm long) expanded at 17 atmospheres. The diagonal branch is no longer visualized. (c) Sub-acute stent thrombosis occurred 12 hours later. This was treated with balloon dilatation but the patient sustained a large myocardial infarction with a peak serum creatine kinase level of 3000 U/L.*

obstructing atherosclerotic plaque, the second is an overlying occlusive thrombus. The thrombus may vary in size, age, and stage of organization. Fresh thrombus, as seen in acute occlusions, is associated with a high recanalization success because it is easily penetrated by a guidewire. Over time the thrombus is reorganized to form loose or dense fibrotic tissue, and eventually it may calcify and make reopening of the vessel more difficult.[49] The thrombus may have a uniform structure, suggesting that a single clot has produced the vessel occlusion, or it may consist of several layers at various stages of organization, implying that multiple plaque ruptures and thrombus formation occurred and eventually caused the vessel occlusion.[48] Spontaneous recanalization of totally occluded vessels may occur with the formation of microchannels through the thrombus.[4,50] The presence of these microchannels through the central, occluding thrombus may facilitate wire crossing. Tapered, short chronic total occlusions have been correlated with the presence of central, loose fibrous tissue, and this angiographic appearance has a high recanalization success rate.[48]

RECANALIZATION TECHNIQUE

THE GUIDING CATHETER

For a successful recanalization procedure, it is essential to have a guiding catheter providing maximum support during advancement of the wire or the balloon. When treating chronic total occlusion, an extra support wire may not compensate for deficient catheter back-up. For the LAD, we first try the standard Judkins or extra-back-up catheters; for the left circumflex artery, we start with an extra support catheter; and for the right coronary artery we use either a standard Judkins, hockey stick, or left Amplatz catheter. The use of small French size catheters allows deep vessel intubation, which increases the support, but it does not allow the use of atherectomy devices and some intravascular ultrasound (IVUS) catheters. We generally use 8 Fr catheters unless debulking is planned, in which case larger catheters are necessary. We prefer to use side holes for occlusions of the right coronary artery in case anterograde collaterals are present. This generally guarantees anterograde flow even during deep catheter intubation, which permits distal opacification during contrast injections but avoids possible ischemia. We cannot overemphasize that spending time to find a guiding catheter with adequate back-up for recanalization procedures is worth the effort.

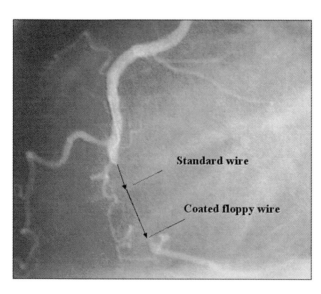

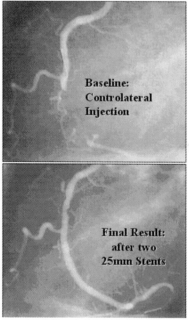

Figure 13.2 *Synergistic two-wire approach to a chronic total occlusion. The occlusion of this right coronary artery was documented angiographically 8 years earlier. The baseline image of the distal vessel was obtained by injecting into the left coronary artery system to opacify the collateral filling of the posterior descending artery. The proximal obstruction was crossed with a stiff, very steerable wire (Athlete Standard, Asahi). Further progression into the distal lumen was obtained with a hydrophilic-coated floppy wire (Choice PT, Scimed) using a 1.5 mm over-the-wire balloon (Ranger, Scimed) for back-up support. The lesion was treated with two 2.5 mm stents (BeStent, Medtronic) expanded to 16 atmospheres with a 4.0 mm balloon.*

CONTRALATERAL INJECTIONS

Another important element that contributes to the success and safety of recanalization procedures in the presence of retrograde collateral flow is the use of contralateral injections. After puncture of the opposite groin, a diagnostic 6 Fr catheter is used to intubate the ostium of the contralateral coronary artery. By visualizing the distal vessel in multiple projections, contralateral injections help to direct the progression of the wire in the occluded segment towards the distal true lumen and confirm the intraluminal position of the wire after crossing the occluded segment.

THE WIRE

The primary recanalization device is the guidewire. Structural differences of wires include tip stiffness, tip form, diameter and coating. Different characteristics of steerability and pushability are specific for the many wires available. Frequently, several wires with different characteristics are necessary to cross the occluded segment. As important as the choice of wire is the correct use and careful handling of the wire. Not only may wires perforate the vessel, but if used incorrectly they may penetrate a false passage and cause dissections, which can easily compromise the crossing.

Chronic total occlusions frequently consist of a hard fibrotic cap proximally, loose fibrotic tissue within the occlusion, and a second hard fibrotic cap distally (the second fibrotic cap is generally the most difficult to cross). In this scenario, stiff wires might be used to penetrate the proximal cap and the distal cap, while floppy, hydrophilic-coated wires with low friction may be preferable to advance within the occlusion.

Figure 13.2 shows a synergistic two-wire approach in a chronic total occlusion in which a stiff wire penetrated the proximal portion and a hydrophilic-coated floppy wire penetrated the distal portion of the occlusion.

Tip stiffness

Floppy wires, as usually used for non-occlusive lesions, are less traumatic and are preferred for acute or recent occlusions. In chronic total occlusions, the success of these floppy wires is lower. An exception to this is the 0.36 mm (0.014-inch) Fast–Dasher wire (Target Therapeutics, San Jose, California, USA), a floppy wire with good steering properties that is especially useful in the presence of tortuosity at the occlusion site.

Stiff wires (intermediate, standard) provide good steerability, shapability, and pushability to allow accurate advancement through hard fibrous tissue and to re-enter the true lumen after subintimal passage. Because of the high risk of vessel perforation with stiff wires, visualization of the distal vessel is extremely important. Widely used stiff wires with good steering characteristics are the Hi Torque ACS standard wires. The recently available Athlete coronary wire (Asahi Intec Co., Seto, Japan) is a 0.36 mm (0.014-inch) diameter wire with optimal steering characteristics and high stiffness, kink resistance, and pushability. The 3 cm radiopaque tip segment has jointless spring coil technology (a one-piece core wire). The Athlete wire has different degrees of tip stiffness expressed as the weight in grams required to cause deflection of the tip (from 2 g to 12 g).

Magnum wire

The Magnum wire (Schneider, Bülach, Switzerland) is a 0.533 mm (0.021-inch) steel wire with a floppy distal end equipped with an olive-shaped tip that is 1 mm in diameter. The blunt ball tip has been designed to avoid subintimal passage or perforation by the highly pushable wire. The crossing success of this wire compares well with other mechanical approaches.[7] A drawback of this wire is that, owing to the large-profile shaft, only a high-profile balloon with a large inner lumen can be used, and exchange of the wire to another wire is practically impossible.

Coated wires

Our first choice wire for most chronic total occlusions is a 0.36 mm (0.014-inch) floppy wire with hydrophilic coating (Choice PT, Scimed). The excellent gliding characteristics and reduced friction of this coated wire allow easy advancement in cases of fresh thrombus or loose fibrous tissue and through intraluminal microchannels. However, the steerability of this wire is poor and the pushability low. Furthermore, the possibility of creating a subintimal passage with subsequent dissection or perforation is relatively high. The hydrophilic-coated floppy wires should cross easily and should not be pushed against resistance. Hydrophilic-coated wires may be used within the occluded segment after breaking the proximal fibrous cap with a stiff wire or may be used to advance within the distal vessel after crossing the occlusion with more traumatic wires. The 0.36 mm (0.014-inch), hydrophilic-coated Crosswire (Terumo) has a high recanalization success despite reduced steerability, although it has good pushability and excellent 'pathfinding' properties. A more recently available coated wire with apparent good crossing properties is the Shinobi wire (Cordis).

Lower-profile wires

The rationale for using lower-profile 0.25 mm (0.010-inch) or 0.30 mm (0.012-inch) wires is the possibility that these wires may pass through intra-arterial microchannels where an 0.36 mm (0.014-inch) wire may not cross. The 0.30 mm (0.012-inch) silk wire (USCI) with floppy tip may advance through tortuous microchannels where coated 0.36 mm (0.014-inch) wires will not cross. A stiff, low-profile alternative is the 0.25 mm (0.010-inch) ACS standard wire, which has been successfully used in our laboratory.

Support wires

After successful crossing with specific wires, it is advisable to change the generally low-support or traumatic crossing wire with a support wire. Exchanges can be made through an open-hole catheter advanced as distally as possible into or past the occlusion using wire extensions or specific wire exchange devices (e.g. Trapper, Scimed; Magnet, Scimed).

Laser wires

The laser guide wire (Spectranetics) consists of a 0.46 mm (0.018-inch) guidewire containing 12 silica fibers with a shapable tip on a 2.5 Fr, coaxial support catheter. As the laser wire progresses, a fluence of 60 mJ/mm^2 at a pulse repetition rate of 25 Hz is applied for 5-second intervals when the wire encounters resistance. In cases of persistent resistance the pulse repetition rate might be increased to 40 Hz. During the procedure, the wire is carefully advanced. It is very important to control the direction of the wire in orthogonal projections. If retrograde collaterals are present, contralateral injections are used to direct the laser wire and to diminish the risk of vessel perforation. The Thoraxcenter (Erasmus University, Rotterdam) experience,[35] with 51 coronary occlusions after a failed attempt at mechanical recanalization,

resulted in a 58% crossing success rate with the laser wire and a procedural success rate (restoring TIMI 3 flow) in 52% of cases.

GUIDEWIRE SUPPORTING SYSTEMS

Over-the-wire systems with end-hole catheters or over-the-wire balloon catheters are used for extra support to cross apparently difficult chronic total occlusions. The purpose of these systems are:

(a) to give support to the guidewire nearly up to its distal end to prevent flexion, kinking and prolapsing of the wire;
(b) to allow wire exchange or wire reshaping without losing any territory gained within the occlusion; and
(c) to allow wire exchange with better support wires after successful crossing with traumatic stiff wires, low-support coated wires, or low-profile wires – the extra support wires facilitate advancement of balloons, atherectomy devices or stents for the rest of the procedure.

A further important characteristic of the wire support systems is the presence of an inner lumen which, after removal of the wire, permits the injection of contrast directly at the occlusion site. This injection should be performed after blood has been aspirated through the catheter to prevent injection of an air bolus. The use of contrast diluted 50% with saline facilitates the injection. Injections should be performed carefully because high pressure could be harmful if the tip of the catheter is positioned within a dissection. If the distal vessel is not opacified after injection through the support catheter, if contrast has been injected into a dissection, or if a side branch is opacified, it may be useful to continue the contrast injection while carefully pulling back the support catheter. This allows the operator to determine at which level of the occlusion the catheter entered a dissection or at which level the catheter deviated into a side branch. After leaving the support catheter in the most distal 'intralumen' position, further attempts with the wire can be performed to work through the occluded segment.

LOW-PROFILE OVER-THE-WIRE BALLOONS

The recent generation of low-profile over-the-wire balloons that are 1.5 mm in diameter (Ranger,

Scimed; Predator, Cordis) are extremely helpful in crossing chronic total occlusions. Compared to low-profile, rapid exchange monorail balloons, over-the-wire catheters require long wires, extensions, or wire exchange devices to be removed after successful recanalization. This drawback is largely overcome by the advantages of increased wire support, quick wire exchange, and the possibility of performing distal contrast injections. Compared to over-the-wire catheters without a balloon, the new balloon catheters provide superior support at a cost of only a slightly increased profile.

Small-diameter balloons allow immediate, careful dilatation of the occluded segment. Most total occlusions should be pre-dilated with small-diameter balloons to confirm anterograde flow after the first dilatation and to reduce the risk of a major perforation, dissection, or potentially dangerous overdilatation of small vessels, side branches, or subintimal passages. Furthermore, an angiogram after a 1.5 mm balloon dilatation generally allows the operator to choose therapeutic strategies such as choice of balloon size, performance of atherectomy, or even discontinuation of the procedure owing to extensive distal disease, dissection, or the small size of the distal vessel. Thus, our preference is to attempt almost all chronic total occlusions with a 1.5 mm over-the-wire balloon to increase the success and safety of the procedure.

END-HOLE CATHETERS

The Transit (Cordis) and Tracker (Target Therapeutics) are flexible end-hole catheters that allow the passage of any 0.46 mm (0.018-inch) guidewire. These catheters give less support and provide less pushability than over-the-wire balloons or probing catheters, but they are more flexible. In the case of occlusions situated at the ostium or immediately distal to bifurcations, or in the presence of a tortuous segment proximal to the occlusion, these catheters may be preferable to over-the-wire balloons. In these cases it may be impossible to direct the less flexible tip of a balloon in the direction of the occlusion. Because the portion of the guidewire advanced in the occluded branch is short and provides little support, the balloon tends to prolapse towards the open branch of the bifurcation. The flexible end-hole catheters may follow the wire more easily into a new direction even if advanced close to the distal tip of the wire.

Probing catheters (Multifunction Probing, Schneider) have two channels, one long over-the-wire channel (proximal) and one short rapid exchange, monorail channel (distal). These catheters allow injections through the proximal channel while the wire is left on the monorail port. They also allow wire exchanges through the proximal channel (over-the-wire system). Drawbacks are the increased profile and the inability to advance the catheter through the occlusion over the wire when placed in the over-the-wire channel since the distal tip may get trapped.

HOW TO DETERMINE SUCCESSFUL WIRE CROSSING

Before any balloon dilatation is performed, it is essential to determine whether the wire has successfully crossed the occlusion and is positioned within the distal vessel lumen. This determination is often easy but in certain cases it can be very difficult. Unimpeded movement of the wire distal to the occluded segment that corresponds to the anatomical direction of the vessel gives the operator enough security to perform balloon dilatations. However, contrast visualization of the distal vessel to confirm the position of the wire within the lumen is preferable. This visualization can be obtained by injections through the guiding catheter if ipsilateral collaterals are present or if a small lumen permitting anterograde flow has been opened. It is sometimes necessary to pull the support system back into the guiding catheter to permit anterograde luminal flow. In the presence of retrograde collateral flow, contralateral injections can be used to determine the position of the wire. Careful contrast injections through an end-hole catheter or an over-the-wire balloon are very useful to confirm the intraluminal position of the catheter. If visualization of the distal lumen is inadequate and the operator is not convinced of the distal position of the wire, a careful, low-pressure 1.5 mm balloon dilatation might be attempted, bearing the risk of vessel perforation well in mind.

SIDE BRANCH TECHNIQUE

The presence of a side branch originating at the occlusion site is generally regarded as a negative predictor for crossing an occlusion, but this can be turned to advantage. If it is impossible to cross the main vessel with the wire, the wire can be positioned into the side

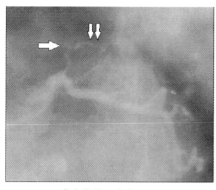
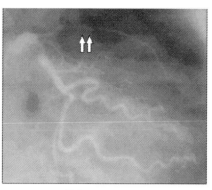

LAO Caudal   RAO Cranial

Baseline

a

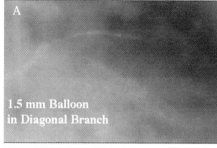
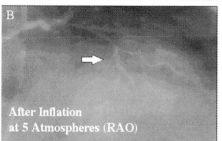
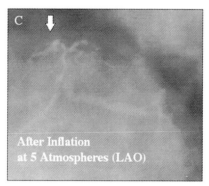

b

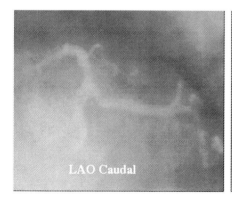
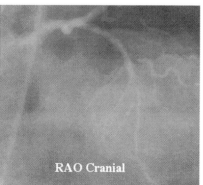

After Placement of Two 18 mm Stents
(3.5mm; 16 atm)

c

Figure 13.3 *(a) Total occlusion of the left anterior descending artery (LAD) angiographically documented 18 months before the procedure. Note the abrupt cut-off of the occluded LAD (single arrow) with a diagonal side branch originating at the occlusion site (double arrow). Recanalization was attempted without success with a floppy hydrophillic-coated wire and with a standard wire. (b) A 1.5 mm over-the-wire balloon was used for support. The floppy wire was then passed into the diagonal branch and the balloon was advanced and inflated at 5 atmospheres (Panel A). Following contrast injection (Panels B and C) the LAD revealed anterograde flow. The occlusion site was crossed easily with the hydrophilic-coated wire. (c) Final result after balloon dilatation and stent implantation using two 18 mm long ACS Duet stents deployed at 16 atmospheres on a 3.5 mm balloon.*

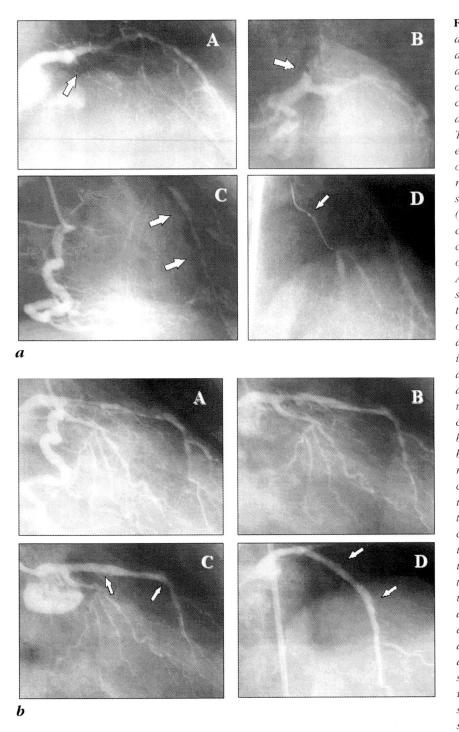

Figure 13.4 *(a) The baseline angiogram in the caudal right anterior oblique view (Panel A) and the caudal left anterior oblique view (Panel B) of a chronic total occlusion of the left anterior descending artery (LAD). The arrows indicate a short, eccentric funnel of the proximal occlusion. Panel C shows retrograde filling of the distal segment and mid-segment (arrows) of the LAD after contralateral injection in the right coronary artery (right anterior oblique view). Panel D shows an Athlete wire within the occluded segment before re-entrance into the distal lumen, which appears opacified with retrograde flow during contralateral contrast injection. The wire is supported by a 1.5 mm over-the-wire balloon advanced close to the tip of the wire. The arrow indicates the central radiopaque marker of the balloon. (b) Panel A shows a bilateral injection in the caudal right anterior oblique view after crossing the occlusion with the wire. The intraluminal position of the wire in the distal artery is confirmed by the contralateral injection. Panel B shows an ipsilateral injection in the same view after balloon angioplasty with a 40 mm × 3.0 mm balloon at 12 atmospheres. Note the long dissection. The caudal right anterior oblique view (Panel C) and the cranial view (Panel D) show the final result after implantation of an 18 mm AVE II stent (distal), a 30 mm Crown stent (mid-segment) and a 16 mm seven-cell NIR stent (proximal), all expanded with a 3.5 balloon at 18 atmospheres. Note the dissection distal to the stented segment (arrow) and the dissection distal to the proximal stent (arrow). (c) Intravascular ultrasound examination after*

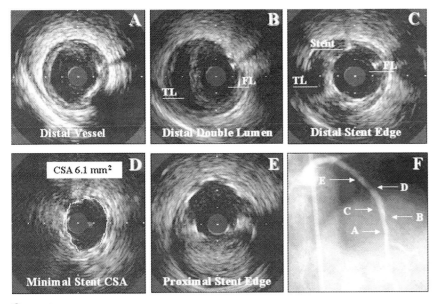

c

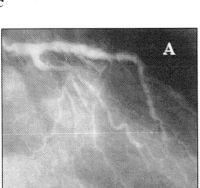 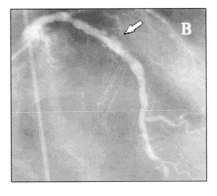

d

stent implantation (pull-back from A to E). Panel A shows the distal, untreated vessel lumen of the left anterior descending artery. Panel B shows the presence of a double lumen just distal to the stented segment. Note the false lumen (FL) through which the ultrasound catheter passed and the parallel true lumen (TL). Panel C shows the distal edge of the stented segment. The stented, newly created, false lumen is bigger than the true lumen. Panel D shows that the minimal cross-sectional area (CSA) within the stented segment measured 6.1 mm². Panel E shows the ultrasound image of the proximal stent edge. Panel F shows the position of the ultrasound cross-sections on the angiographic cranial view. (d) Follow-up angiography 4 months after stent implantation. The caudal right anterior oblique view (Panel A) and the cranial view (Panel B) show persistent patency of the recanalization procedure. Instead of finding restenosis, the angiograms appear to show mild aneurysmal dilatation (arrows) or persistent dissections.

branch and a balloon inflated at the occlusion site. Occasionally the fibrotic cap which occludes the main branch can be broken during the dilatation, allowing subsequent crossing of the occlusion.

Figure 13.3 shows an example of this technique of purposeful side branch dilatation, after which the main vessel could be visualized with anterograde flow and was then easily crossed with a wire.

SUCCESSFUL WIRE CROSSING BUT INABILITY TO ADVANCE THE DILATATION CATHETER

One of the most frustrating situations that may occur during a recanalization procedure is when a wire crosses successfully but it is impossible to advance any device over the wire through the occluded segment. Essential for a successful procedure are superior guiding catheter support, wire support (which is often low since steerable wires do not give high support), and device profile characteristics. It is not necessarily true that the lowest-profile device has the highest probability of crossing. In our experience, low-profile (1.5 mm) over-the-wire balloons combine the increased support of an over-the-wire device (compared to monorail devices) and have increased tip stiffness with better pushability than end-hole catheters despite a slightly higher profile.

If an over-the-wire balloon does not cross the lesion, an end-hole catheter should be attempted, and vice versa. However, before giving up, try repeated, quick forward and backward movements ('dottering') of the balloon, and intermittently adjust the guiding catheter position for deeper intubation. Persistence often leads to success. Further techniques that may help to get the device to cross include exchanging the guiding catheter or crossing the lesion with a second 'buddy' support wire. Another suggestion is to advance the support catheter as distally as possible, pull back the wire that has already crossed the occlusion and try to exchange it with an extra support wire. Crossing the lesion with a second wire may be easier than it was with the first, but it may also fail to cross. A laser catheter can be helpful since it can be advanced on the wire that initially crossed the occlusion. Especially in the presence of calcification, it may be necessary to pull back the wire or exchange it for a rotational atherectomy wire. The Rotablator generally crosses the occlusion easily. The operator should keep in mind that with the Rotablator there is a higher risk of vessel perforation than with the treatment of non-occlusive lesions.

SUBINTIMAL WIRE PASSAGES

Subintimal passage of the wire before re-entrance into the distal lumen is frequently observed during mechanical guidewire recanalization of chronic total occlusions and may result in procedural failure when anterograde flow cannot be established. Without the use of scaffolding stents, a subintimal passage has little chance of remaining patent, especially if the pathway is long. If re-entrance of the wire into the distal true lumen can be achieved, it is possible to create a subintimal conduit using coronary stents that yield long-term vessel patency.[51]

Figure 13.4 provides angiographic and ultrasound documentation of a long subintimal stent conduit in the treatment of a chronic total occlusion. In vitro histologic IVUS imaging of chronic total occlusion arterial segments has been helpful in identifying that guidewires frequently take the path of least resistance through an occlusion.[52] Guidewires often deflect between the plaque and the media, which is a natural dissection plane. This is the same plane that is mechanically dissected during a surgical endarterectomy. For a chronic total occlusion in vivo, the trick is to get the wire to recross from this dissection plane back into the true lumen distally (see Chapter 1, p.19).

TREATMENT AFTER SUCCESSFUL WIRE CROSSING

After a successful wire passage through a total occlusion, we initiate dilatations with the 1.5 mm balloon

that was used initially as the wire support device. In the presence of calcification visible on angiography or during IVUS examination, rotational atherectomy should be considered. For short occlusions with a large, eccentric plaque burden or in the case of occlusion at major bifurcations, directional atherectomy should be performed. Long lesions that require extensive debulking bear an increased risk of complications such as slow flow and reocclusion (*Fig. 13.1*) and they might be better treated by ultrasound-guided spot stenting (see Chapter 20). After debulking or balloon angioplasty, or both, the implantation of a stent is strongly indicated, owing to the improved acute and long-term outcomes compared to balloon angioplasty or debulking alone.[40–45]

THE MILAN EXPERIENCE IN THE MECHANICAL RECANALIZATION OF 322 TOTAL OCCLUSIONS

Between January 1996 and July 1997 interventions on 322 consecutive total coronary occlusions (301 patients) were attempted at our institution according to a standardized protocol (see *Table 13.2*).[6] This protocol consisted of the use of, first, a floppy, hydrophilic-coated wire (Choice PT, Scimed) followed, in cases of failure, with a 0.36 mm (0.014-inch) or 0.25 mm (0.010-inch) standard wire (Athlete, Asahi; Hi-torque, ACS). In all cases, a low-profile (1.5 mm) over-the-wire balloon (Ranger, Scimed; Predator, Cordis) was used to support the wire. The age of occlusion was < 4 weeks in 10% of cases, ≥ 4 weeks and < 3 months in 25%, ≥3 months in 33%, and undetermined in 32%. Bilateral injections when retrograde contralateral filling was present were used in 33% of cases. The overall success of mechanically crossing with a guidewire was 73% (Table 13.1). The floppy wire successfully crossed the occlusion in 45% of cases, a stiff wire in 33%, and the combined use of a floppy and a stiff wire was necessary for crossing the occlusion in 22%. Procedural success with re-established TIMI 3 anterograde flow was achieved in 200 lesions (62%). Stents were used in 79%, rotational atherectomy in 12% of cases, directional atherectomy in 10%, and laser catheter atherectomy in 4%.

Complications (*Table 13.1*) were: one death (0.3%), three urgent coronary artery bypass grafts (1%), two perforations with tamponade (0.6%), two Q-wave MIs (0.6%), 10 non-Q-wave MIs (3%), and 35

Table 13.2
Patient and lesion characteristics in 322 consecutive total coronary occlusions attempted at Milan between January 1996 and July 1997

	n	%
Patients in the study	227	100
Age* (years)	56 ± 4	
Previous myocardial infarction	256	77
Left ventricular ejection fraction* (%)	54 ± 8	
Lesions attempted	322	100
Vessel distribution:		
Left anterior descending artery	110	35
Left circumflex artery	91	30
Right coronary artery	111	35
Age of occlusion* (months)	17 ± 29	
< 1 month	33	10
≥ 1 months and < 3 months	82	25
≥ 3 months	105	33
Undetermined	102	32
Bridging collaterals	65	21
Abrupt occlusion	90	29
Occlusion length ≥ 15 mm	134	43
Side branches at occlusion site	144	45
One or more unfavorable angiographic characteristic	220	71
Contralateral collaterals	145	45

* Mean ± SD.

cases of local contrast staining (11%). Angiographic follow-up was obtained in 134 of 200 lesions (67%). The angiographic restenosis rate was 30% (40 lesions) using a definition of ≥ 50% lumen diameter stenosis.

CONCLUSION

These data suggest that a patient and persistent approach to treating chronic total occlusions can be rewarded with successful recanalization in about 60% of lesions. Although there are potential hazards when aggressive treatment of chronic total occlusions is attempted, the potential for success makes this a reasonable approach for percutaneous techniques. In the future, we may see improved guiding systems, such as with forward-looking ultrasound or coherent reflectometry guiding catheters, which we hope will improve the chance of success.

REFERENCES

1. Ruocco NA, Ring ME, Holubkov R et al. Results of coronary angioplasty of chronic total occlusion (the NHLBI 1985–86 PTCA Registry). *Am J Cardiol* 1992; **69**: 69–76.
2. Puma JA, Sketch MH Jr, Tcheng JE et al. Percutaneous revascularisation of chronic total occlusions: an overview. *J Am Coll Cardiol* 1995; **26**: 1–11.
3. Nowamagbe A, Ellis SG. Chronic total occlusion. In: Ellis SG, Holmes DR, eds. *Strategic Approaches in Coronary Intervention.* Baltimore: Williams and Wilkins, 1996; 380–394.
4. Roberts WC, Virmani R. Formation of new coronary arteries within a previously obstructed epicardial coronary artery (intraarterial arteries): a mechanism for occurrence of angiographically normal coronary arteries after healing of acute myocardial infarction. *Am J Cardiol* 1984; **54**: 1361–1362.
5. Ryan TJ, Baumann WB, Kennedy JW et al. ACC/AHA guidelines for percutaneous transluminal coronary angioplasty: a report of the ACC/AHA task force on assessment of diagnostic and therapeutic cardiovascular procedures. *J Am Coll Cardiol* 1993; **22**: 2033–2054.
6. Reimers B, Kobayashi Y, Akiyama T et al. Mechanical approach in the recanalization of total coronary occlusions: a consecutive series of 322 lesions. *J Am Coll Cardiol* 1998; **31 (suppl)**: 101A.
7. Reimers B, Camassa N, Di Mario C et al. Mechanical recanalization of total coronary occlusions with the use of a new guide wire. *Am Heart J* 1998; **135**: 726–731.
8. Dervan JP, McKay RG, Baim DS. Assessment of the relationship between distal occluded pressure and angiographically evident collateral flow during coronary angioplasty. *Am Heart J* 1987; **114**: 491–495.
9. Flameng W, Schwarz F, Hehrlein FW. Intraoperative evaluation of the functional significance of coronary collateral vessels in patients with coronary artery disease. *Am J Cardiol* 1978; **42**: 187–192.
10. Melchior JP, Doriot PA, Chatelain P et al. Improvement of left ventricular contraction and relaxation synchronism after recanalization of chronic total coronary occlusion by angioplasty. *J Am Coll Cardiol* 1987; **9**: 763–768.
11. Melchior JP, Meier B, Urban P et al. Percutaneous transluminal angioplasty for chronic total coronary arterial occlusions. *Am J Cardiol* 1987; **59**: 535–538.
12. Singh A, Murray RG, Chandler S, Shiu MF. Myocardial salvage following elective angioplasty for total coronary occlusions. *Cardiology* 1987; **74**: 474–478.
13. Finci l, Meier B, Righetti A, Ruitshauser W. Long-term results of successful and failed angioplasty for chronic total coronary arterial occlusion. *Am J Cardiol* 1990; **66**: 660–662.
14. Ivanhoe RJ, Weintraub WS, Douglas JS et al. Percutaneous transluminal coronary angioplasty of chronic total occlusions: primary success, restenosis, and long-term clinical follow-up. *Circulation* 1992; **85**: 106–115.

15. Warren RJ, Black AJ, Valentine PA et al. Coronary angioplasty for chronic total occlusion reduces the need for subsequent coronary bypass surgery. *Am Heart J* 1990; **120**: 270–274.

16. Bell MR, Berger PB, Menke KK, Holmes DR. Balloon angioplasty of chronic total coronary artery occlusions: what does it cost in radiation exposure, time, and materials. *Cathet Cardiovasc Diagn* 1992; **25**: 10–15.

17. Stone G, Rutherford B, McConahay D et al. Procedural outcome of angioplasty for total coronary artery occlusion: analysis of 971 lesions in 905 patients. *J Am Coll Cardiol* 1990; **15**: 849–856.

18. Ellis SG, Shaw RE, Gershony G et al. Risk factors, time course and treatment effect of restenosis after successful percutaneous transluminal coronary angioplasty of chronic total occlusion. *Am J Cardiol* 1989; **63**: 897–901.

19. Seggewiss H, Streck S, Everlein M et al. Successful recanalization of chronically occluded infarct-related arteries in patients with single-vessel disease results in reduction of cardiac events. *Circulation* 1994; **90**: I-435.

20. Kadek C, Burger W, Hartmann D et al. Long-term follow-up in 686 patients with attempted reopening of chronic coronary occlusions. *Circulation* 1993; **88**: II-2722.

21. Bell MR, Berger PB, Bresnahan JF et al. Initial and long-term outcome of 354 patients following coronary balloon angioplasty of total coronary artery occlusions. *Circulation* 1992; **85**: 1033–1041.

22. Katsuragawa M, Fujiwara H, Miyamae M, Sasayama S. Histologic studies in percutaneous transluminal coronary angioplasty for chronic total occlusion: comparison of tapering and abrupt types of occlusion and short and long occluded segments. *J Am Coll Cardiol* 1993; **21**: 604–611.

23. Kinoshita I, Katoh O, Nariyama J et al. Coronary angioplasty of chronic total occlusions with bridging collateral vessels: immediate and follow-up outcome from a large single-center experience. *J Am Coll Cardiol* 1995; **26**: 409–415.

24. Maiello L, Colombo A, Gianrossi R et al. Coronary angioplasty of chronic occlusions: factors predictive of procedural success. *Am Heart J* 1992; **124**: 581–584.

25. Gunnes P, Meyer BJ, Kessler B et al. Magnum wire for angioplasty of total and non-total coronary lesions. *Int J Cardiol* 1997; **60**: 1–6.

26. Meier B, Carlier M, Finci L et al. Magnum wire for balloon recanalization of chronic total occlusions. *Am J Cardiol* 1989; **64**: 148–154.

27. Pande AK, Meier B, Urban P et al. Magnum/magnarail versus conventional system for recanalization of chronic total coronary occlusions: a randomised comparison. *Am Heart J* 1992; **123**: 1182–1186.

28. Hosny A, Lai D, Mancherje C, Lee G. Successful recanalization using a hydrophilic-coated guidewire in total coronary occlusions after unsuccessful PTCA attempts with standard steerable guidewires. *J Intervent Cardiol* 1990; **3**: 225–230.

29. Rees MR, Sivananthan UM, Verma SP. The use of the hydrophilic Terumo glidewire in treatment of chronic coronary total occlusion. *Circulation* 1991; **84 (suppl II)**: II-519.

30. Gray DF, Sivananthan UM, Verma SP et al. Balloon angioplasty of totally and subtotally occluded coronary arteries: results using the hydrophilic Terumo radiofocus guidewire M (Glidewire). *Cathet Cardiovasc Diagn* 1993; **30**: 293–299.

31. Zimarino M, Rasetti G, Venarucci V, Pagliacci M. Terumo guidewire: the wire of choice for chronic total occlusion (letter). *Cathet Cardiovasc Diagn* 1995; **34**: 186–188.

32. Hamm CW, Kupper W, Kuck KH et al. Recanalisation of chronic, totally occluded coronary arteries by new angioplasty systems. *Am J Cardiol* 1990; **66**: 1459–1463.

33. Kaltenbach M, Hartmann A, Valbracht C. Procedural results and patient selection in recanalization of chronic coronary artery occlusions by low speed rotational angioplasty. *Eur Heart J* 1993; **14**: 826–830.

34. Rees MR, Michalis LK. Vibrational angioplasty in chronic total occlusions. *Lancet* 1993; **342**: 999–1000.

35. Hamburger JN, Gijsbers GHM, Ozaki Y et al. Recanalization of chronic total coronary occlusions using a laser guidewire: a pilot study. *J Am Coll Cardiol* 1997; **30**: 649–656.

36. Serruys PW, Hamburger JN, Rutsch W et al. Recanalisation of chronic total coronary occlusion using a Laser guidewire: the European TOTAL Multicentre Surveillance Study. *Eur Heart J* 1996; **17-A**: 516.

37. Kinoshita I, Katoh O, Nariyama J et al. Coronary angioplasty of chronic total occlusions with bridging collateral vessels: immediate and follow-up outcome from a large single center experience. *J Am Coll Cardiol* 1995; **26**: 409–415.

38. Safian RD, McCabe C, Sipperly ME et al. Initial success and long-term follow-up of percutaneous transluminal angioplasty in chronic total versus conventional stenoses. *Am J Cardiol* 1988; **61**: 23G–28G.

39. Holmes DR, Vliestra RE, Reeder GS et al. Angioplasty in total coronary artery occlusion. *J Am Coll Cardiol* 1984; **3**: 845–849.

40. Moussa I, Di Mario C, Moses J et al. Comparison of angiographic and clinical outcomes of coronary stenting of chronic total occlusions versus subtotal occlusions. *Am J Cardiol* 1998; **81**: 1–6.

41. Goldberg SL, Colombo A, Maiello L et al. Intracoronary stent insertion after balloon angioplasty of chronic total occlusions. *J Am Coll Cardiol* 1995; **26**: 713–719.

42. Violaris AG, Melkert R, Serruys PW. Long-term luminal renarrowing after successful elective coronary angioplasty of total occlusions: a quantitative angiographic analysis. *Circulation* 1995; **91**: 2140–2150.

43. Mori M, Kurogane H, Hayashi T et al. Comparison of results of intracoronary implantation of the Palmaz–Schatz stent with conventional balloon angioplasty in chronic total coronary artery occlusion. *Am J Cardiol* 1996; **78**: 985–989.

44. Berger PB, Holmes DR, Ohmann M et al. Restenosis, reocclusion and adverse cardiovascular events after successful balloon angioplasty of occluded versus nonoccluded coronary arteries. Results from the Multicenter American Research trial with Cilazapril after Angioplasty to prevent Transluminal coronary Obstruction and Restenosis (MARCATOR). *J Am Coll Cardiol* 1996; **27**: 1–7.

45. Sirnes PA, Golf S, Myreng Y et al. Stenting in chronic coronary occlusions (SICCO): a randomized, controlled trial of adding stent implantation after successful angioplasty. *J Am Coll Cardiol* 1996; **28**: 1444–1451.

46. Burger W, Kadel C, Keul H et al. A word of caution: reopening chronic coronary occlusions. *Cathet Cardiovasc Diagn* 1992; **27**: 35–39.

47. Leung WH. Coronary vasoconstriction after angioplasty of total coronary occlusions: relation to change in coronary perfusion pressure. *J Am Coll Cardiol* 1993; **22**: 1635–1640.

48. Meier B. Chronic total occlusion. In: Topol EJ, ed. *Textbook of Interventional Cardiology* 2nd edn. Philadelphia: WB Saunders, 1994, 318–338.

49. Myler RK, Shaw RE, Stertzer SK et al. Lesion morphology and coronary angioplasty: current experience and analysis. *J Am Coll Cardiol* 1992; **19**: 1641–1652.

50. Katsuragawa M, Fujiwara H, Miyamae M, Sasayama S. Histologic studies in percutaneous transluminal coronary angioplasty for chronic total occlusion: comparison of tapering and abrupt types of occlusion and short and long occluded segments. *J Am Coll Cardiol* 1993; **21**: 604–611.

51. Reimers B, Di Mario C, Colombo A. Subintimal stent implantation for the treatment of a chronic total occlusion. *G Ital Cardiol* 1997; **27**: 1158–1163.

52. Tobis JM, Smolin M, Mallery J et al. Laser-assisted thermal angioplasty in human peripheral artery occlusions: mechanism of recanalization. *J Am Coll Cardiol* 1989; **13**: 1547–1554.

Chapter 14 **Calcified lesions**

Antonio Colombo and Jonathan Tobis

The severity of calcification within coronary arteries has a significant effect on our ability to correctly deploy coronary artery stents.[1] As coronary artery stenting is applied to more complex lesions and more diffuse disease, the incidence and amount of calcification rises. In our early observations with intravascular ultrasound (IVUS) imaging, we noted that approximately 85% of target lesions had some degree of calcification documented by ultrasound, whereas only 15% appeared to be calcified by angiography. As described in Chapter 1, the exact anatomic position of calcium within the plaque may vary. Calcium may be deposited at the base of the plaque and not have a significant impact on the ability to dilate the artery or place a stent; however, if the calcification is at the interface of the lumen and the plaque, and if the calcification is extensive, then the plaque may be very resistant to balloon dilatation or directional atherectomy. In addition, a sclerotic artery is more resistant and inhibits passage of the stent through the artery to the target lesion. This is especially true of the rigid slotted tubular stents. Even if the stent is delivered correctly to the lesion site, it may not be adequately expanded despite high pressures. Moreover, as higher pressures are required, the risk of rupture increases. A recent review of our data reveals that 30% of lesions have superficial calcium that subtends 180° or more of the plaque circumference.

Examples of these distinctions between degrees of coronary artery calcification are shown in *Fig. 14.1*. When the lumen is narrow and calcium is present for 360°, it is not only difficult to expand the balloon, but it is also usually difficult to pass an IVUS imaging catheter. In the setting of intense calcification, our preference is to use rotational atherectomy and to step up the burr size to provide plaque modification so that we can obtain better expansion of the balloon and eventually achieve a larger stented lumen cross-sectional area. In addition, with the larger burr sizes there is some lesion debulking, which may assist in lowering the rate of restenosis. During pre-dilatation,

< 90° calcium

> 180° calcium

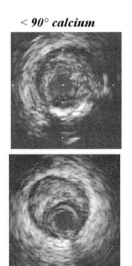

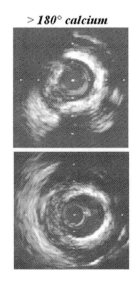

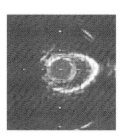

360° IVUS does not cross completely

Figure 14.1 *Intravascular ultrasound images of atherosclerotic plaque demonstrate varying degrees of calcification.*

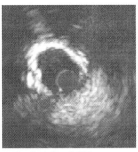

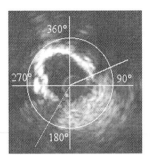

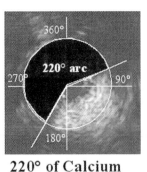

Figure 14.2 *Measuring the degrees of arc of calcified plaque.*

Calcified Plaque   **220° of Calcium**

if there is incomplete balloon expansion despite 12 atmospheres of pressure, we recommend withdrawing the balloon and treating the lesion with rotational atherectomy. The liberal use of pre-intervention IVUS to help assess the need for treatment with rotational atherectomy is also useful. On occasion, what appears to be intense calcification on angiography is due to calcification at the base of the plaque, and it is not necessary to treat this with a Rotablator. When intense calcification is present in large arteries, our preference is to start with a 10 Fr guiding catheter and use progressive burr sizes up to 2.5 mm in diameter. It is helpful in these cases, when a large amount of plaque will be dispersed downstream, to use abciximab before slow flow develops and to use an intra-aortic balloon pump, especially with long lesions.

The method for measuring the amount of plaque calcification is outlined in *Fig. 14.2*. The first panel shows the unedited ultrasound image where there is calcification between 7 o'clock and 3 o'clock, which

is recognized as intense echoes with shadowing peripherally (see Chapter 1). In the second panel, the angles have been identified from the center of the lumen. In this case the calcification subtended an arc of 220°.

Figure 14.3 shows a straightforward LAD lesion that does not appear to be severely calcified on angiography; however, with IVUS imaging, one appreciates 360° of acoustic shadowing consistent with an intensely calcified lesion. This was treated with rotational atherectomy followed by a stent with excellent results.

This ultrasound image should be contrasted with the stenosis in *Fig. 14.4*. Although the plaque is calcified, as documented by IVUS the calcium is at the periphery of the plaque and the lumen is adequate in this region, despite the presence of calcification by angiography.

An example of plaque modification by rotational atherectomy is provided in *Fig. 14.5*. The baseline angiogram shows a mild stenosis, but on ultrasound,

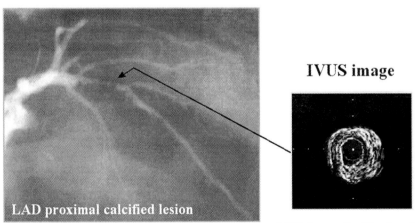

IVUS image

LAD proximal calcified lesion

360° Acoustic Shadowing

Figure 14.3 *Intense calcification with 360° of acoustic shadowing on the IVUS image. The radiograph prior to injection of contrast did not reveal significant calcification.*

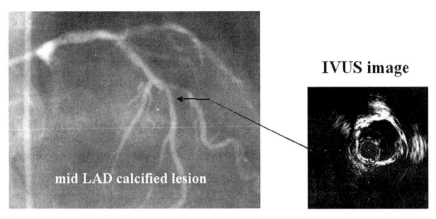

IVUS image

mid LAD calcified lesion

Calcified but not stenotic

Figure 14.4 *Use of IVUS to assess calcified lesions. Although this segment of the artery is calcified, the IVUS image reveals an adequate lumen cross-sectional area with calcification near the media of the artery.*

the plaque completely surrounds the 1.2 mm diameter catheter. After rotational atherectomy with a 1.5 mm and a 1.75 mm burr, a 30 mm Crown stent was deployed at 16 atmospheres with a 3.5 mm balloon. An excellent angiographic and ultrasound result was obtained with a lumen dimension of 3.0 mm × 2.5 mm. The artery is still sclerotic and does not expand to the full dimensions of the balloon, but the result is acceptable and probably better than if plaque modification with rotational atherectomy had not been performed.

In contrast to this satisfactory result, *Fig. 14.6* shows an example of inadequate debulking before stent insertion. The baseline image (Panel A) demonstrates a significant stenosis in an eccentric plaque in the proximal left anterior descending artery (LAD). In this case, no rotational atherectomy was performed but a Multilink stent was delivered and an adequate angiographic result was achieved (Panel B). The IVUS images, however, show less than ideal stent expansion in the proximal portion of the lesion, as shown in Panels C and D, where the minimum cross-sectional area is only 4.5 mm². The result was improved by inserting an AVE stent on a 3.5 mm balloon inflated at 20 atmospheres (*Fig. 14.6b*). The AVE stent has good radial strength but is flexible enough to pass through previously deployed stents. After a final dilatation with a 4 mm balloon, the cross-sectional area increased to 10.7 mm², more than twice the original cross-sectional area.

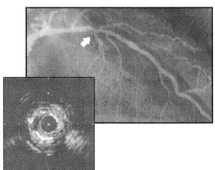

Baseline

After Rotablator 1.5 + 1.75mm 30 mm Crown at 16 Atm 3.5 mm balloon

Figure 14.5 *Plaque modification with rotational atherectomy.*

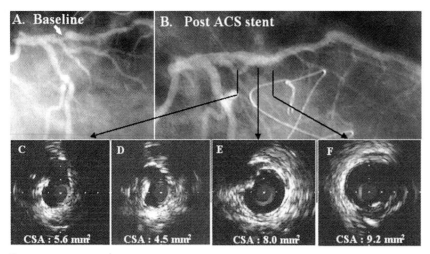

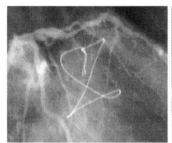

a

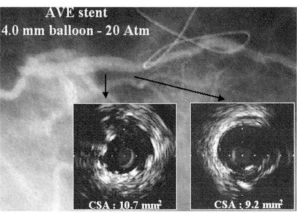

b

Figure 14.6 *Inadequate expansion of a calcified artery. (a) This calcified lesion was stented without rotational atherectomy to modify plaque compliance. The ultrasound images (C and D) demonstrate inadequate expansion of the stent. (b) To treat this problem, a second stent was placed within the first one and the artery was expanded at 20 atmospheres of pressure.*

DIFFERENTIAL CUTTING

Rotational atherectomy is based on the premise that the high-speed diamond drill is more likely to chip rigid calcified tissue than softer tissues that have elastic properties.[2] Softer tissue will be pushed away and not removed. Documentation of this property of differential cutting with rotational atherectomy (i.e. preferential removal of calcified plaque over less rigid material) is shown in *Fig. 14.7*. The baseline angiogram shows severe stenosis in the LAD just after the septal perforator with a 39 mm long lesion by quantitative coronary angiography. The IVUS images in *Fig. 14.7b* are obtained not only at the area of tightest stenosis but also in the section of the lesion that is most heavily calcified. After the use of a 1.5 mm and a 2.0 mm Rotablator burr, the maximum

gain in lumen cross-sectional area occurs at the site of most intense calcification (middle panels). Following dilatation with a 3.5 mm balloon distally and a 4.0 mm balloon in the more proximal half of the lesion, both the angiogram and ultrasound reveal a successful result with a minimum lumen cross-sectional area of 6.4 mm[2] (*Fig. 14.7c*). Based on these observations, a decision was made not to implant a stent in this patient.

ROTATIONAL ATHERECTOMY PLUS STENTING

Figure 14.8 provides an example of how an artery can be dramatically improved with the combination

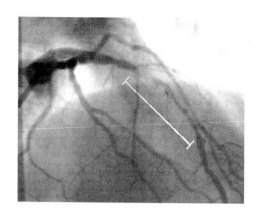

Figure 14.7 *Documentation by IVUS of differential cutting of calcified plaque. After rotational atherectomy with a 1.5 mm and a 2.0 mm burr, the IVUS images in (b) demonstrate that the maximum lumen area gain has occurred at the most calcified zone.*

Baseline Angiography

a

IVUS Results

After RTB with 1.5 mm burr   **After RTB with 2.0 mm burr**

Proximal: LCSA   LCSA

                         1.5 mm²   1.8 mm²

Mid: **Max gain at calcim site**

                1.6 mm²   3.4 mm²

Distal: 2.8 mm²   3.3 mm²

b

After additional balloon angioplasty

Angiography   **IVUS Lumen CSA**

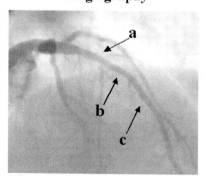

                                                    6.8 mm²

                                                    7.0 mm²

                                                    6.4 mm²

Proximal lesion(a & b) : 4.0 mm 12 atm
Distal lesion(c)   : 3.5 mm 16 atm

c

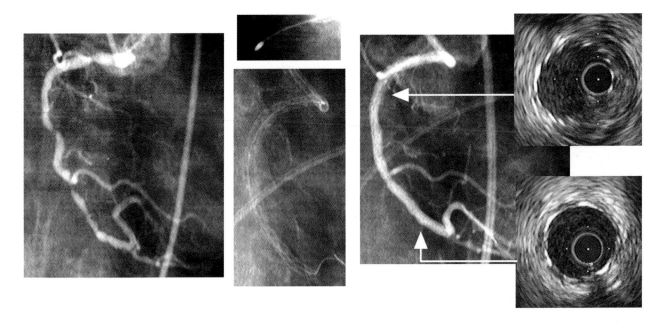

Figure 14.8 *The use of rotational atherectomy to facilitate passage and deployment of coronary stents in a calcified and tortuous vessel.*

of rotational atherectomy and stenting.[3,4] The patient was an 85-year-old female physician who presented with unstable angina. The right coronary artery had diffuse tortuous disease involving the proximal, mid- and distal sections of the artery. The lesion in the mid-segment was a subtotal occlusion because the guidewire would not pass without bringing a transit catheter up to the lesion to provide enough strength to force through the obstruction with a polymer tip (Choice PT) guidewire. Owing to the diffuse disease, rotational atherectomy was initiated with a 1.25 mm burr and then stepped up to 1.5 mm and then a 1.75 mm burr without detriment to blood flow. Balloon dilatation was performed with a 3 mm balloon to provide access for two 30 mm long AVE II Microstents, which were placed in the distal and mid-portion of the artery. The proximal lesion was treated with a 24 mm long AVE II Microstent. The final result showed excellent blood flow with a much larger and smoother arterial bore. By IVUS, the lumen was 3 mm × 3 mm or greater in diameter both proximally and distally.

We have stopped adding nitroglycerin and a calcium channel blocker to the Rotablator flush solution but we still use 10,000 units of heparin per liter. With the use of slower speeds and the technique of pecking at the lesion to permit intermittent flow, we have noticed a decrease in the incidence of slow or no flow phenomena. Removing

the nitroglycerin and calcium channel blocker prevents the marked hypotension that was commonly observed. We prefer to use intermittent boluses of verapamil 100 µg or adenosine 10–20 µg via the guiding catheter.

PRE-INTERVENTION ULTRASOUND IMAGING

The use of IVUS before an intervention frequently alters our approach to the angioplasty. Our initial plan to treat the diffuse disease shown in *Fig. 14.9*, Panel A, was to use a self-expanding Wallstent. Pre-intervention IVUS revealed a large band of calcium surrounding the lumen–plaque interface in the proximal segment, which almost completely encircled the ultrasound catheter (*Fig. 14.9*, Panel A2). On the basis of this observation, rotational atherectomy was performed first. After rotational atherectomy, the lumen was expanded; however, calcified tissue still encircled the lumen (*Fig. 14.9*, Panel B). Since calcium reflects ultrasound so strongly and produces shadowing beyond the surface, it is impossible to know the depth of the calcium or the true size of the vessel in that cross-section (see Chapter 1, *Figs 1.18* and *1.19*) A Wallstent was finally placed in the artery and

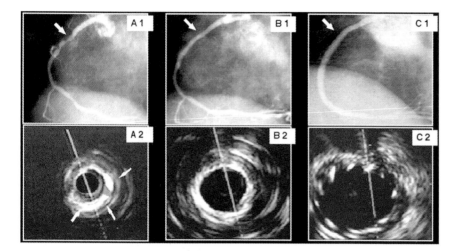

Figure 14.9 *Rotational atherectomy of a severely calcified plaque in preparation for placement of a Wallstent.*

satisfactory expansion was achieved; this would not have been possible without removal of a significant amount of calcified plaque (*Fig. 14.9,* Panel C).

If pre-intervention IVUS is not performed, the amount of calcification and resistance of the plaque may be underestimated. In *Fig. 14.10a,* the circumflex artery is diffusely diseased but it did not appear to be heavily calcified on angiography. An attempt was made to pre-dilate the lesion using a 3 mm diameter balloon. At 12 atmospheres there was still a significant waist in the mid-portion of the balloon (*Fig. 14.10a,* Panel B). Despite the improvement in the angiogram following balloon dilatation (*Fig. 14.10a,* Panel C), our experience has been that if the pre-dilatation balloon is not fully expanded, it will be very difficult to deploy the stent or to expand the stent adequately without risking arterial rupture. Therefore, the balloon was removed and rotational atherectomy was performed with a 1.75 mm burr (*Fig. 14.10b*). The lesion was then redilated with a 30 mm long balloon at 6 atmospheres. Following this, a 25 mm long NIR seven-cell stent was easily placed and was expanded successfully at 16 atmospheres (*Fig. 14.10b*). The corresponding ultrasound images in *Fig. 14.10c* show an adequate result, although the cross-sectional area of 5.7 mm² will place this patient at an increased risk of restenosis.

DILATATION-RESISTANT LESIONS

Another example of an insufficient balloon dilatation despite high pressure is shown in *Fig. 14.11.* The lesion in the mid-right coronary artery did not appear to be extensively calcified on fluoroscopy. Standard balloon angioplasty was initially attempted using a Maxxum 3.5 balloon. The balloon could not pry open the lesion despite 14 atmospheres of pressure (*Fig. 14.11,* Panel B). Rather than continue to crack the lesion at higher pressure, which could potentially result in a ruptured balloon or significant dissection, the decision was made to remove the balloon and use rotational atherectomy (*Fig. 14.11,* Panel C). A 1.25 mm burr was used initially, followed by a 1.5 mm burr. Subsequent balloon inflations were much easier to perform and an AVE GFX 18 mm long stent was placed in the mid-portion of the artery, as well as a second AVE GFX 12 mm long stent in the proximal right coronary artery. These were dilated with a 3.5 mm Titan balloon to 20 atmospheres of pressure without sustaining the kind of resistance that was seen with the initial balloon inflation prior to rotational atherectomy.

REVIEW OF OUR DATABASE: STENTING CALCIFIED LESIONS

The results of our experience with stenting calcified lesions are provided in *Tables 14.1–14.8.* Between April 1993 and September 1997, 476 lesions in 341 patients were considered to have significant calcium by angiography or IVUS. A successful stent impantation was obtained in 99% of cases (*Table 14.2*). The final balloon diameter was 3.7 ± 0.5 mm. The mean

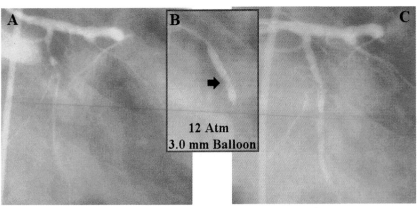

Baseline   Result After Balloon

a

Figure 14.10 *Incomplete balloon expansion in a calcified lesion. The presence of a significant indentation in the balloon at 12 atmospheres indicates the mechanical resistance to expansion. Instead of tearing the artery open at higher pressures, the balloon was removed and rotational atherectomy was performed (b).*

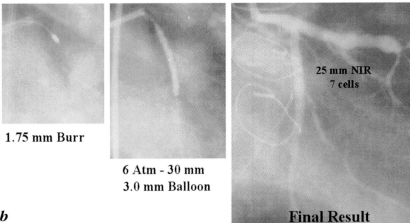

b

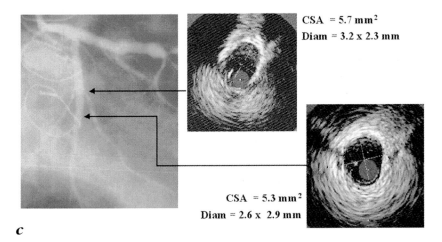

c

final ballooon pressure was 15.9 ± 3.4 atmospheres. Rotational atherectomy was used in 205 lesions (43%). Angiographic follow-up was obtained in 74% of the lesions, with an angiographic restenosis rate of 26%. The indications for stenting presented in *Table 14.3* show that most of the patients had elective procedures and that chronic total occlusion was present in 11% of the cases. Conversely, 18% of 248 chronic total occlusions were designated as calcified by angiography.

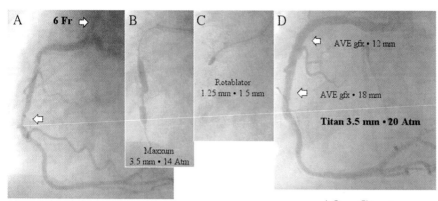

Baseline

After Stent

Figure 14.11 *The use of a Rotablator for an undilatable lesion.*

Table 14.1
Stenting calcified lesions. Patient characteristics

341 patients	*n*	*(%)*
Age (years)	61 ± 10	
Male	294	(86)
Previous MI	180	(53)
Unstable angina	111	(33)
Multivessel disease	220	(65)
LVEF (%)	57 ± 11	

Table 14.3
Stenting calcified lesions. Indications for stenting

	n	*(%)*
Elective	307	(65)
Chronic total occlusion	52	(11)
Suboptimal result	45	(10)
Dissection	32	(7)
Restenosis	28	(6)
Acute closure	6	(1)

Table 14.2
Stenting calcified lesions. Restenosis rate

No. of patients	341
No. of lesions	476
No. of stents	1.5 ± 1.0
Lesion success (%)	473 (99%)
B/V ratio	1.2 ± 0.2
Final balloon size (mm)	3.7 ± 0.5
Final pressure (mmHg)	15.9 ± 3.4
Use of Rotablator (%)	205 (43%)
Angiographic F/U	350 (74%)
Angiographic restenosis	90 (26%)

Table 14.4
Stenting calcified lesions. Lesion distribution

Vessel	*n (%)*	*Lesion*	*n (%)*
LAD	267 (56%)	Ostial	54 (11%)
RCA	96 (20%)	Prox	212 (45%)
LCX	88 (19%)	Mid	175 (37%)
LM	22 (5%)	Distal	35 (7%)

The restenosis rates for the individual stent types are presented in *Table 14.5*. It should be noted that these data are not derived from a randomized trial between the types of stents and that some of the stents were used in more difficult lesion subsets. For example, the AVE Microstent, because of its greater flexibility, was used more frequently in smaller vessels and longer lesions. The angiographic and IVUS descriptive data are presented in *Tables 14.6* and *14.7*. Despite the presence of calcification, a satisfactory lumen cross-sectional area (7.6 ± 2.4 mm²) was obtained in these patients.

Table 14.5

Stenting calcified lesions. Follow-up results

	#Lesions	Angio. F/U (%)	Restenosis (%)
P–S only	164	126 (77%)	19 (15%)
NIR	64	49 (77%)	18 (37%)
AVE Micro	47	31 (66%)	16 (52%)
Combination	45	30 (67%)	10 (33%)
G–R I	31	23 (74%)	10 (43%)
PURA	26	15 (58%)	2 (13%)
BeStent	18	16 (89%)	4 (25%)
Crown	19	16 (84%)	5 (31%)
ACS Multilink	14	11 (79%)	2 (18%)
Wallstent	12	10 (83%)	3 (3%)

Table 14.6

Stenting calcified lesions. Angiographic data

	Pre	Final	Follow-up
Ref. D. (mm)	3.1 ± 0.5	3.2 ± 0.6	3.0 ± 0.6
MLD (mm)	0.9 ± 0.6	3.2 ± 0.6	1.9 ± 1.0
Percentage stenosis	72 ± 17	2 ± 14	37 ± 28
Lesion length (mm)	12 ± 8		

Table 14.7

Stenting calcified lesions. Intravascular ultrasound measurements

Proximal reference LCSA (mm²)	8.6 ± 2.7
Final stent CSA (mm²)	7.6 ± 2.4
Distal reference LCSA (mm²)	7.1 ± 3.0

Procedural complications and clinical events are shown in *Table 14.8*. Although this lesion subset represents a high-risk population with more diffuse disease, the immediate and long-term results were quite acceptable. During a mean follow-up of 6 months, death occurred in 3% of patients and coronary artery bypass surgery was performed in 7% of patients. The procedural incidence of Q-wave and non-Q-wave myocardial infarction (MI) was 7%, with a 2% incidence in the next 6 months.

Table 14.8

Stenting calcified lesions. Procedural complications and clinical events

	Procedural	Early (< 2 months)	Late (> 2 months)
Patients	n = 341		
Acute stent thromb.*	4 (0.8%)		
Subacute stent thromb.*	7 (1.4%)		
Vascular complication	10 (2.9%)		
MI	23 (6.7%)	4	3
CABG	12 (3.5%)	3	9
Death	0	1	8

*per lesion (476)

ROTATIONAL ATHERECTOMY

Many calcified lesions in our series, but not the majority, were treated with rotational atherectomy. A separate analysis of all the lesions treated with a rotablator during the same time period is presented in *Tables 14.9–14.18*. *Table 14.9* presents our indications for using rotational atherectomy. Rotational atherectomy was used in 325 lesions. Not all lesions that were treated by rotational atherectomy were calcified, although the majority (74%) were. Rotational atherectomy was also used for lesions longer than 15 mm in 26% of the cases, diffuse in-stent restenosis (16%), and for debulking bifurcational lesions. Rotational atherectomy is reserved for treatment of more diffuse disease or severe calcification, whereas when a limited amount of calcification is seen on IVUS, then direct balloon dilatation and placement of a stent is used.

Table 14.9

Coronary stenting following rotational atherectomy. Indications for rotablation

	n (%)
No. of lesions	325
Calcified lesions	239 (74%)
Long lesions (>15 mm)	85 (26%)
In-stent restenosis	52 (16%)
Other	48 (15%)

Table 14.10

Coronary stenting following rotational atherectomy.
Patient characteristics

273 patients	n (%)
Age (years)	63 ± 10
Male	222 (86)
Previous MI	133 (49)
Unstable angina	89 (33)
Multivessel disease	203 (75)
LVEF (%)	60 ± 11

Table 14.11

Coronary stenting following rotational atherectomy.
Indications for stenting

Lesions	n = 325 (%)
Elective	237 (73)
Suboptimal result	30 (9)
Chronic total occlusion	23 (7)
Dissection	18 (6)
Restenosis	14 (4)

Table 14.12

Coronary stenting following rotational atherectomy

Stent type		
P–S	90	28%
MR	43	13%
AVE Micro	31	10%
PURA	23	7%
Crown	17	5%
G–R	16	5%
Multilink	17	5%
BeStent	13	4%
Wallstent	10	3%
Wiktor	7	2%
ACT	1	1%
Combination	28	9%

The clinical characteristics of the 273 patients who received rotational atherectomy are described in *Table 14.10*. Of these patients, 33% had unstable angina and 75% of the patients had multivessel disease. The indications for stenting in these 325

Table 14.13

Coronary stenting following rotational atherectomy.
Lesion distribution

Vessel	n (%)	Lesion	n (%)
LAD	181 (56%)	Ostial	48 (15%)
RCA	43 (13%)	Prox	138 (42%)
LCX	40 (12%)	Mid	121 (37%)
LM	24 (7%)	Distal	18 (6%)
Diag.	19 (6%)		
OM	14 (4%)		
Ramus	4 (1%)		

Table 14.14

Coronary stenting following rotational atherectomy.
Procedural data

Lesions	n = 325
Largest burr size (mm)	1.93 ± 0.31
Burr/artery ratio	0.7 ± 0.1
Final balloon size (mm)	3.6 ± 0.5
Balloon/artery ratio	1.2 ± 0.2
Max. inflation pressure (atm)	16 ± 3
Stent length (mm)	28 ± 16
Primary technical success	99%
Clinical success	95%

Table 14.15

Coronary stenting following rotational atherectomy.
Quantitative angiographic measurements

Lesions n = 325	Baseline	Post-procedure
Reference diameter (mm)	3.0 ± 0.5	3.2 + 0.6
Minimum lumen diameter (mm)	0.9 + 0.5	3.1 + 0.6
Percentage diameter stenosis	72 ± 15	2 ± 12
Lesion length (mm)	13.0 ± 9.2	

Table 14.16

Coronary stenting following rotational atherectomy.
Intravascular ultrasound measurements

Lesions	n = 217
Proximal reference LCSA (mm^2)	8.1 ± 2.4
Final stent CSA (mm^2)	7.2 ± 2.3
Distal reference LCSA (mm^2)	6.8 ± 2.5
Final stent MLD (mm)	2.8 ± 0.5

Table 14.17

Coronary stenting following rotational atherectomy. Procedural complications and clinical events

Patients	Procedural n = 273	Early (< 2 months)	Late (> 2 months)
Acute stent thromb.*	2 (0.7%)		
Subacute stent thm.*	2 (0.7%)		
Vascular comp.	10 (4%)		
MI – QMI	6 (2%)	1	4
MI – non-QMI	14 (5%)		
CABG	8 (5%)	2	5
Death	0	3	5

*Based on lesion number (= 325)

Table 14.18

Coronary stenting following rotational atherectomy. Restenosis

No. of lesions	325
Angiographic F/U	227 (70%)
F/U duration (mo)	5.1 ± 1.9
F/U MLD (mm)	1.9 ± 1.1
F/U percentage diameter stenosis	39 ± 28%
Angiographic restenosis	70 (31%)

lesions are shown in *Table 14.11*. The majority of stents (73%) were placed as an elective procedure, but in 9% rotational atherectomy and balloon dilatation yielded a suboptimal result. Chronic total occlusions accounted for 7% of the lesions that were stented after rotational atherectomy. In-stent restenosis represented 4% of the lesions. These were treated with a Rotablator followed by placement of a second stent within the initial one.

The distribution of stent types is described in *Table 14.12*. The vessel and lesion distribution is shown in *Table 14.13*. The frequent use of the Palmaz–Schatz stent reflects the availability of this device at the time of our early experience as well as the preference for this stent, owing to the high radial strength, for ostial and calcified lesions. The specifics of the procedural data are listed in *Table 14.14*. The mean largest burr size was 1.93 mm, which corresponded to a burr-to-

artery ratio of 0.7. The primary technical success rate in this complicated subset of lesions was high, at 99%.

The quantitative angiographic measurements shown in *Table 14.15* revealed a post-procedure minimum lumen diameter of 3.1 ± 0.6 mm, which corresponded to a 2 ± 12% diameter stenosis. The corresponding IVUS measurements in the 217 lesions that had ultrasound studies (67%) revealed a final minimum lumen stent cross-sectional area of 7.2 ± 2.3 mm^2 (*Table 14.16*). The final in-stent minimum lumen diameter (MLD) by IVUS in this subset was 2.8 ± 0.5 mm. The incidence of procedural complications was low except for a 2% incidence of acute Q-wave MI and a 5% incidence of non-Q-wave MI (*Table 14.17*). There was also a higher incidence of emergency coronary artery bypass surgery (5%) than in non-Rotablator cases. These complications yield a final primary clinical success of 95%. Although there were no procedure-related deaths, eight patients (3%) died within 6 months and an additional seven patients (3%) had bypass surgery.

The restenosis data are shown in *Table 14.18*. With a 70% angiographic follow-up of the 325 lesions at 5.1 ± 1.9 months, the mean follow-up MLD was 1.9 ± 1.1 mm. Using the dichotomous definition of angiographic restenosis (> 50% diameter stenosis), this corresponded to a restenosis rate of 31%. For an uncontrolled comparison, the restenosis rate in 1638 lesions treated without the use of a Rotablator during the same time period was 25%. This restenosis rate for rotational atherectomy followed by stenting is not excessive considering that these cases have more diffuse disease with longer lesions.

SUMMARY

There descriptive data of our experience with calcified lesions and rotational atherectomy demonstrate that highly satisfactory results can be obtained with coronary artery stenting when the lesions are approached in a methodical manner. IVUS is an important adjunct in treating these lesions because it helps to define the presence and extent of calcification as well as to direct the sizing of burrs and to determine the final balloon size that may be used. The use of rotational atherectomy has made an enormous impact on the results that can be achieved with coronary artery stenting in these complex lesion subsets.

REFERENCES

1. Henneke KH, Regar E, Konig A et al. Impact of target lesion calcification on coronary stent expansion after rotational atherectomy. *Am Heart J* 1999; **137**: 93–99.
2. MacIsaac AI, Bass TA, Buchbinder M et al. High speed rotational atherectomy: outcome in calcified and noncalcified coronary artery lesions. *J Am Coll Cardiol* 1995; **26**: 731–736.
3. Moussa I, Di Mario C, Moses J et al. Coronary stenting after rotational atherectomy in calcified and complex lesions. Angiographic and clinical follow-up results. *Circulation* 1997; **96**: 128–136.
4. Hoffmann R, Mintz GS, Kent KM et al. Comparative early and nine-month results of rotational atherectomy, stents, and the combination of both for calcified lesions in large coronary arteries. *Am J Cardiol* 1998; **81**: 552–557.

Chapter 15 **Complications**

Antonio Colombo and Jonathan Tobis

Some of the well-documented complications of balloon angioplasty include dissection and acute vessel closure.[1] The use of stents has dramatically improved our ability to treat these undesirable events. The purpose of this chapter is to discuss some of the complications that are more common with coronary artery stenting as distinguished from balloon dilatation alone. These complications include:

(a) dissections proximal or distal to the stent;
(b) arterial rupture;
(c) a lost or dislodged stent;
(d) stent jail;
(e) no or slow flow after stent deployment;
(f) embolization of thrombus; and
(g) side branch occlusion.

Despite these complications, the primary benefit of coronary artery stenting is that it decreases acute vessel closure associated with balloon angioplasty, and thus the overall complication rate is significantly reduced with stents.[2]

When stents were first developed, the high risk of subacute stent thrombosis made some people argue that the immediate benefit of preventing vessel closure during balloon angioplasty was counterbalanced by subsequent vessel closure caused by thrombosis. Now that we understand better how to deploy stents based on the observations of intravascular ultrasound (IVUS), the risk of subacute stent thrombosis should be close to 1%, thereby markedly improving the risk-to-benefit ratio of coronary artery stenting. Despite this improvement in our knowledge and advances in equipment over the past 5 years, we are also treating more complex vessel anatomy. We should expect that complications will continue to occur and evolve with the methodology. In the early days of balloon angioplasty, one of the most instructive parts of Geoffrey Hartzler's courses was entitled 'How To Get In and Out of Trouble'. Just as we

benefited from Geoff Hartzler's masterful technique of balloon dilatation, as well as from the complications that occurred, we hope that this chapter on complications of coronary artery stenting will guide the interventionalist to understand how to avoid situations that are potentially dangerous and how to deal with the complications that might arise.

A list of the complications that have occurred in our laboratory during coronary artery stenting is given in *Table 15.1*. Between April 1993 and June 1998, 3268 lesions were treated in 2337 patients. Successful deployment occurred in 95% of the lesions. Procedure-related myocardial infarction (MI) occurred in 3% of cases (non-Q-wave MI in 2% and Q-wave MI in 1%). Complications that necessitated immediate coronary bypass surgery occurred in 1% and death associated with the procedures occurred in 0.4%. Because none of these patients received coumadin therapy, our vascular complication rate was low, at 1%. In addition, despite the withdrawal of anticoagulation, the rate of subacute thrombosis

Table 15.1

Clinical complications of coronary stenting

April 93 – June 98	n (%)
No. of patients	2337
No. of lesions	3268
Average length stent/lesion (mm)	24.7 ± 16.2
Successful deployment	3120 (95%)
Non-QMI	75 (2%)
QMI	40 (1%)
CABG	43 (1%)
Death	14 (0.4%)
Vascular complication	47 (1%)
Stent thrombosis	
Acute	15 (0.5%)
Subacute	27 (0.8%)

Table 15.2
Angiographic complications of coronary stenting

Total no. of lesions = 3268	n (%)
Dissection from balloon	454 (14%)
Delivery failure	103 (3%)
No or slow reflow	72 (2%)
Wire breakage	58 (2%)
Coronary rupture	43 (1%)
Major side branch closure	33 (1%)
Acute closure	30 (1%)
Other	24 (1%)

was below 1%. A list of the angiographic complications we encountered with coronary artery stenting is shown in *Table 15.2*. These complications include dissection (14%), acute closure (1%), coronary artery rupture (1%), and major side branch closure (1%). A more complete description of these complications and how to avoid them or treat them follows.

DISSECTIONS

In our early experience with IVUS imaging of coronary artery stents, we noted a relatively high incidence of plaque flaps or dissections proximal or distal to the stent. At the time there were no short, high-pressure balloons and we frequently used 20 mm long compliant balloons for 15 mm Palmaz–Schatz stents. These flaps were not often visible on angiography but we thought that they might play a role in subacute stent thrombosis since stent thrombosis frequently occurred in the setting of an adequate angiographic result. On the basis of these observations and hypothesis, we initially recommended that any dissection should be covered with another stent.[3] As we gained more experience, we realized that it is possible to have small flaps near the stent without increasing the risk of subacute stent thrombosis provided that the flow is adequate and that the lumen is not compromised on angiography or ultrasound.[4] The angiogram in *Fig. 15.1* demonstrates a small dissection in the mid-left anterior descending artery (LAD) after placing a 28 mm long PURA stent inflated at 19 atmospheres on a 3.5 mm balloon. This balloon was equal to the distal media-to-media diameter as measured by IVUS. This small dissection as documented by angiography and IVUS would not be covered by another stent in the current era. One way of assessing these dissections is to analyse their physiologic significance by performing a coronary flow reserve study with a Doppler wire. This is described in more detail in Chapters 5 and 20.

An example of a dissection distal to a stent that was not treated with another stent is shown in *Fig. 15.2*. The stent was placed in the proximal diagonal artery at the position of the most severe narrowing (*Fig. 15.2a*). A few millimeters distal to the stent there was tubular narrowing of the lumen but it was not significantly worse than at baseline. After stent expansion at high pressure, there was a linear

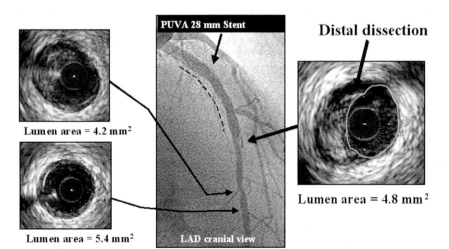

Lumen area = 4.2 mm²

Lumen area = 5.4 mm²

PUVA 28 mm Stent

LAD cranial view

Distal dissection

Lumen area = 4.8 mm²

Figure 15.1 *Small distal dissection after stenting mid LAD.*

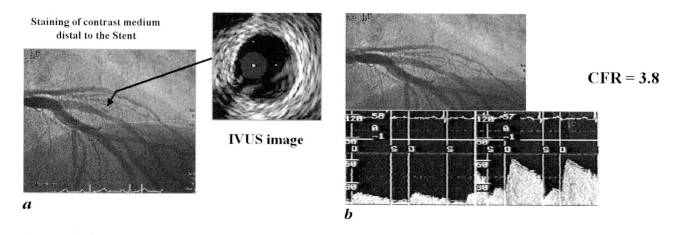

Staining of contrast medium distal to the Stent

IVUS image

CFR = 3.8

a

b

Figure 15.2 *(a) Dissection distal to a stent. (b) Doppler wire analysis of diagonal branch indicates that the dissection is not flow limiting. CFR, coronary flow reserve.*

stain of contrast medium in the wall of the vessel that was consistent with a dissection. This was confirmed by IVUS, which showed torn plaque with an echolucent space behind the plaque flaps between 4 o'clock and 7 o'clock. The lumen was still 2 mm × 2 mm wide and the flaps did not appear to compromise the main lumen. To assess the functional significance of this dissection, a Doppler flow wire analysis was performed (*Fig. 15.2b*). At baseline, the peak flow velocity was below 20 cm/second but following hyperemia with adenosine the velocity increased to over 60 cm/second. The coronary flow reserve (calculated by the peak flow velocity after adenosine divided by baseline) was 3.8. This implies that there was an adequate lumen cross-sectional area to maintain coronary blood flow under conditions of stress. Although in the past we would have placed a second stent to cover this dissection, at the current time we feel confident that the combination of IVUS and Doppler flow reserve provide sufficient information to permit these dissections to go untreated without clinical complications.

Figure 15.3 provides another example of using IVUS to evaluate a dissection distal to a stent. The baseline angiograms show significant stenoses in the proximal LAD at the ostium of the vessel as well as proximal to the bifurcation of a large diagonal branch. This long lesion was treated with a combination of directional coronary atherectomy (DCA) at the ostium and into the bifurcation. A Multilink 25 mm long stent was then placed from the distal left

main artery into the LAD at the level of the bifurcation with the diagonal branch. Following dilatation with a 3.5 mm balloon at 14 atmospheres, a dissection is visible just proximal to the bifurcation with the diagonal vessel on the lateral side of the LAD (*Fig. 15.3b*). As shown by IVUS (*Fig. 15.3c* inset), the dissection appears as an echolucent zone behind the plaque from 3 o'clock to 7 o'clock. There is drop-out of echoes at 6 o'clock owing to shadowing caused by the guidewire. The dissection does not appear to compromise the lumen, which is still > 2 mm in maximum and minimum dimension. Based on this observation, we elected to leave this dissection alone. This dissection did not progress to produce subacute stent thrombosis and the 6-month follow-up angiogram revealed a patent vessel without evidence of restenosis (*Fig. 15.3d*).

In distinction to the relatively small persistent dissections shown in *Figs 15.2* and *15.3*, *Fig. 15.4* reveals the type of dissection for which we would place another stent. Following deployment of a slotted tubular 25 mm long PUVA stent in the proximal LAD, the angiogram reveals a hazy zone with a small lucency in the mid-LAD. The corresponding ultrasound image demonstrates a large flap with a false lumen between 6 o'clock and 12 o'clock. The distal end of the stent is observed as the two struts at 2 o'clock and 4 o'clock. Although on angiography the lumen does not appear to be compromised, this persistent dissection encompasses > 50% of the vessel area and requires an additional stent to prevent propagation and vessel closure.

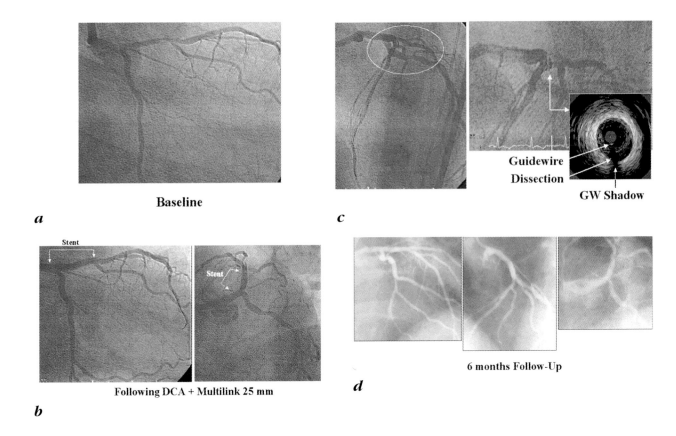

Baseline

a

b

Following DCA + Multilink 25 mm

Guidewire

Dissection

GW Shadow

c

d

6 months Follow-Up

Figure 15.3 *Evaluation of a dissection distal to a stent.*

When a dissection is observed, the decision to place a stent is determined by one or more criteria:

(a) We use IVUS to evaluate the anatomy and to determine the size of the flap and the residual lumen compared to the false lumen. Although we have no absolute criteria for dictating if a second stent should be inserted, in general, if the flap or false lumen encompasses > 50% of the lumen area, we are likely to place a second stent.

(b) Doppler coronary flow reserve (CFR) is often used to assess the effect of a dissection. A CFR > 2.5 implies that the dissection is not hemodynamically compromising the artery. We have refrained from treating these dissections and have noticed no untoward complications.

(c) The third means of assessing the significance of dissection is to measure the pressure gradient across the area of interest. If there is any resting gradient, or if the fractional flow reserve following the administration of adenosine is < 0.75,

then hemodynamic compromise is present and we would place a stent.

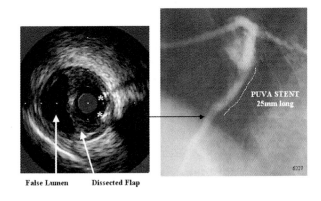

False Lumen   **Dissected Flap**

PUVA STENT 25mm long

Figure 15.4 *A significant dissection by IVUS criteria. Although the angiogram reveals a linear lucency, the true extent of the dissection is seen best on the cross-sectional ultrasound image.*

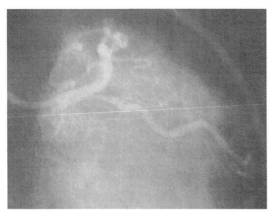

a   **Baseline**

Figure 15.5 *The risk of optimization. Despite pretreatment with large size atherectomy burrs, this artery dissected after stent optimization using a 4.0 mm balloon This type of severe dissection was more common before the introduction of noncompliant balloons that more closely matched the length of the newer stents. RTB, Rotablator.*

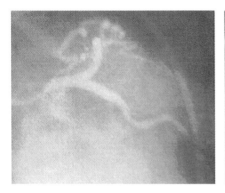
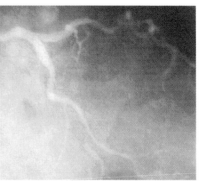

Post RTB + PS 15mm Stent
b   **(1.75, 2.25, 2.5mm burrs)**

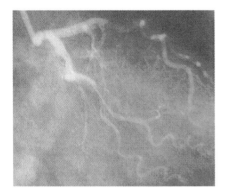
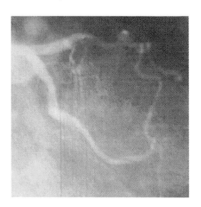

Post Stent Optimization   **Final Result**

c

ACUTE CLOSURE

Although significant benefits have been derived using an aggressive approach of high pressure and large balloons for inserting stents, one of the risks of optimizing the intrastent lumen is potential dissection and vessel closure. An example of how to get 'in and out' of this type of trouble is demonstrated in *Fig. 15.5*. The baseline angiogram reveals

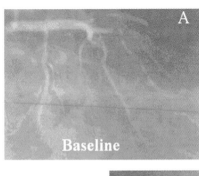

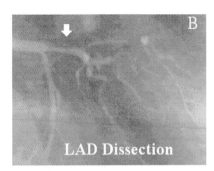

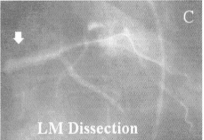

a

Figure 15.6 *Bailout stenting of a left main coronary artery. (a) In an attempt to recanalize an occluded diagonal branch, balloon dilatation created a retrograde dissection into the proximal LAD and left main coronary artery. (b) This was treated successfully by placement of two stents.*

b

significant stenosis at the ostium of the circumflex vessel. This was treated with progressive rotational atherectomy burrs and then placement of a Palmaz–Schatz 153 stent expanded to 4.0 mm at 14 atmospheres at the ostium of the circumflex. There is a tear in the vessel distal to the stent, with diminished blood flow in the distal vessel (*Fig. 15.5b*). This progressed over time to almost complete closure of the vessel with staining of contrast in the wall of the artery (*Fig. 15.5c*). Since guidewire position was maintained in the distal lumen, this complication was treated with repeat balloon dilatations. Following repeat dilatation, a flexible stent

(Gianturco–Roubin II) was placed in the mid- and distal portion of the obtuse marginal vessel (*Fig. 15.5c*). There is still a dissection, which is incompletely covered in the distal portion of the vessel. An attempt was made to pass an AVE Microstent to cover the distal dissection in the obtuse marginal artery but this was unsuccessful. The flow was adequate and the vessel remained patent; however, the patient sustained a large lateral wall MI from losing the inferior branch of the obtuse marginal. Unfortunately, this 77-year-old woman collapsed suddenly 2 days later and succumbed to a myocardial rupture of the lateral wall.

BAIL-OUT STENTING

In the next example, a complication occurred during the initial balloon inflation before inserting a stent. This is an example of a complication associated with balloon angioplasty and how to bail out of threatened closure by using stents. In this case, the dissection progressed in a retrograde direction and compromised the left main coronary artery. In *Fig. 15.6a* the baseline angiogram (Panel A) shows an occlusion of the first diagonal artery. Following guidewire recanalization and balloon dilatation (*Fig. 15.6a*, Panel B) there is compromise of the proximal portion of the LAD (arrow). Subsequent balloon dilatations led to propagation of the dissection in a retrograde direction into the left main coronary artery (*Fig. 15.6a*, Panel C). This was treated by placing a 40 mm long Gianturco–Roubin II stent from the mid-left main artery to the mid-LAD (*Fig. 15.6b*). In addition, a 16 mm long NIR stent was placed in the proximal portion of the left main artery to provide increased radial support. This was dilated to 4 mm. The patient was brought back 12 hours later for a follow-up angiogram which demonstrated a patent left main artery and LAD system. The diagonal branch, which had originally been targeted for treatment, was left untreated as a chronic total occlusion.

Table 15.3

Characteristics of coronary artery perforation

	Rupture	No Rupture	p
n	4	3225	
LAD (%)	48	15	NS
Calcified on fluoro. (%)	19	14	NS
Eccentric (%)	75	78	NS
Bend >45° (%)	16	10	NS
Atherectomy done (%)	14	17	NS
Total occlusion (%)	10	13	NS
Lesion length (mm)	12 ± 8	11 ± 7	NS
Baseline diameter stenosis (%)	70 ± 16	7 ± 15	NS
B2 or C (%)	80	66	< 0.05
Angio reference lumen (m)	29 ± 06	3.1 ± 0.5	< 0.01
Balloon/artery ratio (angio)	126 ± 0.20	1.20 ± 0.20	< 0.05
Balloon/vessel ratio (IVUS)	1.2 ± 0.2	1.0 ± 0.2	< 0.05
Max pressure (atm)	14 ± 4	16 ± 3	< 0.0001
Compliant balloon used (%)	71	24	< 0.00001

CORONARY ARTERY RUPTURE

In an arterial dissection, the tear separates the plaque from the surface of the media. Arterial vessel rupture is distinguished from artery dissection because the tear extends across the media and into or through the adventitia. Examples of the differences between plaque fracture, dissection, and vessel rupture interpreted by IVUS are shown in *Fig. 15.7*. In *Fig. 15.7a*, plaque fracture without dissection occurred following balloon angioplasty. Although the torn plaque protrudes into the lumen at 3 o'clock, there is no continuity between the lumen and the echolucent

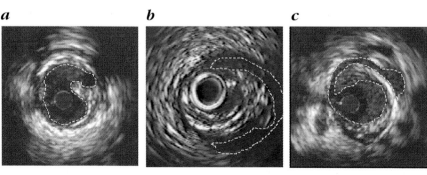

a *b* *c*

Plaque Fracture   **Plaque Dissection**   **Wall Rupture**

Figure 15.7 *Spectrum of plaque and vessel disruption after percutaneous transluminal coronary angioplasty.*

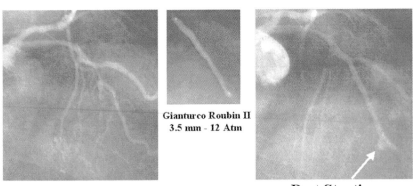

Gianturco Roubin II
3.5 mm - 12 Atm

Pre Intervention

Post Stenting
Distal Vessel Rupture

a

Figure 15.8 *Coronary artery rupture following aggressive balloon expansion of a GR 2 stent. This was treated successfully with prolonged inflation of a perfusion balloon. MLCSA, minimum lumen cross sectional area.*

IVUS during Stenting

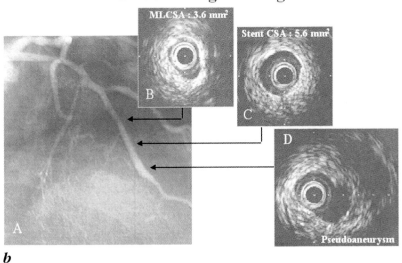

b

media. With a plaque dissection (*Fig. 15.7b*), the plaque is torn at 12 o'clock and also separates from the wall so that the echolucent zone of media is enlarged and is now continuous with the lumen. The dissection extends to 6 o'clock. This pattern is distinguished from a vessel rupture (*Fig. 15.7c*), in which the tear extends beyond the plaque, across the media, and out into the adventitia.

Although arterial rupture may occur with balloon angioplasty alone,[5] the incidence has clearly increased with the aggressive use of larger balloons and higher pressures to optimize the stent cross-sectional area.[6,7] In our series of 3268 lesions, the incidence of vessel rupture was 1%. However, it should be noted that a significant portion of these events occurred early in our experience when we were learning the limits of this technique. In addition, these ruptures occurred when

the balloon technology was less than ideal because the balloons that were used were longer than the stent. We were also using compliant or semi-compliant balloons because non-compliant high-pressure balloons had not yet been developed. A comparison of the arteries that ruptured versus 3225 lesions that did not result in rupture is provided in *Table 15.3*. The characteristics that were different between these two groups included the greater prevalence of grades B2 or C lesions in the ruptured group, smaller artery size, and a larger balloon-to-artery ratio. The greatest statistical difference occurred with the use of a compliant balloon, which was used in 71% of the arteries that ruptured but in only 24% of the arteries that did not rupture.

In this population, the identifiable causes of coronary perforation were balloon rupture 10 (23%), guidewire perforation 3 (7%), DCA 3 (7%), rotational

Baseline angiogram

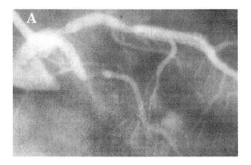

a

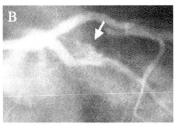

Dissection after PTCA

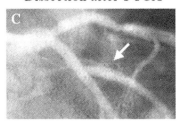

Post Stenting

Figure 15.9 *(a) Vessel rupture following balloon dilatation of a fibrotic lesion. Preparation of the lesion with rotational atherectomy had not been performed in this case. (b) IVUS images at the level of vessel rupture before and after stent insertion to treat this complication.*

Post PTCA   **Post Stenting**

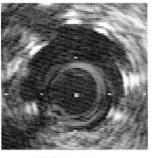

Vessel
rupture

| MLD | 3.9 | | MLD | 3.1 |
| MLA | 3.2 | | MLA | 8.1 |

Minimal lumen diameter = MLD (mm)
Minimal lumen area = MLA (mm²)

b

atherectomy 1 (2%), balloon inflation 25 (57%) and miscellaneous causes 2 (4%). Of the 43 patients with arterial ruptures, 14 (32%) had a major adverse event (a Q-wave MI, coronary artery bypass grafts, or death), which included a 14% mortality as a consequence of the perforation. In conclusion, coronary perforation is associated with a high rate of major adverse event and it most often occurs when oversized compliant balloons are used, especially in smaller vessels with complex lesions.

In *Fig. 15.8a* a long lesion of the mid- to distal LAD was treated with balloon dilatation followed by placement of a 40 mm long Gianturco–Roubin II stent. This was dilated with a 3.5 mm balloon at 12

atmospheres. After expanding the stent, the vessel ruptured at the distal portion of the stent. Although 12 atmospheres is no longer considered a very high pressure, the balloon size was generous for this distal segment of the vessel. This complication was treated with administration of protamine to reverse the heparin and with a low-pressure prolonged (30 minutes) balloon inflation. IVUS imaging was performed (*Fig. 15.8b*). This showed that the most narrowed stented segment has a small cross-sectional area, at 3.6 mm². Another stent was not inserted because of the recent complication. Distal to the stent (*Fig. 15.8b*, Panel D), the vessel was ruptured with a contained tear into the adventitia. Because the media is not clearly seen in this section, it is difficult to identify the extent of the tear, but when it is compared to the proximal segment, it is apparent that there is an aneurysm. The lumen of the vessel is approximately 3 mm × 2 mm in diameter.

Another potential cause of arterial rupture may occur during aggressive debulking, either with rotational atherectomy or DCA. With rotational atherectomy, this complication is usually immediately apparent, with the sudden onset of pain and pericardial staining. With DCA arterial rupture is rare, but deep cuts may result in aneurysm formation, which may only be appreciated several months later.

Although debulking densely calcific or fibrotic arteries has potential complications of vessel rupture,[8] it must be remembered that balloon dilatation alone can occasionally cause rupture, especially if high pressures instead of rotational atherectomy are used in calcified arteries. An example of this is shown in *Fig. 15.9a*, where a subtotal occlusion of an obtuse marginal artery branch was treated with balloon dilatation. This produced rupture of the vessel wall with extravasation of contrast. This complication was treated with a Palmaz–Schatz coronary artery stent (*Fig. 15.9a*, Panel C). The procedure then continued with recanalizing the occluded circumflex artery. The IVUS images of the vessel rupture are shown in *Fig. 15.9b*, Panel A; the containment of the rupture after the stent was placed is shown in *Fig. 15.9b*, Panel B. By compressing the remaining plaque against the wall and expanding the lumen cross-sectional area, the stent is able to help seal the torn artery. Although coronary stenting may not be sufficient to seal a large tear, it was successful in this case. Until plastic-covered stents become available, prolonged inflation, stent insertion, an autologous vein covered stent, and reversal of heparin anticoagulation are the only therapy options short of emergency bypass surgery.

At the present time our approach to treatment of arterial rupture consists of the following therapies:

(a) Heparin should be completely reversed with protamine to achieve an activated clotting time below 120 seconds. If the patient has received abciximab, the dose of protamine that is needed is usually higher. Despite the presence of abciximab, reversing the heparin has a significant impact on diminishing bleeding from the arterial rupture, and platelet transfusion is usually not required.

(b) While the heparin is being reversed, a perfusion balloon should be inserted immediately to tamponade the torn artery while continuing to provide blood flow to the distal myocardium.

(c) Following 15–30 minutes of perfusion balloon inflation, if the vessel is still leaking, we would place a polytetrafluoroethylene (PTFE)-covered stent. Since this stent is experimental at the present time, an alternative would be to deploy a vein-covered stent, as proposed by Stefanardis.[9,10]

(d) Throughout the time course of this emergency following arterial rupture, the patient must be monitored hemodynamically. Echocardiography is helpful to assess the amount of pericardial hemorrhage. A pericardiocentesis tray should be readily available as soon as this complication is appreciated so that pericardial drainage can be initiated promptly if necessary. In addition, some patients do not tolerate prolonged balloon inflations, even with the perfusion balloon, and it may be necessary to proceed with insertion of a stent sooner than expected.

COMPLICATIONS OF DEBULKING AND STENTING

Although aggressive debulking may improve the final stent lumen area, this method also has potential complications. In *Fig. 15.10*, the bifurcation of the distal left main artery with the proximal LAD and the circumflex artery was treated by rotational atherectomy using 1.75 mm, 2.15 mm and 2.38 mm burrs as well as DCA. As shown in *Fig. 15.10*, Panel B, this was followed by a 25 mm long ACS Multilink stent in the LAD and a 15 mm long Palmaz–Schatz stent in the circumflex artery; these stents were placed using the 'V' technique of simultaneous balloon inflations with the two proximal ends of the stents lined parallel to each other in the distal left main (see Chapter 10). Although the results appeared to be satisfactory, the patient was brought back 4 days later after an episode of near-syncope accompanied by sharp chest pain. As shown in *Fig. 15.10a*, Panels C and D, a large pseudoaneurysm was observed caused by vessel wall rupture from the aggressive atherectomy.

Figure 15.10a, Panel D presents the IVUS image of the aneurysm. There is a central stent but there is no apparent wall from the vessel between 9 o'clock and 3 o'clock. The ultrasound markers are 2 mm apart, demonstrating that the diameter of the aneurysm is at least 8 mm. The echo reflections filling this large cavernous aneurysm are due to reflections from blood. This unusual complication was treated by

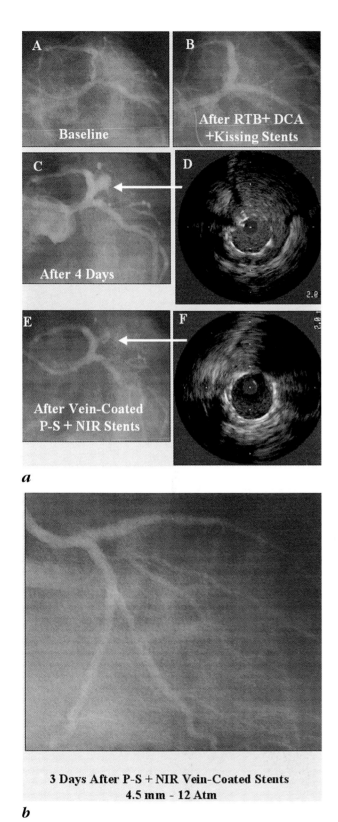

Figure 15.10 *Pseudoaneurysm of LAD following aggressive atherectomy.*

using a segment of autologous vein from the patient and suturing it on to a Palmaz–Schatz 154 stent. The vein-covered stent was then passed inside the previously placed Multilink stent. This did not completely separate the aneurysm from its entry point in the LAD, so a second vein-covered stent, this time on a 9 mm long NIR stent, was placed in the proximal LAD. The final ultrasound study shows the echo reflections from the Multilink stent and the vein-covered NIR stent isolated from the large cavernous aneurysm. Three days later, the angiogram revealed complete isolation of the aneurysm (*Fig. 15.10b*).

VESSEL RUPTURE CAUSED BY INCOMPLETE PREPARATION BEFORE STENTING

Although debulking plaque has potential complications, the underutilization of rotational atherectomy or directional atherectomy may also lead to problems. *Figure 15.11* reveals a series of events that occurred when trying to treat a chronic total occlusion without adequate preparation of the lesion before stent insertion and high-pressure expansion. The artery was recanalized with a guidewire and pre-dilated with a 40 mm long balloon. A 30 mm long Crossflex II stent on a 3.5 mm balloon was deployed in the mid-right coronary artery. After stent deployment, a band-like section of residual narrowing was noted in the mid-right coronary artery (*Fig. 15.11b*). This was treated with a 3.5 mm high-pressure balloon (Unicath Corporation) which was expanded to 25 atmospheres in order to efface the stenosis. At this point the vessel ruptured, with extravasation of contrast into the pericardial space (*Fig. 15.11c*). This was rapidly treated with a long inflation of a 3.0 mm perfusion balloon. In addition, an excimer laser fiber was passed through the torn segment and the laser was excited while injecting contrast in the hope that this might aid in sealing the tear (*Fig. 15.11d*). The final angiograms (*Fig. 15.11e*) demonstrated good flow into the distal vessel without any persistence of contrast extravasation. This type of resistance to high-pressure expansion of the stent usually indicates that the lesion was calcified or intensely fibrotic. The use of IVUS before intervention could have directed us to use rotational atherectomy. This would have lowered the lesion resistance and permitted more uniform expansion at a lower pressure.

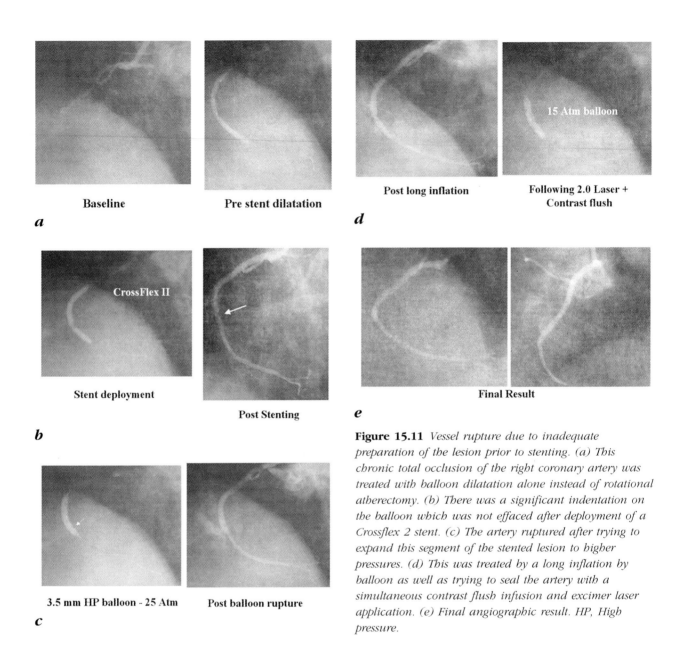

Figure 15.11 *Vessel rupture due to inadequate preparation of the lesion prior to stenting. (a) This chronic total occlusion of the right coronary artery was treated with balloon dilatation alone instead of rotational atherectomy. (b) There was a significant indentation on the balloon which was not effaced after deployment of a Crossflex 2 stent. (c) The artery ruptured after trying to expand this segment of the stented lesion to higher pressures. (d) This was treated by a long inflation by balloon as well as trying to seal the artery with a simultaneous contrast flush infusion and excimer laser application. (e) Final angiographic result. HP, High pressure.*

PTFE-COVERED STENTS FOR TREATING VESSEL RUPTURE OR ANEURYSMS

Although the incidence of vessel rupture or aneurysm is small, there still is a need in interventional cardiology for a covered stent that could separate the lumen from a false aneurysm or seal an arterial rupture. As described in *Fig. 2.49*, the JoMed company (Sweden) has developed a stent that is covered with a plastic sheath of PTFE. An example of the use of this PTFE-covered stent for treating a coronary aneurysm is provided in *Fig. 15.12*. The baseline coronary angiogram reveals an aneurysmal dilatation of the distal section of a long saphenous vein graft. This aneurysm had occurred spontaneously but because of the concern for potential rupture it was decided to treat this percutaneously. In *Fig. 15.12b*, the PTFE-covered stent is shown with the proximal and distal markers centered over the aneurysmal segment. The final result shows successful exclusion of the aneurysm without any contrast entering the aneurysmal cavity. The follow-up

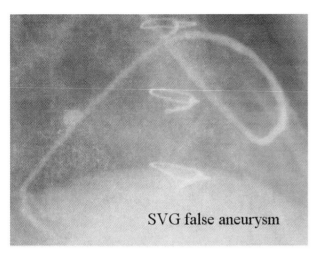

SVG false aneurysm

Baseline : 30-05-97

a

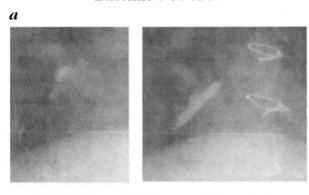

JOMED 20 mm PTFE covered Stent in place

b

Exclusion of SVG false aneurysm with
JOMED PTFE covered stent

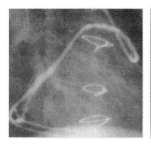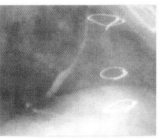

Final Result   **Follow-up : 2 months**

c

Figure 15.12 *An aneurysm in the body of a saphenous vein graft treated with a PTFE covered stent.*

angiogram at 2 months also demonstrates successful exclusion of the aneurysm without evidence of restenosis (*Fig. 15.12c*).

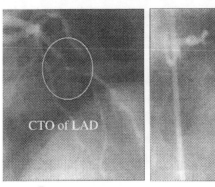

CTO of LAD

Pre treatment   After 1.75 mm rtb

a

Coronary Rupture post Rotational Atherectomy

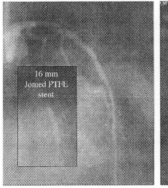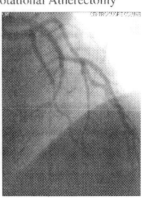

After 1 Jomed PTFE +   6 months Follow Up
2 ACS 15 mm stents

b

Figure 15.13 *(a) Coronary artery rupture after rotational atherectomy for a chronic total occlusion of the mid LAD. (b) This was quickly treated by placement of a 16 mm long PTFE covered stent which prevented any further extravasation of contrast into the pericardium.*

The PTFE-covered stent is also useful during interventional procedures for emergencies such as arterial rupture with extravasation of blood into the pericardium. A dramatic demonstration of the usefulness of a covered stent was provided during the live case demonstration during the 1997 Trans-Cutaneous Therapeutics (TCT) course transmission from Milan. A 65-year-old man with a chronic occlusion of the mid-LAD was pre-treated with a Rotablator before the

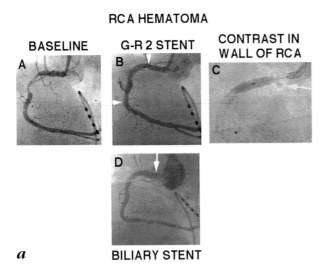

RCA HEMATOMA

BASELINE   G-R 2 STENT   CONTRAST IN WALL OF RCA

A   B   C

D

a   BILIARY STENT

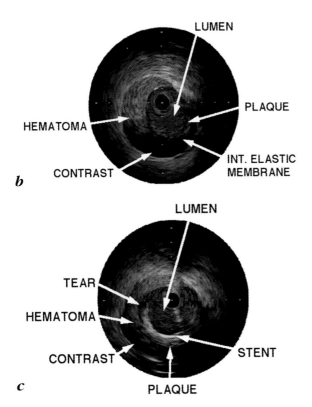

LUMEN

PLAQUE

HEMATOMA

INT. ELASTIC MEMBRANE

b   CONTRAST

LUMEN

TEAR

HEMATOMA

CONTRAST   STENT

c   PLAQUE

Figure 15.14 *Hematoma in the wall of the proximal right coronary artery induced by expanding a Gianturco-Roubin 2 stent.*

planned stent insertion. Although the guidewire crossed the occlusion relatively easily, the passage of a 1.75 mm burr resulted in a perforation of the artery

with active bleeding into the pericardium (*Fig. 15.13a*). The Rotablator was quickly removed and the perforation was temporarily compressed with a 3-minute inflation of a 3.0 mm balloon. After balloon dilatation, there was still evidence of arterial bleeding. A 16 mm long PTFE-covered stent was then placed on a 3 mm balloon and deployed at the site of arterial rupture. Because of the diffuse nature of the disease in this artery, two other 15 mm long ACS stents were also placed. The final result is shown in *Fig. 15.13b*, together with a 6-month follow-up angiogram, which demonstrated minimal restenosis and excellent flow to the distal vessel.

ARTERIAL WALL HEMATOMA

After balloon inflation, a tear into the artery may produce a hematoma within the wall of the vessel. In gradation of severity, a hematoma lies between a linear dissection and rupture of the free wall. It has a distinctive angiographic and ultrasound picture. As shown in *Fig. 15.14a*, a long tubular stenosis in the mid-right coronary artery was treated with a long Gianturco–Roubin II stent. After post-deployment inflation at 12 atmospheres, the angiogram showed puddling of contrast at the ostium of the right coronary artery (*Fig. 15.14a*, Panel C). The IVUS image of this segment is shown in *Fig. 15.14b*. The ultrasound catheter in the center of the image is eccentrically placed in the lumen which is surrounded by a thin layer of plaque. Peripheral to the plaque is a large echolucent space, which is consistent with a dissection except that the large extent of this area is unusual for a dissection. This space consists of an echolucent zone, owing to stagnant contrast, as well as an echogenic zone, owing to reflections of blood from a hematoma within the wall of the artery. There appears to be adequate continuity of the adventitia without evidence of free wall rupture. The lumen became progressively smaller over a 10-minute period.

This large hematoma was treated by placing a Palmaz 104 stent in the proximal right coronary artery that overlapped with the proximal portion of the Gianturco–Roubin II stent (*Fig. 15.14a*, Panel D). After insertion of the biliary stent, the ultrasound image showed a more expanded lumen, which is no longer compromised by the hematoma (*Fig. 15.14c*). The hematoma and the contrast can still be seen but they are externalized by the stent and plaque.

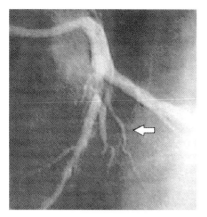
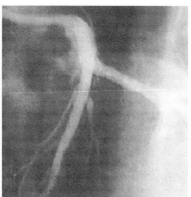

Baseline   After Stenting

Figure 15.15 *Small side branch occlusion after stenting.*

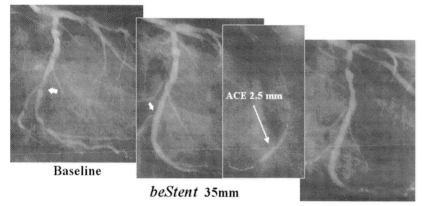

Baseline

beStent 35mm

ACE 2.5 mm

Final Result

Figure 15.16 *Side branch compromise after stenting.*

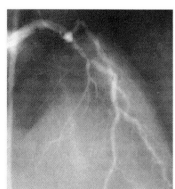
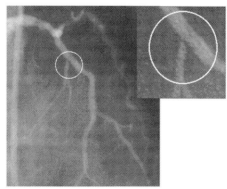

Baseline   After Stenting

Figure 15.17 *Large septal artery compromise following stent insertion in the LAD.*

SIDE BRANCH OCCLUSION AFTER STENTING

When a relatively minor branch is traversed by the main lesion, there is always the potential risk of plaque shifting and closing the side branch (*Fig. 15.15*).[11,12] One needs to make a clinical judgement as to the significance of this vessel and whether it is worth reopening it by dilating through the stent since there is the potential complication of damaging the stent in the main vessel. The ease or difficulty in

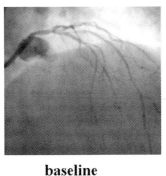
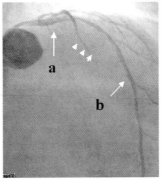

baseline

post stenting at proximal and mid LAD
(arrowheads show occluded septal branch)

a

a : CROSSFLEX
3.5 mm
25 mm
12 atm

b : PURA
3.0 mm
16 mm
6 atm

Figure 15.18 *Large septal artery rupture with hemodynamic compromise. (a) After treating the mid and proximal LAD with coronary artery stents, a large septal perforator artery occluded. (b) During the attempt to reopen the septal perforator with a balloon on a wire, a perforation occurred which led to pericardial tamponade. (c) This was treated with emergency pericardiocentesis. (d) Final angiogram and follow-up study 12 days after the initial procedure.*

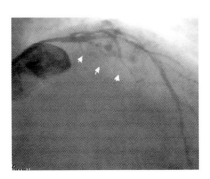

rupture of the septal branch

b

additional stenting after pericardial drainage

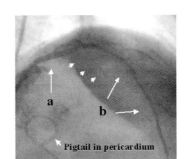

Pigtail in pericardium

arrowheads show disappearance of staining

c

a: Left main
PURA
3.5 mm
16 mm&10 mm (ostium)
10 atm

b: LAD mid & distal
2 CROSSFLEX
3.0 mm
16 mm
12 atm

follow up angiography

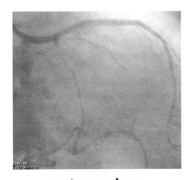
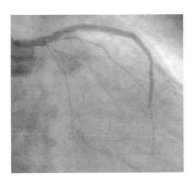

post procedure   **12 days after intervention**

d

traversing the stent into the side branch is dependent on several factors, among which are stent design[13] and the angle of branch origin. If you choose to treat this as a bifurcation lesion and so use a balloon in both vessels, then it is wise to keep a guidewire down the main channel and consider the need for simultaneous balloon inflations to protect the stent in the main branch. In *Fig. 15.16*, the branch vessel was compromised and a decision was made to treat the side branch stenosis. This large circumflex artery was

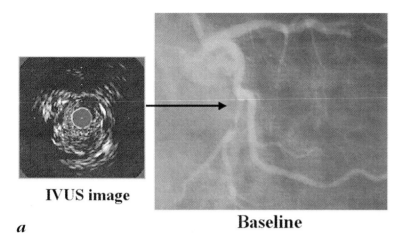

IVUS image

Baseline

a

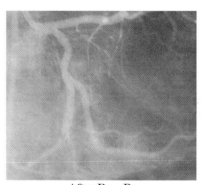

Figure 15.19 *Embolization from a thrombus containing lesion of the mid circumflex into the first obtuse marginal artery.*

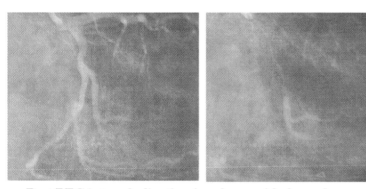

Post PTCA + embolization in a large side-branch

After Reo -Pro

b

c

treated with a 35 mm long BeStent. The small branch vessel was treated using an ACE 2.5 mm balloon. The final result showed adequate flow in the small branch while the main artery remained intact.

Another example of side branch compromise is shown in *Fig. 15.17.* In this example, the proximal LAD was treated with a slotted tubular stent. Following deployment of the stent, there is moderate compromise of a large septal perforator. Since the septal perforator usually takes off at a 90° angle, it is less likely to close during plaque shift, and we tend to leave these stenoses alone unless there is clinical evidence of ischemia.

Even though it is successful on most occasions, the procedure of reopening a side branch occlusion through a stent strut always has the potential for creating more complications. As shown in *Fig. 15.18*, following deployment of a 25 mm Crossflex stent in the proximal LAD on a 3.5 mm balloon, a large septal branch was compromised and eventually

closed. An attempt to open the septal branch with an ACE balloon produced vessel perforation and a hemopericardium that required drainage (*Fig. 15.18b*). It is interesting to note that the vessel rupture occurred just from passing the tip of the balloon on a wire without any balloon dilatation. The patient had received abciximab, which presumably exacerbated the complication and bleeding. Because the location of the vessel perforation was close to the left main coronary artery, the patient did not tolerate a prolonged balloon inflation with a perfusion balloon. Despite this limitation, the rupture was successfully sealed after heparin was reversed with protamine, even though a full dose of abciximab had just been given. Four additional stents were then placed in the distal LAD as well as in the left main artery for this diffusely diseased vessel (*Fig. 15.18c*). The follow-up study 12 days later demonstrated that the artery remained patent without extravasation of contrast.

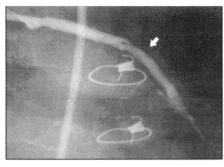

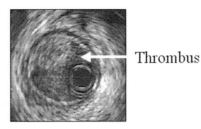

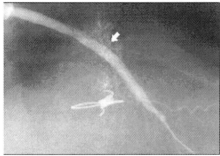

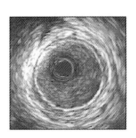

Before AngioJet

Thrombus

After AngioJet

Figure 15.20 *Identification of mobile thrombus inside a saphenous vein graft. This was treated prior to balloon dilatation with the AngioJet thrombectomy device.*

EMBOLIZATION OF THROMBUS WITHIN A LESION

Studies with angioscopy have demonstrated that angiography underestimates the occurrence and extent of thrombus in coronary artery lesions.[14] As discussed in Chapter 1, IVUS may identify thrombus that is not recognized by angiography, but it is not as sensitive as angioscopy.[15] Even when thrombus is appreciated on the angiogram or with pre-intervention ultrasound imaging, a very satisfactory result can be obtained simply with pre-dilatation and stent insertion.

The incidence of distal embolization is remarkably low but this complication can occur (*Fig. 15.19*). The baseline angiogram shows an irregular appearance to the circumflex artery and the ultrasound image was suggestive of thrombus, especially on the real time images. The lesion was dilated in preparation for placement of a stent, but this was complicated by occlusion of the large obtuse marginal branch associated with filling defects seen on angiography (*Fig. 15.19b*). This was treated with intravenous abciximab and dilatation with a 3.0 mm balloon to compress the thrombus; the primary lesion was then successfully stented with a 16 mm long NIR seven-cell stent on a 4.0 mm balloon at 18 atmospheres. The obtuse marginal artery was dilated but not stented (*Fig. 15.19c*).

An alternative way of treating embolization of thrombus is to prevent its occurrence in the first place before the intervention. Early recognition permits the use of one of the thrombectomy devices (*Fig. 15.20*). The filling defect in this saphenous vein graft was imaged with IVUS before intervention. This demonstrated a mobile filling defect within the vein graft, which is observed in the top half of the ultrasound image. The smaller speckled reflections are from blood flow and these are easy to distinguish during real-time imaging from their constant motion or by flushing saline in the guiding catheter while imaging with ultrasound. In this case the thrombus was treated with an AngioJet[16] (Possis Medical Incorporated, Minneapolis, Minnesota, USA) and a 4.0 mm Crown stent with resolution of the thrombus, both angiographically and by IVUS.

TISSUE PROLAPSE THROUGH A STENT

Another potential complication that is unique to coronary artery stenting is the presence of tissue that may prolapse through the intrastrut spaces. If a small amount of tissue prolapses, it provides a cobblestone appearance, which may be seen on angioscopy. However, if a large amount of plaque protrudes

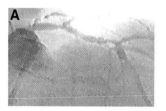
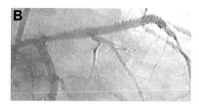
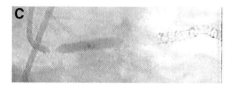
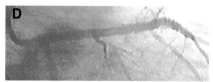

Figure 15.21 *Tissue prolapse through a spiral Palmaz–Schatz stent identified by intravascular ultrasound.*

a

Tissue Inside P-S Stent

Post stent within a stent

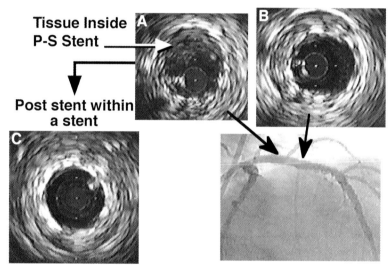

A Second Stent Within the Proximal Stent Compresses the Prolapsed Tissue

b

through the stent, it could compromise the lumen and may cause subacute stent thrombosis. One of the insidious problems with tissue prolapse through a stent is that it is not usually visualized by angiography. This is another area where IVUS may be very useful. *Fig. 15.21a* shows the angiogram of a diffusely diseased LAD that was treated with multiple stents, including a Wiktor stent in the distal segment and a spiral Palmaz–Schatz stent more proximally. Despite an excellent angiographic result (*Fig. 15.21a*, Panel D) the IVUS images reveal prolapse of tissue in the superior aspect between 9 o'clock and 3 o'clock (*Fig. 15.21b*, Panel A). The tissue subtends almost 50% of the available lumen area. On the basis of this

observation, a second stent was placed inside the first one. The repeat ultrasound image (*Fig. 15.21b*, Panel C) shows that the prolapsed tissue has been pushed back behind the stent and that the lumen is now adequately sized at 3 mm × 3 mm.

THE HINGE EFFECT FROM A SLOTTED TUBULAR STENT

When the earlier versions of the slotted tubular stents were being used, an unusual complication called a

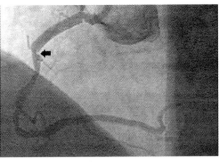
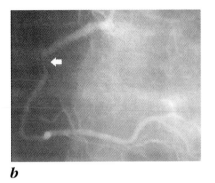

a *b*

Figure 15.22 *(a) The hinge effect from a rigid slotted tube stent. (b) Successful treatment by placement of a more flexible stent at the distal exit of the first stent.*

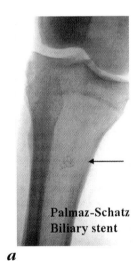
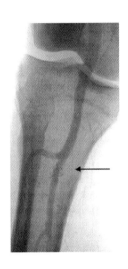
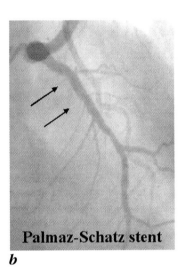

Palmaz-Schatz Biliary stent

Palmaz-Schatz stent

a *b*

Figure 15.23 *Angiograms obtained five years after distal embolization to the peroneal artery of a Palmaz–Schatz biliary stent. (a) Peripheral angiogram. (b) Follow-up angiogram of Palmaz–Schatz stent placed in the proximal LAD.*

'hinge effect' would occasionally be observed. As shown in *Fig. 15.22a* this undesirable effect could occur when a rigid slotted tubular stent is placed into a tortuous segment of vessel. The rigid stent flattens out the curve and forces a new angle between the stented portion and the non-stented segment of the artery. This complication occurs because the stent does not conform to the normal curvature of the sclerotic artery. A new bend or kink in the artery would be observed at the proximal or distal end of the stent and could be exacerbated during motion of the artery with the cardiac cycle. This complication predisposes the artery to restenosis. Now that more flexible stents are available and are used preferentially

for tortuous vessels, the complication of the 'hinge effect' is rarely seen.

RETRIEVAL TECHNIQUES FOR LOST CORONARY ARTERY STENTS

As the materials used for stenting and engineering designs have improved, the incidence of losing a coronary artery stent has diminished significantly. Nevertheless there still is an occasional case in which a stent is hand crimped or in which attempted

The goal is to upsize the introducer to a 10 F sheath

Figure 15.24 *Technique to retrieve a flared stent.*

Cut the proximal Y-Connection of the balloon

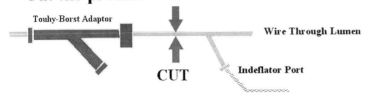

- The wire can be left in place, but pay attention not to cut it
- The wire can be replaced with a platinum plus wire
- If the delivery system is monorail, the wire should be removed

withdrawal of a stent into the guiding catheter results in displacement of an undeployed stent. In most cases the stent remains on the guidewire and can be trapped with a snare device. In other instances the stent is sheered off the delivery balloon and guidewire and the stent embolizes either into a coronary artery or a peripheral artery.

An unusual clinical example of stent embolization is provided in *Fig. 15.23*. This 66-year-old man had stenosis of the proximal LAD, which was treated with balloon dilatation followed by placement of a half (7 mm long) Palmaz–Schatz stent. While attempting to place a second stent, a 10 mm long Palmaz biliary stent that had been hand crimped on to a balloon, could not negotiate the mild tortuous bend in the proximal portion of the artery. The stent and balloon were withdrawn but the stent slipped off of the balloon. To retrieve the stent, the guiding catheter and guidewire were withdrawn to the iliac artery, but in trying to withdraw the stent into the femoral sheath, the stent became dislodged and embolized into the right peroneal–tibial artery. Blood flow to the leg did not appear to be compromised. There was no attempt to retrieve the stent or to flatten it against the wall of the peripheral vessel. Owing to chronic atrial fibrillation, the patient was continued on oral anticoagulant therapy. In addition, aspirin (100 mg/day) was prescribed for 2 weeks.

The patient did well and remained asymptomatic for 5 years, both in terms of his coronary artery disease and the embolized stent. A follow-up cardiac catheterization was performed because of exacerbation of aortic insufficiency. At the time of the follow-up angiogram (*Fig. 15.23b*) the previously stented portion of the proximal LAD demonstrated wide patency. An injection into the right femoral artery revealed excellent flow without obstruction (*Fig. 15.23a*). The stent had not migrated from its original position and there was no evidence of in-stent stenosis, intimal hyperplasia, or luminal compromise.

In 1991, Schatz and colleagues[17] reported a 2.5% incidence of stent embolization without any acute clinical sequelae. In 1996, Alfonso and colleagues[18] reported nine cases of stent embolization. The embolization sites included the femoral artery (three cases), the renal artery (one case), and unknown sites (five cases). All the patients remained free of clinical symptoms during the immediate hospitalization and at 6-month follow-up. One patient had a follow-up aortogram 6 months after the procedure; this revealed that the stent had lodged in a small branch of the right femoral artery that had remained patent.

The case presented in *Fig. 15.23* is unusual in that a follow-up angiogram was obtained 5 years after the procedure and still demonstrated lack of progression of tissue growth around the stent. It raises the question of whether intimal hyperplasia associated with in-stent restenosis is due to the stimulus of the metallic foreign body or to barotrauma caused by the prerequisite balloon dilatation.

The incidence of stent loss depends on the type of stents that are being deployed as well as on the experience of the operator. At the Centro Cuore Columbus in Milan between 1 January 1995 and 31 December 1996, a total of 1788 stents were deployed. Of these, there were 17 stents (0.9%) that embolized in 14 patients. Eight of these were retrieved with either a gooseneck snare (Microvena) or with a Retriever 18 catheter (Target Therapeutics). An additional nine stents were not retrieved, usually because the site of embolization was not known. In all 17 cases there were no complications from either

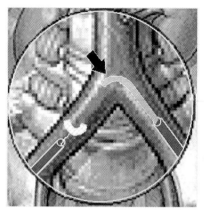

10F contralateral approach

10F guiding catheter across the bifurcation

a

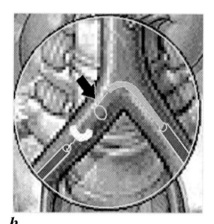

1 Microvena snare or biotome attaches one end of stent

2 Cut the balloon

3 Remove contralaterally

b

Figure 15.25 *Contralateral technique to retrieve a deformed stent.*

the attempted retrieval of the stent or leaving it in its embolized position. The biggest problem that we encounter when trying to retrieve a lost stent is that the 8 Fr guiding catheter is too small to permit the stent to be withdrawn smoothly. The stent is often traumatized in the attempt to retrieve it and the proximal portion may be flared, which exacerbates the problem of withdrawing the stent into the guiding catheter.

It must be emphasized that the best technique for retrieving a lost stent is not to lose it in the first place. Not only does this imply careful technique in deploying the stent but if the stent cannot be deployed in the right place, the best thing to do is deploy the stent proximally, rather than attempt to withdraw the stent back into the guiding catheter. This is more critical with the earlier stent designs, such as the Palmaz–Schatz stent; it is less of a problem with the factory-crimped stents, such as the Multilink, the Gianturco–Roubin II or the AVE stents.

If you are committed to retrieving a stent or if the stent embolizes and you are forced to retrieve it, then the method that we recommend is to upsize the introducer to a 10 Fr sheath. This will permit withdrawal of even a flared stent into the introducer so that it can be removed from the body. Assuming that you have an 8 Fr guiding catheter with a balloon and guidewire system already in place, the method for switching over to a 10 Fr sheath is first to cut the balloon catheter shaft just distal to the 'Y' connection of the balloon (*Fig. 15.24*). Leave the guidewire in place and be careful not to cut the wire when you are cutting the balloon catheter shaft. If the stent is still on the balloon, the wire can be substituted for a stiffer wire, such as a platinum plus wire. If the delivery system is a monorail design then the wire should be removed. Next, remove the 8 Fr guiding catheter and the 8 Fr sheath using the shaft of the balloon as your 'guidewire'. While manual pressure is maintained over the arterial puncture site, the 10 Fr introducing sheath is placed over the proximal end of the cut balloon catheter and advanced into the

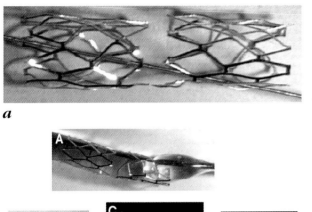

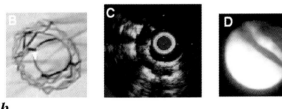

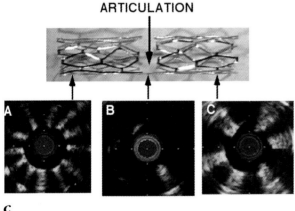

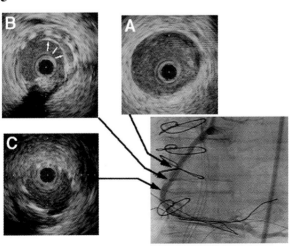

arteriotomy. If the shaft of the balloon will not advance into the dilator of the 10 Fr sheath, the dilator can be cut a few centimeters proximal to its tip, where the lumen is larger. Once the 10 Fr sheath is safely inserted, the balloon with the stent on it can be withdrawn safely into the larger 10 Fr sheath. The sheath and the balloon with the stent are then removed as a unit, keeping the platinum plus guidewire in place. A new 10 Fr sheath can then be inserted and the angioplasty can continue.

RETRIEVAL OF A DAMAGED STENT

If the stent has come off the balloon and is snared but is in an unusual shape, either bent or in the form of a 'U' so that it cannot be withdrawn easily into the guiding catheter or arterial sheath, an alternative method is to retrieve the stent through a second catheter. First, bring the stent down into the iliac artery (*Fig. 15.25*). A puncture of the contralateral artery is then performed using a 10 Fr sheath and guiding catheter. The 10 Fr guiding catheter is passed over a guidewire across the aortic bifurcation and approximates the stent, which resides in the right iliac artery. A Microvena snare or biotome is then extended from the contralateral side. Once the stent is secure in the snare, the balloon that is holding the stent is cut below the balloon's 'Y' connector and then the stent and distal portion of the balloon are removed from the contralateral side through the 10 Fr guiding catheter. Fortunately, with the currently available stents that are bonded to the delivery balloon, the incidence of stent embolization is exceedingly rare.

Figure 15.26 *Deformation of a Palmaz–Schatz stent by re-crossing the guidewire through the side of the stent. (a) and (b) In vitro study to demonstrate how balloon dilatation through the side of a Palmaz–Schatz stent can lead to the IVUS appearance shown in (b, panel C). (c) IVUS images obtained at different cross sections of a Palmaz–Schatz stent demonstrate echo reflections from either 12, 1, or 6 metallic struts. (d) The same IVUS pattern reproduced in the in vitro study was seen in a patient following guide wire re-crossing and balloon dilatation through a Palmaz–Schatz stent (d, panel B)*

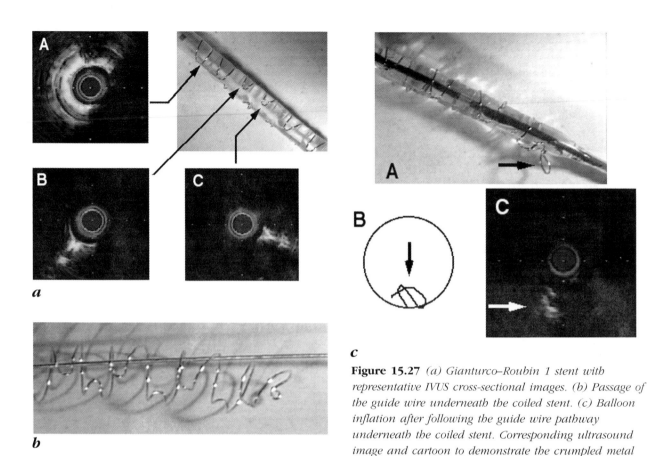

Figure 15.27 *(a) Gianturco–Roubin 1 stent with representative IVUS cross-sectional images. (b) Passage of the guide wire underneath the coiled stent. (c) Balloon inflation after following the guide wire pathway underneath the coiled stent. Corresponding ultrasound image and cartoon to demonstrate the crumpled metal coil which produces the observed ultrasound image.*

COMPLICATIONS OF RECROSSING A STENT

As discussed in Chapter 10, when a stent is placed across a branch vessel it is sometimes difficult to recross the stent and treat the side branch. This was cleverly termed 'stent jail',[19] but this frequently turns out to be less of a problem than originally thought because it is possible to cross through and dilate the stent struts with a balloon to treat the ostium and proximal portion of the branch vessel. This has been described as 'escape from stent jail'.[19] The ease of performing this maneuver depends on the type of stent and the particular anatomy, but if a balloon over a wire will not pass into the side branch, then a balloon on a wire (such as the ACE) frequently can be maneuvered into the side branch. Care should be taken not to pass the entire length of the balloon through the stent because it may be difficult to remove it once the balloon has been inflated and unwrapped.

A related complication can occur when trying to recross a stent with a guidewire. Although it is usually the case that the guidewire is left down the main channel until the entire procedure is completed, on occasion the guidewire gets withdrawn by accident. Alternatively, after intentionally withdrawing the guidewire, an observation of a distal problem requires recrossing the deployed stent. Despite apparent adequate deployment of the stent and apposition against the wall, guidewires have been designed to pick out small channels and can easily slide through the stent strut and pass underneath the stent on its course through the vessel (*Fig. 15.26a*). A low-profile balloon may also pass with limited resistance through this stent strut. If the balloon is then inflated, it will deform the stent struts. Although the lumen may be adequate to prevent subacute stent thrombosis, it seriously impedes passage of other balloons or stents. The deformation of a Palmaz–Schatz stent caused by balloon dilatation through a side strut creates a unique IVUS image (*Fig. 15.26b*). Stent struts are seen in half of the circumference and no stent struts are seen on the other half between 11 o'clock and 4 o'clock in *Fig. 15.26b*, Panel C). There is an unusual semicircle of reflected metal between 4 o'clock and 9 o'clock, which is due to the deformed portion of the stent strut. This was visualized both by IVUS (*Fig. 15.26c*) and by angioscopy (*Fig. 15.26b*, Panel D). The ultrasound pattern was reproduced in vitro by passing a balloon through a side strut and then inflating it (*Fig. 15.26b*, Panels A and B).

This unusual pattern of a Palmaz–Schatz stent should be compared to the typical IVUS image of a Palmaz–Schatz stent (*Fig. 15.26c*). Although the image varies depending on where the cross-section is taken, there is always a circumferential distribution of the struts except at the articulation site.

The best way to prevent this problem when recrossing a stent is to put a large bend on the guidewire and purposely prolapse it through the stented segment. The large knuckle makes it almost impossible to enter underneath the stent and facilitates passing it through the central lumen.

RECROSSING COILED STENTS

The Gianturco–Roubin coiled stent has a different echogenic pattern (*Fig. 15.27a*). Based on the clamshell design, there is no circumferential coverage of the artery. Therefore, as the IVUS device is withdrawn through the stent, the cross-sections of the stented artery show a variable pattern of semicircular arcs and isolated short reflections. If a guidewire recrosses a coiled stent and passes underneath the coils (*Fig. 15.27b*), the balloon will easily follow the guidewire through this passageway and compress the stent following inflation. The in vitro ultrasound image of this phenomenon is shown in *Fig. 15.27c*, where a compressed and crumpled coil is shown as an isolated area of reflection between 6 o'clock and 7 o'clock. Although this decreases the support provided by the stent, further treatment is not necessarily needed and, if recognized, another stent can be passed to provide greater support in the artery.

The second generation of the Gianturco–Roubin coiled stent has been associated with another form of complication, which may occur when attempting to recross the stent with a previously used balloon or a second stent. Since the Gianturco–Roubin II stent has a connecting spine, instead of being compressed against the wall the coils may compress in the longitudinal direction and fold over like an accordion. This can be picked up on fluoroscopy by observing the longitudinal motion of the reference marker on the Gianturco–Roubin II stent.

REFERENCES

1. Holmes DR Jr, Holubkov R, Vlietstra RE et al. Comparison of complications during percutaneous transluminal coronary angioplasty from 1977 to 1981 and from 1985 to 1986: the National Heart, Lung, and Blood Institute Percutaneous Transluminal Coronary Angioplasty Registry. *J Am Coll Cardiol* 1988; **12**: 1149–55.
2. Altmann DB, Racz M, Battleman et al. Reduction in angioplasty complications after the introduction of coronary stents: results from a consecutive series of 2242 patients. *Am Heart J* 1996; **132**: 503–507.
3. Colombo A, Hall P, Nakamura S et al. Intracoronary stenting without anticoagulation accomplished with intravascular ultrasound guidance. *Circulation* 1995; **91**: 1676–1688.
4. Kobayashi N, De Gregorio J, Adamian M et al. New approaches to evaluate coronary dissections post coronary intervention: all dissections are not malignant. *J Am Coll Cardiol* 1999; **33**: 71A.
5. Ajluni SC, Glazier S, Blankenship L et al. Perforations after percutaneous coronary interventions: clinical, angiographic, and therapeutic observations. *Cathet Cardiovasc Diagn* 1994; **32**: 206–212.
6. Nakamura S, Colombo A, Gaglione A et al. Intracoronary ultrasound observations during stent implantation. *Circulation* 1994; **89**: 2026–2034.
7. Alfonso F, Goicolea J, Hernandez R et al. Arterial perforation during optimization of coronary stents using high-pressure balloon inflations. *Am J Cardiol* 1996; **78**: 1169–1172.
8. Warth DC, Leon MB, O'Neill W et al. Rotational atherectomy multicenter registry: acute results, complications and 6-month angiographic follow-up in 709 patients. *J Am Coll Cardiol* 1994; **24**: 641–648.
9. Stefanadis C, Toutouzas P. Percutaneous implantation of autologous vein graft stent for treatment of coronary artery disease (letter). *Lancet* 1995; **345**: 1509.
10. Colombo A, Itoh A, Di Mario C et al. Successful closure of a coronary vessel rupture with a vein graft stent: case report. *Cathet Cardiovasc Diagn* 1996; **38**: 172–174.
11. Fischman DL, Savage MP, Leon MB et al. Fate of lesion-related side branches after coronary artery stenting. *J Am Coll Cardiol* 1993; **22**: 1641–1646.
12. Mazur W, Grinstead WC, Hakim AH et al. Fate of side branches after intracoronary implantation of the Gianturco–Roubin flex-stent for acute or threatened closure after percutaneous transluminal coronary angioplasty. *Am J Cardiol* 1994; **74**: 1207–1210.
13. Kinoshita T, Kobayashi Y, Nameki M et al. Differences in security of stent jail among Palmaz–Schatz stent, NIR stent, and Multi-Link stent: effect of balloon inflation through stent struts. *J Am Coll Cardiol* 1999; **33**: 84A.

14. Teirstein PS, Schatz RA, Denardo SJ et al. Angioscopic versus angiographic detection of thrombus during coronary interventional procedures. *Am J Cardiol* 1995; **75**: 1083–1087.

15. Siegel RJ, Chae JS, Forrester JS, Ruiz CE. Angiography, angioscopy, and ultrasound imaging before and after percutaneous balloon angioplasty. *Am Heart J* 1990; **120**: 1086–1090.

16. Hamburger JN, Serruys PW. Treatment of thrombus containing lesions in diseased native coronary arteries and saphenous vein bypass grafts using the AngioJet Rapid Thrombectomy System. *Herz* 1997; **22**: 318–321.

17. Schatz RA, Baim DS, Leon M et al. Clinical experience with the Palmaz–Schatz coronary stent. Initial results of a multicenter study. *Circulation* 1991; **83**: 148–161.

18. Alfonso F, Martinez D, Hernandez R et al. Stent embolization during intracoronary stenting. *Am J Cardiol* 1996; **78**: 833–835.

19. Caputo RP, Chafizadeh ER, Stoler RC et al. Stent jail: a minimum-security prison. *Am J Cardiol* 1996; **77**: 1226–1229.

20. Hiro T, Leung CY, Russo RJ et al. Intravascular ultrasound identification of stent entrapment in vivo with in vitro confirmation. *Cathet Cardiovasc Diagn* 1996; **40**: 40–45.

Chapter 16 Stenting during acute myocardial infarction

Shunji Kasaoka and Jonathan Tobis

Large randomized trials of thrombolytic therapy in patients with acute myocardial infarction (MI) have demonstrated that early reperfusion can reduce mortality and salvage myocardium.[1–3] However, there are significant limitations of thrombolytic therapy, including:

(a) failure to restore patency in 20–30% of arteries;
(b) an increased incidence of recurrent ischemia (14–17%) and reinfarction (4–13%) compared with placebo;

(c) serious bleeding complications, including intracerebral hemorrhage; and
(d) the fact that many patients who present with acute MI are ineligible to receive treatment.[4]

To overcome these drawbacks, varying strategies of percutaneous transluminal coronary angioplasty (PTCA) in acute MI have been investigated (*Table 16.1*), either as an adjunct to thrombolytic therapy (rescue PTCA) or as a stand-alone procedure without

Table 16.1

Various strategies of using percutaneous transluminal coronary angioplasty in acute myocardial infarction

A Adjunctive strategies (percutaneous transluminal coronary angioplasty (PTCA) in concert with thrombolytic therapy)
1 Immediate PTCA
   Urgent angiography is performed after thrombolytic administration. If a high-grade (less than totally occlusive) residual stenosis is found (present in the majority of patients after successful thrombolysis), PTCA is carried out.
2 Salvage (rescue) PTCA
   Urgent angiography is performed after thrombolytic administration. If the infarct artery remains occluded, PTCA is performed to restore patency.
3 Deferred (delayed) PTCA
   Following thrombolytic therapy, urgent arteriography is deferred. Prior to hospital discharge, cardiac catheterization is electively performed and PTCA is completed if a significant residual stenosis in the infarct artery is identified.
4 Elective PTCA
   Following thrombolytic therapy, patients are treated conservatively unless spontaneous angina, clinical instability, or inducible ischemia develops prior to discharge.
5 Routine predischarge angiography
   Following thrombolytic therapy, patients undergo routine pre-discharge angiography to establish prognosis and identify a high-grade residual stenosis or total occlusion of the infarct artery for further intervention

B Primary (or direct) infarct angioplasty without antecedent thrombolysis
   Patients with evolving acute MI are taken directly to the cardiac catheterization laboratory and undergo left ventriculography and coronary arteriography. Systemic thrombolysis is withheld. Based on clinical, hemodynamic, and anatomic findings, reperfusion of the infarct artery is accomplished by PTCA (or other interventional techniques), bypass surgery, or intracoronary thrombolysis. If spontaneous reperfusion has already occurred at the time of acute arteriography (residual stenosis < 70% with TIMI 3 flow), conservative medical therapy follows. In most prior studies, acute reperfusion was accomplished by PTCA in 90% of patients.

C Primary stenting for acute infarction
   Patients are taken directly to the cardiac catheterization laboratory and undergo coronary arteriography. Reperfusion of the infarct artery is accomplished by direct stent implantation.

Stone GW, Grines CL, Topol EJ: Update on percutaneous transluminal coronary angioplasty for acute myocardial infarction. In: Topol EJ, Serruys PW ed. Current review of interventional cardiology. Philadelphia: Cuurent Medicine, 1995: 2-56.

Table 16.2

Rescue percutaneous transluminal coronary angioplasty during acute myocardial infarction. A compilation of studies

Study	n	Thrombolytic regimen	Success rate (%)	Reocclusion rate (%)	Mortality (%)
Topol	86	t-PA	73	29	10
Calif	15	t-PA	87	15	NA
	25	UK	84	12	NA
	12	t-PA + UK	92	0	NA
Belenkie	16	SK	81	NA	7
Fung	13	SK	92	16	8
Topol	22	t-PA + UK	86	3	0
Grines	12	t-PA + SK	100	8	NA
Holmes	34	SK	71	NA	11
Grines	10	t-PA + SK	90	12	10
O'Connor	90	SK	89	14	17
Baim	37	t-PA	92	26	5
Whitlow	26	t-PA	81	29	NA
	18	UK	89	25	NA
Ellis	109	t-PA	79	20	10
	5	t-PA + UK	80	20	20
	59	SK	76	18	10
Total	560		80	18	11

Ellis SG, Van de Weft F, Riberio-DaSilva E, et al: Present status of rescue coronary angioplasty: current polarization of opinion and randomized trials. *J Am Coll Cardiol* 1992, **19**:681–686.

antecedent thrombolytic therapy (primary PTCA). A variety of these strategies, in vogue since 1980, have produced high success rates and a low incidence of morbidity and mortality.[5] A meta-analysis of rescue PTCA revealed a success rate of 80% in 560 patients with a mortality rate of 11% (*Table 16.2*). *Table 16.3* shows the results of a meta-analysis of three prospective, randomized trials of primary PTCA versus thrombolysis.[6–8] The patients undergoing primary PTCA had lower hospital mortality as well as a lower incidence of reinfarction and recurrent ischemia than the patients undergoing thrombolysis. These initial results were encouraging and suggested that the early and primary use of angioplasty improved the overall results compared to reserving PTCA as a rescue strategy after thrombolysis.

Several limitations of primary PTCA remain to be overcome. After successful PTCA, recurrent ischemia still occurs in 10–15% of patients, which results in hemodynamic and arrhythmic complications that necessitate repeat catheterization and revascularization procedures. This prolongs the hospital stay and increases costs. Infarct-related artery reocclusion develops in 5–10% of vessels, which results in blunted myocardial recovery and excess mortality,

with reinfarction occurring in 3–5% of patients before hospital discharge. Finally, angiographic restenosis has been documented in 37–49% of patients after primary PTCA, with late infarct-related vessel reocclusion in 9–14%. As a result, about 20% of patients require repeat PTCA or bypass surgery within 6 months of discharge.[9,10]

Compared with PTCA, the implantation of coronary stents in the elective setting (i.e. excluding acute MI) has been shown to reduce angiographic restenosis and improve late clinical outcomes.[11,12] However, stenting has historically been contraindicated in thrombus-containing lesions because of the risk of subacute thrombosis. With advances in stent implantation techniques derived from intravascular ultrasound imaging,[13–15] and with the recognition of the importance of adequate platelet inhibition, the incidence of subacute thrombosis has dramatically fallen despite stenting in increasingly complex subsets, including acute ischemic syndromes and thrombus-laden lesions. On the basis of this experience, many interventionalists began inserting stents during an acute MI despite the presence of thrombus. This method has been employed successfully with or without the use of adjunctive thrombolytics (uroki-

Table 16.3

Meta-analysis of the prospective, randomized trials of primary percutaneous transluminal coronary angioplasty (PTCA) versus thrombolysis for acute myocardial infarction

		PAMI Trial (1)		Netherlands (2)		Mayo Clinic (3)		Total	
Patients, n		395		142		108		645	
Thrombolytic agent		t-PA		SK		t-PA			
PTCA success		99%		98%		93%		97%	
Hospital mortality									
	PTCA	2.6%	$p = 0.06$	0.0%	$p = 0.13$	4.3%	NS	2.2%	$p = 0.02$
	Thrombolysis	6.5%		5.6%		3.6%		5.9%	
Reinfarction									
	PTCA	2.6%	$p = 0.06$	0.0%	$p = 0.003$			1.9%	$p = 0.001$
	Thrombolysis	6.5%		12.5%				8.1%	
Recurrent ischemia									
	PTCA	10.3%	$p = 0.001$	8.6%	$p = 0.001$	14.9%	$p = 0.02$	10.6%	$p = 0.0001$
	Thrombolysis	28.0%		37.5%		35.7%		31.4%	

(1) Grines CL, Browne KR, Macro, et al.: A comparison of primary angioplasty with thrombolytic therapy for acute myocardial infarction. *N Engl J Med* 1993, **328**:673-679.
(2) Zijlstra F, DeBoer MJ, Hoorntje JCA, et al.: A comparison of immediate coronary angioplasty with intravenous streptokinase in acute myocardial infarction. *N Engl J Med* 1993, **328**:680-684.
(3) Gibbons RJ, Holmes DR, Reeder GS, et al.: Immediate angioplasty compared with the administration of a thrombolytic agent followed by conservative treatment for myocardial infarction. *N Engl J Med* 1993, **328**:685-691.

nase, tissue plasminogen activator (t-PA)), or platelet inhibitors (abciximab).

Recent studies suggest that intracoronary stenting may improve clinical outcome in patients with acute MI, compared with conventional balloon angioplasty.[16–18] The primary angioplasty for MI (PAMI) stent pilot trial[19] shows that primary stenting is safe and feasible in the majority of patients with acute MI and results in excellent short-term outcomes (*Table 16.4*). The initial report of the complete trial, however, does not show any significant benefit of primary stenting over primary PTCA at 1 month except for a lower rate of target lesion revascularization in the stent group (0.9% versus 3.5%; $p \leq 0.06$). The effect on restenosis and target vessel revascularization at 6 months from the PAMI trial has not been reported at the time of writing. The results from a smaller randomized trial from Italy have been reported.[18] The FRESCO trial randomized 150 patients after successful primary PTCA following an acute MI to elective stenting or to no further intervention. The primary end-point of the trial was composite incidence of clinical events including death, reinfarction or repeat target vessel revascularization within 6 months of randomization. The incidence of these primary end-points was 9% in the stent group and 28% in the PTCA group ($p = 0.003$). In addition, the

Table 16.4

Effect of reperfusion modality on major adverse clinical events (From the PAMI stent pilot trial, *JACC* 1998; **31**: 23-30)

	Stent	Balloon	p value
Patients, n	240	72	
In-hospital			
Death	2 (0.8%)	0	NS
Reinfarction	4 (1.7%)	0	NS
Recurrent ischemia	9 (3.8%)	2 (2.9%)	NS
Repeat PTCA	12 (5.0%)	6 (8.3%)	NS
CABG	7 (2.9%)	9 (12.5%)	0.001
30-day follow-up			
Death	0	0	NS
Reinfarction	0	1 (1.4%)	NS
TVR	1 (0.4%)	5 (6.9%)	0.0004

TVR = target vessel revascularization

incidence of restenosis for reocclusion was 17% in the stent group versus 43% in the PTCA group ($p = 0.001$). The differences in the primary and secondary end-points in this trial were great enough, despite the relatively small number of patients, to show that

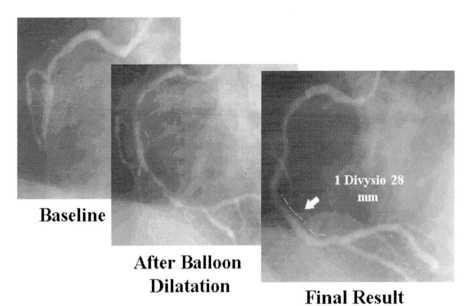

Figure 16.1 *Primary stenting during acute myocardial infarction.*

primary stenting of an infarcted artery compared with primary angioplasty results in a lower rate of major adverse events and a lower rate of angiographic restenosis.

CLINICAL EXAMPLES

Figure 16.1 provides a straightforward example of how coronary stenting facilitates the results achieved with balloon dilatation alone in the presence of an acute MI. A large right coronary artery shown in the first panel was occluded at its mid-portion and it has an irregular hazy appearance consistent with intraluminal thrombus. This was dilated with a 3 mm balloon, which re-established flow to the distal vessels, but the acute margin of the artery had a dissection and probably had residual thrombus. Although this was a successful primary PTCA result, with the establishment of reperfusion, the likelihood that this artery would remain patent is small. The third panel shows the results after placement of one DivYsio 28 mm long stent dilated with a 3.5 mm balloon. Not only is blood flow re-established, but by tacking the plaque up against the wall and improving the cross-sectional lumen area, the chance for maintaining adequate blood flow is increased.

Another benefit of using stents for treatment of acute MI is that more complex angioplasty can be

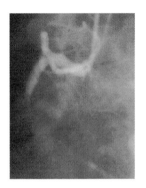 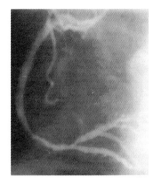

Baseline   **After Balloon Dilatation**

a

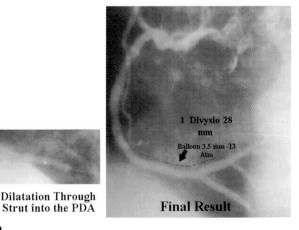

Dilatation Through Strut into the PDA   **Final Result**

b

Figure 16.2 *Primary stenting during acute myocardial infarction. Immediate angioplasty of the occluded vessel permits therapeutic interventions on other stenoses within the same vessel.*

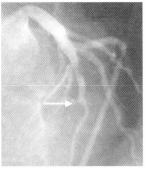
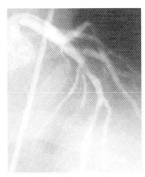

Baseline **After Reopening**

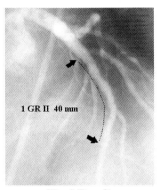

Final Result

Figure 16.3 *Use of a coiled stent to protect sidebranches while stenting the proximal and mid-LAD during acute myocardial infarction.*

performed with increased safety. This is demonstrated in *Fig. 16.2*, where an acute MI from occlusion of the mid-right coronary artery was treated with balloon angioplasty and re-establishment of blood flow to the distal vessel. However, there was disease from the acute margin to the bifurcation of the posterior descending coronary artery. This was treated by

placing one DivYsio 28 mm long stent on a 3.5 mm balloon inflated at 13 atmospheres. The posterior descending artery became compromised after deployment of the stent but this was treated by passing another balloon through the stents into the artery to treat the bifurcation disease (*Fig. 16.2b*).

Another example of treating bifurcation disease during an acute MI is shown in *Fig. 16.3*. In this case there was an occlusion of the mid-left anterior descending artery (LAD) with a more proximal, moderate stenosis just after the bifurcation of the septal perforator. These side branches were protected by placing a 40 mm long Gianturco–Roubin II stent through the occluded segment as well as the more proximal lesion (*Fig. 16.3b*). The coil configuration of the Gianturco–Roubin II stent permits adequate support of dissection post-dilatation as well as easy access to the branch vessels in case they are compromised during the dilatation procedure.

One of the significant benefits of using angioplasty for acute MI is in the subgroup of patients who have the highest mortality, that is those who present with cardiogenic shock. Owing to the poor flow, these patients have a lower incidence of establishing reperfusion after intravenous thrombolytic therapy. In addition, the patients who have slow flow following balloon dilatation may be at a higher risk of developing reocclusion. We prefer to treat these patients by placing an intracoronary stent and to improve blood flow by inserting an intra-aortic balloon pump for 1–2 days. This concept is demonstrated in *Fig. 16.4*: a 69-year-old patient with three-vessel disease presented with acute inferior MI and cardiogenic shock. There was a subtotal occlusion of the proximal right coronary artery with thrombolysis in myocardial infarction (TIMI) 2 blood flow. This was treated with immediate balloon dilatation and placement of a Divysio 15 mm long stent with a 3.5 mm

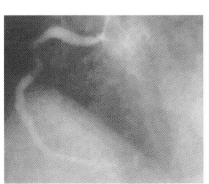
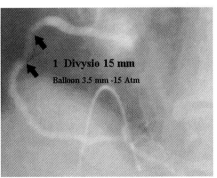

Figure 16.4 *Bail-out stenting in acute myocardial infarction: three-vessel disease and cardiogenic shock.*

Baseline **Final Result**

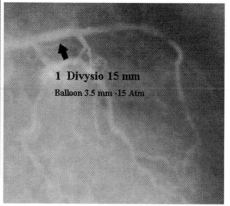

Baseline

Final Result

1 Divysio 15 mm

Balloon 3.5 mm -15 Atm

Figure 16.5 *Acute anterior wall myocardial infarction with occlusion of the ostium of the LAD treated successfully with primary stent deployment.*

balloon inflated at 15 atmospheres. Although this was a tortuous segment of the artery, the flexible DivYsio stent followed the contour of the artery so that there was no visible hinge effect. An intra-aortic balloon pump was placed overnight to treat the heart failure and to assist coronary flow for the first 24 hours.

Even without the presence of cardiogenic shock, treatment of high-risk proximal LAD occlusions can be effected expeditiously with the use of balloon angioplasty. The operator can be reassured that the artery will remain patent with the use of a stent. This is demonstrated in *Figs 16.5* and *16.6*, where a

DivYsio 15 mm long stent was placed in the first patient and a Multilink 15 mm long stent was placed in the second patient. Not only is flow to the proximal LAD re-established, but also balloon dilatation through the side of the stent can be performed to reopen large branches such as the diagonal branch in *Fig. 16.6*. With the Multilink stent, the use of progressive sizes of ACE balloons may be required to dilate through the side struts.

An example of use of a Multilink stent to treat an acute MI with a long lesion and large bifurcating diagonal vessels is shown in *Fig. 16.7*. After re-estab-

Caudal RAO

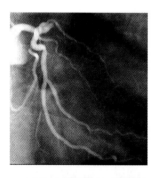

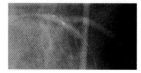

Multilink 15mm stent simultaneous inflations in LAD and Diagonal

Pre

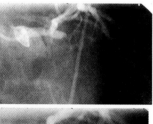

Post

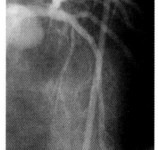

Cranial RAO

Figure 16.6 *Stenting during acute myocardial infarction. The 'Widow Maker'. RAO, right anterior oblique.*

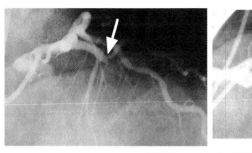

PRE

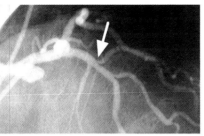

POST

25 mm Multi-Link Stent

Figure 16.7 *Stenting in acute myocardial infarction. Successful treatment of a bifurcation lesion with placement of a single stent and dilatation through the side of the stent into the branch diagonal artery.*

lishing blood flow with balloon dilatation, the large diagonal branch vessel was protected with a second guidewire as the 25 mm Multilink stent was deployed. When it was confirmed that the diagonal artery was still patent, the wire was removed before high-pressure balloon inflation was applied to the stent. The diagonal branch was then recannulated and dilated through the stent.

In addition to maintaining immediate patency, the use of coronary artery stenting rather than balloon dilatation alone for treatment of acute MI may be useful to prevent restenosis. The preliminary findings of the stent PAMI trial were recently reported.[19] In this trial, 900 patients with acute MI were randomized to primary PTCA alone or coronary artery stenting using a heparin-coated stent. The patients received aspirin and ticlopidine in the emergency room and only 5% of patients received abciximab. The mean time from onset of symptoms to emergency room was 160 minutes and the mean time from the emergency room to the catheterization laboratory was 96 minutes. This resulted in a mean emergency room to first balloon inflation time of 135 minutes. The mean time delay associated with these procedures is significant but represents the results from experienced facilities that presumably have more rapid functioning response teams than are generally available. Many of these patients present at night and the data reflect the response time for the catheterization team to return to the hospital. The core laboratory angiographic analysis demonstrated that the minimum lumen diameter (MLD) achieved with stenting was greater than that achieved with PTCA (2.52 mm versus 2.10 mm). However, this MLD for stenting appears to be less than we would expect

with optimally sized balloons. Although it was somewhat surprising, the initial report demonstrated no significant difference in major events at 1 month, including the combination of death, repeat MI or target vessel revascularization. It remains to be seen

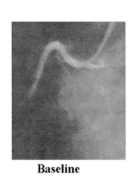

Baseline

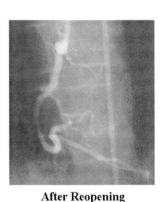

After Reopening

a

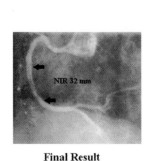

Final Result

6 months F/U

b

Figure 16.8 *Stenting in acute myocardial infarction. Patency documented on six-month follow-up angiogram.*

Table 16.5
Clinical characteristics. Treatment for acute myocardial infarction at UCLA

	Stent	Balloon	CABG	Med-Rx	p value
Number of patients	85	74	46	35	
Age (years)	63 ± 14	67 ± 13	68 ± 11	69 ± 12	NS
Male	67 (79%)	50 (68%)	36 (78%)	24 (69%)	NS
EF (%)	49 ± 9	46 ± 12	42 ± 11	45 ± 12	0.01
Risk factors					
Hypercholesterolemia	33 (39%)	35 (47%)	12 (26%)	15 (43%)	NS
Diabetes	12 (14%)	13 (18%)	12 (26%)	9 (26%)	NS
Hypertension	37 (44%)	42 (57%)	25 (54%)	23 (66%)	NS
Current smoker	17 (20%)	17 (23%)	5 (11%)	5 (14%)	NS
Family history	40 (47%)	22 (30%)	15 (33%)	16 (46%)	NS
Medical history					
Angina	14 (16%)	12 (16%)	9 (20%)	5 (14%)	NS
MI	14 (16%)	16 (22%)	13 (28%)	10 (29%)	NS
PTCA	10 (12%)	9 (12%)	7 (15%)	3 (9%)	NS
CABG	6 (7%)	6 (8%)	3 (7%)	10 (29%)	0.002
Stroke	3 (4%)	2 (3%)	4 (9%)	4 (11%)	NS
MI location					
Anterior	34 (40%)	27 (36%)	21 (46%)	11 (31%)	NS
Inferior	43 (51%)	38 (51%)	13 (28%)	13 (37%)	0.04
Lateral	5 (6%)	3 (4%)	3 (7%)	2 (6%)	NS
Posterior	2 (3%)	6 (8%)	0	0	0.039
Unspecified	0	0	9 (19%)	9 (26%)	< 0.0001
MI type					
Q wave	69 (81%)	57 (77%)	26 (57%)	10 (29%)	< 0.0001
Non-Q wave	16 (19%)	17 (23%)	20 (43%)	25 (71%)	< 0.0001
Killip class					
I	70 (82%)	53 (72%)	27 (59%)	22 (63%)	0.02
II	9 (11%)	4 (5%)	7 (15%)	9 (26%)	0.02
III	3 (4%)	1 (1%)	1 (2%)	1 (3%)	NS
IV	3 (4%)	16 (22%)	11 (24%)	3 (9%)	0.001
Onset-ER time (hours)	4.3 ± 7.8	4.9 ± 7.0	4.6 ± 5.7	4.9 ± 5.6	NS
Length of stay					
CCU/ICU (days)	2.5 ± 2.5	3.4 ± 2.6	6.2 ± 6.7	3.2 ± 4.9	< 0.0001
Hospital (days)	5.2 ± 4.2	6.3 ± 5.3	11.6 ± 10.2	6.9 ± 6.0	< 0.0001

whether the recurrence rate of reinfarction and target vessel revascularization will be different at 6-month follow-up. An example of a patient with an acute MI treated with primary stenting for whom a 6-month follow-up was obtained is demonstrated in *Fig. 16.8*. A 32 mm long NIR stent was placed in the mid-section of the diffusely diseased right coronary artery with an excellent primary result. In addition, at 6 months there was no evidence of restenosis (*Fig. 16.8b*).

SERIAL CHANGES IN INTERVENTIONAL STRATEGIES FOR TREATING PATIENTS WITH ACUTE MI: THE UCLA EXPERIENCE

We evaluated the effect of the changing strategies of how to treat patients with acute MI at the University of California, Los Angeles (UCLA) over the past 4 years. Between 1994 and the end of 1997, 240

Table 16.6

Procedural characteristics. Treatment for acute myocardial infarction at UCLA

	Stent	Balloon	CABG	Med-Rx	p-value
Number of patients	85	74	46	35	
Angiographic success	84 (99%)	66 (89%)			0.009
Number of diseased vessels					< 0.0001
0 vessel	0	0	0	8 (24%)	< 0.0001
1 vessel	51 (60%)	42 (58%)	1 (2%)	3 (9%)	< 0.0001
2 vessels	13 (15%)	15 (20%)	14 (33%)	8 (24%)	NS
3 vessels	21 (25%)	16 (22%)	27 (65%)	14 (42%)	< 0.0001
LM disease	1 (1%)	4 (5%)	6 (14%)	7 (21%)	0.0009
Infarct-related artery					
LAD	34 (40%)	24 (32%)	21 (46%)	6 (17%)	0.04
LCX	16 (19%)	13 (18%)	5 (11%)	3 (9%)	NS
RCA	32 (38%)	33 (45%)	8 (17%)	8 (23%)	0.008
Graft	3 (3%)	4 (5%)	3 (7%)	6 (17%)	NS
Unspecified	0	0	9 (19%)	12 (34%)	<0.0001
Onset–PTCA time					
Mean ± SD (hours)	10.1 ± 12.4	12.7 ± 17.1			NS
<6 hours	44 (55%)	35 (49%)			NS
6–12 hours	15 (19%)	20 (28%)			NS
≥12 hours	21 (26%)	17 (24%)			NS
ER–PTCA time (hours)	2.2 ± 3.42	3.0 ± 1.2			NS
Treated artery					
LAD	34 (40%)	24 (32%)			NS
RCA	31 (36%)	33 (45%)			NS
LCX	17 (20%)	14 (19%)			NS
Graft	3 (4%)	3 (4%)			NS
Max. balloon size (mm)	3.4 ± 0.4	2.8 ± 0.6			< 0.0001
Max. inflation pressure (atm)	18.6 ± 4.2	9.3 ± 2.8			< 0.0001
Type of stent					
Palmaz–Schatz	71 (85%)				
Gianturco–Roubin	6 (7%)				
Combination	4 (5%)				
ACS Multilink	3 (4%)				
Number of stents/lesion	1.5 ± 0.7				
Multiple stents	32 (38%)				
IABP	8 (9%)	23 (31%)	25 (54%)	4 (11%)	< 0.0001
IVUS	10 (12%)	0	–	–	0.002
Abciximab	46 (54%)	7 (9%)	–	–	< 0.0001

patients with acute MI were sent for emergency coronary angiography. During this time period a special response team was established; the team was made up of the cardiology fellow and attending on-call physicians, as well as the catheterization laboratory personnel on rotation. As soon as a diagnosis of acute MI was established in the emergency room, the cardiology fellow and attending physicians were paged and the catheterization laboratory was activated on a 24-hour basis at the discretion of the cardiology fellow. The patients received an intravenous bolus of heparin (5000 units), oral aspirin (325 mg), and intravenous metoprolol (5 mg) in the emergency room as soon as the diagnosis of an acute

Table 16.7

In-hospital adverse events. Treatment for acute myocardial infarction at UCLA

	Stent	Balloon	CABG	Med-Rx	p value
Number of patients	85	74	46	35	
Procedure complications					
Dissection	4 (5%)	3 (4%)	-	-	NS
Coronary perforation	0	1 (1%)	-	-	
Distal embolization	3 (4%)	1 (1%)	-	-	NS
Spasm	4 (5%)	1 (1%)	-	-	NS
VT/VF	2 (2%)	2 (3%)	0	0	NS
Emergent CABG	1 (1%)	5 (7%)	28 (61%)	-	< 0.0001
Death	0	2 (3%)	0	0	NS
Post-procedure events					
Recurrent angina	13 (15%)	9 (12%)	4 (9%)	6 (17%)	NS
Reinfarction	3 (4%)	2 (3%)	3 (7%)	3 (9%)	NS
Repeat PTCA					
Same site	1 (1%)	2 (3%)	-	-	NS
Different site	4 (5%)	0	-	-	
PTCA after Medical Rx	-	-	-	5 (14%)	
Elective CABG	3 (4%)	6 (8%)	18 (39%)	-	< 0.0001
Death	3 (4%)	11 (15%)	4 (9%)	3 (9%)	NS
In-hospital death*	3 (4%)	13 (18%)	4 (9%)	3 (9%)	0.03
With shock	1/3 (33%)	10/16 (63%)	2/11 (18%)	2/3 (67%)	NS
Without shock	2/82 (2%)	3/58 (5%)	2/35 (6%)	1/32 (3%)	NS
Cause of in-hospital death*					
Heart failure	2	10	4	3	
Cardiac rupture	1	1	0	0	
Procedure complication	0	1	0	0	
Non-cardiac	0	1	0	0	

*In-hospital death = [procedural death] + [post-procedural death]

MI was made. The patients were categorized according to the primary therapy delivered. These therapies were:

(a) medical therapy with or without thrombolytic therapy;
(b) balloon angioplasty;
(c) coronary artery bypass surgery; and
(d) insertion of a stent.

Patients were not assigned randomly to these groups, but were treated on the basis of the options available as determined by the admitting attending cardiologist and the interventionalist.

The clinical characteristics of the patients in the four groups is shown in *Table 16.5*. It is of note that the ejection fraction was mildly lower in the patients who were sent for primary bypass surgery (the mean ejection fraction was 42% in this group). Moreover, patients who were treated with medical therapy had a higher incidence of having undergone coronary artery bypass surgery in the past (29%, $p < 0.002$). Patients who received medical therapy also had a higher incidence (71%) of non-Q-wave MI than the other groups ($p < 0.001$). Patients with cardiogenic shock were more likely to have balloon angioplasty alone or coronary artery bypass graft as primary therapy. The time from onset of chest pain to admission to the emergency room averaged between 4.3 and 4.9 hours, although there was no difference between the groups. The length of stay for patients who received a stent was significantly lower, at 5.2 ± 4.2 days ($p < 0.0001$).

The procedural characteristics in the four treatment groups is shown in *Table 16.6*. The number of diseased vessels (diameter stenosis > 50%) was higher

Table 16.8

Serial changes of intervention strategy in acute myocardial infarction patients and clinical outcome at UCLA

Year	1994	1995	1996	1997	p value
Number of patients	49	73	58	60	
Age (yr)	66 ± 12	67 ± 13	64 ± 12	67 ± 15	NS
Male	32 (65%)	59 (81%)	46 (79%)	40 (67%)	NS
EF (%)	45 ± 12	45 ± 11	47 ± 10	46 ± 11	NS
Multivessel disease	27 (55%)	39 (53%)	29 (52%)	34 (56%)	NS
Cardiogenic shock	5 (10%)	11 (15%)	13 (22%)	4 (7%)	NS
Primary therapy					
Stent	0	11 (15%)	33 (57%)	41 (68%)	<0.0001
Balloon	26 (53%)	32 (44%)	9 (16%)	7 (12%)	<0.0001
CABG	10 (20%)	19 (26%)	11 (19%)	6 (10%)	NS
Medical Tx	13 (27%)	11 (15%)	5 (9%)	6 (10%)	0.04
Abciximab	0	0	26 (45%)	27 (45%)	<0.0001
In-hospital adverse events					
Recurrent angina	5 (10%)	13 (18%)	4 (7%)	10 (17%)	NS
Reinfarction	2 (4%)	5 (7%)	0	4 (7%)	NS
Repeat PTCA	0	3 (4%)	0	0	NS
CABG after PTCA	5 (10%)	4 (5%)	3 (5%)	3 (6%)	NS
Cardiac death	7 (14%)	3 (4%)	4 (7%)	8 (13%)	NS
Stent	-	0	0	3	
PTCA	4	2	3	3	
CABG	1	1	1	1	
Med-Tx	2	0	0	1	
In-hospital cardiac death					
With shock	5/5 (100%)	2/11 (18%)	4/13 (31%)	4/4 (100%)	0.002
Without shock	2/44 (5%)	1/62 (2%)	0/45	4/56 (7%)	NS

in patients who were sent to surgery; 65% of these patients had triple-vessel disease ($p < 0.0001$). Although there was no difference in the onset of chest pain to balloon dilatation time in the patients who had stenting or PTCA, it should be noted that the mean value is high because patients who had chest pain for 6–12 hours, or even for more than 12 hours, were included in this analysis. Similar to the findings in the PAMI Stent trial, the mean time from the emergency room to PTCA was 2.2 ± 3.4 hours. Patients who received stents had larger balloons than those who had balloon angioplasty alone (3.4 ± 0.4 mm versus 2.8 ± 0.6 mm) and higher inflation pressures (18.8 ± 4.4 atmospheres versus 9.3 ± 2.9 atmospheres; $p < 0.0001$). The patients who were sent to surgery not only had a greater number of diseased vessels but also had a higher incidence of intra-aortic balloon pumps placed (54% of patients; $p < 0.0001$). Abciximab was used in 54% of the patients who had

stents placed, compared to 9% of patients who had balloon dilatation alone, but this reflects the simultaneous trends of increased use of stents, as well as increased use of abciximab over this time period.

The in-hospital adverse events in the four treatment strategy groups are presented in *Table 16.7*. There was no significant difference in procedural complications between patients who received a stent and those who received a balloon alone. The results revealed no significant difference between the four groups for any post-procedure event, including recurrent angina, reinfarction, repeat PTCA, elective bypass surgery, or death. Although the in-hospital death rate was higher for patients who had PTCA, at 15%, eight of these patients who died had cardiogenic shock on presentation. Four patients who had stents placed as an emergency procedure to treat the occluded artery were brought back electively to the catheterization laboratory for treatment of other lesions.

Table 16.8 provides an analysis of the temporal changes of the intervention strategies for the patients who presented with acute MI between 1994 and 1997 at UCLA. There was a significant trend for increasing use of stents from 0 in 1994 to 68% of patients in 1997 ($p < 0.0001$). This was associated with a complementary decrease in the use of primary PTCA alone. The use of primary bypass surgery also declined, although the trend did not reach statistical significance for the number of cases involved. The use of abciximab was started in 1996, and 45% of the patients received this medication in 1996 and 1997. While the use of abciximab was not assigned on a randomized basis, there was no difference in mortality, repeat PTCA, recurrent angina, and reinfarction in the patients who received this medication. Abciximab tended to be used for more complicated cases of large thrombus burden and no reflow, but it was associated with a greater incidence of vascular bleeding.

Despite these changes in our approach to treatment of patients with acute MI, there was no significant difference in the 4-year period in the incidence of in-hospital adverse events including angina, reinfarction, repeat PTCA, bypass after PTCA, and cardiac death. Although these numbers are relatively small, it appears that the use of stents as the primary intervention strategy for treating patients with acute MI may not significantly improve the short-term clinical outcome compared with the use of PTCA alone. Whether the use of stents in acute MI has any long-term clinical benefit in reducing restenosis or target lesion revascularization over balloon angioplasty alone is currently under analysis.

REFERENCES

1. Verstraete M, Bleifeld W, Brower RW et al. Double-blind randomised trial of intravenous tissue-type plasminogen activator versus placebo in acute myocardial infarction. *Lancet* 1985; **2**: 965–969.

2. Anonymous. Effectiveness of intravenous thrombolytic treatment in acute myocardial infarction. Gruppo Italiano per lo Studio della Streptochinasi nell'Infarto Miocardico (GISSI). *Lancet* 1986; **1**: 397–402.

3. Anonymous. Randomised trial of intravenous streptokinase, oral aspirin, both, or neither among 17,187 cases of suspected acute myocardial infarction: ISIS-2. ISIS-2 (Second International Study of Infarct Survival) Collaborative Group. *Lancet* 1988; **2**: 349–360.

4. White HD, Van de Werf FJ. Thrombolysis for acute myocardial infarction (review). *Circulation* 1998; **97**: 1632–1646.

5. Stone GW, Grines CL, Topol EJ. Update on percutaneous transluminal coronary angioplasty for acute myocardial infarction. In: Topol EJ, Serruys PW, eds. *Current Review of Interventional Cardiology.* Philadelphia: Current Medicine, 1995, 2–56.

6. Grines CL, Browne KF, Marco J et al. A comparison of immediate angioplasty with thrombolytic therapy for acute myocardial infarction. The Primary Angioplasty in Myocardial Infarction Study Group. *N Engl J Med* 1993; **328**: 673–679.

7. Zijlstra F, de Boer MJ, Hoorntje JC et al. A comparison of immediate coronary angioplasty with intravenous streptokinase in acute myocardial infarction. *N Engl J Med* 1993; **328**: 680–684.

8. Gibbons RJ, Holmes DR, Reeder GS et al. Immediate angioplasty compared with the administration of a thrombolytic agent followed by conservative treatment for myocardial infarction. The Mayo Coronary Care Unit and Catheterization Laboratory Groups. *N Engl J Med* 1993; **328**: 685–691.

9. Stone GW, Grines CL, Browne KF et al. Predictors of in-hospital and 6–month outcome after acute myocardial infarction in the reperfusion era: the Primary Angioplasty in Myocardial Infarction (PAMI) trial. *J Am Coll Cardiol* 1995; **25**: 370–377.

10. Brodie BR, Grines CL, Ivanhoe R et al. Six-month clinical and angiographic follow-up after direct angioplasty for acute myocardial infarction. Final results from the Primary Angioplasty Registry. *Circulation* 1994; **90**: 156–162.

11. Serruys PW, de Jaegere P, Kiemeneij F et al. A comparison of balloon-expandable-stent implantation with balloon angioplasty in patients with coronary artery disease. Benestent Study Group. *N Engl J Med* 1994; **331**: 489–495.

12. Fischman DL, Leon MB, Baim DS et al. A randomized comparison of coronary-stent placement and balloon angioplasty in the treatment of coronary artery disease. Stent Restenosis Study Investigators. *N Engl J Med* 1994; **331**: 496–501.

13. Nakamura S, Colombo A, Gaglione A et al. Intracoronary ultrasound observations during stent implantation. *Circulation* 1994; **89**: 2026–2034.

14. Goldberg SL, Colombo A, Nakamura S et al. Benefit of intracoronary ultrasound in the deployment of Palmaz–Schatz stents. *J Am Coll Cardiol* 1994; **24**: 996–1003.

15. Colombo A, Hall P, Nakamura S et al. Intracoronary stenting without anticoagulation accomplished with intravascular ultrasound guidance. *Circulation* 1995; **91**: 1676–1688.

16. Saito S, Hosokawa FG, Kim K et al. Primary stent implantation without coumadin in acute myocardial infarction. *J Am Coll Cardiol* 1996; **28**: 74–81.

17. Stone GW, Brodie BR, Griffin JJ et al. Prospective, multicenter study of the safety and feasibility of primary stenting in acute myocardial infarction: in-hospital and 30–day results of the PAMI stent pilot trial. Primary Angioplasty in Myocardial Infarction Stent Pilot Trial Investigators. *J Am Coll Cardiol* 1998; **31**: 23–30.

18. Antoniucci D, Santoro GM, Bolognese L et al. A clinical trial comparing primary stenting of the infarct-related artery with optimal primary angioplasty for acute myocardial infarction: results from the Florence Randomized Elective Stenting in Acute Coronary Occlusions (FRESCO) trial. *J Am Coll Cardiol* 1998; **31**: 1234–1239.

19. Grines CL, Cox DA, Garcia E et al. Stent PAMI: primary endpoint results of a multicenter randomized trial of heparin coated stenting vs. primary PTCA for AMI. *Circulation* 1998; **98**: 20.

Chapter 17 **The high-risk patient**

Antonio Colombo and Jonathan Tobis

The patient who has already suffered significant myocardial damage presents an unusual challenge for the interventionalist. This situation is all the more difficult if the interventionalist is asked to treat an artery that provides blood to the remaining viable myocardium. The approach to these patients has to be tailored within a framework of high risk where even transient ischemia may produce disastrous hemodynamic compromise. On occasion, an occluded artery may be reopened to provide a conduit for collaterals and thus mitigate the ischemia produced during the intervention.

Between April 1993 and May 1998, we treated 87 lesions in 60 patients with a left ventricular ejection fraction less than 30% (*Table 17.1*). The clinical characteristics of these patients are shown in *Table 17.2*. Bypass surgery had been performed in 40% of the patients, and 34% of these patients had unstable angina patterns. As shown in *Table 17.3*, the majority of the patients had triple-vessel disease and more than one vessel was treated in 28% of the patients. The lesions tended to be complicated with 38% type B2 lesions and 27% type C lesions (*Table 17.4*). The mean lesion length was 13.4 ± 9.0 mm. The number and variety of stents that were used in these 87 lesions is presented in *Table 17.5*. Many of these cases were treated with Palmaz–Schatz stents, which reflects the availability of this device during our early use of stents. The immediate results are provided in *Table 17.6*. Primary success was achieved in 99% of

Table 17.1

Stenting with left ventricular ejection fraction ≤ 30%

Total patients	60
Total lesions	87
Total number stents	102
Stents/lesion	1.17
Mean stent length/lesion	22 ± 12 mm

Table 17.2

Stenting with left ventricular ejection fraction < 30%. Clinical characteristics

		n	%
Patients		60	
Age (years)		63.2 ± 8.9	
Males		48	89
Diabetes		8	13
Prior MI		54	90
Prior CABG		24	40
CCS angina class	I–II	17	36
	III	14	30
	IV	16	34
Ejection fraction (%)		26.8 ± 4.2	

Table 17.3

Stenting with left ventricular ejection fraction ≤ 30%. Angiographic characteristics (60 pts)

	n	%
Lesions treated	87	
lesion/pt	1.5	
Vessel distribution		
Left main	3	3
LAD	32	37
LCX	20	23
RCA	16	18
SVG	10	11
Obtuse marginal	5	6
Diagonal	1	1
Vessel disease		
Single VD	6	10
Two VD	20	34
Three VD	33	56

Table 17.4

Stenting with left ventricular ejection fraction < 30%. Lesion characteristics

		n	%
ACC type	A	5	6
	B$_1$	25	29
	B$_2$	33	38
	C	23	27
Mean ref. diameter (mm)		3.13 ± 0.52	
Lesion length (mm)		13.4 ± 9.0	

ACC, American College of Cardiology

Table 17.5

Stenting with left ventricular ejection fraction < 30%. Type of stent used (total = 102)

	n		n
Palmaz–Schatz	35 (35%)	Div Ysio	2 (2%)
Micro II	9 (9%)	Crossflex LC	2 (2%)
GFX	8 (8%)	JOMED PTFE	2 (2%)
Micro I	7 (7%)	Crown	1 (1%)
MR	6 (6%)	Duet	1 (1%)
G–R (I–I)	5 (5%)	BX	1 (1%)
PURA	5 (5%)	DART	1 (1%)
Wiktor	4 (4%)	TENSUM	1 (1%)
BeStent	4 (4%)	MAC	1 (1%)
Wallstent	3 (3%)	GEX II	1 (1%)
Multilink	3 (3%)		

Table 17.6

Stenting with left ventricular ejection fraction ≤ 30%. Immediate results

	n	%
Primary success	84	97
Death (after emergency CABG)	1	2
Q-wave MI	3	6
Subacute stent occlusion	4	8

the lesions; however, in one patient the artery closed, which produced a Q-wave myocardial infarction (MI). He was sent for emergency coronary bypass surgery but died following the procedure. There was also an 8% incidence of subacute stent thrombosis, which is a much higher rate than our overall population (see Chapter 3).

Table 17.7

Stenting with left ventricular ejection fraction ≤30%. Long-term results. Clinical follow-up (12 months)

	n	%
Death all	9	17
(non-cardiac)	2	4
(probably cardiac)	7	13
Sudden death	3	6
Angiographic F-Up (months)	5.3±1.9	
Lesions studied (72 elegible)	45	63
Restenosis (≥ 50% DS)	13	29

The long-term results in these patients (*Table 17.7*), reflect the poor ventricular function of this population subgroup. During a mean clinical follow-up of 12 ± 16 months, nine patients (17%) died. Only two of these deaths were due to a non-cardiac etiology. Sudden death and heart failure were the primary mode of exodus. In the 65% of lesions that were studied with angiographic follow-up at a mean of 7 months after stent insertion, angiographic restenosis was present in 29%. This restenosis rate is typical for the size of the reference artery, lesion length, and final minimum lumen diameter (MLD). These data indicate that this patient subgroup can be treated with a high primary success rate and an expectation that the restenosis rate will not be higher than that of the general population. The high incidence of cardiac death, and specifically sudden death, is consistent with the underlying dysfunction in this patient population. In appropriate candidates, stenting the remaining artery in patients with low ejection fractions may be beneficial as a bridge to cardiac transplantation. These results are similar to data presented by Welthy and colleagues in 479 patients with previous MI.[1] If the ejection fraction was ≥ 50%, then the 5-year mortality was between 7% and 9%, depending on whether the artery was open or closed. However, in those patients in whom the ejection fraction was < 50%, the 5-year mortality was 20% if the artery was closed.

GENERAL CONSIDERATIONS FOR TREATING HIGH-RISK PATIENTS

Our approach to treating these patients with high-risk lesions has evolved over the past few years. We recommend using an intra-aortic balloon pump prophylactically, which dramatically decreases the stress on both the patient and the operator during the performance of these procedures.[2-4] The use of an intra-aortic balloon pump is especially critical if rotational atherectomy or debulking is part of the treatment strategy.[5] The need to get the artery open and stented quickly needs to be balanced by having an optimal result so that the long-term benefit of the stent can be realized. It is not in the best interest of the patient to treat a heavily calcified artery with balloon dilatation and stent insertion if the residual MLD is such that it poses a high risk of subacute thrombosis. The risk of undertreatment has to be balanced against the potential complications of prolonged ischemia during directional atherectomy or slow flow associated with rotational atherectomy. The intra-aortic balloon pump provides greater force for coronary blood flow in diastole. In addition, if there is a high risk that slow flow may develop, such as with diffuse disease, then we pre-treat with abciximab.

HIGH-RISK PERCUTANEOUS TRANSLUMINAL CORONARY ANGIOPLASTY AND THE USE OF INTRA-AORTIC BALLOON PUMPS

Our experience with using intra-aortic balloon pumps in high-risk patients is presented in *Tables 17.8–17.10*. This patient population includes not only those with a low ejection fraction but also other patients with high-risk lesions, such as left main coronary artery disease or lesions where closure of the treated vessel would result in the patient's demise. In these 168 cases, the mean ejection fraction was 45 ± 21% and intra-aortic balloon pumping was used electively in 128 patients. The procedural

Table 17.8

High-risk percutaneous transluminal coronary angioplasty. Intra-aortic balloon pump (IABP) usage (I). Procedural success

Patients	168	*Success rate*
Males	134 (80%)	
EF%	45±21	
Elective IABP	128 (76%)	95%
Urgent IABP	41 (24%)	68%

Table 17.9

High-risk percutaneous transluminal coronary angioplasty. Intra-aortic balloon pump usage (II). Results in 41 pts with urgent IAPB

Emergency CABG	56%	(23 pts)
Death	19%	(8 pts)
MI	50%	(20 pts)

Table 17.10

High-risk percutaneous transluminal coronary angioplasty. Intra-aortic balloon pump usage (III). Results in 128 pts with elective IAPB

Procedural success	95%
Emergency CABG	0
Death	0.7%
Vascular complic.	4.6%

success rate in these 128 patients was 95%, but in the 41 patients who had a balloon pump placed on an urgent basis because of complications during the procedure, the success rate was only 68%. As shown in *Table 17.9*, of the 41 patients with urgent intra-aortic balloon pump placement, the complication rate was high, with emergency bypass surgery being required in 56% of the patients, death occurring in 19%, and acute MI occurring in 50%. As distinguished from the group of patients in whom intra-aortic balloon pumping was used on an emergency basis for a catastrophic result that occurred in the catheterization laboratory, in the 128 patients in whom an elective balloon pump was placed, the procedural success rate was 95%. No patients required emergency bypass surgery, death occurred in only one patient, and vascular complications associated with the procedure occurred in 4.6% (*Table 17.10*).

THE USE OF ABCIXIMAB IN HIGH-RISK PATIENTS

Between April 1993 and April 1998 we used abciximab in 147 patients. Abciximab was given as a bolus during the procedure in 52 patients and was followed by an infusion over 12 hours in an additional 95 patients. The indications for using abciximab in our patients are presented in *Table 17.11*. Abciximab was

Table 17.11

Abciximab. Indications

	Bolus (n = 52) n (%)	Bolus + infusion (n = 95) n (%)
Elective	25 (48)	13 (14)
Suboptimal PTCA	9 (17)	21 (22)
Dissection	6 (12)	18 (19)
Acute closure	5 (10)	8 (8)
Chronic total occlusion	4 (8)	22 (23)
Acute closure	1 (2)	4 (4)
Slow flow	2 (4)	9 (9)

Table 17.13

Abciximab. Patient characteristics (II)

	Bolus n (%)	Bolus + infusion n (%)	p
Number diseased vessels			NS
1-VD	16 (31)	26 (28)	
2-VD	17 (33)	33 (35)	
3-VD	19 (37)	35 (37)	
Angina class			NS
I	4 (8)	9 (10)	
II	4 (8)	11 (12)	
III	18 (35)	36 (38)	
IV	26 (50)	38 (40)	

used electively during high-risk procedures, such as in patients with triple-vessel disease or long diffuse lesions or in patients in whom a large plaque burden had to be removed with rotational or directional atherectomy. In addition, abciximab was used in the setting of complicated procedures, such as following a suboptimal angioplasty result, arterial dissection, acute closure of a vessel, or chronic total occlusions with diffuse disease, in the presence of acute MI or when there was slow flow following an atherectomy. We also tended to use abciximab when treating saphenous vein grafts if there appeared to be a large amount of thrombus involved. On angiography, if a thrombus was present in the native coronary arteries, our treatment of choice was to compress this with balloon dilatation and place a stent without using abciximab. However, if a large residual thrombus occurred or embolized then we would use abciximab.

The patient characteristics for the groups that received a bolus of abciximab versus the group that received a bolus plus infusion of abciximab are presented in *Tables 17.12* and *17.13*. There was no significant difference in the background of the patients except for the incidence of hypertension and smoking. There was also no significant difference in the location of the artery treated between the two

Table 17.12

Abciximab. Patient characteristics (I)

	Bolus n (%)	Bolus + infusion n (%)	p
Patient number	52	95	
Lesion number	92	174	
Mean age (years)	59 ± 12	61 ± 9	NS
LVEF (%)	60 ± 14	60 ± 12	NS
Male gender (%)	46 (88)	68 (88)	NS
Unstable angina	26 (50)	38 (40)	NS
Hypertension	21 (40)	61 (64)	p <0.01
Diabetes	6 (12)	11 (12)	NS
Prior MI	28 (54)	60 (63)	NS
Smoking	39 (75)	55 (58)	p <0.05

Table 17.14

Abciximab. Treated artery location

	Bolus n (%)	Bolus + infusion n (%)
LAD	41 (45)	71 (41)
Cx	10 (11)	23 (13)
RCA	21 (23)	45 (26)
LM	5 (5)	4 (2)
SVG	1 (1)	15 (9)
Ramus	2 (2)	1 (1)
DIAG	5 (5)	6 (3)
OM	5 (5)	7 (4)
Mamm	1 (1)	0
RCA-PL	1 (1)	2 (1)

p = NS for all

groups (*Table 17.14*). The lesion MLD increased from 0.8 mm to 3.1 mm in both groups (*Table 17.15*). As shown in *Table 17.16* the only difference between the technique for the two groups is that the patients

Table 17.15

Abciximab. Angiographic measurements (I)

	Pre	Final
Bolus (n = 92 lesions)		
Reference diam (mm)	3.1 ± 0.5	3.3 ± 0.5
Lesion MLD (mm)	0.80 ± 0.53	3.14 ± 0.60
Percentage stenosis	73.9 ± 16.9	4.8 ± 10.4
Bolus + infusion (n = 174 lesions)		
Reference diam (mm)	3.1 ± 0.7	3.3 ± 0.6
Lesion MLD (mm)	0.81 ± 0.61	3.12 ± 0.61
Percentage stenosis	74.5 ± 17.1	6.3 ± 11.1

Table 17.16

Abciximab. Angiographic measurements (II)

	Bolus	Bolus + infusion	p
Lesion number	92	174	
Lesion length (mm)	14.7 ± 9.6	15.0 ± 9.4	NS
Max. pressure (atm)	14.0 ± 3.5	15.6 ± 3.8	0.0007
Final balloon diam (mm)	3.67 ± 0.54	3.67 ± 0.61	NS
Stent length	25.0 ± 19.4	27.8 ± 18.6	NS

Table 17.17

Abciximab. Complications

	Bolus (n = 52) n (%)	Bolus+ infusion (n = 95) n (%)	p
Procedural outcome			
Vascular complication	2 (4)	5 (5)	NS
QMI	1 (2)	6 (6)	NS
Non-QMI	3 (6)	5 (5)	NS
Emergency CABG	0	1 (1)	NS
Death	0	0	NS
Post-procedural outcome			
Death	0	1 (1)	NS
CABG	3 (6)	0	NS

who received a bolus plus infusion were treated with higher balloon dilatation pressure (15.6 atmosheres versus 14.0 atmospheres; *p* = 0.0007.

The outcome and complications associated with these two uses of abciximab are presented in *Table 17.17*. There was no statistical difference between the bolus group and the bolus plus infusion group in procedural outcomes, either during hospitalization or within 1 month of the procedure. Our experience with abciximab suggests that it can be used effectively in complex angioplasty situations with a low complication rate.[6] However, owing to the expense of this drug, we reserve it for high-risk patients in whom we expect a greater chance of slow flow or subacute occlusion.

EXAMPLES OF HIGH-RISK LESIONS TREATED WITH CORONARY ARTERY STENTING

Figure 17.1 demonstrates the types of decisions and technical steps that may be necessary to treat complex lesions or complications that arise in high-risk patients. A 66-year-old man had a previous MI with an ejection fraction of 40%. A large circumflex artery was occluded proximally and there was diffuse tubular narrowing in the left main artery and proximal left anterior descending artery (LAD). An intra-aortic balloon pump was placed at the beginning of the procedure and the circumflex artery was recanalized and dilated with a 3.0 mm balloon (*Fig. 17.1a*). Two PURA stents were then placed in the proximal LAD and left main coronary artery. These were expanded with a non-compliant balloon to 3.5 mm at 16 atmospheres. During expansion of the PURA stent, the balloon ruptured at 16 atmospheres. The ostium of the circumflex artery appeared more narrowed owing to plaque shifting, and there was evidence of dissection in the proximal circumflex artery (*Fig. 17.1b*). The patient became asystolic; cardiopulmonary resuscitation was begun and abciximab was administered.

After the patient stabilized, a guidewire was repositioned through the first PURA stent into the circumflex artery and the ostium of the circumflex artery was dilated with a 3.5 mm balloon. Next, a Gianturco–Roubin II stent 2.5 mm in diameter was passed through the PURA stent to the mid-circumflex artery. After successful deployment of the Gianturco–Roubin II stent in the proximal circumflex

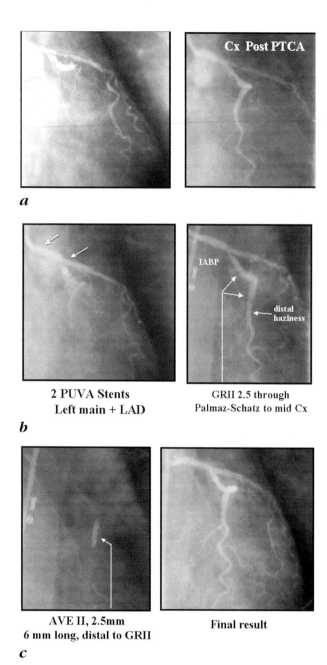

a

b

2 PUVA Stents
Left main + LAD

GRII 2.5 through
Palmaz-Schatz to mid Cx

c

AVE II, 2.5mm
6 mm long, distal to GRII

Final result

Figure 17.1 *Stenting a high-risk, unstable patient. A 66-year-old man with a left ventricular ejection fraction of 40 percent. (a) There is diffuse disease in the left main and proximal LAD arteries. The circumflex was a chronic total occlusion. (b) Balloon rupture during expansion of the stents in the left main artery. The patient became asystolic. Cardiopulmonary resuscitation was begun, an intra-aortic pump was placed, and abciximab was administered. (c) After stabilization, the dissection in the circumflex artery was treated with two stents.*

artery, it became apparent that there was a hazy appearance to the angiogram distal to the stent in the mid-circumflex artery. To tack up this presumed dissection distal to the Gianturco–Roubin II stent, a 2.5 mm AVE II Microstent 6 mm long was passed through the proximal PURA stent and the Gianturco–Roubin II stent. The AVE stent was deployed at the level of the dissection in the mid-circumflex artery (*Fig. 17.1c*).

The final angiogram showed a widely patent left main and proximal LAD–circumflex bifurcation with good flow through the remainder of the vessels. The treatment of this complicated type of anatomy should not be undertaken without proper equipment. The availability of a variety of different stents with enhanced flexibility and hoop strength permits complex cases such as this one to be treated successfully.

Figure 17.2 provides the angiogram of a patient who presented in an extremely grave condition that required expeditious treatment. The patient was an 87-year-old man who had sudden onset of atrial fibrillation. He was cardioverted electrically and was about to be discharged when he developed ventricular tachycardia. While being treated for this, he developed pulmonary edema and there was a mild rise in his troponin level. He was taken to the cardiac catheterization laboratory with the thought that an unstable lesion had extended the zone of ischemic myocardium and precipitated his heart failure. The diagnostic angiograms revealed complete occlusions of all the saphenous vein grafts that had been placed 17 years earlier. His right coronary artery was also completely occluded. The proximal LAD and the circumflex artery both had a severe stenosis (*Fig. 17.2*, Panel A – right anterior oblique cranial view; Panel B – left anterior oblique caudal view). The patient was unable to tolerate the hemodynamic load of the contrast agent and progressed to severe pulmonary edema requiring endotracheal intubation. An intra-aortic balloon pump was inserted to provide hemodynamic support. A cardiac surgeon was consulted but he felt that the patient was too ill for emergency bypass surgery.

Approaching this patient with severe hemodynamic compromise, we felt it was important to limit the amount of ischemic time. Therefore, the LAD lesion was dilated with a 20-second inflation and then a Multilink stent was inserted on a pre-mounted high-pressure balloon to avoid extending the time of the procedure. The use of the high-pressure balloon permitted deployment of the stent and expansion at high pressures without moving the balloon or replac-

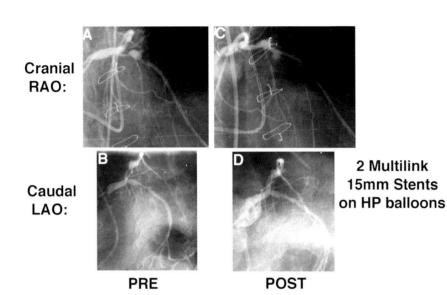

Cranial RAO:

Caudal LAO:

PRE   POST

2 Multilink 15mm Stents on HP balloons

Figure 17.2 *Stenting a high-risk patient. An 87-year-old man with pulmonary edema and edema and ventricular tachycardia. With occluded saphenous vein grafts, the tight stenoses in the LAD and circumflex arteries were treated with rapid deployment of two MultiLink stents on high-pressure balloons.*

ing it with a second device to expand the stent. The LAD stent was expanded at 16 atmospheres with the 3.5 mm delivery balloon for 30 seconds. A second guidewire and dilatation balloon were then passed into the circumflex lesion and the circumflex artery was similarly pre-dilated and then stented with a Multilink high-pressure 3.5 mm balloon and expanded at 16 atmospheres for 30 seconds. With these short inflations and intra-aortic balloon pump support, the patient tolerated the therapeutic intervention.

Over the ensuing days his pulmonary edema resolved with medical therapy and he became hemodynamically stabilized on conventional oral therapy. Owing to his poor left ventricular function and unstable hemodynamic status, we elected not to prolong the procedure by using rotational atherectomy or debulking these lesions. In this instance, the lesions responded well to balloon dilatation and stent insertion alone. Although the restenosis rate may be higher than if we had debulked these lesions, the immediate priority was to provide more blood flow to his ischemic myocardium in order to stabilize this very high-risk patient.

The next case example demonstrates a subset of high-risk patients who have had prior bypass surgery and have significant disease in the native arteries combined with new stenoses in the vein grafts. The angiogram in *Fig. 17.3* is from a 70-year-old man with severe disease in his native vessels. His remaining viable myocardium was jeopardized by an aorto-ostial stenosis in the saphenous vein graft to his obtuse marginal artery. The ejection fraction was below 30% so an intra-aortic balloon pump was placed to provide support during this procedure. As shown in *Fig. 17.3a*, the stenosis at the aorto-ostial junction in the vein graft was treated with balloon dilatation followed by placement of a 19 mm long polytetrafluoroethylene-covered stent using a 3.5 mm balloon inflated at 18 atmospheres. After adequate blood flow was re-established to the circumflex system, treatment of the patient's left main coronary artery was initiated (*Fig. 17.3b*). The diffuse disease in the left main artery was approached by using rotational atherectomy followed by balloon dilatation and placement of a 16 mm long PUVA stent on a 3.5 mm balloon, which was inflated at 18 atmospheres. The combination of using an intra-aortic balloon pump and establishing some collateral flow to the left system decreased the risk of treating the left main coronary artery.

LEFT MAIN ANGIOPLASTY: A HIGH-RISK PROCEDURE DESPITE A NORMAL EJECTION FRACTION

Treatment of left main coronary artery disease is always a high-risk procedure, especially when treating unprotected left main disease in patients who have not had previous bypass surgery. The operator must be aware of complications that could develop into emergency situations. The patient study shown in *Fig. 17.4* is from a 46-year-old woman with signif-

IABP support

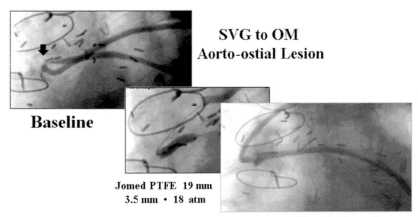

**SVG to OM
Aorto-ostial Lesion**

a

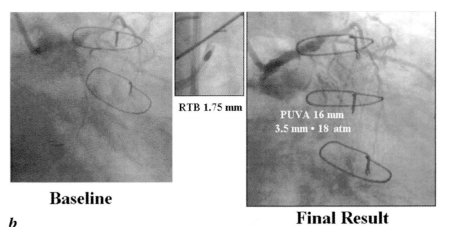

b

Figure 17.3 *Stenting a high-risk patient. A 70-year-old man with severe disease in his saphenous vein graft and native left main artery that supplied his remaining viable myocardium.*

icant effort-induced angina. There was no prior history of MI and her ejection fraction was normal, at 65%. The angiograms show distal left main disease which extends into the bifurcation of the LAD and the circumflex artery. This was treated by debulking the lesion with a 7 Fr atherectomy catheter. Despite the adequate ejection fraction, an intra-aortic balloon pump was placed prophylactically to support the patient during the treatment of her left main artery. After 11 cuts were performed with the atherectomy device, a 15 mm long ACS Multilink stent was placed. The stent was expanded with a 4 mm diameter balloon at 18 atmospheres. The final result (*Fig. 17.4b*) shows no residual filling defect, and the ostium of the LAD and the circumflex artery are not compromised. In addition, the 4-month follow-up angiogram reveals no significant restenosis through-out the length of the stent. A more complete descrip-

tion of stenting left main coronary artery disease is provided in Chapter 10.

Another example of very high-risk angioplasty is provided in *Fig. 17.5*. This procedure was performed during the live demonstration course from Milan in June 1998. This 68-year-old man had severe stenosis of the distal left main artery with an entrance into the LAD that took a retroflexed course with two abrupt 90° bends. Antonio spent close to 30 minutes trying to get a guidewire into the LAD and he was finally successful with a Choice PT Graphix (SciMed, Minneapolis, Minnesota, USA) wire. This wire was exchanged over a 1.5 mm balloon for a rotational atherectomy C wire. Rotational atherectomy was then performed with serial burr sizes from 1.5 mm to 2.5 mm. The baseline angiogram is shown in *Fig. 17.5a*, along with the ultrasound images, which were obtained after rotational atherectomy since the ultra-

Left Main Bifurcational Stenting with IAPB support

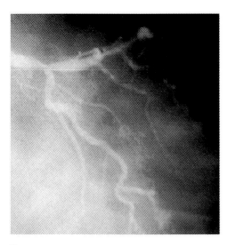

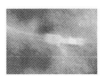

DCA 7 F : 11 cuts

Baseline

a

Left Main Bifurcational Stenting with IAPB support

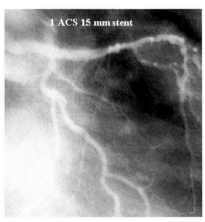

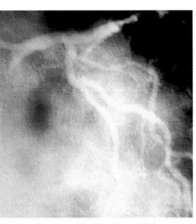

Final Result **4 month Follow-Up**

b

Figure 17.4 *Treating a high-risk patient. This 46-year-old woman had unprotected left main disease. The lesion involved the bifurcation with the LAD and circumflex arteries. This was treated with directional atherectomy followed by placement of an ACS MultiLink stent. There was no evidence of restensosis on the four month follow-up angiogram.*

sound catheter could not be passed initially because of the severe tortuosity and dense calcification of the lesion. The ultrasound image taken at the distal left main artery shows an oblong lumen, 1.5 mm × 3.0 mm in diameter. Sequential balloon dilatation was performed in the circumflex artery and the LAD followed by placement of a 17 mm long Saint Come stent on a 3.5 mm balloon, which was deployed at 17 atmospheres. The stent was placed in the left main artery and extended into the LAD. Dilatation through the side wall of the stent into the circumflex artery was performed with simultaneous inflations (*Fig. 17.5b*). This patient received an intra-aortic balloon pump prophylactically for hemodynamic support during the procedure. In addition, abciximab was given to prevent slow flow and to diminish the risk of acute stent thrombosis.

CONCLUSION

The use of coronary artery stents can be very effective even in high-risk patients with poor ventricular function or with a large amount of myocardium at jeopardy. The likelihood that we would use a prophylactic intra-aortic balloon pump or abciximab

(IABP support + ReoPro)

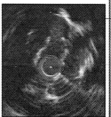

IVUS post RTB

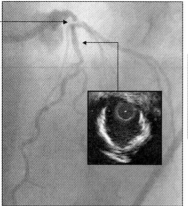

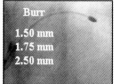

Burr
1.50 mm
1.75 mm
2.50 mm

a **Baseline**

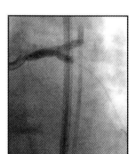

**Saint Come 17 mm Stent
3.5 mm • 17 atm**

b

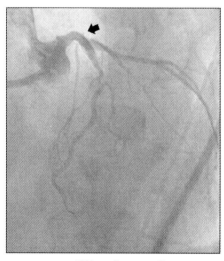

Final result

Figure 17.5 *Treating the high-risk patient. This 68-year-old man had severe, calcified, distal left main disease. He was treated prophylactically by placing an intra-aortic balloon pump and administering abciximab. After significant difficulty, a guide wire was successfully passed into the LAD and sequential rotational atherectomy was performed. The residual left main disease was treated with a single stent and simultaneous balloon inflations into the proximal LAD and circumflex arteries.*

increases in proportion to the degree of risk as assessed by the left ventricular ejection fraction, the extent of myocardium at risk, and the nature of the lesion to be treated.

REFERENCES

1. Welty FK, Mittleman MA, Lewis SM et al. A patent infarct-related artery is associated with reduced long-term mortality after percutaneous transluminal coronary angioplasty for postinfarction ischemia and an ejection fraction < 50%. *Circulation* 1996; **93**: 1496–1501.
2. Talley JD, Ohman EM, Mark DB et al. Economic implications of the prophylactic use of intra-aortic balloon counterpulsation in the setting of acute myocardial infarction. The Randomized IABP Study Group. Intra-aortic Balloon Pump. *Am J Cardiol* 1997; **79**: 590–594.
3. Aguirre FV, Kern MJ, Bach R et al. Intra-aortic balloon pump support during high-risk coronary angioplasty. *Cardiology* 1994; **84**: 175–186.
4. Kahn JK, Rutherford BD, McConahay DR et al. Supported 'high risk' coronary angioplasty using intra-aortic balloon pump counterpulsation. *J Am Coll Cardiol* 1990; **15**: 1151–1155.
5. O'Murchu B, Foreman RD, Shaw RE et al. Role of intraaortic balloon pump counterpulsation in high risk coronary rotational atherectomy. *J Am Coll Cardiol* 1995; **26**: 1270–1275.
6. Kong DF, Califf RM, Miller DP et al. Clinical outcomes of therapeutic agents that block the platelet glycoprotein IIb/IIIa integrin in ischemic heart disease. *Circulation* 1998; **98**: 2829–2835.

Chapter 18 How intravascular ultrasound alters therapeutic decisions

Antonio Colombo and Jonathan Tobis

The examples discussed in this chapter elaborate on how intravascular ultrasound (IVUS) enhances our understanding of coronary artery disease and facilitates therapeutic interventions. The previous chapters concentrate on lesion-specific issues and the approach to their treatment. This chapter highlights some of the general ways that IVUS alters our diagnosis or treatment options and specifically addresses the question, 'Do we need intracoronary ultrasound after high-pressure stent expansion?'

IVUS AS A PRE-INTERVENTION DIAGNOSTIC TOOL

An outline of the benefits of IVUS in coronary stenting is provided in *Table 18.1*. When used before an intervention, IVUS imaging is very helpful in:

(a) determining lesion severity for intermediate stenoses;[1]

(b) assessing the length of artery that needs to be stented;

(c) identifying the amount of calcium present;[2,3]

(d) specifying the position for the stent;

(e) providing a measure of vessel diameter (media to media), which will help in the selection of balloon size;[4]

(f) determining the appropriate device; and

(g) analysing the tissue characteristics of the plaque.[5]

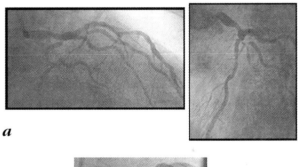

a

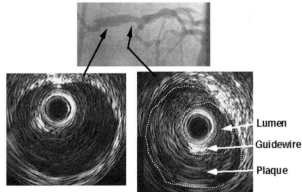

IVUS = 73% CSA STENOSIS, DIAMETER = 2.3 mm

b

Figure 18.1 *The use of IVUS for determining lesion severity. Assessment of this distal left main lesion revealed a lumen of 2.3 mm in diameter. Fibrofatty plaque occupied 73 percent of the available cross-sectional area as outlined at the boundary with the media.*

Table 18.1
Uses of intravascular ultrasound imaging in coronary stenting

Pre-intervention	Post-intervention
1. Lesion severity	1. Stent expansion
2. Lesion length	2. Stent apposition
3. Amount of calcium	3. Edge dissection
4. Precise positioning	4. 'Lost' stent
5. Balloon size	5. Ostial, edge placement
6. Device selection	6. Side branch entrapment
7. Tissue characterization	

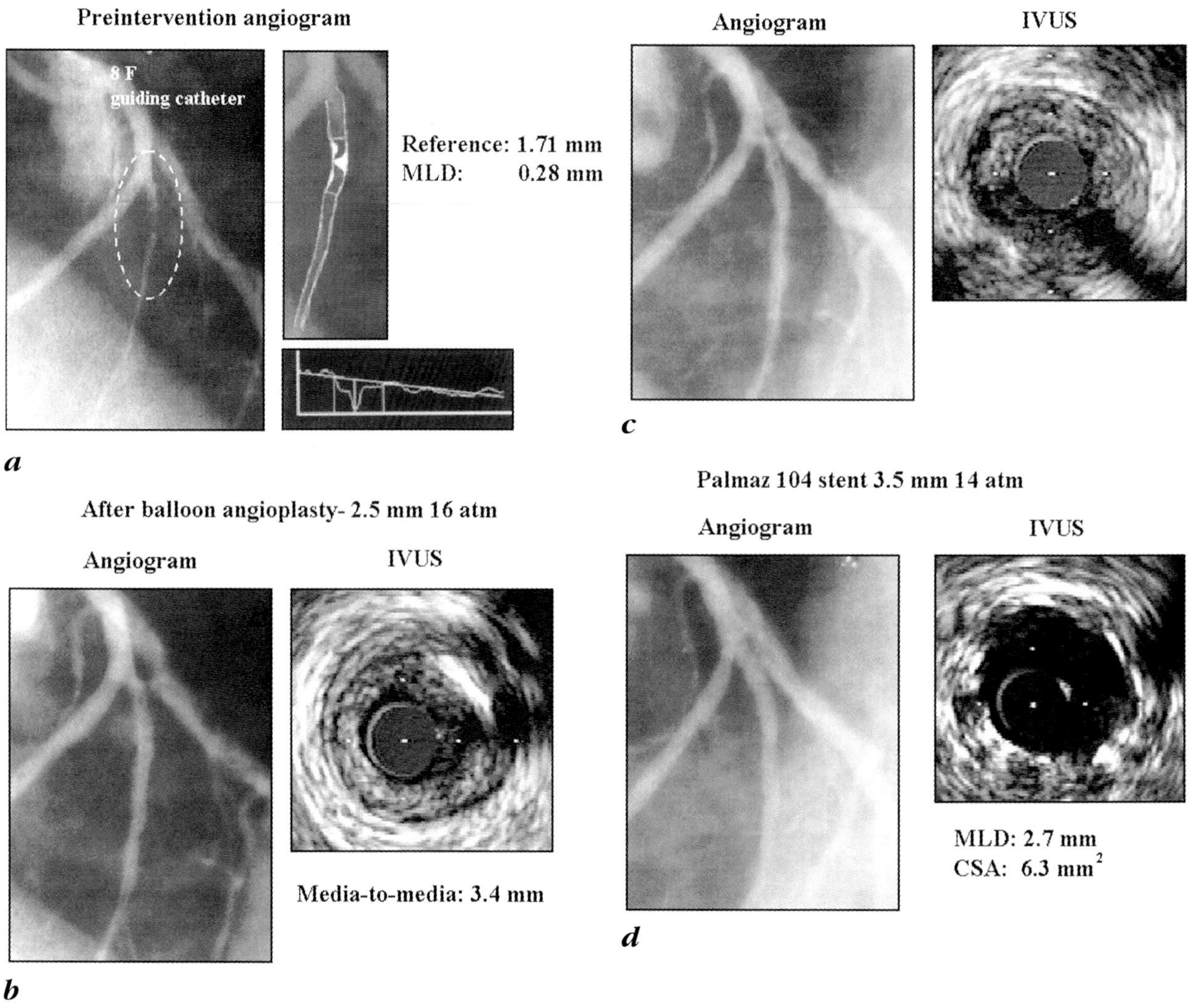

Preintervention angiogram

Reference: 1.71 mm
MLD: 0.28 mm

a

After balloon angioplasty- 2.5 mm 16 atm

Angiogram   IVUS

Media-to-media: 3.4 mm

b

Angiogram   IVUS

c

Palmaz 104 stent 3.5 mm 14 atm

Angiogram   IVUS

MLD: 2.7 mm
CSA: 6.3 mm^2

d

Figure 18.2 *The use of IVUS to optimize the results with balloon dilatation. (a) By quantitative angiography analysis, it was believed that this diagonal artery was a small vessel. (b) By intravascular ultrasound, the media to media measured 3.4 mm. (c) Although the angiogram revealed a satisfactory result after repeat balloon dilatation, the IVUS exam still demonstrated the presence of a small lumen. (d) Based on the IVUS measurements, a Palmaz biliary stent was placed on a 3.5 mm diameter balloon.*

The angiogram in *Fig. 18.1a* is from a patient who was referred because there was disagreement on the form of therapy that should be applied. The cardiologists wanted to perform angioplasty on the diagonal branch, but the surgeons felt that the left main stenosis was greater than 50% and should be treated with a bypass operation. The patient was referred for IVUS (*Fig. 18.1b*) to help clarify the diagnosis.[6] The proximal left main artery was a 4 mm diameter vessel with no intimal thickening, but in the distal left main artery there was a large volume of plaque, which consumes

73% of the available cross-sectional area. The diameter of the remaining lumen was 2.3 mm. Based on this observation of the amount of plaque present in the left main coronary artery, the decision was made to send the patient to surgery. At the present time we might elect to treat this patient with directional atherectomy and a coronary stent. Unfortunately, there is no outcome study to determine what the correct mode of therapy should be. Many of the cases in this chapter represent examples in which the interventionalist had to use his best judgement to make a decision for the patient's treatment despite insufficient scientific data. What the ultrasound imaging provides is a more complete understanding of the anatomy so that a better-informed decision can be reached.

IVUS VERSUS QUANTITATIVE CORONARY ANGIOGRAPHY AS A GUIDE TO STENT SIZE

Quantitative coronary angiography (QCA) has been the gold standard for assessing severity of disease. However, there are many times when QCA may be misleading compared to imaging the cross-sectional anatomy of an artery with ultrasound. The tight stenosis demonstrated in *Fig. 18.2a* measured 0.3 mm by QCA with a reference diameter measurement of 1.7 mm. Based on this measurement, an aggressive balloon size was chosen at 2.5 mm diameter, which was expanded to 16 atmospheres. The angiogram following the initial angioplasty is shown in *Fig. 18.2b*, along with the IVUS image. The angiogram demonstrates a successful angioplasty result, and although there is some haziness around the lumen, the boundary suggests complete effacement of the stenosis. The corresponding ultrasound image reveals that the lumen size has enlarged to 1.5 mm in diameter; however, the vessel diameter from media to media is much larger than expected, at 3.4 mm. The large amount of plaque distributed uniformly throughout the length of the vessel forces QCA to underestimate the true size of this large diagonal branch. On the basis of the ultrasound assessment of vessel diameter, a 3.5 mm balloon was chosen and expanded to 10 atmospheres. The results of this dilatation are shown in *Fig. 18.2c*. Despite the use of a much larger balloon, there is significant recoil and the residual lumen is not much better than that obtained with the 2.5 mm balloon. The angiogram appears to have a wider diameter because there are dissections behind the plaque into which contrast passes, thus making it seem that the diameter of the lumen is larger than it really is.

Based on these ultrasound observations that this artery was not a 'small vessel', a decision was made to proceed with coronary artery stenting. A Palmaz 104 stent was placed in the diagonal branch and expanded with the 3.5 mm diameter balloon at 14 atmospheres (*Fig. 18.2d*). Not only does the angiogram show a more satisfactory result, but the ultrasound cross-section is now 2.7 mm × 3.0 mm and demonstrates a circumferential patent lumen without dissections.

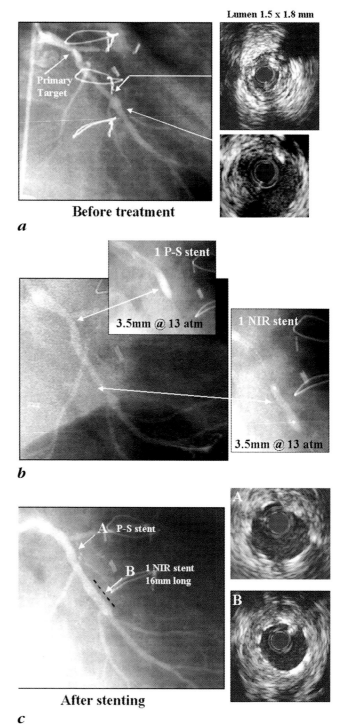

Figure 18.3 *IVUS may identify other stenoses within the target vessel. (a) The primary target was in the proximal circumflex artery but an IVUS exam revealed a tight stenosis in the midportion of the obtuse marginal branch. (b) The proximal and mid lesions were treated with placement of a stent. (c) Final result by angiography and IVUS.*

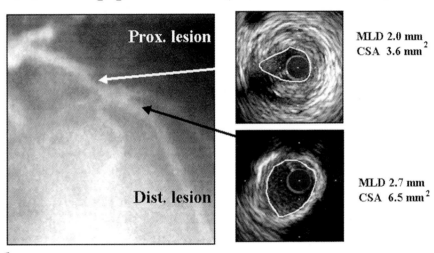

Figure 18.4 *IVUS can be helpful in determining which lesion needs a stent and which lesions can be left alone after balloon dilatation. (a) Baseline angiogram and IVUS study. There is intense calcification of the distal lesion involving the full circumference of the plaque. (b) Following balloon dilatation, the distal calcified lesion has an adequate lumen cross-sectional area but the proximal lesion has significant elastic recoil. (c) Based on this information from the IVUS study, a stent was placed at the proximal lesion only, despite the fact that the distal lesion was a chronic total occlusion.*

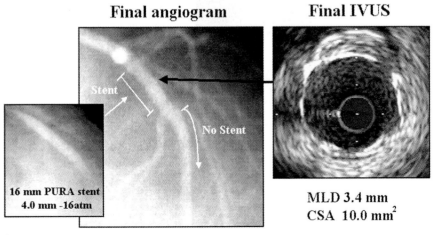

IVUS IDENTIFIES OTHER STENOSES WITHIN THE STENTED VESSEL

IVUS may be helpful during coronary artery stenting to discover other lesions in the vessel that require treatment to obtain an optimal result. In the example shown in *Fig. 18.3a*, there was a significant stenosis in the distal left main artery and the proximal circumflex artery, which was the target lesion to be treated. IVUS was performed before the intervention and, in addition to the recognition of the disease in the proximal artery, it was observed that there was a tight stenosis in the mid-portion of the obtuse marginal artery that was underestimated by angiography. A 16 mm long NIR stent was placed at 13 atmospheres using a 3.5 mm diameter balloon in the mid-portion of the obtuse marginal artery (*Fig. 18.3b*). The proximal lesion was then treated with a Palmaz– Schatz stent deployed on a 3.5 mm balloon at 13 atmospheres. The final angiographic result (*Fig. 18.3c*) reveals a satisfactory lumen in the proximal and mid-portion of the obtuse marginal artery. By ultrasound, the lumen measured 3 mm in diameter.

IVUS CAN HELP DETERMINE WHEN A STENOSIS SHOULD NOT BE STENTED

In addition to using IVUS to help decide what size stent should be used, it can also be used to determine that a stent or angioplasty is not necessary.

Alternatively, IVUS may be helpful in deciding which of several lesions needs a stent and which one does not, despite the angiographic result. This use of IVUS imaging is demonstrated in the case shown in *Fig. 18.4*. This proximal left anterior descending artery (LAD) has a significant stenosis followed by complete occlusion after the bifurcation of the diagonal branch and the first septal perforator.

The lesion was crossed with a guidewire and dilated with a 30 mm long Samba 3.0 mm diameter balloon at 14 atmospheres. The corresponding ultrasound images following recanalization and balloon dilatation at the proximal and distal lesions are shown to the right of the pre-intervention angiogram in *Fig. 18.4a*. Proximally the vessel was about 4 mm in diameter, media to media. The lumen size was still inadequate at 2 mm diameter following the 3 mm balloon dilatation. The distal lesion was intensely calcified, although the majority of the calcium was positioned towards the base or mid-portion of the plaque. Instead of using rotational atherectomy, a larger balloon was chosen. A 20 mm × 4 mm Tacker balloon was expanded at 14 atmospheres. The subsequent angiogram (*Fig. 18.4b*) showed an adequate angioplasty result in both the proximal and distal segments. However, the ultrasound examination revealed an unexpected disparity. The distal lesion, despite being heavily calcified, was expanded adequately by the balloon dilatation, whereas the fibrotic proximal lesion demonstrated more elastic recoil with a minimum lumen diameter (MLD) of only 2 mm. Based on these observations, a 16 mm long PURA stent was placed in the proximal

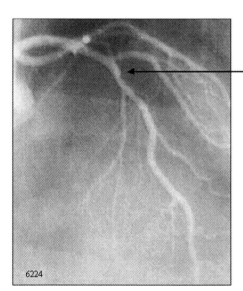

Baseline

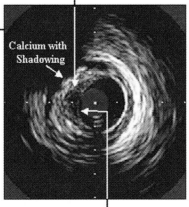

Superficial Lipid Core

Calcium with Shadowing

Thin Fibrous Cap

Figure 18.5 *Tissue characterization using IVUS may help to identify an unstable plaque. This complex plaque has calcium with shadowing at the base between 9 o'clock and 12 o'clock. There is an echo lucent zone just below the surface of the plaque. This is consistent with a lipid filled region. A thin fibrous capsule covers the echo lucent zone.*

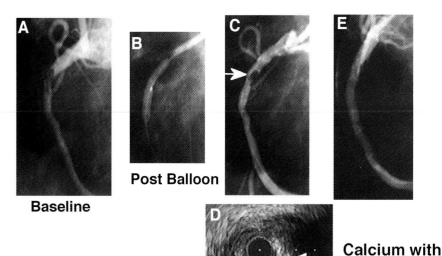

Figure 18.6 *Pseudo thrombus: by angiography this lesion appeared to have a meniscus consistent with thrombus (Panel A). However after balloon dilatation, there was a persistent filling defect which did not respond to repeat balloon dilatation (Panel C). Although the assumption was that this lesion represented residual thrombus, IVUS examination revealed a calcified plaque prolapsing into the lumen.*

lesion but not in the distal lesion, and it was inflated with a 4 mm balloon at 16 atmospheres.

The final angiogram is provided in *Fig. 18.4c*. The final IVUS study showed that the proximal lesion was now 3.4 mm in diameter with a cross-sectional area of 10.0 mm². Results from this and similar cases provided the impetus to treat long lesions with the technique called 'spot stenting' (see Chapter 20).

UNSTABLE PLAQUE MORPHOLOGY

Tissue characterization of plaque composition may be useful for guiding treatment (see Chapter 1). For example, the finding of a large amount of calcium at the lumen–plaque interface may help to determine if rotational atherectomy would be appropriate. *Figure 18.5* reveals a remarkable type of plaque composition that may be diagnosed occasionally by ultrasound and is thought to represent an unstable plaque that is vulnerable to rupture. The angiogram reveals a slit-like stenosis in the proximal LAD before the first septal perforator. Just proximal to the stenosis is an eccentric plaque that appears to have a mixed composition based on tissue characterization. Between 9 o'clock and 12 o'clock there are some intense echo reflections with shadowing peripherally, which are consistent with calcium at the base of the plaque. The majority of the plaque is less intense and consistent with fibrous tissue.

In the central portion of the plaque, between 8 o'clock and 10 o'clock, the plaque is more echolucent with a thin band of echogenic reflection at the lumen surface. Although we do not have the histologic cross-section of this in vivo artery, we may draw conclusions from other histologic and IVUS comparisons.[5]

The interpretation of this ultrasound pattern is that underneath this thin fibrous capsule there is a central core of lipid-laden cells with denser fibrocalcific disease at the base of the plaque. This type of histologic pattern has been described as a likely precursor to acute plaque rupture and thrombus formation that precipitate unstable syndromes or acute myocardial infarction (MI).[7–10] In this case the patient was symptomatic from the associated stenosis and he received a stent based on the clinical evidence of ischemia and the angiographic finding. If this unstable plaque were discovered without being associated with a stenosis, it could potentially be treated medically with aggressive lipid-lowering agents, but the natural history of these plaques, once they are identified by IVUS imaging, is poorly understood.

PSEUDO-THROMBUS – TISSUE CHARACTERIZATION BY IVUS IS SUPERIOR TO ANGIOGRAPHY

Angiography may be misleading in the diagnosis of thrombus formation.[11] This can have significant implications in terms of the type of treatment that is attempted.[12] An example of an apparent thrombus diagnosed by angiography is shown in *Fig. 18.6*. This 60-year-old woman presented with an acute inferior wall MI. Intravenous heparin (5000 mg), intravenous metoprolol (5 mg), and oral aspirin (325 mg) were administered in the emergency room and the patient was immediately brought to the catheterization laboratory. The baseline angiogram revealed a filling defect in the proximal right coronary artery with thrombolysis in MI (TIMI) grade 1 flow and the appearance of a meniscus that is consistent with thrombus. Although it was expected that this lesion would contain soft thrombus, it was difficult to pass a guidewire or follow with a balloon once the guidewire had crossed the lesion. Following initial balloon dilatation, flow was improved but there was still a significant residual filling defect, which had the appearance of thrombus (*Fig. 18.6*, Panel C). It was surprising that this lesion did not efface with repeated balloon dilatations. Rather than proceeding with thrombolytic therapy, transluminal extraction catheter, or AngioJet thrombectomy, an IVUS catheter was passed (*Fig. 18.6*, Panel D). The IVUS image revealed the presence of intense calcification between 1 o'clock and 7 o'clock, with evidence of torn plaque that has also shifted its position at 5 o'clock. Based on this observation, the decision was made not to treat with thrombolytic therapy, but to proceed with stent insertion for this torn calcified plaque. Deployment of an AVE GFX stent produced a satisfactory lumen without the persistent recoil that was seen following balloon dilatation alone (see *Fig. 18.6*, Panel E).

THE USE OF IVUS IMAGING AFTER DEPLOYMENT OF A CORONARY STENT

As outlined in *Table 18.1*, there are several uses of IVUS after a stent has been inserted. IVUS is more precise than angiography for determining that the stent is optimally expanded and completely apposed to the wall of the artery and that any edge dissections do not compromise the lumen. In addition, IVUS imaging may help find a misplaced or undeployed stent, assist in correct placement for ostial or bifurcation lesions, and reveal if a side branch lumen at a bifurcation is adequate or is entrapped by the stent edge. Examples of the first three uses of IVUS are presented throughout this book; the following cases describe some additional situations where IVUS may help after an intervention.

IVUS DISCOVERY OF UNDEPLOYED OR LOST STENTS

One of the more dramatic examples of a situation in which IVUS imaging has been essential for understanding complications that occur with coronary artery stenting is the discovery of a stent that has slipped off the delivery balloon and is sitting in the artery in an undeployed state. Early in our experience, when a variety of flexible stents was still not available, it could require significant force to coax a Palmaz–Schatz stent around a bend in an artery. An

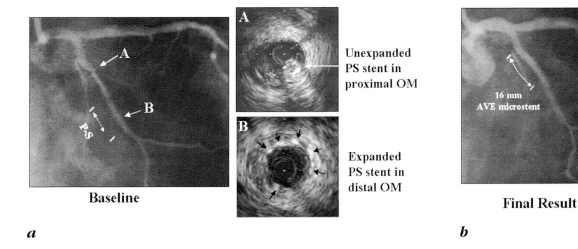

a   *b*

Figure 18.7 *(a) Intravascular ultrasound (IVUS) imaging reveals an undeployed stent in proximal circumflex. (b) Treatment for an undeployed stent. P–S, Palmaz–Schatz; OM, obtuse marginal.*

example of this is provided in *Fig. 18.7*. A Palmaz–Schatz stent was placed with great difficulty in the distal portion of the obtuse marginal artery. During the struggle to place a second Palmaz–Schatz stent in the proximal segment, the guiding catheter and guidewire suddenly flipped out of the artery. When the balloon was examined, the stent was not present. We did not know if the stent was stripped off in the coronary artery or embolized in the aorta. The guidewire was repositioned and an ultrasound catheter was passed into the obtuse marginal artery. The ultrasound image (*Fig. 18.7a*, Panel A) showed an unusual pattern whereby the echogenic stent struts were seen at 4 o'clock in a collapsed state to the side of the ultrasound catheter. No stent strut reflections appeared anywhere else around the circumference of the lumen. For comparison, the IVUS image in *Fig. 18.7a*, Panel B reveals the circumferential struts of the adequately placed first Palmaz–Schatz stent in the distal section of the artery.

This IVUS study documented that the second Palmaz–Schatz stent had slipped off the delivery balloon and had lodged in the proximal obtuse marginal artery. To treat this complication, a new 16 mm AVE stent was placed in the main lumen of the artery, external to the undeployed stent, and it was expanded with a 3.5 mm balloon at 10 atmospheres. This compressed the Palmaz–Schatz stent to the side and provided adequate expansion and support of the proximal and mid-vessel (*Fig. 18.7b*).

STENT UNDEREXPANSION

The recognition of inadequate stent expansion was one of the earliest and most significant observations by IVUS to improve results of coronary artery stenting.[13,14] As shown in *Fig. 18.8*, a 58-year-old man had a Palmaz–Schatz stent placed for a tight stenosis in the mid-right coronary artery. Following stent implantation with a 3.0 mm balloon inflated at 16 atmospheres, there was a satisfactory angiographic result (*Fig. 18.8b*). However, the ultrasound study (*Fig. 18.8b*, Panel D) revealed an asymmetrically deployed stent with dimensions of 2 mm × 2.5 mm. On the basis of these findings, a 3.5 mm balloon was chosen and the stent was redilated at 16 atmospheres. The final angiogram in (*Fig. 18.8b*, Panel F) showed mild improvement compared to the angiogram in *Fig. 18.8b*, Panel B. However, the ultrasound showed a more dramatic change, with an increase in symmetry of the vessel as well as expansion of the lumen to 3 mm × 3 mm.

A Short RCA Stenosis

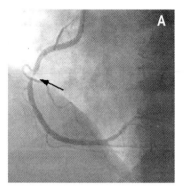

Baseline Stenosis

a

IVUS Demonstrates Stent Under-Expansion

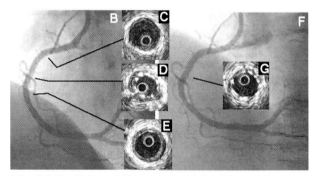

After P-S Stent 3.0mm at 16atm   After 3.5mm at 16atm

b

Figure 18.8 *The use of intravascular ultrasound to guide the operator in maximizing lumen cross-sectional area following stent insertion.*

In the future, stent underdeployment may be diagnosed during the initial stent implantation with IVUS imaging by using an imaging wire.[15] *Figure 18.9a* shows the IVUS images obtained with an imaging core device placed within a dilatation catheter during balloon inflation of a 3.5 mm Titan balloon expanded at 16 atmospheres. This imaging core is currently being developed by Boston Scientific and has a 30 MHz ultrasound transducer at the tip of a 0.46 mm (0.018-inch) motor drive shaft. This can be inserted into catheters that accept 0.46 mm (0.018-inch) guidewires to obtain ultrasound cross-sectional images through the shaft of the balloon during inflation. In this case the distal stent was adequately expanded to 3 mm but the mid-portion of the stent was underexpanded, with a diameter of 2.1 mm × 2.8 mm, despite

Distal stent   **Mid stent**

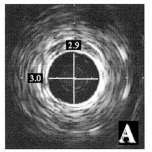   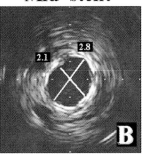   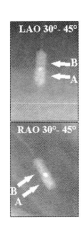

CSA = 6.7 mm²   CSA = 4.9 mm²

Cordis 3.5 mm Titan Balloon 16 atm

a

Figure 18.9 *An 0.018 inch ultrasound imaging transducer on a wire was used to produce these images during balloon deployment of a stent. Despite the use of 16 atmospheres pressure, the IVUS imaging core documented inadequate expansion in the mid-portion of the stent.*

Cordis 3.5 mm Titan Balloon 24 atm

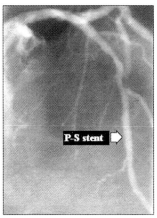   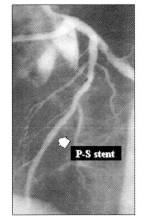

Final Result

b

the relatively large size of the balloon and a pressure of 16 atmospheres. The corresponding radiographs of the inflated balloon are shown in the panels of *Fig. 18.9a.* Some indentation of the proximal portion of the balloon can be appreciated only in the right anterior oblique cranial projection. On the basis of the ultrasound findings, the balloon was inflated to 24 atmospheres without changing its position or obtaining another angiogram. The cross-sectional area by ultrasound improved, as it did on the final angiogram (*Fig. 18.9b*).

INCOMPLETE PLAQUE COVER

IVUS may be very useful in guiding the treatment of bifurcation or ostial lesions (see Chapter 10). An example of a situation in which the ultrasound findings altered our therapeutic approach to an ostial lesion is demonstrated in *Fig. 18.10.* In this case pre-intervention ultrasound imaging was not performed. The angiograms at baseline show a significant stenosis in the proximal LAD in this 64-year-old symptomatic woman. There did not appear to be any obstruction in the distal left main artery. A Palmaz–Schatz stent was placed at the ostium of the LAD, with careful attention paid so as not to place the stent across the entrance of the circumflex artery.

The angiograms shown in *Fig. 18.10a*, bottom panels, indicated that a satisfactory angiographic result had been obtained. The ultrasound images, however, told a different story. As shown in *Fig. 18.10b*, Panel A, the ultrasound image in the body of the left main artery showed a 4 mm lumen with

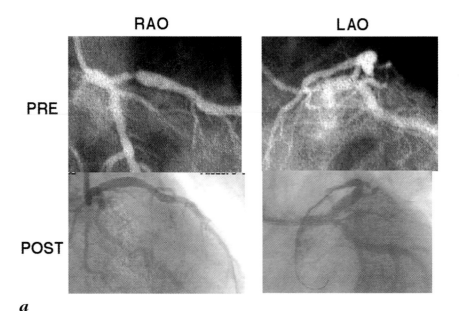

a

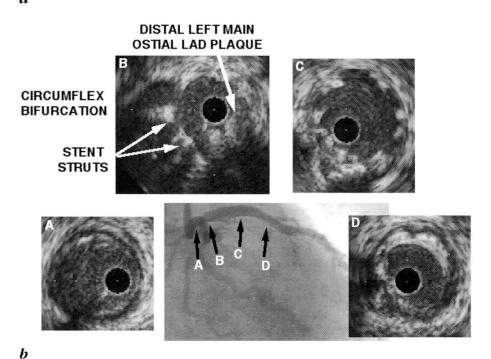

b

Figure 18.10 *IVUS guidance in treating ostial LAD disease. (a) Angiograms before and after placement of a Palmaz–Schatz stent. (b) IVUS documented correct placement of the stent but the disease process extended into the left main artery which was not appreciated by angiography.*

only trivial intimal hyperplasia. The ultrasound image in *Fig. 18.10b*, Panel B was taken at the bifurcation of the circumflex artery and the LAD. It shows that there are stent struts at the bifurcation between 7 o'clock and 9 o'clock, which do not approximate the wall. This demonstrates that the proximal end of the stent was placed slightly extending into the bifurcation. The stent struts are not seen in a uniform circumference because the tube of the stent and the IVUS catheter are not exactly coaxial. Despite this

correct position of the stent, the opposite wall of the artery (between 2 o'clock and 6 o'clock) has a moderate amount of plaque without any stent support. This implies that the plaque actually extended from the LAD back into the distal left main coronary artery. The stent in the proximal LAD was adequately expanded at 3.5 mm (*Fig. 18.10b*, Panel C).

We would not recommend leaving such a large plaque proximal to a stented zone and would recom-

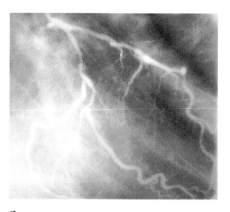

a

Post Rotational Atherectomy

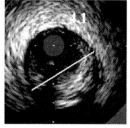
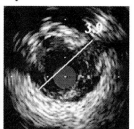

Proximal Reference   **Lesion**   **Distal Reference**

b

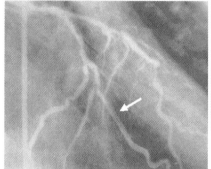
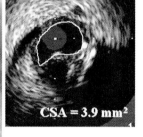

CSA = 3.9 mm²

c

Figure 18.11 *Intravascular ultrasound (IVUS) for decision making. (a) Pre-intervention angiography. (b) Vessel size determined by IVUS. (c) Distal dissection post PTCA. (d) Discovery of plaque prolapse. (e) Final result.*

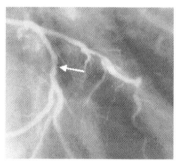
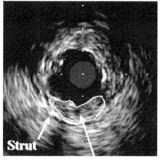

BeStent 4.0mm 16atm   Strut   **Plaque prolapse**   *d*

Inside BeStent 4.0mm at 18 atm

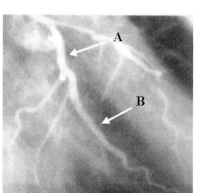
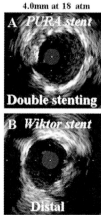

A   *PURA stent*

Double stenting

B   *Wiktor stent*

Distal

4.0mm at 12 atm   *e*

mend treating this distal left main artery either with implantation of a bifurcation stent or with surgery if the operator did not feel comfortable performing elective left main stenting.

IVUS IS MOST EFFECTIVE WHEN USED AS AN ITERATIVE PROCESS

A summary of how IVUS can be helpful during multiple stages of complex coronary artery stenting is exemplified in *Fig. 18.11*. The lesson to be learned from this case is that IVUS provides the most information for complex cases when it is utilized repeatedly, in an iterative fashion, for pre-intervention diagnosis and device selection, then after balloon dilatation to determine where the stent needs to be placed, and then after stent insertion to ensure optimal expansion and that appropriate results are achieved.

Figure 18.11a reveals diffuse disease in the LAD and circumflex systems. For the current purpose, we will focus on treatment of the circumflex artery. An IVUS examination was attempted before intervention but the ultrasound device could not pass through the tortuous vessel. The inability to pass the ultrasound device is typical of calcified lesions and is best treated with rotational atherectomy, since these lesions tend to be very resistant to balloon dilatation and this results in incomplete stent expansion if the lesions are not pre-treated with atherectomy. Following rotational atherectomy with a 2.0 mm and 2.5 mm burr, the lumen diameter was still quite small, at 1.7 mm; however, the ultrasound image also revealed that the media-to-media dimension of the vessel was close to 4 mm (*Fig. 18.11b*). On the basis of this finding the artery was treated with directional atherectomy to remove more tissue, and then it was dilated with a 3.5 mm balloon. After balloon dilatation, the obtuse marginal artery had a dissection with a small cross-sectional area documented by ultrasound (*Fig. 18.11c*). Based on the ultrasound observation, we would feel uncomfortable leaving this result with balloon dilatation alone; therefore, a Wiktor stent was placed in the obtuse marginal artery. In addition, a BeStent stent was placed in the proximal circumflex artery and expanded with a 4.0 mm balloon at 16 atmospheres. Despite a satisfactory angiographic result, the ultrasound image in *Fig. 18.11d* demonstrates that there was prolapse of tissue through the stent struts, which diminished the effective lumen cross-sectional area. A PURA stent

was placed in the proximal circumflex artery to treat the tissue prolapse through the BeStent. The proximal stent was dilated at 18 atmospheres with a final balloon size of 4.0 mm, and it attained a 3.5 mm × 3.5 mm diameter lumen (*Fig. 18.11e*). This complex coronary artery stenting requires an interventionalist who can operate with patience and persistence, but by using the information that IVUS provides, one can achieve results that are superior to those obtained with angiographic guidance alone.

DO WE NEED INTRACORONARY ULTRASOUND AFTER HIGH-PRESSURE STENT EXPANSION?

Background

Following the initial observations with IVUS of the benefits derived from using larger balloons and higher pressures during coronary artery stenting, several groups adopted this technique but without using ultrasound guidance.[16] These authors showed that by using the method of high-pressure inflations and larger balloons, the incidence of subacute stent thrombosis is significantly reduced even without using ultrasound guidance. Although we agree that this approach dramatically reduces the incidence of subacute thrombosis to approximately 1%, we feel that there are other benefits of using ultrasound guidance during coronary stenting. In addition to improving the diagnosis before or after stent deployment, we believe that IVUS, when appropriately used, also lowers the incidence of restenosis.

To assess this hypothesis, we reviewed 584 lesions in 504 patients treated between April 1993 and July 1996, who had high-pressure balloon inflations within coronary stents that were then assessed with IVUS imaging. Following high-pressure final stent dilatation of ≥ 16 atmospheres and a balloon-to-artery ratio of 1.0, there was an angiographic residual stenosis of < 10% in all of these cases. The lesions then underwent IVUS evaluation. If the stented lesion met the criteria for optimal expansion by IVUS, no further dilatation was performed. If the criteria were not achieved, the stented zone underwent further dilatation, and repeat IVUS evaluation was performed until optimal dilatation was achieved or no further improvement could be obtained. The definition of optimal stent expansion that was used in this analysis was:

(a) circumferential stent apposition to the vessel wall of all the stent struts; and

Table 18.2

IVUS reference table. For choosing PTCA balloon size from IVUS measurements

Balloon diameter (mm)	Nominal CSA (mm²)	70% of balloon CSA (mm²)
2.5	4.9	3.4
2.75	5.9	4.2
3.0	7.1	5.0
3.25	8.3	5.8
3.5	9.6	6.7
3.75	11.0	7.7
4.0	12.6	8.8
4.25	14.2	9.9
4.5	15.9	11.1

CSA: cross-sectional area

Table 18.3

Intravascular ultrasound (IVUS) guided high-pressure stent insertion. Effect of further dilatation in Group One

	After ≥16 atm	Final result	p value
Balloon diameter (mm)	3.37 ± 0.33	3.62 ± 0.44	$p < 0.001$
Max. pressure (atm)	17.9 + 1.7	18.5 + 1.7	$p < 0.001$
IVUS			
In-stent MLD (mm)	2.50 ± 0.42	2.80 ± 0.44	$p < 0.001$
In-stent CSA (mm²)	7.00 ± 1.80	8.18 + 2.22	$p < 0.001$
Symmetry index	0.85 ± 0.11	0.86 ± 0.10	NS
Balloon/vessel ratio	1.12 ± 0.17	1.21 ± 0.20	$p < 0.001$

MLD: Minimum lumen diameter

(b) the smallest cross-sectional area within the stent was > 60% of the average of the proximal and distal reference vessel cross-sectional areas.

The balloon was chosen by having a reference table of the different sized balloons, and the expected cross-sectional area obtained at nominal inflation pressures (*Table 18.2*). After balloon inflation at nominal pressures, IVUS measurements reveal that the usual cross-sectional area achieved is only 70% of the calculated balloon cross-sectional area expected at full expansion. The ultrasound images were measured on line and an average of the proximal and distal reference cross-sectional areas was obtained.

This was then compared with the look-up table and an appropriately sized balloon was chosen. The criterion of 60% of the reference vessel area was chosen because 60% of the area bounded by the media corresponds to the average reference lumen cross-sectional area. In patients with coronary artery disease, most angiographically normal segments have 30–40% of the vessel cross-sectional area filled with atherosclerotic plaque (see Chapter 1). By using the vessel area instead of the reference lumen, we were trying to account for any disease in the reference zones that might compromise the lumen.

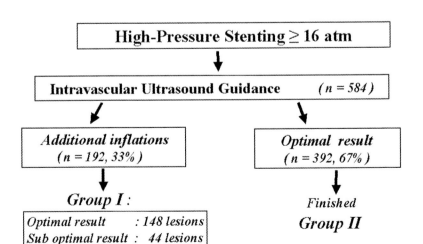

Figure 18.12 *Protocol for using intravascular ultrasound as a guide to optimize the lumen cross-sectional area within a stent.*

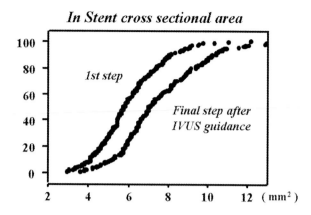

Figure 18.13 *Frequency distribution curve of the in stent lumen cross-sectional area comparing the result after the initial high-pressure inflation with the final result after IVUS guidance.*

IVUS guidance and restenosis

The protocol outline and patient groups for high-pressure ultrasound-guided stenting are shown in *Fig. 18.12.* After high-pressure stenting (≥ 16 atmospheres) IVUS imaging was performed in 584 patients, and an optimal result was obtained in 392 (67%) of the patients. These patients did not receive any further treatment and were designated as Group Two. In the other 192 patients (33%), who did not initially achieve the IVUS criteria for an optimal result, additional inflations were performed. This group was defined as Group One. An optimal result was eventually achieved in 148 lesions (77% of Group One lesions). A suboptimal result was left in 44 lesions where we felt that higher pressures or a larger balloon could potentially be detrimental. The quantitative measurements that were effected by further dilatation in Group One patients are shown in *Table 18.3.*

On the basis of the IVUS results, the balloon diameter that was used to treat the lesion increased from 3.37 mm to 3.62 mm ($p < 0.001$) and the maximum pressure increased from 17.9 atmospheres to 18.5 atmospheres ($p < 0.001$). The MLD by IVUS increased in these lesions from 2.5 mm to 2.8 mm ($p < 0.001$) and the in-stent cross-sectional area increased from 7.0 mm^2 to 8.2 mm^2 ($p < 0.001$). The frequency distribution curve for the stent cross-sectional area between the initial and final treatment steps is demonstrated in *Fig. 18.13,* which shows the improvement in lumen cross-sectional area obtained by IVUS-guided stent expansion.

Table 18.4

Intravascular ultrasound (IVUS) guided high-pressure stent insertion. Patient characteristics

	Group One (n=174)	Group Two (n=330)	p value
Gender (male %)	89.1%	87.6%	NS
Mean age (years)	58.4 ± 10.1	58.2 ± 9.4	NS
Family history (%)	48.3%	53.0%	NS
Hypertension (%)	43.1%	41.5%	NS
Hyperlipidemia (%)	56.3%	52.7%	NS
Diabetes (%)	13.8%	11.8%	NS
Smoking (%)	67.8%	73.3%	NS
Prior MI (%)	50.6%	57.6%	NS
Prior CABG (%)	9.8%	13.9%	NS
Unstable angina (%)	28.7%	29.4%	NS
Multivessel disease (%)	50.0%	44.8%	NS

Table 18.5

Intravascular ultrasound (IVUS) guided high-pressure stent insertion. Lesion characteristics before intervention

	Group One (n=192)	Group Two (n=392)	p value
Type of lesion (%)			NS
A	4.1%	4.8%	
B1	36.5%	29.6%	
B2	41.7%	46.2%	
C	17.7%	19.4%	
Calcified lesion (%)	13.8%	10.1%	NS
Eccentricity (%)	80.8%	77.4%	NS

In addition, there were no distinguishing baseline characteristics between the patients who did or did not obtain optimal stent expansion. The comparison between Group One and Group Two for baseline clinical characteristics showed no significant difference between the groups (*Table 18.4*). Similarly, a comparison of lesion characteristics revealed no differences (*Table 18.5*). The quantitative angiographic analysis between Group One and Group Two showed no difference with respect to reference vessel size, pre-treatment MLD, or lesion length (*Table 18.6*). The number of stents per lesion was

Table 18.6

IVUS guided high pressure stent insertion. Quantitative angiographic analysis

	Group One (n = 192)	Group Two (n = 392)	p value
Reference vessel (mm)	3.0 ± 0.5	3.1 ± 0.5	
Pre MLD (mm)	0.9 ± 0.5	0.9 ± 0.5	NS
Pre % stenosis (%)	70.8+16.8	69.3 ± 17.8	NS
Lesion length (mm)	10.7+6.9	11.2 ± 7.0	NS
Stents per lesion	1.7 ± 1.0	1.6 ± 1.1	NS
Post MLD (mm)	3.1 ± 0.5	3.0 ± 0.5	p = 0.025
Post % stenosis (%)	−2.2 ± 14.1	1.2 ± 11.5	p = 0.026

Table 18.7

Intrvascular ultrasound (IVUS) guided high pressure stent insertion. Follow-up results

	Group One (n = 192)	Group Two (n = 392)	p value
Angiography (%)	62.7%	61.8%	NS
FU MLD (mm)	2.1 ± 1.0	2.1 ± 1.0	NS
FU % stenosis (%)	30.7 ± 30.0	29.8 ± 28.6	NS
Restenosis rate (%)	26.6%	23.5%	NS

FU: Follow-up

Table 18.8

Comparison between optimal and suboptimal subsets in Group One

	Optimal (n = 148)	Suboptimal (n = 44)	p value
Reference diameter (mm)	3.1 ± 0.5	3.0 ± 0.4	NS
Lesion length (mm)	10.3 ± 5.9	12.6 ± 7.6	p < 0.05
Pre MLD (mm)	0.8 ± 0.5	0.9 ± 0.5	NS
Pre % stenosis	72.5 ± 16.1	68.0 ± 18.1	NS
Final MLD (mm)	3.2 ± 0.5	3.0 ± 0.5	p < 0.01
Final % stenosis	−3.7 ± 13.7	3.4 ± 14.1	p < 0.01
IVUS			
Final in-stent CSA (mm²)	7.8 ± 2.1	6.5 ± 1.6	p < 0.001
Final in-stent MLD (mm)	2.9 ± 0.4	2.5 ± 0.4	p < 0.001
Symmetry index	0.86 ± 0.09	0.83 ± 0.12	p = 0.028

Table 18.9

Comparison between optimal and suboptimal subsets in Group One

	Optimal (n = 148)	Suboptimal (n = 44)	p value
Balloon/vessel ratio	1.2 ± 0.2	1.2 ± 0.2	NS
Final balloon diam. (mm)	3.6 ± 0.5	3.6 ± 0.4	NS
Final pressure (atm)	17.8 ± 1.7	18.4 ± 1.4	NS
FU angiography (%)	67.4%	68.3%	NS
FU MLD (mm)	2.0 ± 1.0	2.2 ± 1.1	NS
FU % stenosis	27.6 ± 29.5	31.6 ± 30.2	NS
Restenosis rate (%)	23.8%	41.5%	p < 0.01

also similar. There was a small but statistical difference in post-treatment MLD between Group One (3.1 mm) and Group Two (3.0 mm) ($p = 0.025$).

The 6-month follow-up angiographic results are shown in *Table 18.7*. Angiographic follow-up was approximately 62% in both groups. There was no difference in the mean value of MLD (2.1 ± 1.0 mm) or the follow-up percentage diameter stenosis (30 ± 29%). The restenosis rate was also not statistically different between the two groups: 27% in Group One and 24% in Group Two. However, Group One consisted of patients who had an optimal result only after further ultrasound-guided balloon dilatation and 44 patients who had a suboptimal result based on the pre-determined IVUS criteria. The differences between these two subsets of Group One are shown in *Table 18.8*.

The IVUS optimized patients had a shorter lesion length, a larger final MLD, and a lower final percentage diameter stenosis than the patients in the suboptimal group. It should be noted that the measurements in the suboptimal group are quite acceptable results for coronary stenting with a final MLD of 3.0 ± 0.5 mm and final percentage diameter stenosis of 3.4 ± 14%. As expected, the final IVUS measurements also were statistically significant between these two subgroups with respect to MLD and cross-sectional area. The restenosis rate between those patients from Group One who achieved an optimal result versus those who did not was significantly different (*Table 18.9*). The restenosis rate in the optimal group was 23.8%, which was not different from the patients in Group Two who achieved an optimal result after initial therapy. However, the patients who achieved a suboptimal result based on the ultrasound criteria had a significantly higher restenosis rate, at 41.5%.

We derive the following conclusions from this analysis of our data.

(a) Routine high pressure inflation of coronary artery stents using visual angiographic comparisons with the reference lumen diameter corresponds to obtaining an optimized IVUS result in only 67% of unselected lesions.

(b) In the group of patients that did not achieve an optimized result after initial treatment, there were no clinical or angiographic predictors to identify which of these lesions would require further inflations. Only the IVUS measurements revealed that repeat dilatation was indicated.

(c) The restenosis rate corresponded to the final lumen cross-sectional area result that was achieved. The highest restenosis rate was seen in the subgroup of patients in which an optimal final result could not be achieved despite repeat balloon inflations, higher pressures, or larger balloons.

Let us put this information into the perspective of a busy clinician's practice. This analysis suggests that in an unselected group of patients treated with high-pressure inflations but without IVUS guidance, an optimal result would be achieved in two-thirds of the cases and these patients with an optimal result would have a restenosis rate of 24%. One-third of the patients, however, would have a suboptimal result despite an angiographic appearance of success, with a restenosis rate of approximately 42%. The total overall restenosis rate would presumably be a weighted average of these two figures. Moreover, in 77% of patients who did not achieve an initial optimal result, the stented lumen cross-sectional area could have been improved if the procedure had been guided by ultrasound imaging. This would lower the restenosis rate back to that achieved in the group of patients who obtained an initial optimal result. Although this was not a prospective randomized trial, we believe the data support the hypothesis that the use of IVUS to optimize stent expansion has a positive impact in reducing post-stent restenosis.

STENTING WITH IVUS GUIDANCE REDUCES RESTENOSIS

A second study supports our hypothesis that stenting with IVUS guidance minimizes the restenosis rate. Patients from our service in Milan were compared with a similar group of patients who were treated at the Center for Cardiology Othmarschen in Hamburg with high-pressure inflations but without the use of IVUS guidance.[17] From each institution, 173 lesions were matched for sex, history of diabetes mellitus, prior percutaneous transluminal coronary angioplasty, vessel treated, reference diameter ± 0.3 mm, baseline MLD ± 0.1 mm, and number ± 0.5 of stents deployed. Only patients who received Palmaz stents or Palmaz–Schatz stents were included. In Hamburg, post-dilatation was performed with non-compliant balloons, closely sized to the angiographic lumen diameter by visual estimate, and inflated at 14 to 21 atmospheres. In Milan, the criteria for a successful result evolved; before September 1993, most post-dilatations were performed with minimally compliant balloons, usually 9 mm long, (about 0.5 mm larger than the reference lumen diameter), which were inflated at 8–20 atmospheres. Subsequently, most post-dilatations were performed with non-compliant balloons that approximated the size of the angiographic lumen diameter and were inflated at 14–20 atmospheres. IVUS examination was then performed and the stent was redilated until the following IVUS criteria were met:

> Between March and September 1993 (the early phase), the target for defining a successful result was the achievement of a stent lumen cross-sectional area of 60% of the average of the proximal and distal vessel cross-sectional areas (measured at the media). This target criterion was chosen to accommodate compensatory dilatation at the reference sites. If the target lumen size was not reached initially, a larger balloon or higher pressure was employed. The balloon size was chosen close to the distal vessel media-to-media diameter measured by IVUS.
>
> In September 1993, the IVUS criterion was altered (late phase), the goal now being to achieve a stent lumen cross-sectional area equal to or greater than the distal reference lumen cross-sectional area.

This change in technique resulted in a decrease in the balloon-to-artery ratio from 1.3 in the early phase to 1.1 in the late phase ($p < 0.001$) (*Fig. 18.14*).

Although the late loss in MLD was similar in all groups, the net gain was higher (1.6 mm versus 1.1 mm) and the loss index was lower (0.38 versus 0.51) in the early phase of the IVUS-guided group from Milan compared to the angiographically guided group from Hamburg (*Table 18.10*). This resulted in a significantly lower restenosis rate in the early phase (9.2% versus 22.3%; $p = 0.04$) for the IVUS-guided

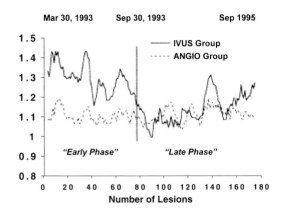

Figure 18.14 *A comparison of the balloon-to-artery ratio used in the early versus late phase of our experience with IVUS guided stenting. Bigger balloons were used initially which resulted in larger cross-sectional areas and a lower restenosis rate but with a slight increase in complications.*

group compared with the angiographically guided group. However, in the late phase, using criteria that resulted in a similar balloon-to-artery ratio, the restenosis rate was similar between IVUS and angiographic guidance (22.7% versus 23.7%).

The balloon size was altered in September 1993 because of an increased incidence of vessel rupture (3%) with the oversized balloons (*Table 18.11*). However, these complications occurred in a low percentage of cases in which the balloon was significantly larger than the distal reference media-to-media diameter. In Milan, a more aggressive dilation strategy for stent optimization was used in the early phase than in the late phase, with final balloon size selected to match the IVUS average proximal and distal vessel media-to-media diameter. This resulted in an (angiographically) oversized choice of balloon. This strategy was initially used to maximize protection against stent thrombosis in our early experience of patients who were undergoing stent implantation without subsequent anticoagulation. Although this

Table 18.10

Comparison of quantitative angiographic and intravascular ultrasound (IVUS) results of the matched lesions in the IVUS (Milan) and angiography (Hamburg) groups during the early and late phases of the Milan experience

	Early phase (n = 76)		Late phase (n = 97)	
	IVUS group	*Angiography group*	*IVUS group*	*Angiography group*
Reference vessel diameter (mm)	3.04 ± 0.34	3.01 ± 3.0	3.00 ± 0.35	2.96 ± 0.34
Minimum lumen diameter (mm)				
Pre	0.80 ± 0.34	0.80 ± 0.33	0.80 ± 0.36	0.79 ± 0.35
Post	3.43 ± 0.48	2.95 ± 0.45	3.10 ± 0.40	2.85 ± 0.38
Follow-up	2.41 ± 0.77	1.85 ± 0.71	2.06 ± 0.87	1.85 ± 0.81
No. of pts c̄ % DS at F/U > 50%	7/76	17/76	22/97	23/97
Final balloon size (mm)	3.93 ± 0.44	3.32 ± 0.30	3.40 ± 0.39	3.29 ± 0.33
Range	(3.0–5.0)	(3.0–4.0)	(2.5–4.5)	(3.0–4.5)
Final balloon/artery ratio	1.30 ± 0.15	1.11 ± 0.11	1.14 ± 0.15	1.12 ± 0.10
Maximal inflation pressure (atm)	14.6 ± 2.9	17.11 ± 1.94	16.3 ± 2.9	16.8 ± 1.56
	(9–20)	(10–20)	(8–20)	(12–20)
Difference in MLD				
Acute gain (mm)	2.62 ± 0.57	2.15 ± 0.57	2.29 ± 0.54	2.06 ± 0.51
Relative gain	0.84 ± 0.16	0.71 ± 0.16	0.76 ± 0.16	0.69 ± 0.14
Late loss (mm)	1.01 ± 0.77	1.10 ± 0.80	1.04 ± 0.85	1.00 ± 0.70
Relative loss	0.33 ± 0.26	0.36 ± 0.24	0.35 ± 0.29	0.34 ± 0.26
Net gain	1.61 ± 0.79	1.05 ± 0.70	1.25 ± 0.90	1.06 ± 0.87
Net gain index	0.53 ± 0.27	0.35 ± 0.23	0.41 ± 0.30	0.35 ± 0.29
Loss index	0.38 ± 0.30	0.51 ± 0.31	0.46 ± 0.39	0.51 ± 0.38

Pre = before stent implantation; Post = after intervention; F/U = at 6-month follow-up; pts = patients; % DS = percent diameter stenosis.

Table 18.11

Comparison of in-hospital (< 24 hours) and post-discharge events in the patients in the intravascular ultrasound (IVUS) (Milan) and angiography (Hamburg) groups

	IVUS group (n = 158) n (%)	Angiography group (n = 154) n (%)	p value
Stent thrombosis	0	0	–
Q-wave MI			
In-hospital (< 24 h)	1 (0.6)	0	.99
Post-discharge	2 (1.3)	0	–
Non-Q-wave MI			
In-hospital (< 24 h)	2 (1.3)	0	.49
Post-discharge	0	0	–
CABG			
In-hospital (< 24 h)	0	0	–
Post-discharge	3 (1.9)	0	–
Repeat PTCA intervention	8 (5.1)	18 (11.6)	.05
Death	0	0	
Acute vascular complications	2 (1.3)	1 (0.6)	–

CABG = coronary artery bypass graft; F/Up = follow-up

strategy was protective against stent thrombosis, in this phase a higher procedural complication rate with a higher incidence of intracoronary vessel rupture was observed; this was possibly related to the use of compliant balloons.

In the late phase, with the experience gained from IVUS imaging together with an evaluation of the clinical results, the final balloons selected were smaller than in the early phase, with a size slightly larger than the IVUS lumen diameters (not angiographically oversized), and higher pressures were used to provide adequate expansion within the stented segment. This adjustment in the balloon dilation strategy resulted in a lower intraprocedural complication rate without increasing the incidence of stent thrombosis. In Hamburg, the balloon dilation strategy did not change over time: balloon size was selected to match the angiographic lumen diameter.

These results indicate that restenosis can be reduced by achieving as large an MLD as possible and that IVUS guidance is better than angiographic guidance in achieving this goal. Angiography underestimates the extent of atherosclerotic disease in coronary arteries that undergo compensatory enlargement,[18,19] thus leading to underestimation of the size of the final balloon that can be selected to expand the stent safely and to maximize the stent lumen cross-sectional area. The use of IVUS guidance allows one to oversize the balloon (compared to angiography) and to obtain a larger final MLD than would be achieved by inflating a smaller balloon at higher pressure. The operator should avoid choosing a balloon that is larger than the vessel diameter even when it is not possible to obtain an adequate stent lumen cross-sectional area, because this strategy increases the risk of vessel rupture, especially in hard, fibrocalcific lesions. In these resistant lesions, plaque pre-treatment with rotational atherectomy is a better strategy than trying to use force to overcome the lesion with a bigger balloon inflated at high pressure.

THE CRUISE STUDY: A RANDOMIZED TRIAL OF IVUS GUIDANCE

In addition to our own data and the comparison with the group from Hamburg, there are few randomized trials of IVUS guidance for coronary artery stenting. The initial results from the CRUISE (Can Routine Ultrasound Influence Stent Expansion?) study, which was a substudy of the STARS (Stent Anticoagulation Restenosis Study) trial, were reported in March 1998.[20] This substudy included 299 randomized patients who received a Palmaz–Schatz stent under angiographic guidance alone versus 270 patients who received a Palmaz–Schatz stent under IVUS guidance. The end-points were angiographic and IVUS dimensions post-stenting, the 30-day primary clinical end-points of major adverse clinical events, and the 9-month incidence of target vessel revascularization. The patients who received IVUS-guided coronary stenting had a 23% greater cross-sectional area (9.6 mm² versus 7.47 mm²) and a 44% lower target vessel revascularization rate than the angiographic guidance group. Target vessel revascularization was 15.3% in the angiography-guided group and 8.5% in the IVUS-guided group. These figures were very similar to those that were obtained in Milan and in the comparison study with the angiographic guidance group from Hamburg.

The combination of the results from these studies encourages us to keep using IVUS guidance to optimize the cross-sectional area during coronary artery stenting with the expectation that the restenosis rate for our patients will be lowered commensurately. In addition, we have learned that longer stents increase the risk of restenosis, and IVUS guidance is exquisitely helpful in identifying the cases in which a stent is necessary and the cases in which excessive metal length can be avoided (see Chapter 20).

REFERENCES

1. Ehrlich S, Honye J, Mahon D et al. Unrecognized stenosis by angiography documented by intravascular ultrasound imaging. *Cathet Cardiovasc Diagn* 1991; **23**: 198–201.

2. Tuzcu EM, Berkalp B, De Franco AC et al. The dilemma of diagnosing coronary calcification: angiography versus intravascular ultrasound. *J Am Coll Cardiol* 1996; **27**: 832–838.

3. Mintz GS, Pichard AD, Popma JJ et al. Determinants and correlates of target lesion calcium in coronary artery disease: a clinical, angiographic and intravascular ultrasound study. *J Am Coll Cardiol* 1997; **29**: 268–274.

4. Moussa I, Moses J, De Gregorio J et al. The discrepancy between quantitative coronary angiography and intravascular ultrasound in determining true vessel size: a homogeneous or a selective phenomenon? *J Am Coll Cardiol* 1999; **33 (suppl A)**: 76A.

5. Tobis JM, Mallery J, Mahon D et al. Intravascular ultrasound imaging of human coronary arteries in vivo. Analysis of tissue characterizations with comparison to in vitro histological specimens. *Circulation* 1991; **83**: 913–926.

6. Pande AK, Tardif JC, Doucet S et al. Intravascular ultrasound for diagnosis of left main coronary artery stenosis. *Can J Cardiol* 1996; **12**: 757–759.

7. Fuster V, Badimon L, Badimon JJ, Chesebro JH. The pathogenesis of coronary artery disease and the acute coronary syndrome (2). *N Engl J Med* 1992; **326**: 310–318.

8. Davies MJ. Pathology of arterial thrombosis. *Br Med Bull* 1994; **50**: 789–802.

9. Falk E, Shah PK, Fuster V. Coronary plaque disruption. *Circulation* 1995; **92**: 657–671.

10. Fuster V. Elucidation of the role of plaque instability and rupture in acute coronary events. *Am J Cardiol* 1995; **76**: 24C–33C.

11. Teirstein PS, Schatz RA, DeNardo SJ et al. Angioscopic versus angiographic detection of thrombus during coronary interventional procedures. *Am J Cardiol* 1995; **75**: 1083–1087.

12. Hamburger JN, Serruys PW. Treatment of thrombus containing lesions in diseased native coronary arteries and saphenous vein bypass grafts using the AngioJet Rapid Thrombectomy System. *Herz* 1997; **22**: 318–321.

13. Nakamura S, Colombo A, Gaglione A et al. Intracoronary ultrasound observations during stent implantation. *Circulation* 1994; **89**: 2026–2034.

14. Goldberg SL, Colombo A, Nakamura S et al. Benefit of intracoronary ultrasound in the deployment of Palmaz–Schatz stents. *J Am Coll Cardiol* 1994; **24**: 996–1003.

15. Di Mario C, Akiyama T, Moussa I et al. First experience with imaging core wires. *Semin Interv Cardiol* 1997; **2**: 69–73.

16. Kastrati A, Schuhlen H, Hausleiter J et al. Restenosis after coronary stent placement and randomization to a 4-week combined antiplatelet or anticoagulant therapy: six-month angiographic follow-up of the Intracoronary Stenting and Antithrombotic Regimen (ISAR) Trial. *Circulation* 1997; **96**: 462–467.

17. Albiero R, Rau T, Schluter M et al. Comparison of immediate and intermediate-term results of intravascular ultrasound versus angiography-guided Palmaz–Schatz stent implantation in matched lesions. *Circulation* 1997; **96**: 2997–3005.

18. Mintz GS, Painter JA, Pichard AD et al. Atherosclerosis in angiographically 'normal' coronary artery reference segments: an intravascular ultrasound study with clinical correlations. *J Am Coll Cardiol* 1995; **25**: 1479–1485.

19. Moussa I, Moses J, De Gregorio J et al. Effects of arterial remodelling on the degree of discrepancy between quantitative coronary angiography and ultrasound imaging in determining true vessel dimensions. *J Am Coll Cardiol* 1999; **33**: 78A.

16. Hayase M, Oshima A, Cleman M et al. Relation between target vessel revascularization and minimum stent area by intravascular ultrasound (CRUISE Trial). *J Am Coll Cardiol* 1998; **31**: 386A.

Chapter 19 Debulking: removal of plaque prior to stenting

Issam Moussa, Jeffrey Moses and Antonio Colombo

PLAQUE BURDEN IS AN IMPORTANT PREDICTOR OF NEOINTIMAL HYPERPLASIA DEVELOPMENT

Prospective randomized clinical trials have demonstrated the superiority of coronary stents in reducing angiographic restenosis and clinical events compared to percutaneous transluminal coronary angioplasty (PTCA) in focal de novo lesions in native coronary arteries.[1,2,3] However, restenosis remains a problem when stents are implanted in complex lesion subsets such as long lesions,[4] ostial lesions,[5,6,7] chronic total occlusions,[8,9,10] and bifurcational lesions.[11] Restenosis after implantation of slotted tube stents occurs mainly as a result of neointimal proliferation.[12] It has been postulated that the degree of neointimal hyperplasia after stenting is stimulated by the degree of vessel wall stretch.[13] The stretching force needed to expand the vessel is proportional to the vessel wall resistance, which depends on the amount and the consistency of the plaque. Therefore, it is likely that the maximal stretching force needs to be applied where the plaque volume is largest in order to achieve an adequate lumen gain. Theoretically, this stretching effect could lead to more neointimal hyperplasia at the original stenosis site.

Preliminary experimental data in animal models[14] support this concept. In humans, observational intravascular ultrasound (IVUS) data[15,16] indicate that a larger pre-intervention plaque burden leads to a higher rate of late lumen loss after stenting. In addition, angiographic data[17] indicate that, after stent implantation, restenosis tends to occur at the original lesion site (where the plaque burden is largest). On the basis of these observations, we propose that removal of atherosclerotic plaque prior to stenting may lead to a reduction in neointimal hyperplasia, therefore reducing the incidence of restenosis.

MORE AGGRESSIVE PLAQUE REMOVAL WITH DIRECTIONAL ATHERECTOMY HAS LED TO AN IMPROVEMENT IN OUTCOME BUT THE RESTENOSIS RATE REMAINS HIGH

The efficacy of interventional devices in excising the atherosclerotic plaque depends primarily on whether the plaque is non-calcified or calcified. Directional coronary atherectomy (DCA) using the Simpson Coronary AtheroCath (Devices for Vascular Interventions, Temecula, California, USA) has been shown to be the most effective technique for removing fibrotic non-calcified plaque,[18] thus transforming the atherosclerotic arterial wall to a more elastic structure that is more amenable to dilatation.[19] Despite the reduction in restenosis with 'optimal' directional atherectomy compared to PTCA, the restenosis rate remains at 30% with no difference in the need for repeat revascularization at 1-year follow-up.[20]

ROTATIONAL ATHERECTOMY IS A VALUABLE TECHNIQUE FOR REMOVING CALCIFIED PLAQUE; ALTHOUGH WHEN USED AS A STAND-ALONE STRATEGY IT IS STILL ASSOCIATED WITH A HIGH RESTENOSIS RATE

Rotational atherectomy, as compared with directional atherectomy, has been shown to be the preferred strategy for ablating calcified plaque.[21] Despite the high procedural success rate, significant restenosis rates of 37–57% have been observed after stand-alone rotational atherectomy.[22,23] A recent histopathologic study demonstrated that the presence of calcium is a powerful predictor of the amount of plaque burden in atherosclerotic arteries.[24] In addition, in vivo IVUS studies have demonstrated that coronary calcium is an important determinant of decreased wall compliance,[25] and leads to a high incidence of dissections when these lesions are dilated[26] and a high rate of suboptimal expansion when stents are used.[27]

Therefore, the failure of stand-alone debulking or stand-alone stenting to reduce restenosis in complex lesion subsets[28,29] highlights the need to explore the synergistic role of combining both techniques to reduce restenosis. This chapter reviews the available relevant data and the potential clinical implications.

DCA BEFORE STENT IMPLANTATION

To examine the feasibility, safety, and efficacy of DCA before stent implantation we conducted a pilot prospective registry between February 1996 and January 1998. A total of 128 patients with 168 lesions were enrolled. Inclusion criteria were:

(a) clinical or functional evidence of ischemia;
(b) no myocardial infarction (MI) within 48 hours;
(c) reference diameter ≥ 2.75 mm;
(d) diameter stenosis > 70 %; and
(e) lesion length > 15 mm by visual estimate.

Ostial and bifurcational lesions were considered for enrollment regardless of vessel size and lesion length. Restenotic lesions and chronic total occlusions were also included. Directional atherectomy was performed using methods previously described.[18] The end-point of the atherectomy procedure was to achieve a < 20% residual diameter stenosis by visual estimate. A 7 Fr GTO cutter was used in 96% of lesions with an average of 14 ± 7 cuts per lesion. Coronary stenting was performed with the goal of achieving a near-zero angiographic residual stenosis. Only slotted tube stents were used:

(a) the Multilink stent (15 mm, 25 mm) (Advanced Cardiovascular Systems Inc., Temecula, California, USA) was used in 51 lesions (30%);
(b) the Palmaz–Schatz stent (Johnson and Johnson

Table 19.1
Patient and lesion characteristics

Patients	*n = 128*
Age	58 ± 10
Male	118 (92%)
Smoking (past or current)	77 (60%)
Hypertension	53 (41%)
Diabetes mellitus	10 (8%)
Hyperlipidemia	74 (58%)
Prior MI	54 (42%)
Unstable angina	23 (18%)
LVEF	61 ± 11%
Number of vessels diseased	
1 vessel	60 (47%)
2 vessels	31 (24%)
3 vessels	37 (29%)
Lesions	n = 168
Artery treated	
Left anterior descending	102 (61%)
Left circumflex	27 (16%)
Right coronary	32 (19%)
Left main	7 (4%)
Lesion location	
Ostial	26 (15%)
Proximal	72 (43%)
Mid-artery	55 (33%)
Distal	15 (9%)
Lesion type	
A	1 (0.6%)
B1	34 (20%)
B2	97 (58%)
C	36 (21.4%)
Chronic total occlusion	13 (8%)
Major bifurcations	40 (23%)
Restenotic lesions	18 (11%)

Interventional Systems, Warren, New Jersey, USA) in 45 lesions (27%);
(c) the NIR stent (16 mm, 19 mm, 25 mm, 32 mm) (SciMed Inc., Minneapolis, Minnesota, USA) in 26 lesions (15%); and
(d) other slotted tube stents in 46 lesions (28%).

The AVE Microstent (18 mm, 24 mm, 39 mm) (Arterial Vascular Engineering, Santa Rosa, California, USA) was used in situations were other stents could not be

Table 19.2
Quantitative angiographic and intravascular ultrasound measurements.

	Pre-intervention	Post DCA	Post Stenting
Angiographic measurements	n = 168	n = 168	n = 168
Reference diameter (mm)	3.25 ± 0.54 (*3.18 ± 0.50)	3.37 ± 0.50	3.50 ± 0.57
Minimum lumen diameter (mm)	0.84 ± 0.48	2.42 ± 0.64	3.51 ± 0.53
Percentage diameter stenosis	74 ± 14	28 ± 16	0.04 ± 9
Lesion length (mm)	12.80 ± 7.66 (*13.8 ± 7.6)	–	–
Stent length (mm)	–	–	22 ± 13
IVUS measurements	n = 100	n = 116	n = 142
Minimum lumen cross-sectional area (mm²)	2.57 ± 1.07	6.59 ± 2.08	8.85 ± 2.15
Vessel cross-sectional area (mm²)	13.23 ± 4.12	14.88 ± 4.24	–
Percentage plaque area	80 ± 7	54 ± 14	–

* Ostial lesions excluded.

delivered. IVUS guidance was used in a subset of patients before intervention, after DCA, and after stenting. All patients were discharged on oral aspirin (325 mg qid) and oral ticlopidine (250 mg bid) for 2 weeks. Clinical follow-up was obtained in all patients at 1 month and 1 year after the procedure.

RESULTS

The patients' clinical profile and baseline angiographic characteristics are shown in *Table 19.1*. IVUS-guided stent implantation was used in 95% of lesions. Stents were expanded using a balloon-to-artery ratio of 1.19 ± 0.16 and an inflation pressure of 16 ± 4 atmospheres. The quantitative angiographic and IVUS measurements are shown in *Table 19.2*. Mean residual percentage plaque area after DCA was 54 ± 14 %, but about 30% of lesions had a residual percentage plaque area > 60% (*Fig. 19.1*). Clinical success was achieved in 96% of patients.

Major procedural and in-hospital complications occurred in four patients (3.2%): emergency bypass surgery was required in two patients (1.6%), both of whom died during hospitalization; and two other patients (1.6%) had non-fatal Q-wave MI. Non-Q-wave MI occurred in 17 patients (13.3%). No other events had occurred by 1-month follow-up.

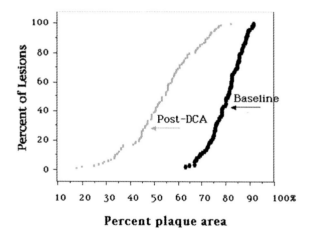

Figure 19.1 *Frequency distribution curves for percentage plaque area pre-intervention and after directional coronary atherectomy (DCA).*

Angiographic follow-up was performed in 132 out of 164 eligible lesions (80%) at 5.3 ± 1.4 months. Binary angiographic restenosis occurred in 18 lesions (13.6%): intrastent in 11 lesions (8.3%), and at stent borders in seven lesions (5.3%). The majority of these restenotic lesions were focal and only 14 lesions (8%) needed repeat intervention (PTCA in 13 patients and coronary artery bypass grafts in one patient) at long-term follow-up (12 ± 5 months). The cumulative composite end-point of major adverse cardiac events (MACE) (death, non-fatal Q-wave MI, and repeat revascularization) occurred in 18 patients (14%).

IS THE COMBINATION OF DCA AND STENTING SAFE?

When an alternative approach is proposed to improve clinical outcome after catheter-based coronary interventions, safety has to be established first. In this study, a major adverse clinical event occurred in four patients (3.2%) in the first 30 days after intervention. This is not significantly different from what has been reported in clinical trials using stent alone or DCA alone in a more selected patient population. In the Stress Restenosis Study (STRESS) trial,[2] MACE at 1 month post-intervention occurred in 4.9% of patients (Q-wave MI in 2.9% of patients and emergency bypass surgery in 2% of patients). In the OARS[18] and BOAT[20] optimal atherectomy trials, MACE occurred in 2.5% and 2.8%, respectively. When comparing these data with the current study, it must be recalled that we primarily included high-risk lesions such as long lesions, ostial lesions, and bifurcational lesions. It appears that combining atherectomy and stenting does not increase the major procedural complications that are encountered with either procedure alone.

The high incidence of non-Q-wave MI remains a concern. In this study, non-Q-wave MI occurred in 13.3% of patients, which is similar to what has been reported in both the OARS trial[18] (14%) and the BOAT trial[20] (16%). However, the impact of non-Q-wave MI following an otherwise successful procedure on long-term outcome is still the subject of ongoing investigation. Cutlip and colleagues[30] recently reported the results of a prospective, randomized multicenter data set of 3,387 patients treated with various interventional devices, pooled from the BOAT, STARS, and Study To Determine Rotablator And Transluminal Angioplasty Strategy (STRATAS) trials. In this analysis, the authors found no association between cardiac enzyme elevation and mortality at 1-year follow-up. On the other hand, Simoons and colleagues[31] also reported the results of a prospective, randomized multicenter data set of 4,762 patients pooled from the Chimeric c7E3 Antiplatelet Therapy in Unstable REfractory angina (CAPTURE), Evaluation of 7E3 for the Prevention of Ischemic Complications (EPIC), and

Evaluation in PTCA to Improve Long-Term Outcome with abciximab GPIIb/IIIa blockade (EPILOG) trials. In this analysis, the authors found an association between the degree of rise in creatine kinase MB isoenzyme levels and mortality at 6-month follow-up. Furthermore, in a subset analysis of the EPIC trial[32] the use of the IIb–IIIa receptor antagonist abciximab was shown to reduce the incidence of non-Q-wave MI in patients undergoing directional atherectomy from 15.4% in the placebo arm to 4.5% in the abciximab arm. No conclusions can be drawn from the present study with respect to the effect of abciximab on the incidence of MI with debulking before stenting since this agent was not used in this cohort. However, the majority of patients who developed MI in our study underwent aggressive debulking for several lesions in the same procedure. Perhaps the use of GPIIb-IIIa receptor antagonists may be of benefit when aggressive debulking is anticipated.

Our conclusion from the analysis of our experience is that directional atherectomy before stent implantation does not increase the incidence of major procedural complications. However, similar to DCA alone, this combined technique results in a high rate of non-Q-wave MI. Two strategies may decrease the frequency of non-Q-wave MI:

(a) the use of IIb–IIIa platelet receptor antagonists; and
(b) not treating more than one lesion in a given procedure to decrease the amount of potential embolic material.

DOES DIRECTIONAL ATHERECTOMY BEFORE STENT IMPLANTATION LOWER THE INCIDENCE OF ANGIOGRAPHIC RESTENOSIS AND THE NEED FOR REPEAT INTERVENTIONS?

In the absence of a control arm of patients who had stent implantation without prior atherectomy, matching study patients with reference patients with similar characteristics may compensate for some of the limitations of a non-randomized study. Matching was performed with respect to presence of diabetes mellitus, previous PTCA, reference vessel diameter, lesion length, lesion severity, type of stent, and total length of stents implanted. All the 132 lesions from the study group with angiographic follow-up were matched

Table 19.3

A matched group comparison of stenting after directional coronary atherectomy (DCA) versus stenting alone

	DCA plus stenting n = 132	Stenting alone n = 132	p value
Baseline measurements			
Reference diameter (mm)	3.22 ± 0.53	3.21 ± 0.35	NS
Minimum lumen diameter (mm)	0.83 ± 0.47	0.76 ± 0.34	NS
Percentage diameter stenosis	74 ± 13	76 ± 11	NS
Lesion length (mm)	12.34 ± 7.35	12.28 ± 5.93	NS
Post-intervention measurements			
Reference diameter (mm)	3.48 ± 0.52	3.27 ± 0.38	0.001
Minimum lumen diameter (mm)	3.47 ± 0.57	3.28 ± 0.48	0.003
Percentage diameter stenosis	−0.1 ± 10	−0.6 ± 12	NS
Stent length (mm)	21 ± 10	22 ± 11	NS
Follow-up measurements			
Reference diameter (mm)	3.21 ± 0.48	3.07 ± 0.50	0.02
Minimum lumen diameter (mm)	2.43 ± 0.92	2.09 ± 0.86	0.002
Percentage diameter stenosis	25 ± 25	32 ± 25	0.02
Loss index	0.39 ± 0.35	0.48 ± 0.35	0.04
Restenosis (%)	18 (13.6%)	31 (23.5%)	0.04
Focal in-stent	5 (3.8%)	11 (11.4%)	
Focal edge	7 (5.3%)	2 (1.5%)	
Diffuse	3 (2.3%)	10 (7.6%)	
Reocclusion	3 (2.3%)	4 (3%)	

Table 19.4

Predictors of restenosis by multivariate logistic regression analysis

Study population	Variable	B coefficient ± SE	p value
DCA plus stent group (n = 64)	Residual percentage plaque area post-DCA	8.52 ± 3.88	0.03
	Intrastent MLCSA	−0.50 ± 0.29	0.08
DCA plus stent group and stent alone group (n = 264)	Stent length	0.05 ± 0.02	0.0003
	DCA performed	−0.35 ± 0.17	0.047

* Only patients who had post-DCA and post-stent IVUS and who returned for angiographic follow-up are included.
† All lesions in the study group and the control arm are included.
MLCSA = minimum lumen cross-sectional area.

with 132 lesions in patients who underwent stenting alone (*Table 19.3*). The directional atherectomy plus stent group had a loss index of 0.39 ± 0.35, which was significantly lower than the loss index in the stent alone group (0.48 ± 0.35; *p* = 0.04). This equated to a restenosis rate of 13.6% in the atherectomy plus stent group compared with 23.5% in the stent alone group (*p* = 0.04).

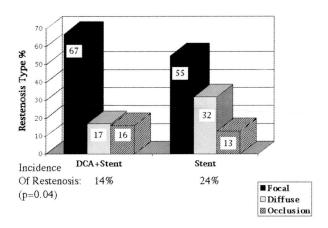

Figure 19.2 *Difference in restenosis type between the atherectomy plus stent group and the control arm (stent alone group).*

The role of debulking in reducing restenosis was shown to be independent of other factors as determined by a multivariate logistic regression analysis (*Table 19.4*). In the combined population of 264 lesions, the only independent predictors of restenosis were stent length and the use of DCA. The performance of DCA predicted a lower probability of restenosis, and stent length predicted a higher probability of restenosis. Other common variables, such as reference diameter, final minimum luminal diameter (MLD), or lesion length, were not independent predictors of restenosis. Notably, in the atherectomy plus stent group not only was the incidence of restenosis lower but the restenotic lesions were also more often focal and more often outside the stented segment (*Fig. 19.2*).

The lower late lumen loss in the DCA plus stent group is also illustrated in *Fig. 19.3*. In this figure, the frequency distribution curves after DCA and at follow-up almost overlap both for MLD and percentage diameter stenosis. In other words, it appears that stent placement after plaque removal may 'conserve' the lumen gain achieved with debulking.

It is difficult to perform a meaningful comparison between the current study and the randomized trials that test the efficacy of stents alone because these trials have traditionally included patients with short lesions and excluded patients with total occlusions, restenotic, ostial, and bifurcational lesions. Instead, it may be more meaningful to compare the current study to other retrospective series with heterogeneous patient populations. In vessels < 3.25 mm, Mehran and colleagues[33] reported a target lesion revascularization (TLR) rate of 22% after stenting lesions 10–15 mm long and a TLR rate of 28% in lesions longer than 15 mm. However, TLR was 14% in lesions longer than 10 mm in vessels > 3.25 mm. Kornowsky and colleagues[34] reported on the clinical outcome of patients who had stent implantation in 3.25 mm vessels. In that study, TLR varied according to whether lesions were de novo or restenotic (14% versus 23%, respectively). In the present study, repeat intervention during the first year after the index procedure (DCA plus stent) was needed only in 8% of lesions.

These findings strongly suggest that plaque removal before stenting attenuates the intensity of neointimal hyperplasia traditionally encountered with coronary stenting alone. This is better illustrated in *Fig. 19.4*, where it appears that for every given amount of acute gain there is less late lumen loss (neointimal hyperplasia) when atherectomy is used before stenting

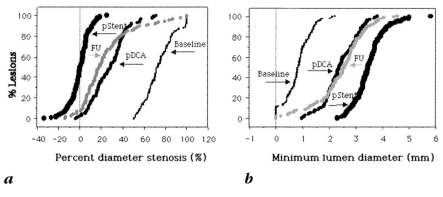

Conservation of lumen gain achieved by stenting after DCA

Figure 19.3 *(a) Frequency distribution curves for angiographic percentage diameter stenosis pre-intervention, after DCA (pDCA), after stenting (pStent), and at follow-up. (FU). (b) Frequency distribution curves for angiographic minimum lumen diameter (MLD) pre-intervention, after directional coronary atherectomy (DCA), after stenting, and at follow-up. Note that the curves for MLD and percentage diameter stenosis at follow-up overlap those after atherectomy for the majority of lesions.*

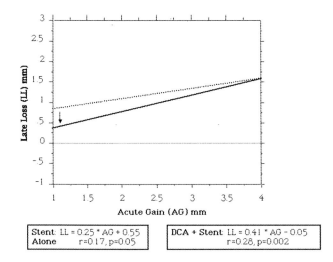

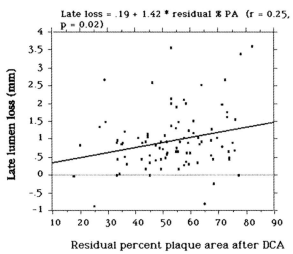

Figure 19.4 *Simple linear regression lines of late loss (LL) plotted versus acute gain (AG) for the atherectomy stent group (solid line) and the stent alone group (dotted line). Note the downward shift in the regression line.*

Figure 19.5 *Simple linear regression of late lumen loss after stent placement versus residual percentage plaque area (PA) after directional coronary atherectomy (DCA). Note that the larger the residual plaque burden is before stent implantaion, the higher the late lumen loss is at follow-up.*

(note the downward shift in the regression line). However, the regression lines converge and intersect when large acute lumen gain is achieved. This may suggest that in vessels in which large acute lumen gain can be achieved with stenting alone, such as large vessels, the addition of DCA might be of less benefit. Alternatively, perhaps more plaque removal in these lesions might have maintained the favorable balance between acute gain and late loss. These observational data support the hypothesis that directional atherectomy before stent implantation reduces late lumen loss, with subsequent reduction in restenosis and the need for repeat interventions

These findings are in accordance with another report on the use of DCA before stenting in different lesion subsets. Keitz and colleagues[35] reported on 44 patients treated with DCA before stenting using the Palmaz–Schatz stent. A total of 51 stents were deployed in 47 vessels. Aorto-ostial lesions were present in 14 patients (32%). The diameter stenosis increased from 73.6 ± 9.6% at baseline to 30.7 ± 13.6% after DCA and to –8.2 ± 12.6% after stenting. Bramucci and colleagues[36] reported on 68 patients (71 lesions) who underwent DCA before elective Palmaz–Schatz stent implantation. This cohort included focal lesions that required a single Palmaz–Schatz stent. Similar to our series, at 6-month follow-up, TLR was needed in only 7% of patients.

WHY SHOULD PLAQUE REMOVAL BEFORE STENT IMPLANTATION REDUCE RESTENOSIS?

It has been previously demonstrated that restenosis after coronary stent implantation is a multifactorial process in which patient, lesion, and post-procedural factors[37,38] interact to produce a given outcome. To understand the role of plaque removal in this complex process we matched the lesions for known clinical, angiographic, and procedural factors between the DCA plus stent group and the stent alone group. Despite matching for baseline characteristics, the post-procedure lumen dimensions were significantly larger in the DCA plus stent group. This is theoretically expected since plaque removal facilitates stent expansion, which in turn would translate into larger lumen gain. Restenosis was significantly lower in the DCA plus stent group.

An important question arises: Is the lower restenosis rate in the atherectomy plus stent group entirely due to the acute lumen gain achieved or is it also due to the attenuation of late lumen loss because of plaque removal? To answer this question we performed multivariate logistic regression analysis in the group of patients that had IVUS interrogation post-DCA and post-stenting and who returned for angiographic follow-up (see *Table 19.4*). In this model, only a lower residual plaque burden after DCA and a larger lumen area after stenting predicted a lower probability of restenosis. A larger lumen area after stenting had only a trend ($p = 0.08$) towards predicting a lower probability of restenosis. Interestingly, the influence of residual plaque burden after DCA (before stent implantation) on the probability of restenosis was more prominent than that of post-procedure lumen cross-sectional area. *Figure 19.5* further illustrates the positive linear relationship between residual plaque burden after DCA and late lumen loss despite placing a stent after atherectomy. These findings add further support to the concept that the residual plaque burden after catheter-based coronary interventions[15,16,39,40] is a risk factor for restenosis. Furthermore, plaque removal before stent implantation reduces restenosis in proportion to the amount of plaque removed. DCA before stent implantation reduces restenosis by two mechanisms:

(a) facilitating stent expansion, thus leading to a large post-procedure lumen; and
(b) more importantly, reducing the propensity for late neointimal hyperplasia; this effect is proportional to the magnitude of plaque removal.

ROTATIONAL ATHERECTOMY BEFORE STENT IMPLANTATION IN CALCIFIED AND UNDILATABLE LESIONS

Elective use of stents in calcified lesions was not extensively applied initially, owing to the concern that the stent could not be fully expanded because of lesion rigidity. When coronary stenting was applied to calcified arteries, an incomplete and asymmetrical expansion occurred in up to 50% of patients.[27] Even balloon pressures exceeding 20 atmospheres may be insufficient to overcome the vessel wall resistance imposed by a severely calcified plaque. In addition, attempts to obtain full expansion of a stent may cause vessel rupture instead of further enlarging the stent.[41] An alternative to using larger balloons with greater force is to use rotational atherectomy to reduce the calcified plaque burden.

To examine the role of rotational atherectomy before stenting in the treatment of calcified or undilatable lesions, we studied 75 consecutive patients with 106 lesions who underwent this combined approach between March 1993 and June

1995.[42] Calcified, uncrossable or undilatable lesions were present in 90% of cases and lesions > 15 mm were present in 10% of cases. The majority of patients had IVUS-guided stenting followed by oral antiplatelet therapy. Procedural success was achieved in 93% of lesions. Acute stent thrombosis occurred in two lesions (1.9%) and subacute stent thrombosis occurred in one lesion (0.9%). Angiographic follow-up was performed in 83% of lesions at 4.6 ± 1.9 months with an angiographic restenosis rate of 22.5%. Clinical follow-up was performed in all patients at 6.4 ± 3 months.

TLR was needed in 18% of lesions. In this study, we performed a comparative analysis between calcified lesions that underwent elective Palmaz–Schatz stenting with and without rotablation over the same time period. The stent alone approach without rotational atherectomy was used for shorter lesions in larger vessels (*Table 19.5*). After adjusting for vessel size, the rotational atherectomy plus stenting group had a lower residual angiographic percentage diameter stenosis and higher ratio of minimum stent cross-sectional area to vessel cross–sectional area and a higher symmetry index. In addition, three out of 41 patients (7%) in the stent alone group had to undergo emergency bypass surgery because of occlusive dissections after stenting.

The role of rotablation prior to stenting in calcified lesions has also been studied by other investigators. Comparing calcified lesions in vessels > 3.0 mm treated with rotational atherectomy and stenting to lesions treated with rotational atherectomy alone or stenting alone, Hoffmann and colleagues[43] showed a greater acute lumen gain (2.17 ± 0.60, 1.12 ± 0.61 and 1.81 ± 0.66 mm, respectively; $p < 0.01$) and a lower TLR in lesions treated with rotational atherectomy and stenting (12.2%, 31.6%, and 24.5% respectively; $p < 0.05$).

Several observational studies demonstrate that when the culprit lesion is calcified or undilatable, the performance of rotational atherectomy facilitates stent deployment and expansion, which may have a positive impact on late outcome. However, it remains unclear whether more aggressive debulking would yield superior long-term results. Using rotational atherectomy alone, Kaplan and colleagues[44] showed a higher TLR rate with burr-to-vessel ratio < 0.6 or > 0.85 after rotational atherectomy. They explained their results by stating that the significant undersizing of the burr might not ablate enough plaque or calcium to allow effective balloon expansion during adjunctive angioplasty. Alternatively, significant burr oversizing might increase the risk of vessel dissection or increase the stimulus for smooth muscle cell

Table 19.5

A comparison between elective Palmaz–Schatz stenting alone versus Palmaz–Schatz stenting after rotablation for calcified lesions

Lesions	Rotablation + stent (n = 71)	Stent alone n = 46	p value
Angiographic measurements			
Proximal reference diameter (mm)	3.24 ± 0.51	3.50 ± 0.61	0.01
Post-procedure MLD (mm)	3.25 ± 0.55	3.29 ± 0.58	NS
Post-procedure percentage diameter stenosis	−3 ± 13	2 ± 10	0.03
IVUS measurements *			
Stent minimum lumen cross-sectional area (mm²)	7.60 ± 1.94	8.25 ± 2.07	NS
Symmetry index	0.87 ± 0.11	0.83 ± 0.09	0.05
Average reference vessel cross-sectional area (mm²)	11.18 ± 3.96	15.14 ± 4.78	<0.0001
Ratio of stent minimum lumen cross-sectional area to vessel cross-sectional area	0.71 ± 0.32	0.57 ± 0.32	0.03
Procedural data			
Stents per lesion	1.9 ± 1.1	1.3 ± 0.9	0.003
Balloon-to-vessel ratio	1.15 ± 0.18	1.11 ± 0.17	NS
Balloon inflation pressure (atmospheres)	16 ± 3	15 ± 3	NS

* IVUS performed in 65 lesions in the rotastent group and 43 lesions in the stent alone group; values are presented as mean±standard deviation.

proliferation, leading to an increased restenosis rate. However, no comparable data are available when rotablation is followed by stent implantation.

In an attempt to address the issue of whether aggressive debulking improves long-term outcome, we evaluated the short-term and long-term outcome of 126 consecutive patients (162 lesions) who underwent stenting following rotational atherectomy between May 1995 and February 1997 because of the presence of severe calcification on fluoroscopy or IVUS (95%). All the lesions were type B2 or type C, and 39% were longer than 15 mm, necessitating a long stent or multiple stents. Lesions were divided into two groups:

(a) Group 1 (56 lesions), in which aggressive rotational atherectomy was performed (defined as the use of a final burr size ≥ 2.25 mm and/or a final burr-to-vessel ratio ≥ 0.8);
(b) Group 2 (106 lesions), in which less aggressive rotational atherectomy was performed; the objective was to alter vessel wall compliance and allow better balloon expansion.

Most of the patients underwent optimization of stent deployment with high-pressure final balloon dilata-

tion and received oral antiplatelet therapy with ticlopidine and aspirin. Particular attention was paid to patients who had no reflow that did not resolve promptly. In these patients, intra-aortic balloon pumping was initiated or abciximab was used. These may be important adjuncts to prevent subacute stent thrombosis when stenting is performed after rotational atherectomy.[42]

Patients in the aggressive rotational atherectomy group had a higher incidence of procedural Q-wave MI (8.9% versus 1.9%; $p < 0.05$) and non-Q-wave MI (11% versus 1.9%; $p < 0.05$). Although there was no significant difference in MLD after the procedure (3.11 ± 0.68 mm versus 2.99 ± 0.48 mm) between the aggressive and less aggressive group, a greater MLD was observed at follow-up in the lesions treated with aggressive rotational atherectomy (2.12 ± 1.31 mm versus 1.56 ± 0.89 mm; $p < 0.01$). Restenosis rates were 30.9% in the lesions treated with aggressive rotational atherectomy and 50.0% in those treated without aggressive rotational atherectomy ($p < 0.05$). In addition, lesions treated with aggressive rotational atherectomy had a lower incidence of diffuse restenosis than lesions treated with less aggressive rotational atherectomy (9.5% versus 25.0%; $p < 0.05$) despite similar lesion and stent lengths.

THE IMPACT OF THE AGGRESSIVENESS OF ROTABLATION ON ACUTE SAFETY

As with DCA, the incidence of creatine kinase-MB elevation with rotational atherectomy remains a concern. Procedural MI occurred more frequently in lesions treated with aggressive rotational atherectomy. Coronary arteries that are treated with rotational atherectomy have calcification or complex atherosclerotic plaques, or both, and MI has been presumed to be caused by embolic atherosclerotic particles plugging the capillaries.[45] Previous studies[22,23] have shown that the incidence of non-Q-wave MI after rotational atherectomy was 2–5% and that of Q-wave MI was 0–4.8%. In the present study, although rotational atherectomy was performed with a stepped burr approach and particular attention was paid to avoid any drop in rotational speed and long passes, higher incidences of non-Q-wave (11%) and Q-wave (8.9%) myocardial infarction were observed with aggressive rotational atherectomy. This finding may reflect the volume of microparticulate debris produced by aggressive rotational atherectomy. A strategy to limit MI is needed to make this aggressive technique more applicable. It is interesting to speculate that a more liberal prophylactic usage of abciximab might have significantly decreased the occurrence of MI.[46]

In summary, very aggressive rotablation before stent implantation is associated with an unacceptably high incidence of Q-wave MI and should not be used in long lesions or in patients with a low ejection fraction. A potential use for this technique may be in focal severely calcified lesions or in ostial lesions.

DOES AGGRESSIVE ROTABLATION BEFORE STENTING HAVE AN IMPACT ON THE INCIDENCE OF ANGIOGRAPHIC RESTENOSIS?

In the present study, although stenting after aggressive rotational atherectomy reduced the restenosis rate compared to stenting after less aggressive atherectomy, the restenosis rate was still moderately high at 30.9%. The fact that the restenosis rate is lower in the aggressive atherectomy group despite the absence of a difference in the angiographic and IVUS dimensions immediately following stenting may suggest that plaque ablation has a favorable impact on late loss. It is possible that plaque removal may decrease the chronic arterial wall stretch following stent placement, removing a stimulus for intimal hyperplasia. Further large-scale studies, possibly with follow-up IVUS evaluation, may help to clarify this issue. Interestingly, the incidence of diffuse restenosis was significantly lower, at 9.5%, in lesions treated with aggressive rotational atherectomy followed by stenting. Previous studies have shown that the need for repeat interventions after balloon angioplasty of lesions with diffuse restenosis is significantly higher than that of focal restenosis.[47] Therefore, even though a number of lesions treated with aggressive rotational atherectomy followed by stenting needed a subsequent intervention, a second recurrence is probably less likely because the restenotic lesions are frequently focal and therefore more amenable to treatment by PTCA.

Unlike the negative impact on procedural safety, aggressive rotablation may lead to a reduction in late lumen loss after stent implantation. A challenge for the future would be to design an interventional device that is able to ablate calcium with a lower rate of embolization.

CASE STUDIES

CASE 1

A 62-year-old man who was an active smoker and had a history of hypertension and hyperlipidemia presented with progressive exertional angina. Coronary angiography demonstrated the presence of two obstructive lesions in the distal segment of the right coronary artery (RCA) and the proximal segment of the left anterior artery (LAD).

Figure 19.6a shows the distal RCA lesion located at the bifurcation of the posterior descending artery (PDA) and the posterolateral (PL) branch. The interpolated reference diameter on quantitative coronary angiography was 2.87 mm (towards the PDA) and 2.88 mm (towards the PL branch). Two high-support coronary wires were used to cannulate both the PDA and the PL branches. DCA was then performed using a 7 Fr GTO cutter towards the PDA and the PL branch (*Fig. 19.6b*). Two Multilink ACS stents were implanted at the bifurcation and both stents were expanded simultaneously using the 'kissing balloon' technique (balloon diameter 3.5 mm inflated to 10 atmospheres in both branches). The final result is shown in *Fig. 19.6c*.

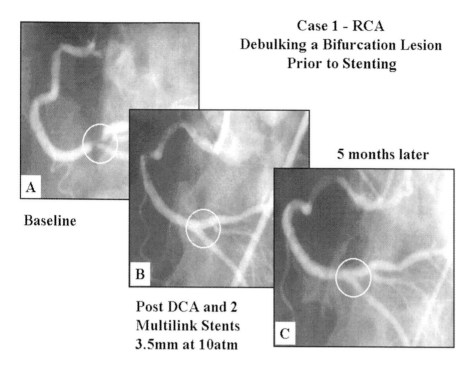

**Case 1 - RCA
Debulking a Bifurcation Lesion
Prior to Stenting**

5 months later

A

Baseline

B

**Post DCA and 2
Multilink Stents
3.5mm at 10atm**

C

Figure 19.6 *(a) Baseline angiogram of the right coronary artery (RCA) shows a bifurcational lesion at the crux. (b) Post-procedure angiogram after directional coronary atherectomy (DCA) and implantation of two Multilink stents in a V-shaped fashion. (c) Coronary angiogram at 5-month follow-up.*

The lesion in the proximal segment of the LAD was calcified on angiography and measured 30 mm in length, with a reference diameter of 2.98 mm (*Fig. 19.7a*). An attempt was made to perform pre-intervention IVUS, but the IVUS catheter could not cross the lesion. The decision was then made to perform rotablation, and an intra-aortic balloon pump was inserted. Rotational atherectomy was performed using a stepped burr approach. The first burr used was 2.0 mm burr followed by a 2.25 mm and then a 2.38 mm burr. IVUS imaging after rotablation showed a large residual plaque burden. Therefore, DCA was

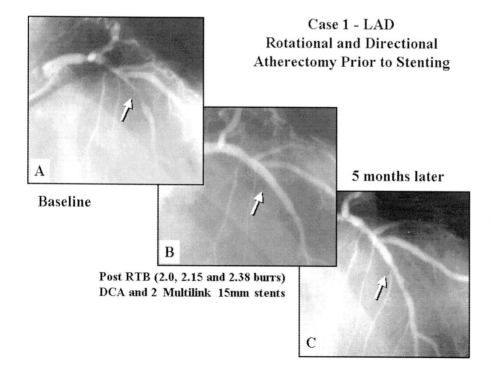

**Case 1 - LAD
Rotational and Directional
Atherectomy Prior to Stenting**

A

Baseline

B

5 months later

**Post RTB (2.0, 2.15 and 2.38 burrs)
DCA and 2 Multilink 15mm stents**

C

Figure 19.7 *(a) Baseline angiogram of the left anterior descending artery (LAD) shows a long, heavily calcified lesion in the mid-segment (white arrow). (b) Post-procedure angiogram after rotablation, directional coronary atherectomy (DCA) and, implantation of two Multilink stents. (c) Coronary angiogram at 5-month follow-up.*

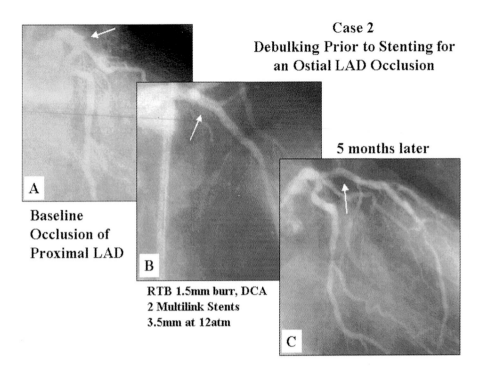

Case 2
Debulking Prior to Stenting for
an Ostial LAD Occlusion

5 months later

Baseline
Occlusion of
Proximal LAD

RTB 1.5mm burr, DCA
2 Multilink Stents
3.5mm at 12atm

Figure 19.8 *(a) Coronary angiogram of the left coronary artery system in the right anterior oblique projection shows a totally occluded ostial left anterior descending artery (LAD) (white arrow). (b) Post-procedure angiogram in the anteroposterior cranial projection after rotational atherectomy, directional coronary atherectomy (DCA), and implantation of two ACS Multilink stents, each 15 mm long (white arrow). (c) Coronary angiogram 5 months post-intervention. RTB, rotablator.*

then performed using a 7 Fr GTO cutter. Slow flow developed during this intervention, so the atherectomy was stopped and abciximab was initiated. Then, two ACS Multilink stents were implanted and expanded using a 3.5 mm balloon inflated at 11 atmospheres (*Fig. 19.7b*). This patient sustained a Q-wave MI (peak creatine kinase level 1200 U/l MB 14%) but he had an uneventful recovery.

The patient returned for follow-up angiography at 5 months. As shown in *Figs 19.6c* and *19.7c*, both treatment sites (one in the RCA and one in the LAD) were free of restenosis. Clinical follow-up was performed 16 months post-procedure, and the patient remained free from angina and other cardiac events.

CASE 2

A 69-year-old man with history of hypertension and hyperlipidemia presented with unstable angina. There was no evidence for MI by cardiac enzymes or new Q-waves on electrocardiogram. Coronary angiography showed a total occlusion of the proximal LAD (*Fig. 19.8a*). After recanalizing the vessel, an attempt was made to perform IVUS imaging but the IVUS catheter could not cross the lesion. Rotational atherectomy was performed with a 1.5 mm burr followed by DCA using a 7 Fr GTO cutter. The percentage diameter stenosis after rotational atherec-

tomy and DCA was 28%. (This is not considered to be aggressive debulking.) The reference diameter at the lesion site by angiography measured 3.08 mm. Two Multilink ACS stents (30 mm) were implanted and then expanded using a 3.5 mm balloon inflated to 12 atmospheres (*Fig. 19.8b*). The patient was discharged after 24 hours with no in-hospital events. *Figure 19.8c* shows the follow-up angiography at 5 months, which demonstrated the absence of restenosis. Late clinical follow-up was performed at 16 months; the patient was free of angina or other cardiac events.

CASE 3

A 57-year-old man with history of hypertension presented with unstable angina. Coronary angiography showed a distal left main artery stenosis (*Fig. 19.9a*) with a reference diameter of 3.53 mm. IVUS interrogation was performed; it showed a fibrotic non-calcified plaque. An intra-aortic balloon pump was inserted and DCA was performed using a 7 Fr GTO cutter (12 cuts). One Multilink ACS stent was implanted towards the LAD. A 'kissing balloon' technique was used for final stent expansion: a 4.0 mm balloon inflated to 20 atmospheres towards the LAD and a 3.5 mm balloon inflated to 10 atmospheres towards the left circumflex artery (*Fig.*

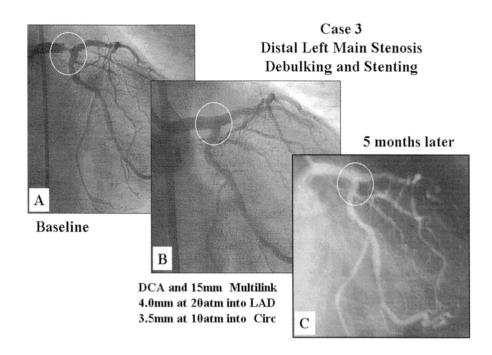

Case 3
Distal Left Main Stenosis
Debulking and Stenting

5 months later

Baseline

DCA and 15mm Multilink
4.0mm at 20atm into LAD
3.5mm at 10atm into Circ

Figure 19.9 *(a) Coronary angiogram of the left coronary artery system in the right anterior oblique projection shows an unprotected distal left main coronary artery stenosis (white circle). (b) Post-procedure angiogram after directional coronary atherectomy (DCA) (12 cuts) and implantation of one ACS Multilink stent towards the left anterior descending artery (LAD). (c) Coronary angiogram 5 months post-intervention; note the minimal late lumen loss. Circ, circumflex artery.*

19.9b). The patient was discharged after 24 hours with no in-hospital events. *Figure 19.9c* shows the follow-up angiogram at 5 months, which demonstrated the absence of restenosis. Late clinical follow-up was performed at 11 months; the patient was free of angina or other cardiac events.

CASE 4

A 63-year-old man with a history of hypertension presented with unstable angina. The patient had normal cardiac enzymes but coronary angiography showed a total occlusion of the proximal RCA (*Fig. 19.10a*). After recanalization, a very long segment of the artery appeared diseased (*Fig. 19.10b*). DCA was

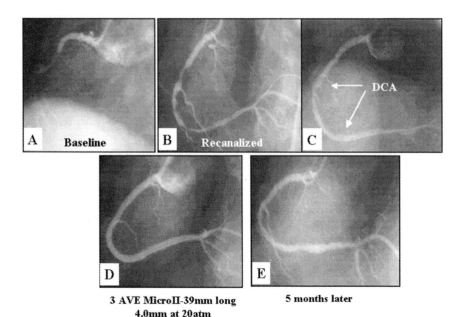

A   Baseline   B   Recanalized   C   DCA

D   3 AVE MicroII-39mm long
4.0mm at 20atm

E   5 months later

Figure 19.10 *(a) Baseline angiogram of the right coronary artery shows a proximal total occlusion. (b) Angiogram after vessel recanalization. (c) Angiogram after directional coronary atherectomy (DCA) (40 cuts). (d) Angiogram after implantation of three 39 mm long AVE II stents expanded with a 4.0 mm balloon inflated to 20 atmospheres. (e) Coronary angiogram at 5-month follow-up.*

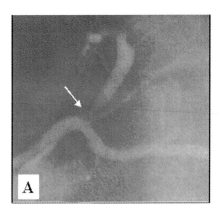
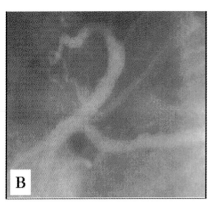

Figure 19.11 *(a) Coronary angiogram of the left coronary artery system in the left anterior oblique (LAO) caudal projection shows an ostial left anterior descending artery (LAD) stenosis (white arrow). (b) Angiogram after directional coronary atherectomy (DCA) (26 cuts) and placement of 15 mm Palmaz–Schatz stent expanded with a 4.0 mm balloon to 22 atmospheres (white arrow).*

Baseline - Caudal LAO   **Post DCA, 15mm PS stent, 4.0mm at 22atm**

performed using a 7 Fr GTO cutter (40 cuts) (*Fig. 19.10c*). Three 39 mm long AVE II Microstents were implanted and expanded using a 4.0 mm balloon inflated to 20 atmospheres (*Fig. 19.10d*). The patient had no in-hospital events. *Figure 19.10e* shows the follow-up angiography at 5 months, which demonstrated the absence of restenosis despite the extensive length of the stents. Late clinical follow-up was performed at 10 months; the patient was free of angina or other cardiac events.

CASE 5

A 57-year-old man presented with unstable angina pectoris. Coronary angiography showed an ostial LAD stenosis (*Fig. 19.11a*). DCA was performed using a 7 Fr GTO cutter (26 cuts). One 15 mm Palmaz–Schatz stent was implanted and expanded using a 4.0 mm balloon inflated to 22 atmospheres (*Fig. 19.11b*). The patient had no in-hospital events and was asymptomatic at his 18-month clinical follow-up.

CLINICAL IMPLICATIONS OF DEBULKING BEFORE STENT IMPLANTATION

In summary, debulking before stent implantation is an approach that is based on sound theoretical, experimental, and clinical observations. Preliminary non-randomized experience has shown the feasibility of this approach and its favorable long-term outcome

in selected patients. However, several issues have to be addressed:

(a) the risk of Q-wave MI is unacceptably high when aggressive rotablation is used in severely calcified and long lesions, a fact that limits the clinical utility of this approach;

(b) the incidence of non-Q-wave MI is also increased with both rotational atherectomy and DCA compared to PTCA or stent alone. Despite the controversy concerning the impact of this event on long-term clinical outcome, this remains a limitation that has to be addressed by the use of potent antiplatelet agents or the development of new atherectomy devices that produce a lower rate of embolization, or both; and

(c) considering the increased procedural time and cost, this approach has to be applied in selected patient subsets in whom debulking or stenting as a stand-alone strategy is associated with a high restenosis rate.

Randomized clinical trials testing this approach using the various debulking devices are currently in progress. Until the results of such randomized clinical trials are available, this approach may serve an important clinical purpose when applied selectively. DCA before stenting is best used in non-calcified lesions located in vessels > 2.75 mm in diameter that have any of the following characteristics:

(a) aorto-ostial location;
(b) bifurcations;
(c) chronic total occlusions; or
(d) the need for two or more stents.

On the other hand, rotablation before stenting is best used for lesions located in native coronary arteries > 2.5 mm in diameter that have any of the following characteristics:

(a) moderate to severe calcification;
(b) uncrossable with low-profile balloon catheters; or
(c) undilatable with moderate balloon inflation pressures (12 atmospheres).

REFERENCES

1. Serruys P, Jaegere P, Kiemeneij F et al. A comparison of balloon expandable stent implantation with balloon angioplasty in patients with coronary artery disease. *N Engl J Med* 1994; **331**: 489–95.
2. Fischman DL, Leon MB, Baim D et al. A randomized comparison of coronary stent placement and balloon angioplasty in the treatment of coronary artery disease. *N Engl J Med* 1994; **331**: 496–501.
3. Macaya C, Serruys PW, Ruygrok P et al. for the Benestent Study Group. Continued benefit of coronary stenting compared to balloon angioplasty: one year clinical follow-up of the Benestent trial. *J Am Coll Cardiol* 1996; **27**: 255–261.
4. Itoh A, Hall P, Maiello L et al. Coronary stenting of long lesions (greater than 20 mm): a matched comparison of different stents (abstract). *Circulation* 1995; **92 (suppl I)**: I-688.
5. Zampieri P, Colombo A, Almagor Y et al. Results of coronary stenting of ostial lesions. *Am J Cardiol* 1994; **73**: 901–903.
6. Rocha-Singh K, Morris N, Wong SC et al. Coronary stenting for treatment of ostial stenoses of native coronary arteries or aorto-coronary saphenous vein grafts. *Am J Cardiol* 1995; **75**: 26–9.
7. Mehran R, Mintz GS, Bucher TA et al. Aorto-ostial instent restenosis: mechanisms, treatment, and results. A serial quantitative angiographic and intravascular ultrasound study. *Circulation* 1996; **94 (suppl I)**: I-200.
8. Goldberg SL, Colombo A, Maiello L et al. Intracoronary stent insertion after balloon angioplasty of chronic total occlusions. *J Am Coll Cardiol* 1995; **26**: 713–719.
9. Sirnes P, Golf S, Myreng Y et al. Stenting in chronic coronary occlusion (SICCO): a randomized, controlled trial of adding stent implantation after successful angioplasty. *J Am Coll Cardiol* 1996; **28**: 1444–1451.
10. Moussa I, Di Mario C, Moses J et al. Comparison of angiographic and clinical outcome of coronary stenting of chronic total occlusions versus subtotal occlusions. *Am J Cardiol* 1998; **81**: 1–6.
11. Colombo A, Maiello L, Itoh A et al. Coronary stenting of bifurcational lesions: immediate and follow-up results (abstract). *J Am Coll Cardiol* 1996; **27**: (suppl A): 277A.
12. Hoffmann R, Mintz G, Dussaillant G et al. Patterns and mechanisms of in-stent restenosis: a serial intravascular ultrasound study. *Circulation* 1996; **94**: 1247–1254.
13. Rogers C, Edelman E. Endovascular stent design dictates experimental restenosis and thrombosis. *Circulation* 1995; **91**: 2195–3001.
14. Carter AJ, Farb A, Laird J et al. Neointimal formation is dependent on the underlying arterial substrate after coronary stent placement (abstract). *J Am Coll Cardiol* 1996; **February special issue**: 320A.
15. Moussa I, Di Mario C, Moses J et al. The impact of preintervention plaque area as determined by intravsacular ultrasound on luminal renarrowing following coronary stenting (abstract). *Circulation.* 1996; **94**: 1528.
16. Hoffman R, Mintz GS, Mehran R et al. Intravascular ultrasound predictors of angiographic restenosis in lesions treated with Palmaz–Schatz stents. *J Am Coll Cardiol* 1998; **31**: 43–49.
17. Corvaja N, Moses J, Moussa I et al. Stent restenosis: where does it occur? An angiographic analysis (abstract). *Eur Heart J* 1997; **18**: P2193.
18. Simonton CA, Leon MB, Baim DS et al. 'Optimal' directional coronary atherectomy: final results of the Optimal Atherectomy Restenosis Study (OARS). *Circulation* 1998; **97**: 332–339.
19. Ibrahim A, Kronenberg M, Boor P et al. Atherectomy and angioplasty improve compliance and reduce thickness of iliac arteries – an in vitro ultrasound study (abstract). *Circulation* 1994; **90**: I-534.
20. Baim DS, Cutlip D, Sharmin SK et al. for the BOAT Investigators. Final results of the Balloon versus Optimal Atherectomy Trial (BOAT). *Circulation* 1998; **97**: 322–331.
21. MacIsaac AI, Bass TA, Buchbinder M et al. High speed rotational atherectomy: outcome in calcified and noncalcified coronary artery lesions. *J Am Coll Cardiol* 1995; **26**: 731–736.
22. Warth D, Leon M, O'Neill W et al. Rotational atherectomy multicenter registry: acute results, complications and 6–month angiographic follow-up in 709 patients. *J Am Coll Cardiol* 1994; **24**: 641–648.
23. Reifart N, Vandormael M, Krajcar M et al. Randomized comparison of angioplasty of complex coronary lesions at a single center. *Circulation* 1997; **96**: 91–98.
24. Sangiorgi G, Rumberger J, Severson A et al. Arterial calcification and not lumen stenosis is highly correlated with atherosclerotic palque burden in humans: a histologic study of 723 coronary artery segments using nondecalcifiying methodology. *J Am Coll Cardiol* 1998; **31**: 126–133.
25. Alfonso F, Macaya C, Goicolea J et al. Determinants of coronary compliance in patients with coronary artery disease: an intravascular ultrasound study. *J Am Coll Cardiol* 1994; **23**: 879–884.
26. Fitzgerald P, Ports T, Yock P. Contribution of localized calcium deposits to dissection after angioplasty. An observational study using intravascular ultrasound. *Circulation* 1992; **86**: 64–70.
27. Fitzgerald P, STRUT Registry Investigators. Lesion composition impacts size and symmetry of stent expansion: initial report from the strut registry (abstract). *J Am Coll Cardiol* 1995; **February special issue**: 49A.
28. Mintz GS, Popma JJ, Hong MK et al. Intravascular ultrasound to discern device-specific effects and mechanisms of restenosis. *Am J Cardiol* 1996; **78 (suppl 3A)**: 18–22.

29. de Vrey E, Mintz GS, Kimura T et al. Arterial remodeling after directional coronary atherectomy: a volumetric analysis from the Serial Ultrasound Restenosis (SURE) Trial (abstract). *J Am Coll Cardiol* 1997; **February special issue**: 280A.

30. Cutlip DE, Chauhan M, Senerchia C et al. Influence of myocardial infarction following otherwise successful coronary intervention on late mortality (abstract). *Circulation* 1997; **96**: 162.

31. Simoons ML, Harrington R, Anderson KM et al. Small, non-Q-wave myocardial infarctions during PTCA are associated with increased 6 months mortality (abstract). *Circulation* 1997; **96**: 163.

32. Lefkovits J, Blankenship JC, Anderson KM et al. Increased risk of non-Q-wave myocardial infarction after directional atherectomy is paletelet dependent: evidence from the EPIC trial. *J Am Coll Cardiol* 1996; **28**: 849–855.

33. Mehran R, Hong M, Lansky A et al. Vessel size and lesion length influence late clinical outcomes after native coronary artery stent placement (abstract). *Circulation* 1997; **96**: 1520.

34. Kornowsky R, Mehran R, Hong M et al. Procedural results and late clinical outcomes after placement of three or more stents in single coronary lesions. *Circulation* 1998; **97**: 1355–1361.

35. Kiesz R, Rozek MM, Mego DM et al. Device synergy: directional atherectomy and stenting significantly reduces residual stenosis (abstract). *Eur Heart J* 1996; **17**: P974.

36. Bramucci I, Angoli L, Merlini PA et al. Acute results of adjunct stents following directional coronary atherectomy (abstract). *J Am Coll Cardiol* 1997; **February special issue**: 415A.

37. Kastrati A, Schomig A, Elezi S et al. Predictive factors of restenosis after coronary stent placement. *J Am Coll Cardiol* 1997; **30**: 1428–1436.

38. Kuntz RE, Safian RD, Joseph P et al. The importance of acute luminal diameter in determining restenosis after coronary atherectomy or stenting. *Circulation* 1992; **86**: 1827–1835

39. Mintz GS, Popma JJ, Pichard AD et al. Intravascular ultrasound predictors of restenosis after percutaneous transcatheter coronary revascularization. *J Am Coll Cardiol* 1996; **27**: 1678–1687.

40. The GUIDE trial investigator. IVUS-determined predictors of restenosis in PTCA and DCA: final report from the GUIDE trial, phase II (abstract). *J Am Coll Cardiol* 1996; **29**: 156A.

41. Nakamura S, Colombo A, Gaglione S et al. Intracoronary ultrasound observations during stent implantation. *Circulation* 1994; **89**: 2026–2034.

42. Moussa I, Di Mario C, Moses J et al. Coronary stenting following rotational atherectomy in calcified and complex lesions: angiographic and clinical follow-up results. *Circulation* 1997; **96**: 128–136.

43. Hoffmann R, Mintz GS, Kent KM et al. Comparative early and nine-month results of rotational atherectomy, stents, and the combination of both for calcified lesions in large coronary arteries. *Am J Cardiol* 1998; **81**: 552–557.

44. Kaplan BM, Safian RD, Mojares JJ et al. Optimal burr and adjunctive balloon sizing reduces the need for target artery revascularization after coronary mechanical rotational atherectomy. *Am J Cardiol* 1996; **78**: 1224–1229.

45. Hansen DD, Auth DC, Vracko R et al. Rotational arterectomy in atherosclerotic rabbit arteries. *Am Heart J* 1988; **115**: 160–165.

46. Braden GA, Applegate RJ, Young TM et al. Abciximab decreases both the incidence and magnitude of creatine kinase elevation during rotational atherectomy (abstract). *J Am Coll Cardiol* 1997; **29**: 499A.

47. Christophe B, Banos J, Belle EV et al. Six-month angiographic outcome after successful repeat percutaneous intervention for in-stent restenosis. *Circulation* 1998; **97**: 318–321.

Chapter 20 Intravascular ultrasound-guided percutaneous transluminal coronary angioplasty with spot stenting

Joseph DeGregorio

The concept of 'spot stenting' has evolved as a method to address the high restenosis rate associated with stenting long lesions. As described in Chapter 4, one of the strongest independent predictors of in-stent restenosis is the length of the stent that is deployed. This evidence provides the rationale for limiting the stent length when treating a long lesion. Although there is a higher rate of restenosis with balloon dilatation alone than with stenting in specific lesion subsets, there are some lesions which do exceedingly well with percutaneous transluminal coronary angioplasty (PTCA) alone. 'Spot stenting' is an attempt to optimize the benefits of balloon angioplasty and focal stenosis stenting using intravascular ultrasound (IVUS) guidance in long lesions or small vessels, in which extensive use of stents alone or PTCA alone does not provide satisfactory results.

HISTORICAL RESULTS IN TREATING LONG LESIONS

The treatment of long lesions and lesions in small vessels has historically yielded poor immediate and long-term results when approached with traditional balloon angioplasty.[1-5] Angiographic restenosis rates for these lesions have ranged from 41% to 55%. In the STRESS subanalysis,[3] smaller vessels treated with PTCA had a restenosis rate of 53%.

The treatment of focal lesions with coronary stenting in vessels ≥ 3.0 mm in diameter reduces restenosis when compared to balloon angioplasty.[6-8] However, apart from the intrinsic lesion characteristics that predispose to restenosis, the length of the

deployed stent and the number of stents implanted in long lesions have been implicated as contributing factors for increased restenosis rates.[9-11] IVUS-guided PTCA with spot stenting is a new approach for difficult lesion subsets. It is a synergistic strategy utilizing PTCA, stents, and IVUS for the treatment of long lesions and lesions located in small vessels. It is a combined method that seeks to maximize the results of balloon dilatation by adopting pre-determined IVUS criteria and to use stents when necessary while restricting stent length. This approach is based on the premise that IVUS guidance of the coronary intervention will allow the operator to:

(a) maximize the probability of achieving a pre-specified criterion of lumen enlargement with balloon angioplasty, therefore minimizing or removing the need for stenting; and
(b) identify the particular segment or segments of a lesion where the luminal result is not optimal and to implant a focal stent only at those specific sites.

Theoretically, this approach may provide a reduction in restenosis by the attainment of an optimal minimum luminal diameter (MLD) with balloon dilatation while simultaneously limiting the length of stented artery so as to diminish the stimulus for intimal hyperplasia.

Improvements in stent implantation technique and technology, along with alterations in post-procedural pharmacological management that reduce stent thrombosis and bleeding complications,[2-14] have led to the broader application of coronary stenting to more complex lesions, such as long lesions and lesions located in small vessels. Initial reports on the use of coronary stenting in these lesion subsets (in which the lesion is covered from the proximal normal segment to the distal normal segment) indicate improved immediate outcome compared to balloon angioplasty in terms of a low incidence of acute and subacute occlusion, but they still demonstrate deficient long-term results.[3–5,15–19] A Benestent subanalysis that examined the results of treating small vessels showed a 7-month major adverse clinical event (MACE) rate of 48% in lesions treated with PTCA and a MACE rate of 36% with stenting.

The use of other contemporary devices, such as rotational atherectomy, directional coronary atherectomy (DCA) and laser angioplasty in the treatment of long lesions has produced disappointing results. Although recent studies with the Rotablator have shown a procedural success rate of about 92% in lesions 16–25 mm in length, there is also an increased risk of Q-wave myocardial infarction (MI), non-Q-wave MI, coronary artery perforation, and restenosis.[20–25] With regards to DCA, increased lesion length (> 20 mm) has been associated with a high rate of procedural failure (26%) and an increased complication rate (10.8%).[26] In addition, directional atherectomy cannot be applied easily to small vessels or vessels with diffuse disease. In another study, in de novo lesions > 10 mm in length, the rate of major complications was 12.5% and the procedural success rates was 84%.[27] An early report by Robertson and colleagues[28] showed a restenosis rate of 62.5% in lesions > 20 mm treated with DCA.[28] Randomized trials of devices for long lesions have compared excimer laser coronary angioplasty (ELCA) to PTCA (the AMRO trial[29]) and ELCA versus PTCA versus Rotablator (the ERBAC trial[30]) The AMRO trial showed that there was no difference in procedural success rate or late clinical events, but in the ELCA group there were more acute closures (8% versus 0.8%) and a trend towards more restenosis (52% versus 41%). In the ERBAC trial, both Rotablator and ELCA resulted in a better immediate lumen enlargement, but there was no difference in 6-month restenosis rates.

THE CONCEPT OF IVUS-GUIDED PTCA

Several studies employing the concept of IVUS-guided PTCA without stenting in the treatment of coronary lesions have produced promising results.[31–33] Stone and colleagues[31] reported the early angiographic and clinical results of IVUS-guided PTCA in the CLOUT pilot trial. On the basis of the

vessel size and extent of plaque burden in the reference segment as evaluated by IVUS post-initial dilatation, 73% of the lesions required balloon upsizing (final balloon-to-artery ratio 1.30 ± 0.17) even after achieving an optimal angiographic result with the initial balloon. The success rate of IVUS-guided PTCA was 99%. This angiographic oversized balloon angioplasty with IVUS guidance resulted in a large final MLD without increased rates of significant dissections or ischemic complications.

The Washington Hospital Center reported a pilot work of IVUS-guided balloon angioplasty using balloons sized according to the media-to-media diameter as determined by IVUS.[32] The end-point used in this study was the achievement of a minimum lumen cross-sectional area of more than 70% of the average reference vessel area with no lumen-compromising dissections. Cross-over to stenting was needed in 61% of lesions. The final lumen area in the PTCA group was 6.0 ± 2.0 mm² and there was no incidence of abrupt vessel closure. Target lesion revascularization (TLR) was needed in 17% of lesions. Frey and colleagues[33] reported on a total of 269 patients (358 lesions), who were randomized to IVUS-guided intervention or angiographically guided intervention in the SIPS trial.[33] Stenting was performed in about 50% of lesions in both groups. MACE during hospitalization occurred less often with the IVUS-guided interventions. Cumulative in-hospital MACE, including myocardial infarction (MI), coronary artery bypass grafts, and death, included 14 cases in the IVUS-guided group but 46 cases in the standard angiographically guided group ($p < 0.07$).

IVUS-GUIDED SPOT STENTING

On the basis of these preliminary data, we hypothesized that the restenosis rate for long lesions and diffuse disease could be reduced if IVUS-guided PTCA could be used as the primary modality while reserving coronary stents to those segments of a lesion in which the lumen dimensions after dilatation did not meet pre-specified IVUS criteria. Instead of traditional stenting, in which a lesion is covered from a proximal normal segment to a distal normal segment, the concept behind the spot stenting approach is to avoid stenting long segments even if small dissections are left behind, provided that the dilated sections have an adequate lumen cross-sectional area on IVUS.

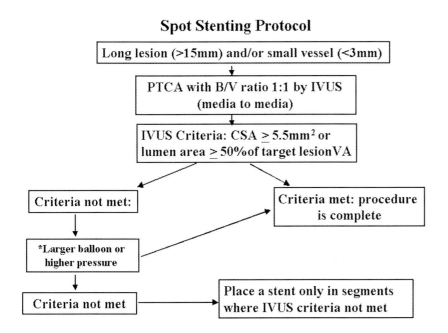

Spot Stenting Protocol

Figure 20.1 *Protocol guidelines and criteria for performing spot stenting. CSA, cross sectional area; B/V, balloon to vessel ratio; VA, vessel area.*

THE PROCEDURE AND THE MILAN EXPERIENCE

We tested this approach by applying the technique in a prospective study performed between April 1997 and May 1998. This study included 109 consecutive patients with 160 lesions. The flow diagram for this study is depicted in *Fig. 20.1*. Long lesions (> 15 mm) or lesions located in small vessels (< 3 mm in diameter) are approached with primary PTCA using a balloon-to-vessel ratio of 1:1. The vessel size is defined as the reference media-to-media diameter measured by a pre-intervention IVUS study. However, if extensive calcium is present, rotablation may be performed before PTCA, or if extensive eccentric plaque or thrombus is apparent, DCA or thrombectomy may be carried out before PTCA. If the IVUS criteria are met in all segments of the lesion after initial balloon dilatation, the procedure is considered complete. IVUS criteria for success are defined as:

(a) achievement of a lumen cross-sectional area ≥ 50% of the vessel cross-sectional area at the lesion site; or
(b) a minimum lumen cross-sectional area ≥ 5.5 mm².

These success criteria are defined independently of the presence of dissection as long as the cross-sectional area of the true lumen is greater than the cross-sectional area of the false dissection lumen and angiographic flow of TIMI grade 3 is present. If the IVUS criteria are not met, the operator would consider using a larger balloon, higher pressure, or an adjunctive device if this was deemed possible on the basis of lesion morphology and vessel measurements. If this is not possible, a stent is implanted focally only in the segment or segments of the lesion where the IVUS criteria have not been achieved, and care is taken to use the shortest stent length necessary to obtain an optimal result. There is no particular device that is considered most favorable for the technique of spot stenting; rather, the operator should use whichever devices are deemed necessary for that particular lesion in order to optimize the lumen and achieve the IVUS criteria. If extensive calcium is present, rotablation may be performed before PTCA, and if extensive eccentric plaque or thrombus is apparent, DCA or thrombectomy may be carried out before PTCA. Rotablation was used as an adjunct in about 10% of these 160 lesions approached with spot stenting. The cutting balloon was also used in a number of cases in which very resistant or fibrotic lesions were encountered. IVUS is performed at the end of the procedure to ensure achievement of IVUS criteria and to document final lumen dimensions.

The majority of patients treated with this approach had a history of previous MI, and 94% had multivessel

Table 20.1

Patient characteristics

	Total (n = 106)
Age (years)	59 ± 10
Male, n (%)	96 (91)
Risk factors	
Hypertension, n (%)	52 (49)
Hypercholesterolemia, n (%)	65 (61)
Diabetes, n (%)	10 (10)
Smoker, n (%)	60 (57)
Family history, n (%)	56 (52)
Prior myocardial infarction, n (%)	55 (52)
Previous angioplasty, n (%)	26 (25)
Previous coronary bypass, n (%)	14 (13)
LVEF (%)	59 ± 12
Unstable angina, n (%)	28 (27)
Multivessel disease, n (%)	101 (94)
Antiplatelet therapy	
Ticlopidine + aspirin, n (%)	62 (58)
Aspirin alone, n (%)	44 (42)

LVEF indicates left ventricular ejection fraction.

disease (*Table 20.1*). Angiographic and procedural characteristics are shown in *Table 20.2*. Of the 160 lesions treated, 78 (49%) achieved minimum IVUS criteria with PTCA alone while 82 (51%) required spot stenting. The vessel in which the lesion was located and its location within the vessel had no influence on whether a stent would eventually be required. Most of the lesions approached were located in the left anterior descending artery (LAD) and were proximal to mid-artery in location. Seventy-three percent of the lesions were complex (type B2 and type C); the lesion types that were more likely to require adjunctive stenting were type C lesions and calcified lesions. Rotablator was used adjunctively before PTCA only for cases in which severe calcification was present (11%). The lesions that were approached with IVUS-guided PTCA and spot stenting had an average reference vessel diameter of 2.94 ± 0.5 mm and a lesion length of 20.6 ±12 mm (*Table 20.3*). In general, larger-diameter vessels and longer lesions were more likely to require placement of at least one stent. The approach to these difficult lesions included an average balloon size of 3.63 ± 0.5 with an average pressure of 14.5 atmospheres.

Table 20.2

Angiographic and procedural characteristics

	Total (n = 160)	Balloon (n = 78)	Stent (n = 82)	p value
Stented vessel, n (%)				NS
LAD	73 (46)	34 (44)	39 (48)	
RCA	46 (29)	26 (33)	20 (24)	
LCX	39 (24)	18 (23)	21 (26)	
Left main	2 (1)	0 (0)	2 (2)	
Lesion site, n (%)				NS
Ostial	8 (5)	3 (4)	5 (6)	
Proximal	61 (38)	30 (38)	31 (38)	
Mid-vessel	66 (41)	27 (35)	39 (48)	
Distal	25 (16)	18 (23)	7 (6)	
Modified AHA/ACC lesion type, n (%)				< 0.05
A	3 (2)	2 (3)	1 (1)	
B1	40 (25)	30 (39)	10 (12)	
B2	62 (38)	28 (35)	34 (42)	
C	55 (35)	18 (23)	37 (45)	
Calcified lesion, n (%)	46 (29)	17 (22)	29 (35)	0.06
Rotablation, n (%)	18 (11)	9 (12)	9 (11)	NS
Length of stents (mm)	–	–	18.7 ± 10	–
Final balloon size (mm)	3.63 ± 0.5	3.51 ± 0.5	3.74 ± 0.5	< 0.05
Final B/A ratio (mm)	1.24 ± 0.2	1.26 ± 0.2	1.22 ± 0.2	NS
Maximal inflation pressure (atm)	14.5 ± 3.5	13.6 ± 3.7	15.2 ± 3.2	< 0.05

Data presented are mean value ± SD or number (%) of lesions; LAD, left anterior descending; RCA, right coronary artery; LCX, left circumflex artery; AHA/ACC, American Heart Association/American College of Cardiology; B/A, balloon-to-artery ratio.

Table 20.3

Quantitative angiographic measurements

	Total (n = 160)	Balloon (n = 78)	Stent (n = 82)	p value
Pre-intervention				
Reference vessel diameter (mm)	2.94 ± 0.5	2.86 ± 0.5	3.12 ± 0.5	< 0.05
Minimal lumen diameter (mm)	0.73 ± 0.5	0.78 ± 0.5	0.69 ± 0.6	NS
Diameter stenosis (%)	76 ± 12	74 ± 13	78 ± 17	NS
Lesion length (mm)	20.6 ± 12	18.7 ± 10	22.6 ± 14	< 0.05
Post-intervention				
Reference vessel diameter (mm)	3.17 ± 0.5	3.08 ± 0.5	3.25 ± 0.60	< 0.05
Minimal lumen diameter (mm)	2.83 ± 0.7	2.47 ± 0.5	3.16 ± 0.7	< 0.01
Stenosis (%)	11 ± 16	19 ± 14	3 ± 15	< 0.01
Acute gain (mm)	2.08 ± 0.77	1.69 ± 0.60	2.51 ± 0.65	< 0.01

Given that stents were being placed and the arteries were larger, larger balloons and higher pressures were utilized in the arm that advanced to stent placement (*Table 20.2*). Average stent length utilized in the lesions that did not meet IVUS criteria by PTCA alone (n = 82) was 18.7 ± 10 mm, which is in fact shorter than the average lesion length. *Table 20.3* also shows that significantly better angiographic results were achieved in the stenting arm. The balloon-to-vessel ratio, which was determined by IVUS, resulted in an angiographic balloon-to-artery lumen ratio of 1.24. This aggressive balloon sizing resulted in an acute gain of 2.10 mm in all lesions; acute gain was 1.69 mm for

the lesions that were treated with PTCA alone and 2.51 mm for the lesions that received a stent. The immediate results achieved with IVUS guidance obtained in the PTCA-alone group (1.69 mm) are similar to the acute gain achieved in the stent arms of both the BENESTENT and STRESS trials (1.40 mm and 1.72 mm, respectively) (*Fig. 20.2*). Final IVUS measurement data (*Table 20.4*) concur with the quantitative coronary angiography (QCA) results in displaying more favorable lumen dimensions in the stent arm of the trial. This is not a surprising finding, given that stents were placed in slightly larger vessels and that stents provide greater wall expansion and support.

Table 20.4

Final intravascular ultrasound quantitative measurements

	Total n = 160	PTCA n = 78	Stent n = 82
Proximal reference			
Lumen CSA	7.99 ± 2.54	7.84 ± 2.69	8.18 ± 2.37
Vessel CSA	13.12 ± 4.15	12.68 ± 4.64	13.65 ± 3.43
Lesion site			
Lumen CSA	6.46 ± 2.51	5.73 ± 2.04*	7.19 ± 2.72*
Vessel CSA	12.01 ± 4.12	11.72 ± 4.01	12.35 ± 4.25
Distal reference			
Lumen CSA	6.86 ± 2.13	6.91 ± 2.33	6.81 ± 1.92
Vessel CSA	10.54 ± 4.06	10.16 ± 3.94	10.92 ± 4.17

*p <0.01; PTCA, percutaneous transluminal coronary angioplasty; CSA, cross-sectional area (mm²).

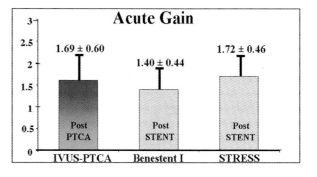

Figure 20.2 *Intravascular ultrasound (IVUS) guided percutaneous transluminal coronary angioplasty (PTCA) without stent assistance compared to prior stent trial results.*

Before procedure

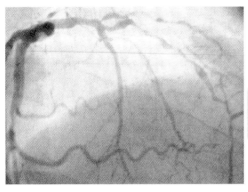

QCA

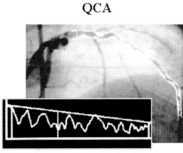

Lesion length = 82.0 mm

Ref. diameter = 3.05 mm
MLD = 0.98 mm
% diameter stenosis = 67.7%

a

After balloon angioplasty

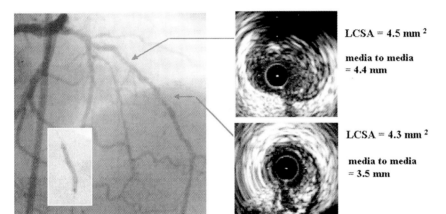

LCSA = 4.5 mm ^{2}

media to media
= 4.4 mm

LCSA = 4.3 mm ^{2}

media to media
= 3.5 mm

MAXXUM : 2.5 mm 30 mm 10 atm

b

After cutting balloon angioplasty

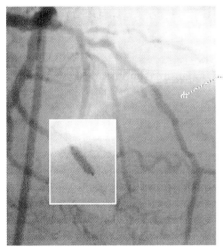

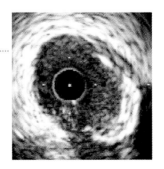

LCSA = 8.4 mm ^{2}

Cutting balloon : 2.75 & 3.5 mm
10 mm 12 atm

c

Figure 20.3 *IVUS guided spot stenting. (a) Baseline coronary angiogram of a diffusely diseased left anterior descending artery. By QCA the diseased segment was 82 mm long. (b) Following balloon dilatation with a cutting balloon, the lumen cross-sectional area does not meet the IVUS criteria of > 5.5 mm squared. (c) Repeat balloon dilatation with different size cutting balloons produces significant benefit in cross-sectional area. (d) Two stents were placed in focal areas of the mid LAD where the lumen cross-sectional area was still inadequate after balloon dilatation. (e) Angiograms comparing the LAD before and after sport stenting identifies the position of the stents and where balloon angioplasty or cutting balloon angioplasty was performed. QCA, quantitative coronary angiography; LCSA, lumen cross sectional area; MLD, minimum lumen diameter.*

After stent placement

Figure 20.3 *continued*

Stent

**Balloon angioplasty
4.0 mm 12 atm**

LCSA = 8.1 mm²

LCSA = 11.1 mm²

**2 Crown Stent 15 mm
4.0 mm 12 atm**

LCSA = 9.2 mm²

d

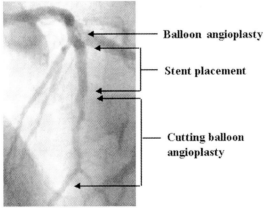

Summary

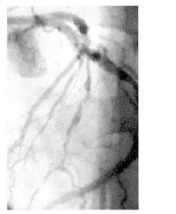

Balloon angioplasty

Stent placement

Cutting balloon
angioplasty

Before procedure   **After procedure**

e

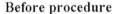

CLINICAL EXAMPLES

CASE 1

The LAD lesion treated with spot stenting in *Fig. 20.3* is typical of the cases in this series. The LAD was diffusely diseased, and the initial treatment was with a long balloon followed by IVUS evaluation. The mid-segment in this lesion remained inadequate by IVUS criteria after initial inflation (*Fig. 20.3b*). The next step was to apply two different-sized cutting balloons: 3.5 mm in the long mid-segment and 2.75 mm in the more distal part of the LAD. The

lumen cross-sectional area improved significantly in the distal portion of the mid-lesion (*Fig. 20.3c*), but most of this segment remained suboptimal. Therefore, two 15 mm Crown stents were placed in the mid-LAD and dilated with a 4.0 mm balloon to 12 atmospheres (*Fig. 20.3d*). *Figure 20.3e* shows a summary of this case before and after treatment; balloon angioplasty was adequate for the proximal LAD, stents were necessary in the mid-LAD, and a cutting balloon sufficed for the distal LAD. In this instance, an 82 mm long lesion was adequately treated with 30 mm of stent length. Limiting stent length in this manner while still obtaining an optimal

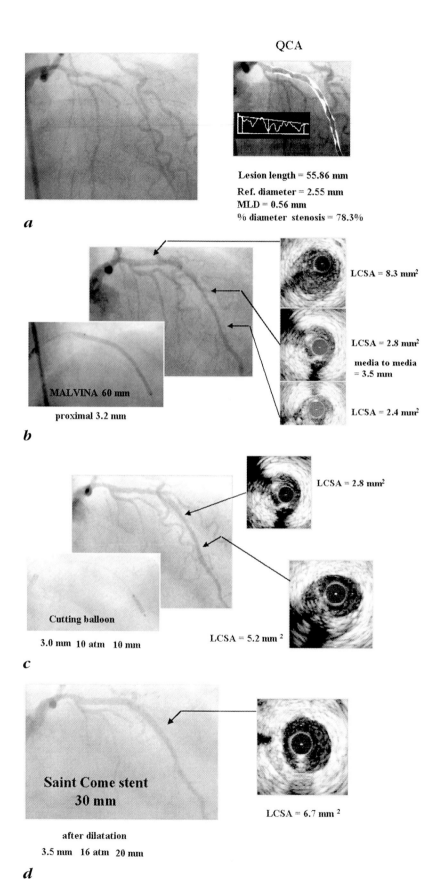

QCA

Lesion length = 55.86 mm
Ref. diameter = 2.55 mm
MLD = 0.56 mm
% diameter stenosis = 78.3%

a

LCSA = 8.3 mm²

LCSA = 2.8 mm²
media to media
= 3.5 mm

LCSA = 2.4 mm²

MALVINA 60 mm

proximal 3.2 mm

b

LCSA = 2.8 mm²

Cutting balloon

3.0 mm 10 atm 10 mm

LCSA = 5.2 mm²

c

Saint Come stent
30 mm

LCSA = 6.7 mm²

after dilatation

3.5 mm 16 atm 20 mm

d

Figure 20.4 *Intravascular ultrasound (IVUS)-guided spot stenting. (a) Before procedure. (b) After balloon angioplasty. (c) After cutting balloon angioplasty. (d) After stent placement. LCSA, lumen cross-sectional area; QCA, quantitative coronary angiography; MLD, minimum lumen diameter.*

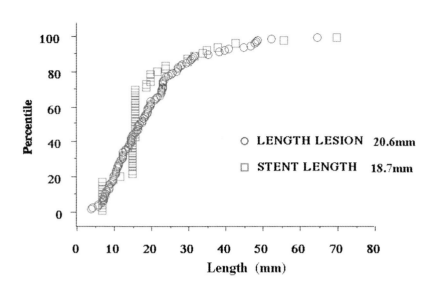

Figure 20.5 *Spot stenting: IVUS guided PTCA with stent assistance. Frequency distribution curve of stent length vs. lesion length.*

result throughout the rest of the lesion is the basis behind spot stenting. We expect that this combined approach will improve long-term outcome.

CASE 2

This case is another example of the type of lesion that might benefit from the spot stenting approach. *Fig. 20.4a* depicts another diffusely diseased LAD in which not many treatment options are available. If spot stenting were not utilized here, long stents might be able to be placed or rotational atherectomy might be performed. However, the suboptimal results that have been reported from such approaches in this lesion subset render them unfavorable options. This lesion was 56 mm in length and the reference lumen diameter measured 2.55 mm by QCA. Quantitative angiographic measurements in sizing vessels have been demonstrated to be less accurate than IVUS measurements, especially in small vessels and vessels with diffuse disease. As is often the case with diffuse disease, the vessel tapers significantly in the distal portion. Therefore, a long tapering balloon was used for pre-dilatation; this balloon was 60 mm in length and tapered from 3.2 mm in diameter in the proximal portion to 2.0 mm in the distal portion. After the first inflation to 8 atmospheres, IVUS showed that the lesion in the mid- to distal segment of the artery was fibrocalcific in nature and that the media-to-media diameter in the distal lesion was 3.2 mm (*Fig. 20.4b*). On the basis of these observations, a 3.0 mm cutting balloon was applied only in the mid- to distal

segment of the lesion, where the lumen cross-sectional area did not meet our minimal criteria. The cutting balloon was effective in achieving the minimal criteria in the more distal segment, where the lumen by IVUS now measured > 50% of the reference vessel area (*Fig. 20.4c*). In the mid-portion, the luminal result was still unsatisfactory, with a cross-sectional area of 2.8 mm², so a stent was deployed only in the mid-segment, where the inadequate result was present. This stent was 30 mm in length and it was post-dilated with a 3.5 mm balloon to 16 atmospheres. The final angiogram shows an excellent result and the IVUS measurement demonstrates the new cross-sectional area in the mid-portion to be 6.7 mm² (*Fig. 20.4d*).

RESULTS OF SPOT STENTING

The mean stent length used in the 82 stented lesions was 18.7 ± 10 mm. *Figure 20.5* portrays a frequency distribution curve of the relationship between lesion length and stent length with the spot stenting approach. These curves are virtually overlapping. This denotes something which is very different from our usual experience. As can be noted from previous studies such as the BENESTENT I and II and STRESS trials,[6,7] it is usual for the stent length to exceed the lesion length significantly. However, with the spot stenting approach, stent length is actually shorter than the lesion length (18.7 ± 10 mm versus 20.6 ±

Table 20.5

Stent length, lesion length and restenosis

	Group I (n=565)	Group II (n=278)	Group III (n=247)
Stent length	≤ 20 mm	> 20 mm & ≤ 35 mm	> 35 mm
	(avg. 15 ± 3)	(avg. 30 ± 3)	(avg. 52 ± 16)
Lesion length	9.5 ± 5 mm	12.4 ± 7 mm	13.5 ± 8 mm
Restenosis	23.9%	34.6%	47.2%

Kobayashi Y, De Gregorio J, Reimers B, et al. J Am Coll Cardiol 1998 (abstract) (725 consecutive patients, 1090 lesions)

12 mm). This is an important concept, since evidence shows that the length of deployed stent is a major contributing factor to restenosis[9–11] (see Chapter 4). *Table 20.5* demonstrates the significant relationship between stent length, lesion length and restenosis rates. In an analysis from our laboratory that included 1090 lesions in 725 patients, the restenosis rate for all lesion types was 24% when a relatively short lesion (9.5 mm ± 5 mm) was treated with a short stent (15 mm ± 3 mm). The restentosis rate increased to 35% when a 12.4 ± 7 mm lesion was treated with a stent of 30 ± 3 mm. Restenosis continued to increase, up to 47%, when a 13.5 ± 8 mm lesion was treated with a long stent (52 ± 16 mm). Multivariate logistic regression analysis of these lesion subsets showed stent length to be the strongest independent predictor of restenosis.

Subsequent evidence to support the concept that longer stent length contributes to restenosis in long lesions is brought out in further analyses from our laboratory.[34] Lesions were divided into two groups: one group with stent length less than lesion length (n = 103) and a second group with stent length greater than lesion length (n = 166). These groups were matched for vessel size (3.02 ± 0.65 mm versus 3.10 ± 0.60 mm; *p* not significant) and lesion length (27.9 ± 8.5 mm versus 27.3 ± 6.9 mm; *p* not significant). Stent lengths differed significantly (19.0 ± 7.01 mm versus 44.3 ± 16.4 mm; *p* < 0.05). Restenosis rates in the group in which stent length was less than lesion length was 18% but the restenosis rate was 41% in the group in which stent length was greater than lesion length (*p* < 0.05).

In order to provide further testimony of the negative impact of long stent lengths, we performed a direct matched comparison of long lesions treated by spot stenting versus traditional stenting (in which the lesion is covered from proximal normal segment to distal normal segment). Seventy patients with 87 lesions in the spot stenting group were matched for baseline clinical and lesion characteristics, including lesion complexity and vessel size, with 688 patients (769 lesions) in the traditional stenting group. The only difference in baseline characteristics was that the spot stenting group had a higher percentage of calcified lesions (31% versus 17%; *p* < 0.05) and significantly longer lesions (28 ± 11 mm versus 23 ± 8 mm; *p* < 0.01). The mean stent length used for these groups was very different: 21 ± 13 mm in spot stenting versus 29 ± 17 mm in traditional stenting (*p* < 0.05). Short-term event rates did not differ between the two groups, with no difference in stent thrombosis or procedural MACE. However, long-term outcome was significantly different with angiographic restenosis of 25% in the spot stenting group versus 39% in the traditional stenting group (*p* < 0.05) and TLR of 17% in the spot stenting group versus 31% in the traditional stenting group (*p* < 0.05).

The concept of spot stenting is that stents are limited to the shortest length that will achieve an adequate lumen throughout the treated segment. In spite of these shorter stent lengths, there was a high procedural success rate of 96% with a commensurate low rate of acute and subacute complications with this approach: procedural Q-wave MI 1.9%, procedural coronary artery bypass grafts 0%, procedural death 0.9%, acute closure 0 %, acute thrombosis 0%, and subacute thrombosis 0.6%.

PROCEDURAL SAFETY

Historically, balloon angioplasty performed with 'oversized' balloons without IVUS guidance has been reported to be associated with a poor outcome.[35,36] In addition, placing a stent without fully 'covering' the lesion has been viewed as dangerous because of the theoretical risk of acute and subacute stent thrombosis, owing to the potential flow disturbance and lesion reactivity. However, when IVUS is used to guide the intervention, any flow-limiting segments or dissections can be more accurately assessed and a more educated decision can be made as to whether such segments can be left untreated. The rate of major procedural complications in this study does not differ significantly from what has been reported with traditional coronary stenting in less complicated and more focal lesions. In the STRESS trial, Q-wave MI occurred in 2.9% of patients and emergency bypass surgery in 2% of patients.[1] The cumulative incidence of acute and subacute thrombosis in our spot stenting trial was 0.6%, a rate of incidence that is as low as or lower than any of the major stent trials. Therefore, it appears that spot stenting does not increase the incidence of major procedural complications or subacute events despite treating a more complex lesion subset.

IMPLICATIONS FOR MANAGEMENT OF DISSECTIONS AFTER CORONARY INTERVENTIONS

Traditionally, dissections after PTCA have been considered a predictor of acute closure. This concept was extended to include coronary stenting, for which an additional stent was recommended even for small edge dissections that were detected only by IVUS because of the fear of subacute stent thrombosis. However, inducing dissections is an integral part of lumen enlargement with PTCA and most dissections do not proceed to occlusion. A dissection represents an adverse event when it compromises the lumen. We concur that a dissection should be treated when it is associated with TIMI flow < 3. When a dissection is associated with flow of TIMI grade 3, further evaluation beyond angiographic assessment should be considered, e.g. IVUS interrogation or coronary flow measurements. A recent study that compared angiography and IVUS has reported a large discrepancy between these two modalities particularly when dissections are present.[37]

In the IVUS-guided PTCA with spot stenting strategy, residual dissections evaluated by IVUS were present and left untreated in 44% of lesions (82% type B dissections), both in the angioplasty alone group and the spot stenting group (*Table 20.6*). These dissections were all associated with flow of TIMI grade 3 and met the IVUS criteria with the true lumen being > 50% of the vessel area at the dissection site. These dissections were not associated with an increased risk of acute or subacute adverse events in either group. In addition, leaving these dissections untreated allowed further limitation of stent length. Abciximab was used in only 12 of these 109 patients (11%). Although abciximab was more likely to be used for the most complicated cases, there was no difference in the outcome (either immediately or at 6

Table 20.6

Residual angiographic type of dissection after spot stenting

	Total n = 160	Balloon n = 78	Stent n = 82	p
Dissections	71 (44%)	34 (44%)	37 (45%)	NS
Type A, n (%)	3 (4)	1 (3)	2 (6)	
Type B, n (%)	58 (82)	29 (85)	29 (78)	
Type C, n (%)	10 (14)	4 (12)	6 (16)	
Type D, n (%)	0	0	0	

months) in the patients who received abciximab and those who did not.

CASE 3

An example of a long lesion in which a dissection was evaluated by IVUS and left untreated during spot stenting is shown in *Fig. 20.6*. This was a 49 mm long lesion located in the right coronary artery in a patient with previous bypass graft surgery. If traditional stenting were performed in this lesion, the long stent length that would be required to cover it would significantly increase the probability of restenosis. QCA measurement of this artery showed a reference lumen size of 2.67 mm; however, the IVUS media-to-media measurement at the lesion site indicated a diameter of close to 4.0 mm (see *Fig. 20.6a*). The lesion, which measured > 49 mm in length by QCA, was initially treated with a 40 mm long balloon, 3.75 mm in diameter inflated to 14 atmospheres (*Fig. 20.6b*). Although the angiographic result was acceptable, IVUS measurements showed an inadequate result at site A, where the lumen cross-sectional area (CSA) was 3.5 mm² (*Fig. 20.6c*). All other segments of the lesion met minimum IVUS criteria, including site B, where a non-flow-limiting dissection was present. This type of dissection commonly occurred in long lesions with an aggressive balloon approach. IVUS evaluation enabled us to classify this as a benign dissection that could therefore go untreated. The next step was to implant one 16 mm slotted tubular stent only at site A and post-dilate it with a 4.0 mm balloon to 10 atmospheres (*Fig. 20.6d*).

Pre-intervention angiogram

IVUS

QCA

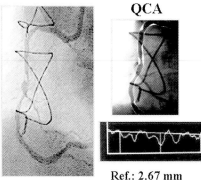

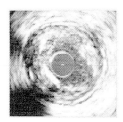

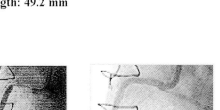

Ref.: 2.67 mm
MLD: 0.98 mm
Lesion length: 49.2 mm

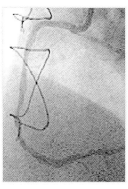

Balloon size: 3.75 mm

a

Figure 20.6 *IVUS guided spot stenting. (a) Baseline angiogram of a right coronary artery with diffuse disease. (b) Angiogram after balloon dilatation. (c) IVUS after balloon angioplasty demonstrates that some areas are more successfully dilated than others. (d) Focal placement of a 16 mm long stent in the proximal RCA. (e) Final angiogram and IVUS study demonstrate that the lumen cross-sectional area satisfies the criteria of being > 5.5 mm². QCA, quantitative coronary angiography; LCSA, lumen cross sectional area.*

Balloon angioplasty

D: 3.75 mm
L: 40 mm
P: 14 atm

After balloon angioplasty

Pre-intervention

b

IVUS after balloon angioplasty

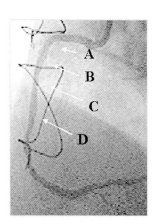

A
B
C
D

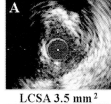

LCSA 3.5 mm²

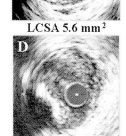

LCSA 5.6 mm²

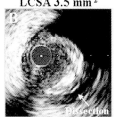

LCSA 7.3 mm²

LCSA 6.3 mm²

c

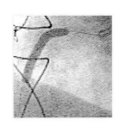

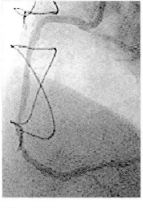

After balloon angioplasty

Stent: DART 16 mm

Post dilatation balloon
D: 4.0 mm
L: 20 mm
P: 10 atm

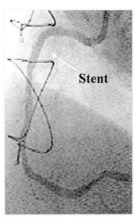

Stent

After spot stenting

d

Figure 20.6 *continued*

IVUS after final procedure

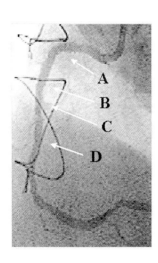

A B C D

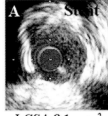

A Stent

LCSA 8.1 mm²

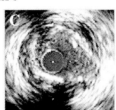

C

LCSA 6.6 mm²

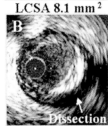

B

Dissection

LCSA 10.2 mm²

LCSA 7.7 mm²

e

In summary, this long lesion was successfully treated with only one short stent to cover the segment that had an inadequate IVUS result. The final IVUS evaluation (*Fig. 20.6e*) confirms the achievement of an acceptable lumen cross-sectional area at all sites. Of note is the dissection at site B, which is not apparent angiographically. The true lumen cross-sectional area is 10.2 mm², which meets the IVUS criteria. In addition, the false lumen of the dissection does not compromise the true lumen as it is < 50% of the vessel area and is associated with TIMI grade 3 flow. The dissection was therefore left untreated.

LONG-TERM OUTCOME

The incidence of restenosis, TLR, and MACE at 6 months after IVUS-guided spot stenting is provided in *Table 20.7*. Considering that the lesions treated with the IVUS-guided spot stenting approach had a mean vessel diameter of 2.94 mm and a mean length of 20.6 mm, an incidence of angiographic restenosis of 17.4%, TLR rate of 13%, and 6-month MACE rate of 22% is very encouraging when compared to what has been reported for treatment of small vessels and long lesions.[7,8,12–14,18,19,38]

Table 20.7

Angiographic and clinical follow-up

	Total	PTCA	Stent	P value
Angiographic follow-up, n* (%)	86 (78)	40 (76)	46 (81)	NS
Minimum lumen diameter (mm)	1.93 ± .76	1.75 ± .67	2.06 ± .80	NS
Mean reference diameter (mm)	2.94 ± .05	2.79 ± .45	3.05 ± .53	< 0.05
Diameter stenosis (%)	34.9 ± 22	37.4 ± 21	33.2 ± 22	NS
Late lumen loss (mm)	0.92 ± 0.77	0.61 ± 0.77	1.15 ± 0.69	0.0012
Loss index	0.43 ± 0.45	0.35 ± 0.58	0.49 ± 0.31	NS
Restenosis, n (%)	15 (17.4)	9 (23)	6 (13)	NS
TLR, n (%)	14 (13)	9 (17)	5 (9)	NS
MACE 6-month, n (%)	16 (22)			

TLR is target lesion revascularization; * number of eligible lesions (n = 110).

CASE 4

The 6-month follow-up data are typified in this case example (*Fig. 20.7*). As in the previous examples, this is a diffusely diseased vessel. In this case there was a subtotal occlusion in the right coronary artery in a patient who had previously undergone bypass surgery. The initial approach was to use balloon angioplasty, which was followed by a cutting balloon with a good angiographic result. IVUS interrogation showed that there was an inadequate cross-sectional area in the mid-portion (< 5.5 mm², which was < 50% of the reference vessel area at the lesion site) even though there was a satisfactory angiographic result (*Fig. 20.7b*). The cross-sectional area in the distal portion of the right coronary artery measured 4.5 mm²; however, the vessel area at this site was only 8.8 mm² and thus the lumen met the minimal criteria of being greater than 50% of the vessel area. The final step was to place a 15 mm slotted tubular stent only at the specific site with an inadequate result in the mid-portion of the vessel. The 6-month angiographic follow-up showed an excellent long-term result with minimal recoil and little intimal hyperplasia (*Fig. 20.7c*).

This case exemplifies the basis of this technique: to allow maximal lumen optimization while limiting stent length. This approach confines short-term complications and maximizes long-term outcome by permitting the largest lumen possible to compensate for remodeling while at the same time minimizing the foundation for intimal hyperplasia.

CONCLUSIONS

The major concepts brought out by this technique include:

(a) treatment of small vessels and long lesions with IVUS-guided balloon angioplasty assisted with focal stenting has a procedural success rate that is higher than historical success rates reported with traditional PTCA alone and is similar to success rates reported with contemporary coronary stenting (in which the lesion is covered from a proximal normal segment to a distal normal segment);

(b) acute and subacute complication rates with this approach are similar to those for contemporary stenting;

(c) long-term follow-up data suggest that the angiographic restenosis and the need for TLR with this approach are significantly better than with either traditional PTCA alone or traditional stenting when applied to small vessels and long lesions; and

(d) angiographic dissections with preserved lumen dimensions as documented by IVUS could be left unstented without increased risk of acute or subacute closure.

IVUS-guided balloon angioplasty assisted by spot stenting permits safe treatment of long lesions and lesions in small vessels. This strategy requires the use

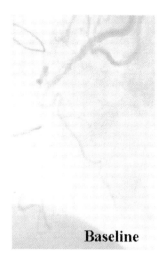

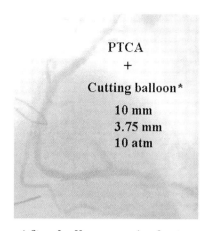

PTCA
+
Cutting balloon*
10 mm
3.75 mm
10 atm

Baseline

After balloon angioplasty

(*final procedure before stenting)

a

Figure 20.7 *IVUS guided spot stenting. (a) Baseline angiogram reveals diffuse disease in this RCA. (b) Following balloon dilatation and cutting balloon dilatation, the IVUS study demonstrates focal areas with an inadequate lumen cross-sectional area. (c) A 15 mm long BX stent was placed in the mid-RCA. The six-month follow-up angiogram demonstrates minimal restenosis despite the extensive disease at baseline.*

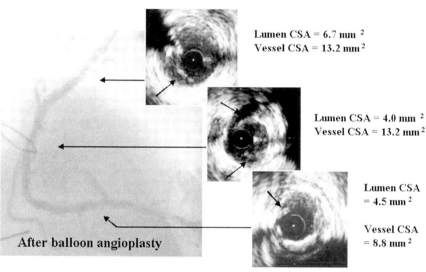

Lumen CSA = 6.7 mm²
Vessel CSA = 13.2 mm²

Lumen CSA = 4.0 mm²
Vessel CSA = 13.2 mm²

Lumen CSA
= 4.5 mm²

Vessel CSA
= 8.8 mm²

After balloon angioplasty

b

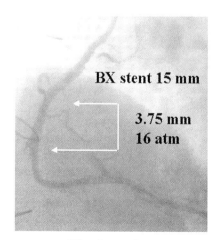

BX stent 15 mm

3.75 mm
16 atm

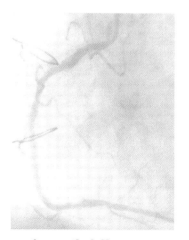

Final result

6 month follow-up

c

of stents in half the cases; most of the stents used are shorter than the original lesions. Both short-term events and long-term outcome, including 6-month MACE (22%), target lesion revascularization (13%), and angiographic restenosis (17%) appear to be superior to the results achieved in historical controls that use balloon angioplasty alone or traditional stenting, in which the lesion is covered from normal segment to normal segment.

REFERENCES

1. Ellis S, Roubin G, King SI et al. Importance of stenosis morphology in the estimation of restenosis risk after elective percutaneous transluminal coronary angioplasty. *Am J Cardiol* 1989; **63**: 30–34.

2. Tenaglia A, Zidar J, Jackman J et al. Treatment of long coronary artery narrowings with long angioplasty balloon catheters. *Am J Cardiol* 1993; **71**: 1274–1277.

3. Savage MP, Fischman DL, Rake R et al. Efficacy of coronary stenting vs balloon angioplasty in small coronary arteries. Stent restenosis study (STRESS) investigators. *J Am Coll Cardiol* 1998; **31**: 307–11.

4. Fernandez-Ortiz A, Perez-Vizcayno MJ, Goicolea J et al. Should we stent small coronary vessels? Comparison with conventional balloon angioplasty (abstract). *Eur Heart J* 1997; **18 (suppl)**: 286.

5. Keane D, Azar AJ, de Jaegere PP et al, on behalf of the BENESTENT investigators. Clinical and angiographic outcome of elective stent implantation in small coronary vessels: an analysis of the BENESTENT trial. *Semin Interven Cardiol* 1996; **1**: 255–262.

6. Fischman DL, Leon MB, Baim D et al. A randomized comparison of coronary stent placement and balloon angioplasty in the treatment of coronary artery disease. *N Engl J Med* 1994; **331**: 496–501.

7. Serruys P, Jaegere P, Kiemeneij F et al. A comparison of balloon expandable stent implantation with balloon angioplasty in patients with coronary artery disease. *N Engl J Med* 1994; **331**: 489–95.

8. Garcia E, Serruys PW, Dawkins K et al. BENESTENT II trial: final results of visit II & III: a 7–months follow-up (abstract). *Eur Heart J* 1997; **18 (suppl)**: 1960.

9. Kobayashi Y, DeGregorio J, Reimers B et al. The length of the stented segment is an independent predictor of restenosis (abstract). *J Am Coll Cardiol* 1998; **31**: 306A

10. Moussa I, Di Mario C, Moses J et al. Single versus multiple Palmaz–Schatz stent implantation: immediate and follow-up results. *J Am Coll Cardiol* 1997; **(Suppl)**: 276A.

11. Kobayashi Y, DeGregorio J, Reimers B et al. Immediate and follow-up results following implantation of the long and short NIR stent. Comparison with the Palmaz–Schatz stent. *J Am Coll Cardiol* 1998; **31**: 312A.

12. Colombo A, Hall P, Nakamura S et al. Intracoronary stenting without anticoagulation accomplished with intravascular ultrasound guidance. *Circulation* 1995; **91**: 1676–1688.

13. Schomig A, Neumann FJ, Kastrati A et al. A randomized comparison of antiplatelet and anticoagulant therapy after the placement of coronary artery stents. *N Engl J Med* 1996; **334**: 1084–1089.

14. Karrillon GJ, Morice MC, Benveniste E et al. Intracoronary stent implantation without ultrasound guidance and with replacement of conventional anticoagulation by antiplatelet therapy. *Circulation* 1996; **94**: 1519–1527.

15. Chan CN, Tan AT, Koh TH et al. Intracoronary stenting in the treatment of acute or threatened closure in angiographically small coronary arteries (< 3.0 mm) complicating PTCA. *Am J Cardiol* 1995; **75**: 23–25.

16. Lau KW, He Q, Ding ZP, Johan A. Safety and efficacy of angiography guided stent placement in small native coronary arteries of < 3.0 mm. *Clin Cardiol* 1997; **20**: 711–716.

17. Akiyama T, Reimers B, Moussa I et al. Angiographic and clinical outcome following coronary stenting of small vessels: a comparison with coronary stenting of large vessels. *J Am Coll Cardiol* 1998; **32**: 1610–1618.

18. Itoh A, Hall P, Maiello L et al. Coronary stenting of long lesions (greater than 20 mm): a matched comparison of different stents (abstract). *Circulation* 1995; 92 **(suppl I)**: I-688.

19. Yokoi H, Nobuyoshi M, Nosaka H et al. Coronary stenting for long lesions (lesion length > 20 mm) in native coronary arteries: comparison of three different types of stents (abstract). *Circulation* 1996; **94**: 4006.

20. Warth D, Leon MB, O'Neill W et al. Rotational atherectomy multicenter registry: acute results, complications and 6 month angiographic follow-up in 709 patients. *J Am Coll Cardiol* 1994; **24**: 641–648.

21. Ellis S. Popma J, Buchbinder M et al. Relation of clinical presentation stenosis morphology and operator technique to the procedural results of rotational atherectomy-facilitated angioplasty. *Circulation* 1994; **89**: 882–892.

22. Reisman M, Cohen B, Warth D et al. Outcome of long lesions treated with high speed rotational ablation (abstract). *J Am Coll Cardiol* 1993; **21 (suppl)**: 443A.

23. Tierstein PS, Warth DC, Haq N et al. High speed rotational coronary atherectomy for patients with diffuse coronary artery disease. *J Am Coll Cardiol* 1991; **18**: 1694–1701.

24. Cohen BM, Weber VJ, Bass TA et al. Coronary perforation during rotational ablation: angiographic determinants and clinical outcome. *J Am Coll Cardiol* 1994; **March special issue: (Suppl)** 354A.

25. Leguizamon JH, Chambre DF, Torresani EM et al. High-speed coronary rotational atherectomy. Are angiographic factors predictive of failure, major complications or restenosis? A multivariate analysis (abstract). *J Am Coll Cardiol* 1995; **March special issue: (Suppl)** 95A.

26. Baim D, Hinohara T, Holmes D et al., and the US Directional Atherectomy Investigator Group. Results of directional coronary atherectomy during multicenter preapproval testing (abstract). *Am J Cardiol* 1993; **72 (suppl)**: 6E–11E.

27. Hinohara T, Rowe MH, Tcheng JE et al. Effect of lesion characteristics on outcome of directional coronary atherectomy. *J Am Coll Cardiol* 1991; **17**: 1112–1120.

28. Robertson G, Selmon M, Hinohara T et al. The effect of lesion length on outcome of directional coronary atherectomy. *Circulation* 1990; **82**: III–623.

29. Foley DP, Appleman YE, Piek JJ. Comparison of angiographic restenosis propensity of excimer laser coronary angioplasty and balloon angioplasty in the

Amsterdam Rotterdam (AMRO) trial (abstract). *Circulation* 1995; **92 (suppl)**: I–477.

30. Appleman YE, Piek J, Redekop WK et al. Excimer laser angioplasty versus balloon angioplasty in longer coronary lesions: a multivariate analysis (abstract). *Circulation* 1995; **92 (suppl)**: I–74.

31. Stone GW, Hodgson JM, St Goar FG et al, for the Clinical Outcomes With Ultrasound Trial (CLOUT) investigators. Improved procedural results of coronary angioplasty with intravascular-ultrasound guided balloon sizing. *Circulation* 1997; **95**: 2044–2052.

32. Abizaid A, Mehran R, Pichard AD et al. Results of high pressure ultrasound-guided 'over-sized' balloon PTCA to achieve 'stent-like' results. *J Am Coll Cardiol* 1997; **29 (suppl A)**: 280A.

33. Frey AW, Muller Ch, Hodgson J, Roskamm H. Fewer acute major adverse cardiac events (MACE) by ultrasound guided interventions: findings from the strategy of intracoronary ultrasound guided PTCA and stenting (SIPS) trial (abstract). *Eur Heart J* 1997; **18 (suppl)**: 862.

34. Kobayashi N, De Gregorio J, Kobayashi Y et al. Effect of varying stent length on outcome in the treatment of long lesions with subanalysis of small and large reference vessels. *Circulation* 1998; **98 (suppl):** 1486.

35. Roubin GS, Douglas JS, King SB et al. Influence of balloon size on initial success, acute complications, and restenosis after percutaneous transluminal coronary angioplasty. *Circulation* 1988; **78**: 557–565.

36. Nichols AB, Smith R, Berke AD et al. Importance of balloon size in coronary angioplasty. *J Am Coll Cardiol* 1989; **13**: 1094–1100.

37. Ozaki Y, Violaris A, Kobayashi T et al. Comparison of coronary luminal quantitation obtained from intracoronary ultrasound and both geometric and videodensitometric quantitative angiography before and after balloon angioplasty and directional atherectomy. *Circulation* 1997; **96**: 491–499.

38. Mehran R, Hong M, Lansky A et al. Vessel size and lesion length influence late clinical outcomes after native coronary artery stent placement (abstract). *Circulation* 1997; **96**: 1520.

Chapter 21 Mechanisms of in-stent restenosis: the effect of high-pressure inflations and large balloons in the deployment of intracoronary stents

Steven L Goldberg

INTRODUCTION

Despite the early promise of stent technology as an adjunct to coronary angioplasty, the initial experience with stents was associated with a 10–30% incidence of subacute thrombosis. This complication often led to a devastating myocardial infarction (MI) and carried a high mortality risk.[1] To reduce this complication, aggressive anticoagulation strategies were adopted, including prolonged heparinization and routine use of warfarin, aspirin, and dextran. Although these strategies appeared to lessen the likelihood of stent thrombosis, the incidence remained approximately 5%, still high given the important clinical consequences. Additionally, bleeding complications were common, especially at vascular access sites, with an incidence of 10–20% of stent cases. The prolonged hospitalization needed for anticoagulation, as well as the management of bleeding and vascular complications, significantly increased the cost of stenting compared to angioplasty alone.[2] These disadvantages to stenting partly offset their important benefits, which include the successful treatment of acute or threatened closure resulting from balloon angioplasty and a reduction in the incidence of the common problem of restenosis.

Although some initial investigators, in particular Richard Schatz, proposed using oversized balloons to expand coronary stents more fully, this strategy was not universally applied. In late 1992, based on information from intravascular ultrasound (IVUS) imaging, we recognized that angiography could be misleading after stent insertions.[3,4] IVUS revealed several patterns of inadequate stent deployment, including poor apposition to the arterial wall, inadequate expansion resulting from insufficient plaque compression, and incomplete plaque or dissection coverage, despite acceptable angiographic appearances. Limitations of angiography arise because angiography is a two-dimensional imaging modality whereas the coronary tree is a complex three-dimensional structure.[5]

It was hypothesized that stent thrombosis may partly be the result of inadequate stent expansion with insufficient plaque compression and a small residual lumen. Less optimal blood flow or inadequate lesion coverage could create relative stasis or turbulence, which might also promote thrombus formation. It was theorized that if full stent expansion could be achieved, the resultant brisk blood flow should minimize stent thrombosis even without anticoagulation. To improve stent expansion, larger balloons were used and later high-pressure inflations were added, with IVUS employed to document and guide the results. Using these more aggressive stent implantation techniques, standard anticoagulant regimens were abandoned and replaced with the antiplatelet agent ticlopidine along with aspirin.[6]

This approach was associated with stent thrombosis rates under 1%, with a significant decrease in bleeding complications and hospital stays. This led to lower costs of the stent procedure resulting from the decreased rates of complications and shorter hospitalizations. Owing to these benefits, high-pressure balloon inflation has become the current standard of stent implantation, along with the post-procedure regimen of aspirin and ticlopidine. As a consequence of the ease of this approach and the predictable results achieved, stent use has flourished; stents are now used in over 50–70% of coronary angioplasty procedures world-wide. However, questions have been raised on the need for high-pressure techniques and, in particular, whether these more aggressive techniques may lead to more exuberant scarring within the stent, resulting in greater rates of restenosis or more aggressive restenosis.

TWO CONFLICTING THEORIES OF RESTENOSIS

Two somewhat contradictory theories regarding promotion of restenosis after coronary angioplasty have emerged. In the first theory, deep wall injury is hypothesized to lead to an aggressive healing process with a greater amount of scar formation and restenosis.[7-11] The other theory is based upon the observation that 'bigger is better', that is, the rate of restenosis decreases as the final lumen size increases after an angioplasty procedure.[12-14] Proponents of the first theory try to minimize trauma to the arterial wall, whereas those who subscribe to the 'bigger is better' approach seek to achieve as large a lumen as possible without regard to deep wall injury. One caveat is that the greater the increase in lumen dimensions achieved from an angioplasty procedure, the more late loss (reduction in minimum lumen diameter (MLD) from the end of the procedure until follow-up) is realized (i.e. a greater 'tax' is imposed).[7,15] Additionally, the insertion of a stent is associated with a greater late loss than non-stent angioplasty procedures. Although this is in part due to the effect of the tax of the greater acute gain, there appears to be increased intimal proliferation after stenting, perhaps resulting from a biological reaction to a foreign body.[16-20] Inflammation, thrombus formation, and compression of various components of the arterial wall have been implicated in the mechanism of stent-induced fibrous tissue proliferation.

VESSEL WALL INJURY AND THE HEALING PROCESS

Compression of the arterial wall by angioplasty devices causes destruction of the vasa vasorum in the arterial adventia, resulting in the potential for arterial wall hypoxia inducing a healing response.[21] Increased platelet activation may occur, owing to

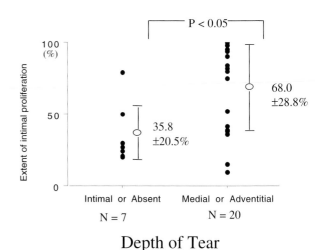

Figure 21.1 *Relation between depth of the pathologically identified coronary tear and extent of intimal proliferation in 27 lesions. Deep arterial injury is associated with more extensive intimal proliferation. From Nobuyoshi et al.,[30] with permission.*

deep arterial wall injury.[9] Compression of the media results in smooth muscle cell injury and subsequent increased DNA synthesis.[21] Studies in some animal models have demonstrated that the degree of coronary artery injury leads to a proportional increase in neointimal proliferation and restenosis.[8,23–24] In a porcine overstretch model of in-stent restenosis, the extent of vascular injury was correlated with the amount of neointimal formation.[8] Rupture of the internal elastic lamina and medial injury were related to an increased proliferative response (*Fig. 21.1*). Similarly, a graded in-stent neointimal response was seen in response to worsening histological injury in a porcine model reported by Frimerman and colleagues.[23] In addition, neointimal thickness has been related to the maximum stent strut penetration into the vessel wall in porcine coronary arteries.[25] However, other animal studies have not shown a consistent relationship between amount of stress applied to the arterial wall and subsequent neoproliferative response.[26,27] Carter and colleagues[26] described greater neointimal thickening at stent wire sites with underlying plaque but not at sites of internal elastic lamina rupture in an atherosclerotic rabbit model. The same investigators, however, did find a relationship between elastic lamina rupture and

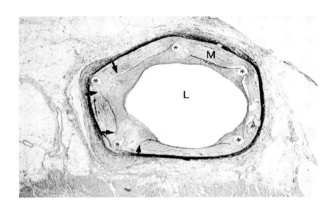

Figure 21.2 *Histological image from a porcine coronary artery 28 days after a coil stent was implanted and dilated with an oversize balloon. An increased neointimal response is seen at the site of internal elastic membrane rupture (arrows). M, media; L, lumen. From Schwarz et al.,[26] with permission.*

increased neointimal growth in a porcine coronary artery model.[24] Vorwerk and colleagues[27] evaluated two types of self-expanding Wallstents in a non-atherosclerotic canine model in iliac arteries. One type of Wallstent has about twice the force of the other type; however, the degree of neointimal proliferation was similar at 6 months between the two stent types.

Animal models of restenosis may be misleading. Recent data have demonstrated different mechanisms of restenosis after balloon angioplasty or atherectomy in animal models from humans. Whereas intimal proliferation is the primary mechanism of restenosis in animal models, vascular remodeling or chronic recoil is an important contributor to the restenosis process after non-stent angioplasty procedures in humans.[16,28] This calls into question the clinical significance of animal studies of restenosis.

There are few data relating the level of deep arterial wall injury to restenosis in humans. In a postmortem study of 20 patients who had restenosis, greater intimal proliferation was found when deep arterial injury (media or adventitial) was found (*Fig. 21.2*).[29] This small study seems to support a potential relationship between deep arterial injury and neointimal tissue growth in humans. Different investigators

have examined histological specimens obtained from directional coronary atherectomy with divergent conclusions. Garratt and colleagues[11] reported a slightly higher recurrent restenosis rate when tissue from the media or adventitia were obtained from restenotic lesions, but not from de novo atherosclerotic lesions. However, Kuntz and colleagues[14] found that restenosis was not adversely affected by the retrieval of subintimal elements. In fact, restenosis was actually lower when adventitia was recovered from atherectomy specimens. The effect of deep wall injury alone does not appear to have a strong effect on the restenosis process.

MINIMIZING DEEP ARTERIAL TRAUMA AND RESTENOSIS: NON-STENT TRIALS

Several trials of coronary interventions using atherectomy devices have attempted to incorporate strategies that would minimize the degree of vascular compression with the hope that less vascular scar formation would ensue.[30-33] In the CAVEAT (Coronary Angioplasty Versus Excisional Atherectomy Trial)[30] a minimalist strategy of directional atherectomy was used, which included avoidance of adjunctive balloon angioplasty to reduce vascular barotrauma, under the impression that this avoidance would lead to less intimal proliferation. This strategy of directional atherectomy was shown to have a modest, clinically insignificant restenosis benefit compared to balloon angioplasty. However, the OARS[34] and BOAT[35] trials employed aggressive strategies of directional atherectomy, including the use of adjunctive balloon angioplasty. These trials demonstrated significant reductions in restenosis, both compared to balloon angioplasty as well as the results seen with the minimalist directional atherectomy approach tried in CAVEAT.

Similarly, the STRATAS trial[32,33] was designed to compare the results of two different strategies of rotational atherectomy. A strategy of using large rotational atherectomy burrs with subsequent avoidance of the barotrauma of adjunctive balloon angioplasty was compared with a strategy of maximizing the acute results with adjunctive balloon angioplasty following a less aggressive rotablation strategy. Despite avoiding the barotrauma of adjunctive balloon angioplasty, the first strategy was not associated with more favorable rates of restenosis.

THE 'BIGGER IS BETTER' APPROACH

In contrast to the paucity of data relating the degree of induced vascular injury to subsequent restenosis, several investigators have noted a strong relationship between the final luminal result achieved after a coronary intervention and the risk of restenosis.[12,13,15,21,36] This relationship remains whether the intervention being performed is an atherectomy procedure, a stent implantation, or a stand-alone balloon angioplasty, although differences may exist between devices.[37] This association is confounded in part by the strong inverse relationship between vessel size and restenosis[38] (i.e. small vessel size is associated with higher rates of restenosis). Despite this, multivariate logistic regression analyses have consistently demonstrated a relationship between the final luminal result achieved and follow-up lumen diameter, independent of reference lumen arterial diameter.

MECHANISM OF IN-STENT RESTENOSIS

Some differences exist between the causes of restenosis when stents are used and when angioplasty is performed without the use of stents. Arterial remodeling, or chronic recoil of the balloon-injured artery, contributes significantly to the restenosis process in non-stented lesions, with neointimal proliferation playing a secondary role.[16,28,39] After placement of a rigid stent, such as the Palmaz–Schatz stent, chronic recoil remodeling is essentially abolished at the stent site, and restenosis is entirely due to neointimal tissue growth.[18,40,41] Recoil may contribute to restenosis occurring at the stent borders and at the articulation of the Palmaz–Schatz stent.[41] Whether chronic remodeling is abolished with other stent types, in particular the coil stents, is not known. Some remodeling may occur as a result of their decreased radial strength. Tissue prolapse may also contribute to restenosis in coil stents, which have larger gaps between metal struts than the slotted tube stents.

RESTENOSIS AT STENT BORDERS

Although one of the important benefits of stents is the prevention of recoil, this advantage is offset in part by an increased production of new tissue compared to lesions treated only with angioplasty.[19,20] Restenosis at the stent borders comprises approximately one-third of cases of stent restenosis.[42] The edges of stents are potentially exposed to a dual mechanism for restenosis: remodeling and increased proliferative response. However, in one study of serial IVUS examinations after stent implantation, vascular remodeling was present without progression of disease in the reference segments.[43] Animal studies have suggested that neointimal proliferation may be directly related to the amount of underlying atherosclerotic plaque.[24,26] IVUS evaluations have shown that plaque volume is an important predictor of restenosis in both stenting and non-stenting procedures.[44–47] Therefore, the smaller plaque volume present at the edge of the stent compared with the more significantly stenosed part of the artery may lead to less intimal proliferation at this location than at the site of the original lesion. This lack of intimal proliferation at the stent borders suggests that the barotrauma caused by the high-pressure balloon inflation does not, by itself, induce a hyperproliferative response. Rather, the increased intrastent neointimal response is probably related to the increased plaque burden at the original lesion location and the hyperproliferative reaction to a foreign body.

DATA SUGGEST INCREASED INTRASTENT RESTENOSIS FROM AGGRESSIVE STENT DEPLOYMENT TECHNIQUES

Some investigators have suggested that the use of aggressive techniques to expand stents may lead to a greater restenosis reaction by stimulating a more profound healing response. In addition, aggressive techniques may lead to more stent edge restenosis by promoting more intimal tissue growth or negative vascular remodeling or by leading to dissections that require additional stenting. Some observers have noted a relationship between the use of very high pressures and increased restenosis.[48–53] Mehran and colleagues[48] constructed an injury score to assess balloon-to-artery ratios and inflation pressures as contributing factors to in-stent restenosis. They evaluated the quantitative coronary angiography parameters of acute gain, late loss, and the loss index, as well as the degree of neointimal proliferation identified by IVUS imaging. Acute gain is defined as the increase in the minimum lumen diameter from the original stenosis to the result achieved at the end of the stenting procedure. The late loss is the subsequent decrease in MLD from the end of the stent procedure until the follow-up angiogram. The loss index is the late loss divided by the acute gain, a measurement of the 'tax' imposed by the intervention, and it is independent of the size of the initial result achieved. In this retrospective analysis, greater neointimal proliferation and a higher loss index were seen in the arteries with larger injury scores. However, they also noted an inverse relationship between increasing injury scores and treated vessel size (i.e. more aggressive techniques were used in smaller vessels).

Savage and colleagues[49] performed a subgroup analysis of data from the Saphenous Vein De Novo (SAVED) trial, which evaluated the use of intracoronary stents in saphenous vein grafts. They noted that the use of high-pressure balloon inflations was initiated during the course of the trial, and they therefore compared the angiographic outcomes between lesions treated with pressures < 16 atmospheres (88 patients) and those treated with ≥ 16 atmospheres (31 patients). Despite similar minimum intrastent lumen diameters at the end of the stenting procedure, the MLD at 6 months was considerably lower in the lesions treated with higher pressures (1.26 mm versus 1.91 mm; $p < 0.01$), owing to greater late loss (1.47 mm versus 0.91 mm; $p < 0.01$).

One limitation of this evaluation is a trend towards larger arteries in the low-pressure group (3.23 mm versus 3.03 mm; $p = 0.09$ using a standard deviation of 0.56 mm seen from the trial overall)[54] suggesting that there may have been significant underlying differences between the two groups. It is not clear from this analysis how many lesions treated with < 16 atmospheres of pressure were in the earlier time period and how many were in the later time period, or if an important percentage of patients in the low-pressure group were in fact in the later time period. If an excellent result is achieved with 12–15 atmospheres of pressure, this may represent a compliant lesion in contrast to the lesions treated with high pressures, which may have been more refractory. In addition, the effect of balloon size was not accounted for. It was not reported if larger balloons or higher balloon-to-artery ratios were employed in the low-pressure group. Finally, the selection of 16 atmospheres as the division between high and low pressures appears to be somewhat arbitrary. In the BENESTENT (Belgian–Netherland Stent) trial, the mean inflation pressure to expand

stents was 10 ± 18 atmospheres.[55] Therefore, an analysis of high-pressure stenting should compare strategies using pressures larger than those used during previous periods. By selecting the higher end of the pressures, more refractory lesions may be selected, creating a bias against the use of higher pressures.

Hausleiter and colleagues[50] also evaluated the impact of high inflation pressures on late luminal loss and restenosis. They compared 435 stented lesions treated with pressures > 15 atmospheres (mean pressure 17 ± 2 atmospheres) to 622 lesions treated with pressures < 15 atmospheres (mean pressure 12 ± 2 atmospheres). These investigators found a greater acute gain but also a greater late loss in the group treated with higher pressures, resulting in a similar follow-up MLD, loss index, and restenosis rate. The relative increase in late loss is consistent with the previously described effect of larger initial gain (i.e. the tax that is imposed is a function of the size achieved). This is reflected in the identical loss index, and therefore restenosis does not appear to be a function of inflation pressure used. In addition, there were important baseline differences between the two groups. The high-pressure group had smaller baseline MLDs and higher percentage diameter stenoses, suggesting greater plaque volume. Reference arterial diameters and lesion lengths are critical baseline parameters and unfortunately were not reported.

Fernandez-Aviles and colleagues,[51] reporting on 225 lesions treated with coronary stenting, noted a direct relationship between maximum deployment pressure and late loss. Lesions treated with ≤ 12 atmospheres had a late loss of 1.0 ± 0.8 mm, whereas when > 12 atmospheres of pressure was used the late loss was 1.3 ± 0.8 mm ($p = 0.01$). Important variables, including reference artery diameters, acute gain, and baseline and final MLD, were not reported, however. These same investigators expanded this analysis to include 411 type A or B lesions in 362 patients; they found maximum deployment pressure to be predictive of late loss and loss index (the late loss divided by the acute gain) by multivariate analysis.[56]

Werner and colleagues[57] noted a direct relationship between the relative amount of vessel stretch and the relative amount of neointimal tissue at follow-up. This reflects the increased 'tax' imposed on larger lumen gain. This points to a potentially deleterious effect of overexpanding the vessel; however, the final overall luminal result was not addressed by this study and it is not clear how much vessel size confounded these observations.

Metzger and colleagues[59] performed coronary blood flow reserve measurements using a Doppler-tipped guidewire and intracoronary injections of adenosine in 14 patients undergoing intracoronary stent insertions. The implantation of a stent deployed to 9 atmospheres led to an increase in coronary flow reserve compared to the results after pre-dilatation but before stent implantation. However, after further inflations within the stent to 15 atmospheres, there was a decrease in coronary flow reserve, despite an improvement in angiographic dimensions. The clinical significance of this finding is unclear, however, because the measurements were performed only immediately after stent deployment and they may have reflected a transient phenomenon (e.g. diffuse spasm after the high-pressure inflation or distal embolization). The strong correlation of final MLD and subsequent freedom from restenosis, combined with the improved lumen diameters achieved after the higher-pressure inflations, argues against the authors' assertion that the measured drop in coronary flow reserve is clinically relevant.

A strategy of high-pressure stent deployment as is practiced currently (mean pressure 14 ± 3 atmospheres) was compared with the routine use of very high pressures (20 atmospheres) by Urestsky and colleagues.[53] In this non-randomized study of 97 patients, those treated with 20 atmospheres of pressure did not achieve statistically significantly larger final lumen dimensions. However, they did have a higher incidence of major adverse cardiac events after the index hospitalization, including death, MI, subsequent percutaneous transluminal coronary angioplasty, and coronary artery bypass graft surgery (32% versus 12%; $p = 0.025$).

Yokoi and colleagues[58] retrospectively evaluated 212 discrete (<15 mm) lesions in vessels > 3.0 mm in diameter. They compared angiographic and clinical outcomes based on the final pressure used to dilate the stent: < 10 atmospheres, 10–14 atmospheres or > 14 atmospheres.[58] Slightly larger MLDs at the end of the procedure were seen in the medium- and high-pressure groups, but the difference was not statistically significant. A trend towards greater MLD at follow-up was seen with progressive balloon inflation pressures, but the restenosis rate was 13% in all three groups. Of note is the fact that the three groups had similar balloon-to-artery ratios. This study therefore failed to support a benefit or a detriment of high-pressure balloon inflations, although a trend towards improved follow-up MLD with increasing pressures suggests that a benefit might have been seen with larger numbers.

A randomized trial comparing low pressures (9 ± 3 atmospheres) to high pressures (14 ± 2 atmospheres) has been reported by Glogar and colleagues,[59] using Wiktor stents in 187 patients. These investigators reported no difference in initial success, MLD at the end of the procedure and follow-up, rate of restenosis or clinical events between the two groups. The balloon-to-artery ratios were not reported, however. It is not clear if larger stent sizes were selected for the lower pressure group, which would have made a significant impact on the acute lumen results obtained. The inability to achieve a larger initial result in the high-pressure group may have been a reflection of smaller balloon sizes or of a possible lack of benefit of higher pressures for this stent type. Despite similar initial lumen results using low and high pressures, there were no differences in the 6–month angiographic diameters. This does not support, therefore, the presence of any deleterious effects of the high-pressure inflations on the induction of intimal proliferation. Improved outcomes would not be expected if larger acute lumen results were not obtained.

Other investigators have failed to find a relationship between inflation pressures or balloon-to-artery ratios and subsequent tissue proliferation.[60-62]

AGGRESSIVE STRATEGIES FOR RESISTANT LESIONS

There are several limitations to the analyses presented above. In most of these studies, the authors were comparing different levels of high pressures. The choice of pressure was at the discretion of the interventionalist. It is likely that the highest pressures were used in the most resistant lesions. Lesions resistant to expansion are associated with higher rates of restenosis.[63] Therefore, such analyses suffer from comparing different types of lesions rather than comparing different strategies. Furthermore, there is usually an inverse relationship between pressure used and balloon sizes, especially when the balloon sizes are normalized for reference artery size. This complex interaction of arterial size, balloon-to-artery ratio, pressure, and plaque resistance limits the ability to dissect the precise impact of a specific technique.

HISTORICAL COMPARISON OF STRATEGIES

In an attempt to circumvent some of the limitations mentioned above, we performed an analysis on outcomes from intracoronary stent insertions. We compared two different time periods when divergent strategies were employed for stent deployment at Centro Cuore Columbus Hospital in Milan, Italy.[64] Before 1993, stents were routinely deployed using a balloon-to-artery ratio of 1.0:1 and 1.1:1, with 6–8 atmosphere inflations, when a < 30% diameter stenosis was considered successful. From early in 1993, IVUS was used to guide the stent deployment to ensure optimal stent expansion. Initially, larger balloons were used to maximize stent expansion; however, a few cases of catastrophic vessel rupture occurred, when we used balloons larger than the vessel dimensions identified by IVUS. As an alternative to such oversized balloons, high-pressure inflations (> 12 atmospheres) became routine, with IVUS used in more than 80% of cases to ensure maximal stent expansion.

For analysis of the effects of aggressive stent implantations, 688 lesions in 614 patients were divided into two chronological groups: the lesions treated before 1993 (Group A, 212 vessels in 194 patients) and the lesions treated in 1993 and 1994 (Group B, 476 vessels in 420 patients). To minimize the effect of an early learning curve of stent implantation, the first 150 patients treated with stents at this institution were not included in the analysis.

Lesion characteristics were generally well matched between the two groups, although there were some important differences.[64] Whereas all lesions in Group A were treated with Palmaz–Schatz stents, 14% of the lesions in Group B were treated with other stent types, including Wiktor stents and Gianturco–Roubin Flexstents. Longer lesions were seen in Group B, and the lesions in Group B were more frequently located in the left anterior descending artery.

Early (30-day) complication rates were similar between the two groups but less stent thrombosis was seen in Group B (0.7% versus 4.4%; $p < 0.05$). (However, patients in Group A were treated with warfarin after the procedure, whereas the majority in Group B were treated with aspirin and ticlopidine. Less stent thrombosis occurs with aspirin and ticlopidine than with warfarin.[65–76]) The rate of early complications was higher in the first 6 months of our experience with Group B than later, suggesting a learning curve in the use of aggressive stent implantation (11.3% in the first 6 months versus 5.4% thereafter and 10.4% in Group A, $p < 0.03$ for both comparisons).

Angiographic follow-up was achieved in 79% of Group A and in 81% of Group B patients (p not significant). A greater acute gain was obtained in Group B (2.4 ± 0.7 mm versus 2.1 ± 0.7 mm; $p < 0.001$), resulting in a larger final MLD (2.2 ± 0.9 mm versus 1.9 ± 0.9; $p < 0.01$). Neither late loss nor loss index were significantly different between the groups. There was a trend towards increased net gain in Group B compared to Group A (1.4 ± 0.9 mm versus 1.2 ± 0.9; $p = 0.08$). Group B had a lower rate of restenosis (20% versus 29%; $p < 0.05$).

Group B lesions were treated with 'aggressive' stent deployment (balloon-to-artery ratios > 1.15:1 or dilating pressure ≥ 12 atmospheres) 88% of the time, compared with 56% of the time in Group A ($p < 0.0001$). Lesions treated with 'aggressive' stent deployment had a lower percentage diameter stenosis on the follow-up angiogram (28% versus 37%; $p < 0.01$) and a lower rate of restenosis (20% versus 33%; $p < 0.01$).

The following parameters were identified as univariate predictors of restenosis from the overall population: Group A (pre-1993) lesion, longer lesion, smaller reference artery, smaller baseline MLD smaller final MLD, complex lesion (type B2 or C), a restenotic narrowing, or not using an 'aggressive' stent deployment. Stepwise logistic regression analysis was performed using these variables. Group A remained an independent predictor of restenosis when the final MLD was not included in the calculation, but it was not significant when the final MLD was included. Not using 'aggressive' stent deployment techniques remained an independent predictor of restenosis except when the group of the patient was included in the regression formula. Therefore, the benefits of being in Group B or of the use of 'aggressive' stent deployment techniques were entirely due to the achievement of larger final lumen diameters.

Clinical evidence of restenosis (death, MI, or the need for target lesion revascularization at least 1 month after the procedure) was reduced in Group B patients compared to those in Group A (17% versus 26%; $p < 0.02$). There were fewer non-fatal MIs in Group B patients (0% versus 1.9%; $p < 0.05$) with a trend towards lower target lesion revascularization (16% versus 22%; $p = 0.1$). Freedom from any clinical occurrence, including both early and follow-up events, was more favorable in Group B (78% versus 70%; $p < 0.03$).

This study suggests that freedom from restenosis is primarily dependent on the lumen achieved and that this does not appear to be altered when aggressive attempts to optimally expand stents are employed. The important concept is that restenosis is affected by the final lumen achieved and not necessarily by the

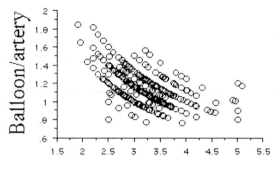

Figure 21.3 *A regression plot between the reference artery diameter and the balloon-to-artery ratio selected. The balloon-to-artery size was inversely related to the reference artery diameter.*

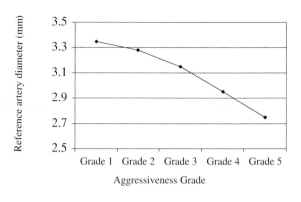

Figure 21.4 *The relationship between the level of aggressiveness of stent implantation and the reference artery diameter. More aggressive strategies are used in smaller arteries.*

technique used to obtain this result. A number of randomized studies are now in progress to evaluate the effect on late outcome of a particular associated technique, such as IVUS to guide and optimize stent deployment. The conclusions of these studies need to be interpreted not in the light of the particular technique used but with consideration of the final results achieved with that particular approach.

In attempting to use the same data set to analyse the effects of aggressive techniques on late loss and restenosis, limitations similar to those described above for other centers remain. In particular, there are inter-relationships between vessel diameter, balloon-to-artery ratio, and pressure. Larger balloon-to-artery ratios are selected for smaller arteries, for example (*Fig. 21.3*). An 'aggressiveness scoring system' was devised to combine balloon-to-artery ratios and inflation pressures. Balloon-to-artery ratios were segregated as < 1.1:1, between 1.1:1 and 1.3:1, or > 1.3:1. Balloon pressures were similarly segregated as ≤ 10 atmospheres, between 10 and 15 atmospheres, or ≥ 15 atmospheres. These groups were combined into a graded scale from minimally aggressive (Grade 1) to maximally aggressive (Grade 5). *Figure 21.4* demonstrates an inverse linear relationship between aggressiveness grade and arterial size (i.e. more aggressive strategies were employed for less favorable lesions). Therefore, measurements of lumen diameter changes, such as acute gain, late loss, and net gain, must be normalized for the reference artery diameter in order to be

meaningful. The acute gain normalized for reference artery size increases with greater levels of aggressiveness, reflecting greater stent expansion (*Fig. 21.5a*). However, the loss index is not affected (*Fig. 21.5b*), with a resulting favorable effect on the normalized net gain (*Fig. 21.5c*). A diminished follow-up percentage diameter stenosis and rate of restenosis is seen as the aggressiveness grades is increased, reflecting the effect of the greater acute gain achieved with more aggressive therapies (*Fig. 21.6*).

DATA ON RESTENOSIS FROM RANDOMIZED STENT TRIALS

More aggressive stent deployment techniques have been employed in the most recent clinical trials. If high-pressure inflations led to increased late loss and restenosis, then current trials should reflect worse outcomes compared with the results from earlier trials, such as STRESS and BENESTENT.[55,68] However, the outcomes are considerably better than the results from the earlier trials (*Fig. 21.7*).[69,70] Although heparin-coated stents were used in BENESTENT II,[71] in both BENESTENT I[55] and BENESTENT II[69] Palmaz–Schatz stents were deployed in focal lesions (< 15 mm) in large vessels (≥ 3 mm). In BENESTENT

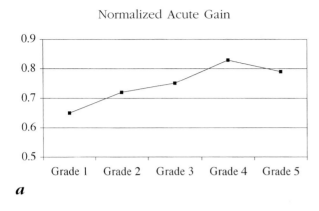

a

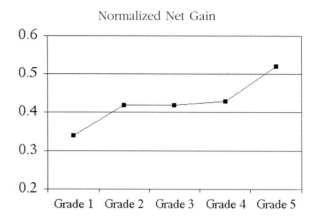

c

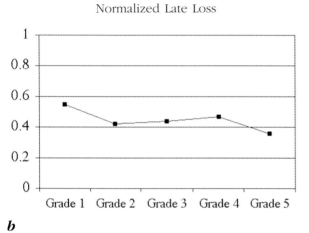

b

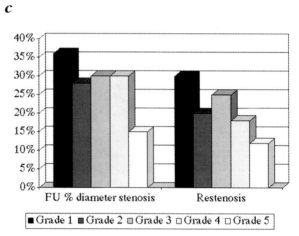

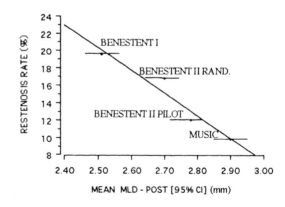

Figure 21.5 *(a) Effect of aggressiveness grade on the normalized acute gain. The acute gain is the difference in minimum lumen diameter (MLD) of the arterial narrowing from the beginning of the procedure and the final result obtained. The normalized acute gain is the acute gain divided by the reference artery diameter. Larger gains were achieved with more aggressive strategies (p < 0.001). (b) The effect of aggressiveness grade on loss index. The loss index is the late loss divided by the acute gain, which is independent of vessel diameter. Loss index was not affected by aggressive grade. (c) The effect of aggressiveness grade on the normalized net gain. The net gain is the improvement in MLD within the arterial narrowing from before the procedure to the follow-up angiogram; it is the difference between the acute gain and the late loss. The normalized net gain is the net gain divided by the reference arterial diameter. A trend towards improvement in the normalized net gain is seen with more aggressive strategies (p = 0.1).*

Figure 21.6 *Effect of aggressiveness grade on follow-up (FU) percentage diameter stenosis and rate of restenosis. More favorable results are seen with increasing grades of aggressiveness.*

Figure 21.7 *Relationship of minimal lumen diameter (MLD) after stenting to the restenosis rate in four trials and 804 lesions with comparable demographic baseline characteristics. Across these trials, the bigger the lumen achieved at the time of stenting, the better the rates of restenosis. From Serruys et al.[69]*

Table 21.1

Differences in immediate and follow-up angiographic and clinical outcomes in the stent arms of the BENESTENT I and II trials

	BENESTENT I *(n = 259)*	*BENESTENT II* *(n = 414)*	*p value*
Reference artery diameter (mm)	2.99 ± 0.45	2.96 ± 0.48	NS
Minimum lumen diameter (pre-intervention) (mm)	1.07 ± 0.33	1.09 ± 0.28	NS
Minimum lumen diameter (post-intervention) (mm)	2.48 ± 0.39	2.69 ± 0.37	< 0.0001
Minimum lumen diameter (follow-up) (mm)	1.82 ± 0.64	1.89 ± 0.65	NS
Percentage diameter stenosis (pre-intervention)	64 ± 10	63 ± 10	NS
Percentage diameter stenosis (post-intervention)	22 ± 8	16 ± 7	< 0.001
Percentage diameter stenosis (follow-up)	38 ± 18	35 ± 17	0.07
Restenosis rate (%)	22	16	0.06
Acute gain (mm)	1.40 ± 0.44	1.61 ± 0.39	< 0.0001
Late loss (mm)	0.65 ± 0.57	0.80 ± 0.54	< 0.001
Net gain (mm)	0.75 ± 0.66	0.80 ± 0.62	NS

Based on numbers presented in the BENESTENT I randomized trial and BENESTENT II randomized trial (in press). Angiographic follow-up rates were achieved in 93% of patients, however, in BENESTENT II only 50% of patients enrolled were assigned to have angiographic follow-up.
NS, not significant

I, stents were deployed using balloon-to-artery ratio of 1.12:1 and an inflation pressure of 10 ± 8 atmospheres, whereas in BENESTENT II, balloon-to-artery ratio of 1.18:1 and an inflation presure of 15 ± 3 atmosphere were used. *Table 21.1* shows the difference in immediate and follow-up angiographic and clinical outcomes comparing the stent arms of each trial. The use of more aggressive strategies in BENESTENT II led to a larger initial acute gain, lower follow-up percentage diameter stenosis, and less restenosis. Additionally, lower follow-up clinical event rates were seen in the stent arm of BENESTENT II than in BENESTENT I (13% versus 20%; *p* < 0.01). Although this analysis is confounded by the use of warfarin sodium in BENESTENT I and the use of heparin-coated stents and ticlopidine in BENESTENT II, the findings remain consistent with the 'bigger is better' theory and do not support the theory that more aggressive stent deployment strategies lead to increased restenosis.[70]

The STRESS III trial[72] was a non-randomized, prospective study of 250 patients that compared current stent implantation techniques (high-pressure balloon inflations and the use of aspirin and ticlopidine instead of warfarin) to the results achieved in

the original STRESS trial. Similar restenosis rates were seen in the STRESS III trial and the stent arm of STRESS I (31% versus 32%). However, the arteries in STRESS III were smaller (2.84 versus 3.03; *p* < 0.05) and therefore more prone to restenosis.

IVUS-GUIDED STENT TRIALS

A subset analysis evaluating the effect of IVUS was performed as part of STRESS III.[73] The use of IVUS was optional and was incorporated into 43% of the lesions treated. Although stent thrombosis occurred in three out of 132 patients who did not have IVUS guidance and none of 100 patients whose treatment was guided by IVUS, this difference was not statistically significant. There were no reported differences in reference arterial size or lesion length between the two groups. The group with IVUS guidance had larger balloons, higher pressures, and more stents implanted. These more aggressively treated lesions were found to be associated with a trend towards more late loss (1.02 mm versus 0.84 mm; *p* = 0.06)

Table 21.2

The MUSIC criteria guidelines for optimal stent expansion

- Complete apposition of the stent over its complete length.
- In-stent minimal lumen area $\geq$ 90% of the average reference area or $\geq$ 100% of the lumen area of the reference segment with the smallest lumen area; this criterion is modified (80% average reference area and 90% lumen area of the reference segment with the smallest area) if the minimal lumen area inside the stent $\geq$ 9.0 mm²; in-stent lumen area of proximal stent entrance $\geq$ 90% of proximal reference lumen area.
- Symmetric stent expansion, defined by the ratio of the minimum-to-maximum lumen diameter $\geq$ 0.7.

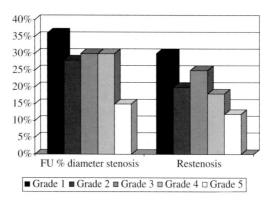

Figure 21.8 *Relationship of aggressiveness grade and diffuse restenosis as a percentage of total restenosis. Although not statistically significant, there is a trend towards less diffuse restenosis using less aggressive techniques. This is confounded by the relationship between aggressiveness grade and vessel size, as demonstrated in Figure 21.4.*

and higher rates of angiographic restenosis (40% versus 23%; p = 0.01). This non-randomized trial therefore suggested a potential detrimental effect of IVUS and aggressive techniques to guide stent deployment.

Moussa and colleagues[63] evaluated the impact of incremental lumen gain on the probability of angiographic restenosis, using IVUS guidance. If vessel stretch were detrimental, then additional balloon inflations based on information gained from IVUS after an acceptable angiographic result has been obtained should lead to enhanced intimal proliferation and higher rates of restenosis, as described above in the study of Werner and colleagues.[57] However, there was a decrease in restenosis as lumen area increased, resulting from the IVUS information. As the lumen gain increased, the probability of restenosis decreased.

Two prospective trials evaluating the effect of IVUS guidance of stent implantation on clinical outcomes argue against the theory that aggressive techniques promote restenosis. In the Multicenter Ultrasound guided Stent Implantation in the Coronaries (MUSIC) trial,[74] strict IVUS criteria were used to ensure maximal stent expansion would be attained (*Table 21.2*). Using these strategies, with a mean stent inflation pressure of 15.8 atmospheres, the remarkably low angiographic restenosis rate of 7% was achieved.

In the CRUISE (Can Routine Ultrasound Influence Stent Expansion) substudy[75] of the STARS trial, the value of IVUS in guiding stent deployment was evaluated in 499 patients. In this trial, the use of IVUS guidance was associated with a statistically significant

39% decrease in target vessel revascularization, from 14.9% to 8.9%. The primary role of IVUS has been to identify suboptimally expanded stents in order to select higher inflation pressures or larger balloons. The improved outcomes with IVUS guidance are inconsistent with detrimental effects of high-pressure balloons and support the benefits of achieving a maximal intrastent lumen.

EFFECT OF AGGRESSIVE STENT IMPLANTATION TECHNIQUES ON TYPE OF RESTENOSIS

Recently, interest in restenosis has been directed to the idea that the type of restenosis has potential clinical relevance. Yokoi and colleagues[42] identified that diffuse restenosis (as defined as stenoses > 10 mm in length) responded poorly to repeat balloon angioplasty, with recurrent restenosis in 85%. Focal restenosis, however, had a significantly lower recurrent restenosis rate whether the restenosis was within the stent (12%) or at the stent border (19%). Worse subsequent clinical outcomes when diffuse restenosis is found have been observed by other investigators as well,[76,77] although not universally.[78]

This has led to the search for different predictors of diffuse in-stent restenosis as well as angioplasty methods that may be more successful in treating this more malignant process. Speculation has centered on whether aggressive strategies may be associated with increased diffuse restenosis. A more recent retrospective analysis from Centro Cuore Columbus identified 455 restenotic lesions, which were characterized as diffuse or focal. These lesions were evaluated for the effect of aggressiveness on type of restenosis. The percentage of restenotic lesions presenting as diffuse restenosis was evaluated for the level of aggressiveness, using a grading system as described above. Diffuse restenosis appears to be diminished when minimally aggressive strategies are used (*Fig. 21.8*). These data are confounded by the compliance of the atherosclerotic artery as well as the relationship of arterial size and aggressiveness employed, as mentioned above. By logistic regression analysis, aggressiveness grade was not an independent predictor of diffuse restenosis.

ARE HIGH PRESSURES OR AGGRESSIVE TECHNIQUES NEEDED?

The predominant attractiveness of more aggressive stent deployment strategies was to minimize the risk of stent thrombosis, with a reduction in restenosis also hoped for, although this was less important. Coincident with the initiation of the use of routine high-pressure stent deployment techniques was the adoption of stronger antiplatelet instead of antithrombotic agents. Some investigators have questioned if the perceived benefit of aggressive stent deployment techniques were not in fact due to the simultaneous use of the more powerful antiplatelet therapy, ticlopidine.[79,80] A low incidence of stent thrombosis when ticlopidine is used has been reported even without IVUS or routine high-pressure inflations inside the stents.[79,81] It is not clear if relatively larger balloon sizes (a powerful means of increasing stent dimensions and contributing to vascular barotrauma) were used in these patients. Schomig and colleagues[81] have just conducted a randomized trial comparing inflation pressures of 11 atmospheres with 18 atmospheres in implanting stents. In 900 patients who were randomized to receive one of the two inflation pressures, similar 30-day outcomes were seen, including stent occlusion rates of 1.8% and 1.6% respectively (not significant). Larger luminal results were seen in the high-pressure group, but the impact on restenosis is not available at the time of writing.

OPTIMAL INTRASTENT LUMINAL DIMENSIONS VERSUS AGGRESSIVE TECHNIQUES

The ability to achieve a maximum intrastent luminal result and the means used to achieve those results are highly dependent. This interdependence may obscure the relative contribution of these features to a reduction in restenosis. Because the achievement of larger lumens is inversely related to the rates of restenosis, it is logical to expand the stent maximally. However, when such expansion requires higher pressures and larger balloon-to-artery ratios, less optimal results may be expected, owing to the resistant plaque. Studies that have examined strictly aggressive strategies independent of luminal results achieved have reported worse outcomes,[49] whereas when the achievement of an optimal lumen was a goal, the outcomes have generally been improved.[43] Therefore, it is likely that the important parameter is the achievement of an optimal lumen. It is not clear if further attempts at expansion after the lumen has been optimized may induce other less favorable results, such as alterations in flow or hyperstimulation of a healing response. Some of the conflicting results reported in the literature may reflect the importance of aggressive techniques in optimizing the intrastent lumen, balanced by potential deleterious effects after the lumen has already been optimized. Thus, the trials using IVUS, which have relied on the intrastent lumen achieved as the indication for stopping further expansion, have usually shown improved results, whereas studies comparing atmosphere pressures used without regard to results achieved have shown inferior results. Additionally, some patients may have a predilection for an increased proliferative response after stent implantation.[83-85] This predilection may be independent of the technique used to implant the stent, or it may be an exaggerated response to vessel wall barotrauma. Such patients may therefore not respond favorably to aggressive stent implantation techniques, whereas others may enjoy the larger luminal benefits resulting from larger balloons or higher-pressure inflations.

CONCLUSIONS

Randomized trials are currently being performed specifically to compare strategies of stent deployment, but the data are not yet available. Current data suggest that contemporary strategies do not lead to greater late loss compared to historical strategies, but are instead associated with less restenosis and improved outcomes. It remains unclear if, once maximal stent expansion is achieved, further vascular barotrauma leads to higher rates of restenosis or more aggressive restenosis. There may be an important relationship between the resistance to stent expansion and the likelihood of restenosis. If this relationship does exist, the need for aggressive stent expansion techniques may reflect a marker but not a cause for restenosis. Obtaining optimal lumen dimensions is currently the best way of achieving low rates of restenosis in stented lesions.

REFERENCES

1. Schatz RA, Goldberg S, Leon M et al. Clinical experience with the Palmaz–Schatz coronary stent. *J Am Coll Cardiol* 1991; **17 (Suppl B)**: 155B–159B.
2. Cohen DJ, Breall JA, Ho KKL et al. Evaluating the potential cost-effectiveness of stenting as a treatment for symptomatic single-vessel coronary disease. Use of a decision–analytic model. *Circulation* 1994; **89**: 1859–1874.
3. Goldberg SL, Colombo A, Nakamura S et al. Benefit of intracoronary ultrasound in the deployment of Palmaz–Schatz stents. *J Am Coll Cardiol* 1994; **24**: 996–1003.
4. Nakamura S, Colombo A, Gaglione A et al. Intracoronary ultrasound observations during stent implantation. *Circulation* 1994; **89**: 2026–2034.
5. Ehrlich S, Honye J, Mahon D et al. Unrecognized stenosis by angiography documented by intravascular ultrasound imaging. *Cathet Cardiovasc Diagn* 1991; **23**: 198–201.
6. Colombo A, Hall P, Nakamura S et al. Intracoronary stenting without anticoagulation accomplished with intravascular ultrasound guidance. *Circulation* 1995; **91**: 1676–1688.
7. Beatt KJ, Serruys PW, Luijten HE et al. Restenosis after coronary angioplasty: the paradox of increased lumen diameter and restenosis. *J Am Coll Cardiol* 1992; **19**: 258–266.
8. Schwartz RS, Huber KC, Murphy JG et al. Restenosis and the proportional neo-intimal response to coronary artery injury: results in a porcine model. *J Am Coll Cardiol* 1992; **19**: 267–274.
9. Lam JYT, Chesebro JH, Steale PM et al. Deep arterial injury during experimental angioplasty: relation to a positive indium-111–labeled scintigram, quantitative platelet deposition and mural thrombus. *J Am Coll Cardiol* 1986; **8**: 1380–1386.
10. Liu MW, Roubin GS, King SB. Restenosis after coronary angioplasty: potential biological determinants and role of intimal hyperplasia. *Circulation* 1989; **79**: 1374–1387.
11. Garratt KN, Holmes DRJ, Bell MR et al. Restenosis after directional coronary atherectomy: differences between primary atheromatous and restenosis lesions and influence of subintimal tissue resection. *J Am Coll Cardiol* 1990; **16**: 1665–1671.
12. Kuntz RE, Safian RD, Carrozza JP et al. The importance of acute luminal diameter in determining restenosis after coronary atherectomy or stenting. *Circulation* 1992; **86**: 1827–1835.
13. Farb A, Virmani R, Atkinson JB, Anderson PG. Long-term histologic patency after percutaneous transluminal coronary angioplasty is predicted by the creation of a greater lumen area. *J Am Coll Cardiol* 1994; **24**: 1229–1235.
14. Kuntz RE, Hinohara T, Safian RD et al. Restenosis after directional coronary atherectomy. Effects of luminal diameter and deep wall excision. *Circulation* 1992; **86**: 1394–1399.
15. Kuntz RE, Baim DS. Defining coronary restenosis. Newer clinical and angiographic paradigms. *Circulation* 1993; **88**: 1310–1323.
16. Mintz GS, Popma JJ, Pichard AD et al. Arterial remodeling after coronary angioplasty. A serial intravascular ultrasound study. *Circulation* 1996; **94**: 35–43.
17. Hoffman R, Mintz GS, Mehran R et al. Late tissue proliferation both within and surrounding Palmaz–Schatz stents is associated with procedural vessel wall injury (abstract). *J Am Coll Cardiol* 1997; **29 (suppl)**: 397A-3970.
18. Mintz GS, Pichard AD, Kent KM et al. Endovascular stents reduce restenosis by eliminating geometric arterial remodeling: a serial intravascular ultrasound study (abstract). *J Am Coll Cardiol* 1995; **25 (suppl)**: 36A–360.
19. Karas SP, Gravanis MB, Santoian EC et al. Coronary intimal proliferation after balloon injury and stenting in swine: an animal model of restenosis. *J Am Coll Cardiol* 1992; **20**: 467–474.
20. Chronos N, Dleinman ME, Cipolla GD et al. Stent implantation induces late arterial wall cellular proliferation compared to angioplasty in normal rabbits (abstract). *Eur Heart J* 1997; **18 (suppl)**: 451.
21. Dangas G, Fuster V. Management of restenosis after coronary intervention. *Am Heart J* 1996; **132**: 428–436.
22. Kornowski R, Hong MK, Tio FO et al. In-stent restenosis: contributions of inflammatory responses and arterial injury to neointimal hyperplasia. *J Am Coll Cardiol* 1998; **31**: 224–230.
23. Frimerman A, Litvack F, Makkar R, Eigler N. Neointimal in-stent proliferation is related to the degree of strut induced arterial wall injury (abstract). *J Invas Cardiol* 1997; **9**: 71C.
24. Carter AJ, Farb A, Laird JR, Virmani R. Neointimal formation is dependant on the underlying arterial substrate after coronary stent placement (abstract). *J Am Coll Cardiol* 1996; **27**: 320A.
25. Gunn J, Malik N, Shepherd L et al. In-stent restenosis: relationship to strut protrusion and asymetrical deployment (abstract). *Eur Heart J* 1997; **18**: 451.
26. Carter AJ, Farb A, Gould K et al. Neointimal formation is dependent on the arterial morphology and plaque compression after stent placement in atherosclerotic arteries (abstract). *Am J Cardiol* 1997; **80**: 10S.
27. Vorwerk D, Redha F, Neuerburg J et al. Neointima formation following arterial placement of self-expanding stents of different radial force: experimental results. *Cardiovasc Intervent Radiol.* 1994; **17**: 27–32.
28. Kimura T, Kaburagi S, Tamura T et al. Remodeling of human coronary arteries undergoing coronary angioplasty or atherectomy. *Circulation* 1997; **96**: 475–483.

29. Nobuyoshi M, Kimura T, Ohishi H et al. Restenosis after percutaneous transluminal coronary angioplasty: pathologic observations in 20 patients. *J Am Coll Cardiol* 1991; **17**: 433–439.

30. Topol EJ, Leya F, Pinkerton CA et al. A comparison of directional atherectomy with coronary angioplasty in patients with coronary artery disease. The CAVEAT Study Group. *N Engl J Med* 1993; **329**: 221–227.

31. Holmes DRJ, Topol EJ, Califf RM et al. A multicenter, randomized trial of coronary angioplasty versus directional atherectomy for patients with saphenous vein bypass graft lesions. CAVEAT-II Investigators. *Circulation* 1995; **91**: 1966–1974.

32. Whitlow PL, Cowley MJ, Kuntz RE et al. Study to determine rotablator and transluminal angioplasty strategy (STRATAS): acute results (abstract). *Circulation* 1996; **94 (suppl)**: I-435–I-430.

33. Bass TA, Whitlow PL, Moses JW et al. Acute complications related to coronary rotational atherectomy strategy: a report from the STRATAS trial (abstract). *J Am Coll Cardiol* 1997; **29 (suppl)**: 68A–680.

34. Simonton CA, Leon MB, Baim DS et al. 'Optimal' directional coronary atherectomy. Final results of the Optimal Atherectomy Restenosis Study (OARS). *Circulation* 1998; **97**: 332–339.

35. Baim DS, Cutlip DE, Sharma SK et al, for the BOAT Investigators. Final results of the Balloon versus Optimal Atherectomy Trial (BOAT). *Circulation* 1998; **97**: 322–331.

36. Ellis SG, Savage M, Fischman D et al. Restenosis after placement of Palmaz–Schatz stents in native coronary arteries. Initial results of a multicenter experience. *Circulation* 1992; **86**: 1836–1844.

37. Foley DP, Melkert R, Umans VA et al. Differences in restenosis propensity of devices for transluminal coronary intervention. A quantitative angiographic comparison of balloon angioplasty, directional atherectomy, stent implantation and excimer laser angioplasty. CARPORT, MERCATOR, MARCATOR, PARK, and BENESTENT Trial Groups. *Eur Heart J* 1995; **16**: 1331–1346.

38. Foley DP, Melkert R, Serruys PW. The influence of coronary vessel size on luminal renarrowing and late angiographic outcome after successful coronary balloon angioplasty. *Circulation* 1994; **90**: 1239–1251.

39. Luo H, Nishioka T, Eigler NL et al. Coronary artery restenosis after balloon angioplasty in humans is associated with circumferential coronary constriction. *Arterioscler Thrombosis Vasc Biol* 1996; **16**: 1393–1398.

40. Painter JA, Mintz GS, Wong SC et al. Serial intravascular ultrasound studies fail to show evidence of chronic Palmaz–Schatz stent recoil. *Am.J.Cardiol.* 1995; **75**: 398–400.

41. Mudra H, Regar E, Klauss V et al. Serial follow-up after optimized ultrasound-guided deployment of Palmaz–Schatz stents. In-stent neointimal proliferation without significant reference segment response. *Circulation* 1997; **95**: 363–370.

42. Yokoi H, Kimura T, Nakagawa Y et al. Long-term clinical and quantitative angiographic follow-up after the Palmaz–Schatz stent restenosis (abstract). *J Am Coll Cardiol* 1996; **27**: 224A-2240.

43. Mudra H, Sunamura H, Figulla H et al. Six month clinical and angiographic outcome after IVUS guided stent implantation (abstract). *J Am Coll Cardiol* 1997; **29**: 171A–1710.

44. Hoffmann R, Mintz GS, Mehran R et al. Intravascular ultrasound predictors of angiographic restenosis in lesions treated with Palmaz–Schatz stents. *J Am Coll Cardiol* 1998; **31**: 43–49.

45. Hoffmann R, Mintz GS, Kent KM et al. Serial intravascular ultrasound predictors of restenosis at the margins of Palmaz–Schatz stents. *Am J Cardiol* 1997; **79**: 951–953.

46. Mintz GS, Popma JJ, Pichard AD et al. Intravascular ultrasound predictors of restenosis after percutaneous transcatheter coronary revascularization. *J Am Coll Cardiol* 1996; **27**: 1678–1687.

47. The GUIDE Trial Investigators. IVUS-determined predictors of restenosis in PTCA and DCA: final report from the GUIDE trial, Phase II (abstract). *J Am Coll Cardiol* 1996; **27**: 156A.

48. Mehran R, Mintz GS, Pichard AD et al. Impact of vessel wall injury on in-stent restenosis: a serial quantitative angiographic and intravascular ultrasound study (abstract). *Circulation* 1996; **94 (suppl)**: I-262–I-263.

49. Savage MP, Fischman DL, Douglas JS et al. The dark side of high pressure stent deployment (abstract). *J Am Coll Cardiol* 1997; **29 (suppl)**: 368A–3680.

50. Hausleiter J, Schuhlen H, Elezi S et al. Impact of high inflation pressures on six-month angiographic follow-up after coronary stent placement (abstract). *J Am Coll Cardiol* 1997; **29 (suppl)**: 369A–3690.

51. Fernandez-Aviles F, Alonso JJ, Duran JM et al. High pressure increases late loss after coronary stenting (abstract). *J Am Coll Cardiol* 1997; **29 (suppl)**: 369A–3690.

52. Metzger JP, Catuli D, Le Feuvre C et al. Impact of high pressure inflation on coronary stent deployment: an intracoronary blood flow analysis (abstract). *Circulation* 1997; **96 (suppl)**: I-403–I-400.

53. Urestsky BF, Estella P, Lerakis S et al. Very high pressure stent deployment is associated with an increase in long-term major adverse cardiac events (abstract). *Circulation* 1997; **96 (suppl)**: I-403–I-400.

54. Savage MP, Douglas JSJ, Fischman DL et al. Stent placement compared with balloon angioplasty for obstructed coronary bypass grafts. *N Engl J Med* 1997; **337**: 740–747.

55. Serruys PW, de Jaegere P, Kiemeneij F et al, for the Benestent Study Group. A comparison of balloon expandable stent implantation with balloon angioplasty in patients with coronary artery disease. *N Engl J Med* 1994; **331**: 489–495

56. Fernandez-Aviles F, Alonso JJ, Duran JM et al. High pressure impairs restenotic process after coronary stenting (abstract). *Circulation* 1997; **96 (suppl)**: I-87.

57. Werner F, Regar E, Henneka KH et al. Vessel stretching is an important factor for neointima proliferation after stent implantation: an investigation with intravascular ultrasound (abstract). *Circulation* 1997; **96 (suppl)**: I-583.

58. Yokoi H, Nosaka H, Kimura T et al. Influence of high-pressure stent dilatation on late angiographic and clinical outcomes of Palmaz–Schatz stent implantation (abstract). *J Am Coll Cardiol* 1997; **29**: 312A.

59. Glogar D, Yang P, Hassan A et al. Does high-pressure balloon post-dilatation improve long-term results of Wiktor coil stent? (Austrian Wiktor Stent Trial) (abstract). *J Am Coll Cardiol* 1997; **29**: 313A.

60. Schofer J, Rau T, Golestani R, Mathey DG. Procedural vessel wall injury is not associated with late tissue proliferation within stents (abstract). *Circulation* 1997; **96 (suppl)**: I-402.

61. Mehran R, Popma JJ, Baim DS et al. Routine high pressure post-stent dilatation did not influence clinical restenosis in STARS (abstract). *J Am Coll Cardiol* 1998; **31**: 80A.

62. Prati F, Lioy E, Loschiavo P et al. Is late in-stent endothelial hyperplasia related to the technique of implantation? Assessment with three-dimensional intracoronary ultrasound (abstract). *Circulation* 1997; **96 (suppl)**: I-583.

63. Moussa I, Tobis JM, Moses JW, Collins M. Does incremental lumen gain with intravascular ultrasound-guided stenting have an impact on the probability of angiographic restenosis (abstract)? *Circulation* 1997; **96 (suppl)**: I-409.

64. Goldberg SL, di Mario C, Hall P, Colombo A. Comparison of aggressive versus nonaggressive balloon dilatation for stent deployment on late loss and restenosis in native coronary arteries. *Am J Cardiol* 1998; **81**: 708–712.

65. Schomig A, Neumann FJ, Kastrati A et al. A randomized comparison of antiplatelet and anticoagulant therapy after the placement of coronary-artery stents. *N Engl J Med* 1996; **334**: 1084–1089.

66. Leon MB, Baim DS, Gordon P et al. Clinical and angiographic results from the Stent Anticoagulation Regimen Study (STARS) (abstract). *Circulation* 1996; **94 (suppl)**: I-685.

67. Bertrand ME, Legrand V, Boland J et al. Full anti-coagulation versus ticlopidine plus aspirin after stening implantation: a randomized multicenter European study: the FANTASTIC trial (abstract). *Circulation* 1996; **94 (suppl)**: I-685.

68. Fischman DL, Leon MD, Baim DS et al. A randomized comparison of coronary stent placement and balloon angioplasty in the treatment of coronary artery disease. *N Engl J Med* 1994; **331**: 496–501.

69. Serruys PW, Emanuelsson H, van der Giessen W et al. Heparin-coated Palmaz–Schatz stents in human coronary arteries. Early outcome of the Benestent-II Pilot Study. *Circulation* 1996; **93**: 412–422.

70. Serruys PW, Kootstra J, Melkert R et al. Peri-procedural QCA following Palmaz–Schatz stent implantation predicts restenosis rate at 6 months: result of a meta-analysis of BENESTENT-I, BENESTENT-II Pilot, BENESTENT-II and MUSIC (abstract). *J Am Coll Cardiol* 1998; **31**: 64A.

71. Serruys PW, Benestent Study Group. BENESTENT-II Pilot Study: 6 months follow-up of phase 1, 2 and 3 (abstract). *Circulation* 1995; **92 (suppl)**: I-542.

72. Fischman DL, Savage MP, Penn I et al. High pressure inflation in conjunction with ticlopidine and aspirin following coronary stent placement: results of the STRESS III trial (abstract). *J Am Coll Cardiol* 1997; **29**: 171A.

73. Strain JE, Fischman DL, Savage MP et al. More restenosis with IVUS-guided stenting: STRESS III IVUS Substudy results (abstract). *Circulation* 1997; **96 (suppl)**: I-408.

74. de Jaegere P, Mudra H, Figulla H et al. Intravascular ultrasound-guided optimized stent deployment. Immediate and 6 months clinical and angiographic results from the Multicentre Ultrasound Stenting in Coronaries Study (MUSIC Study). *Eur Heart J* 1998; **19**: 1214–1223.

75. Fitzgerald PJ, Hayase M, Mintz GS et al. CRUISE: can routine intravascular ultrasound influence stent expansion? Analysis of outcomes (abstract). *J Am Coll Cardiol* 1998; **31 (suppl)**: 396A.

76. Bauters C, Banos JL, Van Belle E et al. Six-month angiographic outcome after successful repeat percutaneous intervention for in-stent restenosis. *Circulation* 1998; **97**: 318–321.

77. Mehran R, Ito S, Abizaid A et al. Does lesion length affect late outcome of patients with in-stent restenosis? Results of the multicenter Laser Angioplasty for Stent Restenosis (LARS) registry (abstract). *J Am Coll Cardiol* 1998; **31 (suppl)**: 142A.

78. Reimers B, Moussa I, Akiyama T et al. Long-term clinical follow-up after successful repeat percutaneous intervention for stent restenosis. *J Am Coll Cardiol* 1997; **30**: 186–192.

79. Barragan P, Sainsous J, Silvestri M et al. Coronary artery stenting without anticoagulation, aspirin, ultrasound guidance, or high balloon pressure: prospective study of 1051 consecutive patients. *Cathet Cardiovasc Diagn* 1997; **42**: 367–373.

80. Morice MC, Zemour G, Benveniste E et al. Intracoronary stenting without coumadin: one month results of a French multicenter study. *Cathet Cardiovasc Diagn* 1995; **35**: 1–7.

81. Dirschinger J, Schuehlen J, Hausleiter J et al. A randomized trial of low versus high balloon pressure for coronary stent placement: analysis of early outcome (abstract). *Circulation* 1997; **96 (suppl)**: I-653.

82. Mehran R, Mintz GS, Pichard AD et al. Morphologic and procedural predictors of diffuse in-stent restenosis (abstract). *J Am Coll Cardiol* 1997; **29**: 76A–77A.

83. Ribichini F, Steffenino G, Dellavalle A et al. Plasma activity and insertion/deletion polymorphism of angiotensin I-converting enzyme: a major risk factor and a marker of risk for coronary stent restenosis. *Circulation*. 1998; **97**: 147–154.

84. Ribichini F, Steffenino G, Dellavalle A et al. The pattern (focal/diffuse) of angiographic in-stent restenosis is associated to the I/D polymorphism of the angiotensin converting enzyme gene (abstract). *Circulation* 1997; **96 (suppl)**: I-87.

85. Kastrati A, Elezi S, Schuhlen H et al. Intrapatient dependence of restenosis between lesions treated with intracoronary stenting (abstract). *J Am Coll Cardiol* 1998; **31**: 140A.

Chapter 22 **Treatment of in-stent restenosis**

Steven L Goldberg

INTRODUCTION

With the explosion in the use of intracoronary stents in recent years, the problem of in-stent restenosis has been receiving increased attention. Stents are currently implanted in approximately 70% of coronary angioplasties. In 1997 an estimated 900,000 stents were implanted worldwide in approximately 600,000 lesions. If the clinical restenosis rate is estimated to be 15%, nearly 100,000 cases of in-stent restenosis can be expected to have occurred. Yokoi and colleagues[1] identified that diffuse restenosis, which they defined as ≥ 10 mm in length, has a significantly worse outcome after treatment than focal restenosis. Diffuse restenosis, which occurs in approximately 30–50% of coronary angioplasties, is found in approximately 30,000 to 45,000 angioplasties yearly, and the number is increasing.

Historically, in-stent restenosis has been treated with medical therapy, balloon angioplasty, or coronary artery bypass surgery. Balloon angioplasty is highly successful acutely when treating in-stent restenosis and is associated with a very low incidence of complications.[2–7] In particular, stent thrombosis is not known to occur after angioplasty for in-stent restenosis. However, the follow-up results are less predictable, and high restenosis rates have been reported in selected subsets.[1,2,6,8]

MECHANISM OF IN-STENT RESTENOSIS

After the implantation of a rigid slotted tube stent, neointimal proliferation occurs in response to the barotrauma applied to the vessel wall as well as the persistent irritation of the foreign body.[9,10] This mechanism of restenosis differs from that after balloon angioplasty or atherectomy, in which there is

an initial insult followed by a healing response characterized by acute recoil, vascular remodeling (chronic recoil or dilatation), and neointimal growth.[11,12] Ideally, the management of in-stent restenosis should address not only the new tissue growth, but also the predilection for the exuberant proliferative response that is present in such lesions, in order to minimize further recurrences.

Pseudo-in-stent restenosis may also occur if the stent is not properly expanded at the time of implantation. In this circumstance a stent may slip off a balloon and be incompletely expanded. If the stent is not radio-opaque this may not be appreciated unless intravascular ultrasound (IVUS) is performed (*Fig. 22.1*). If recoil of the arterial wall occurs, it may

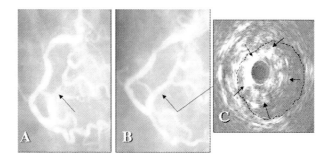

Figure 22.1 *Angiogram and intravascular ultrasound (IVUS) of inadequate stent expansion, not seen angiographically. (a) Baseline stenosis in the posterolateral branch of a right coronary artery. (b) Angiogram after a Palmaz–Schatz stent implantation. An acceptable result is seen. (c) IVUS image demonstrating unsuccessful stent expansion at this site. The dotted line outlines the lumen border. The arrows point out the struts of the stent. Because the stent is porous, the contrast streams outside the stent struts giving the illusion by angiography of a well-expanded stent. If this is not recognized and recoil of the artery upon the stent occurs, an appearance of stent collapse may be interpreted at follow-up but this would actually be a stent pseudorestenosis.*

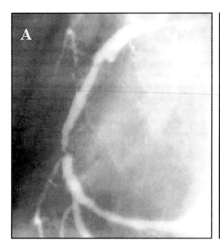

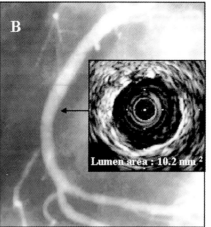

Baseline   **Post Stent**

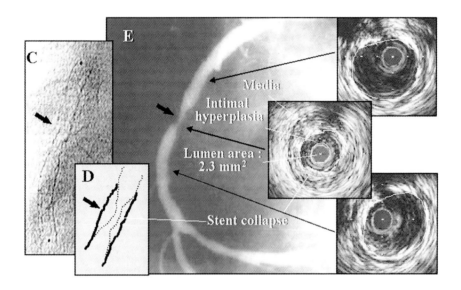

Figure 22.2 *A narrowing in the right coronary artery treated with a BeStent. (A) Baseline. (B) After stenting with an acceptable angiographic and intravascular ultrasound (IVUS) image. (C) Fluoroscopic outline of the stent demonstrating partial stent collapse. (D) A cartoon outlining the stent as seen in (C). (E) Angiogram showing the stent restenosis at the site of the partial stent collapse. IVUS images are seen at the site of stent restenosis showing a smaller intrastent area than seen at the time of stent implantation, as well as some intimal proliferation. IVUS images of the stent proximal and distal to the site of restenosis reveal no evidence of stent collapse or intimal proliferation.*

present as pseudo-in-stent restenosis. True stent compression has rarely been described with the Palmaz–Schatz stent but it may possibly occur with other types of stent that have less radial strength (*Fig. 22.2*).[13]

MEDICAL MANAGEMENT OF IN-STENT RESTENOSIS

In the early series by Baim and colleagues,[2] medical management was used in 30% of patients with in-stent restenosis (these patients had less severe restenosis and symptoms than those treated with repeat revascularization). Performing routine follow-up angiography after initial stent implantation, Fernandez-Aviles[14] reported that 59% of angiographic in-stent restenoses were not associated with symptoms. Asymptomatic recurrences are usually less severe and associated with less ischemia on stress testing than when there are associated symptoms.[14] Nibler and colleagues[15] found a 98% event-free survival at 1 year in 122 patients who had been treated medically for asymptomatic in-stent restenosis.

These investigators, and others, have also reported a lack of progression or an improvement in angio-

6 Months PostStent

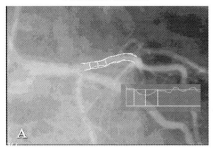

24 Months PostStent

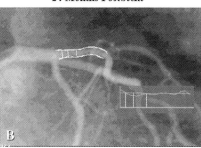

Reference Diameter2.26 mm
MLD   1.43 mm
Diameter Stenosis   36.6 %

Reference Diameter   2.47 mm
MLD   1.94 mm
Diameter Stenosis   21.5 %

Figure 22.3 *Quantitative coronary angiography 6 months and 2 years after stenting of a left anterior descending coronary artery. An increase in minimum lumen diameter and a decrease in percentage diameter stenosis has occurred between 6 months and 2 years. MLD, minimum lumen diameter.*

graphic dimensions with a further 6 months' observation (*Fig. 22.3*).[1,15–17] Another series of patients with asymptomatic restenosis had a less favorable event-free survival rate (69%) when treated with angioplasty or surgery.[14] Finally, patients in the BENES-TENT II trial[18] who had routine follow-up angiography had more subsequent clinical events than patients who were not assigned to routine follow-up angiography, and this was more marked in patients who received stents than in those treated with balloon angioplasty alone.[18] Similar findings were demonstrated in ASCENT (ACS Multilink Clinical Equivalence Trial),[19] which compared the ACS Multilink stent to the Palmaz–Schatz stent. This reinforces the impression that, particularly after stenting, it is better to avoid interventions unless the patient manifests symptoms of ischemia.

BALLOON ANGIOPLASTY FOR IN-STENT RESTENOSIS

The earliest observations regarding the treatment of in-stent restenosis noted the safety of treating this particular lesion subtype.[2] Balloon angioplasty leaves a smooth angiographic appearance when used for in-stent restenosis, with a low incidence of dissections and virtually no stent thrombosis. Restenosis recurs, however, to a varying degree. In the initial series reported by Baim and colleagues,[2] the recurrent rate of angiographic restenosis was 54%, although this number was probably artificially high owing to a low

(47%) incidence of repeat follow-up angiography. Recurrent angiographic restenosis was found in 37% by Yokoi and colleagues.[1] Clinical recurrence (death, myocardial infarction (MI), repeat target lesion revascularization) was seen in 17% by Reimers and colleagues[4] in 124 patients from the Centro Cuore Columbus in Milan, Italy. This incidence may be low partly because of the use of routine angiographic follow-up after initial stent implantation but not after treatment of in-stent restenosis. Asymptomatic patients

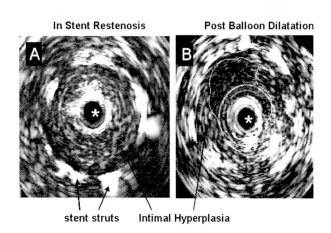

Figure 22.4 *Intravascular ultrasound (IVUS) appearance of in-stent restenosis before and after balloon angioplasty. (a) In-stent restenosis is characterized by tissue growth inside the stent, which is completely surrounding the IVUS catheter (*). (b) After balloon angioplasty is performed there is less in-stent tissue seen, although it is still present.*

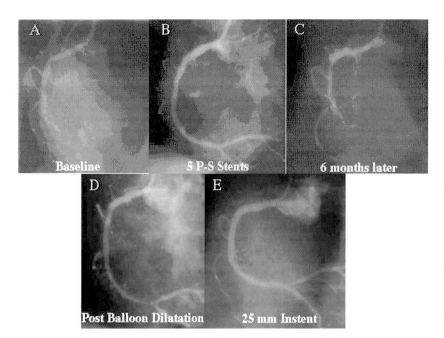

Figure 22.5 *Treatment of in-stent restenosis with additional stent placement. (a) The original lesion is a diffusely diseased right coronary artery with a mid-artery total occlusion. (b) After placement of five Palmaz–Schatz stents to cover lesion and a proximal dissection. (c) Six months later, there is diffuse in-stent restenosis with a total occlusion. (d) Angiographic appearance after balloon angioplasty for in-stent restenosis. The lumen is not as large as that achieved at the time of original stent implantation. (e) After placement of a 25 mm long Instent, the angiographic appearance is improved compared to (d) and similar to that achieved at the time of original stent implantation.*

may lower the incidence of clinical events after treatment of in-stent restenosis using this strategy.

The mechanism of balloon angioplasty in treating in-stent restenosis has been evaluated in the slotted tube Palmaz–Schatz stent with serial IVUS imaging by the Washington Hospital group, and others.[20-22] According to the Washington Hospital group,[20] further expansion of the stent accounts for 56% of the subsequent increase in lumen dimensions, with tissue extrusion leading to an additional 44% increase. Importantly, the lumen dimensions achieved are not as large as seen after the initial stent implantation is performed (*Fig. 22.4*). Other investigators have noted that the original post-stent dimensions are not achievable using balloon angioplasty to treat in-stent restenosis,[21,22] but they have found no significant tissue extrusion or removal, with further stent expansion the only mechanism of increasing the in-stent lumen.

Part of this discrepancy between investigations may be explained by the dynamic process of tissue movement through the stent struts. Shiran and colleagues[23] at the Washington Hospital Center have reported a 23% decrease in in-stent minimal lumen area studied with IVUS immediately after treatment of in-stent restenosis and then again 45 minutes later. The decrease in neointimal tissue that is seen immediately after balloon angioplasty (or ablative therapy) was not present after a waiting period; these investigators have termed this 'instant' in-stent restenosis. Whether this is tissue re-extrusion or new tissue (e.g. platelet deposition) is not known. The

lack of stent thrombosis when treating this condition argues against significant platelet or thrombus deposition being a likely cause.

The use of additional stents to treat in-stent restenosis has been tried by several investigators.[24-30] We found that the addition of a new stent made it possible to attain the lumen result achieved at the time of original stent implantation as assessed by quantitative coronary angiography (QCA) (*Fig. 22.5*).[27] Using intravascular ultrasound, Mehran and colleagues[28] demonstrated that the additional stent primarily compressed or extruded the neointimal tissue through the previous stent. Despite these favorable results on acute lumen dimensions, the subsequent event rate has been high after repeat stent implantation to treat in-stent restenosis (see below).

PREDICTORS OF RECURRENT IN-STENT RESTENOSIS

Recently, more attention has been paid to characteristics that may be predictive of additional recurrence when using balloon angioplasty to treat in-stent restenosis. Although the acute results are usually acceptable, certain cases of in-stent restenosis are refractory to favorable long-term results when treated with balloon angioplasty. In the study presented by Yokoi and colleagues,[1] the recurrence rate for diffuse restenosis was 85% after being treated with balloon angioplasty, as opposed to 12% when the lesion was focal, and 19% when the lesion was at the stent border. Similarly, other investigators have found a significantly worse clinical outcome when lesions longer than 20 mm are treated with a repeat intervention (balloon angioplasty or laser atherectomy).[31,32] Previous in-stent restenosis has been considered a likely marker of recurrent restenosis after balloon angioplasty. Reimers and colleagues[4] found four characteristics predictive of a subsequent event after treating in-stent restenosis. They included:

(a) in-stent restenosis in a bypass graft;
(b) a short time interval (< 3 months) in the development of in-stent restenosis;
(c) multivessel disease; and
(d) a depressed ejection fraction.

Some investigators have hypothesized that a hyperproliferative response to endothelial injury may be predicted by a specific polymorphism of the angiotensin converting enzyme (ACE) gene.[33,34] They theorize that patients with the D/D phenotype have higher levels of ACE, which activates angiotensin-II; this in turn induces cellular proliferation and so leads to in-stent restenosis. Additionally, ACE blocks the cellular proliferation, inhibiting effects of bradykinin. These investigators found that the D/D genotype was found in 80% of patients with diffuse in-stent restenosis (> 10 mm) but in only 36% of patients with focal restenosis, whereas the I/I genotype was found in only 3% of diffuse lesions but in 6% of focal lesions.[34] The mixed type I/D was seen in 17% of diffuse lesions and 58% of focal lesions.

Because of the recognition that some cases of in-stent restenosis are refractory to effective long-term management with balloon angioplasty, increased attention has recently been directed to alternate strategies of treating in-stent restenosis for more refractory subsets of lesions. These strategies have focused on debulking with various atherectomy devices, the placement of additional stents, or inhibiting further intimal proliferation with radiation, as well as a combination of techniques.

ATHERECTOMY OF IN-STENT RESTENOSIS

Various atherectomy devices have been used to treat in-stent restenosis. Both laser and rotational atherec-

tomy devices have been evaluated with multicenter registries.[35–38] The Laser Atherectomy Restenosis Study (LARS) examined the acute results of the use of this device with adjunctive balloon angioplasty in 414 vessels with diffuse in-stent restenosis (mean length 19 ± 13 mm).[35] Procedural success (defined by the investigators as the achievement of < 50% stenosis with the laser device alone or the successful pass of a 2.0 mm or 1.7 mm eccentric laser catheter) was seen in 92% of lesions. Complications from the laser device, including dissections or minor perforations, occurred in 13.8% of lesions, with an additional 10.9% of complications occurring after adjunctive balloon angioplasty, primarily dissections. Additional stents were implanted in 16% of patients. In-hospital complications included six deaths, two Q-wave MIs, and 10 non-Q-wave MIs. Follow-up on this patient population is currently pending.

The mechanism of excimer laser coronary angioplasty in treating in-stent restenosis was examined using QCA and IVUS in 107 restenotic lesions by Mehran and colleagues.[39] Using volumetric analysis obtained from IVUS information, these investigators determined that tissue ablation from the laser device accounted for 29% of lumen enlargement, with 31% caused by tissue extrusion, and 40% caused by additional stent expansion after adjunctive balloon angioplasty. Forty-seven lesions with in-stent restenosis treated with laser atherectomy and adjunctive balloon angioplasty were matched for vessel and lesion dimensions, with 45 lesions treated with balloon angioplasty alone. Compared to balloon angioplasty alone, the combination of laser and adjunctive balloon angioplasty resulted in greater lumen gain, more removal of intimal hyperplasia by ablation or extrusion, and a larger lumen cross-sectional area as seen by IVUS. A trend was also noted towards less subsequent target vessel revascularization in the group undergoing laser atherectomy in this matched population (21% with laser angioplasty versus 38% with balloon angioplasty alone; p = 0.08).

The same investigators performed another matched comparison and found that rotational atherectomy was more efficient in tissue ablation than the non-eccentric excimer laser.[40] Examining the volume of intrastent tissue by IVUS before and after atherectomy with similarly sized devices, they noted that rotational atherectomy removed 44 ± 8 mm^3 of tissue in 10 patients compared with only 19 ± 10 mm^3 after excimer laser in 14 patients. There were increases in lumen volume commensurate with the decrease in tissue volume. It is not known if the newer, larger

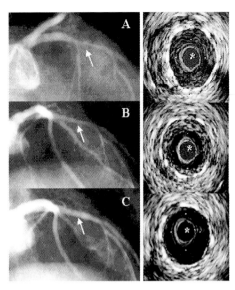

Baseline
In-stent Restenosis

2.25 mm RTB burr

Adjunctive Balloon
Dilatation
3.5 mm @ 18 atm

Figure 22.6 *Angiographic and intravascular ultrasound (IVUS) images of a lesion with in-stent restenosis treated with rotational atherectomy and adjunctive balloon angioplasty. (A) Baseline in-stent restenosis. The stent is filled with material which completely surrounds the IVUS catheter (*). (B) After treatment with a 2.25 mm rotational atherectomy burr, improvement in the angiographic appearance may be appreciated. By IVUS there is less intrastent tissue. (C) After treatment with adjunctive balloon angioplasty. A 3.5 mm balloon was inflated to 18 atmospheres. An excellent angiographic result is seen. No intrastent tissue can be appreciated on the IVUS image owing to tissue extrusion through the stent struts or tissue compression, or both.*

eccentric laser devices might be more effective in tissue removal.

ROTATIONAL ATHERECTOMY

Rotational atherectomy has been used to treat in-stent restenosis with a low incidence of complications and a high early success rate (*Fig. 22.6*).[36–38,40–47] The Balloon Angioplasty versus Rotational Atherectomy for Stent Restenosis (BARASTER) registry was created to assess the safety and efficacy of rotational ablation in treating diffuse intrastent restenosis.[36,37] Centers with experience in rotational atherectomy were invited to contribute the results of their initial series

of patients who had Rotablator therapy for in-stent restenosis; the results were to include acute and follow-up outcomes.

Clinical success was defined as achieving a < 50% residual diameter stenosis, with or without adjunctive balloon angioplasty, without the development of a complication. (This definition of success is slightly different than used for the LARS registry, as outlined above.) Clinical success was achieved in 174 of 179 lesions (97%) in 172 patients in this initial series of in-stent restenosis treated with rotational atherectomy. Baseline and procedural characteristics are shown in *Table 22.1*. Although occasionally a burr would not cross a lesion, possibly owing to the guidewire passing through a stent strut, burr entrapment did not occur. Slow flow, reported to occur in 8–15% of patients undergoing rotational atherectomy of non-stented lesions,[47,48] was not noted in this series of patients.

Techniques of intervention were left to the discretion of the investigators; however, two general strategies were adopted by the operators. The first strategy consisted of rotational atherectomy as a stand-alone intervention or with a 1 atmosphere balloon inflation to smooth out the angiographic appearance; this was performed in 26% of lesions in this registry. This

Table 22.1

BARASTER registry – baseline characteristics of lesions treated

Lesions (n)	179
Patients (n)	173
Age (years)	61 ± 11
Female (%)	33
Prior therapy for in-stent restenosis (%)	21
Reference artery diameter (mm)	2.8 ± 0.5
Baseline minimum lumen diameter (mm)	0.7
Baseline percentage stenosis	76 ± 12
Lesion length (mm)	21 ± 12
Diffuse restenosis (> 10 mm) (%)	85
Intravascular ultrasound guidance (%)	38
No adjunctive balloon or 1 atmosphere only (%)	28
Adjunctive balloon angioplasty (%)	72
Additional stents implanted (%)	7
Final burr size (mm)	2.1 ± 0.3
Burr-to-artery ratio	0.74 ± 0.18
Final balloon size (mm)	3.4 ± 0.4
Inflation pressure (atmospheres)	9.0 ± 6.1

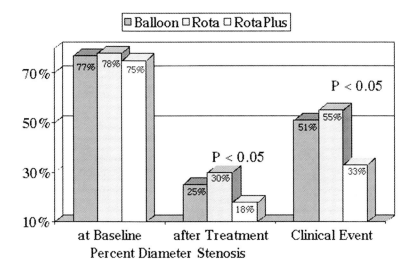

Figure 22.7 *Percentage diameter stenosis of lesions with in-stent restenosis being treated with balloon, rotational atherectomy alone, or at most 1 atmosphere balloon inflation pressure or with rotational atherectomy and adjunctive balloon angioplasty. There is no difference in baseline percentage diameter stenosis between the three groups, but the group treated with rotational atherectomy and adjunctive balloon angioplasty achieved the lowest percentage diameter stenosis at the end of the procedure and had fewer clinical events (death, myocardial infarction, or target lesion revascularization) with follow-up.*

approach was used with the intention of minimizing barotrauma to the arterial wall, according to the hypothesis that this would be less likely to stimulate a healing response and subsequent restenosis.[49] The other strategy was to perform rotational atherectomy and subsequent adjunctive balloon angioplasty with the intention of creating as large a lumen as possible, incorporating the philosophy that 'bigger is better' in reducing restenosis.[51]

To compare the angiographic and clinical results of rotational atherectomy with stand-alone balloon angioplasty, the results of the BARASTER registry were compared to cohorts of consecutive patients (n = 117) with in-stent restenosis treated with balloon angioplasty from two centers (the Mayo Clinic, Rochester, Minnesota, USA and Beth Israel Hospital, Boston, Massachusetts, USA). The lesions treated with rotational atherectomy were divided into two groups:

(a) those treated with stand-alone rotational atherectomy or 1 atmosphere balloon inflation; and
(b) those treated with rotational atherectomy and adjunctive balloon angioplasty.

The group treated with the combination of rotational atherectomy and adjunctive balloon angioplasty had the most favorable final angiographic results. This angiographic benefit translated into better freedom from follow-up clinical events, which included death, MI and target vessel revascularization (*Fig. 22.7*).

Although the group treated with rotational atherectomy plus adjunctive balloon angioplasty had improved outcomes relative to the other treatment groups, even in this group the follow-up clinical event rate remained rather high, at 33%, indicating that improvements are required. It is possible that the use of larger burr sizes may be more effective. Operators in this series were somewhat cautious with burr sizing, owing to the lack of available information on the potential for burr entrapment or slow flow in these diffusely diseased vessels. The lack of these complications in this series suggests that it may be possible to use larger burr sizes. Stents are usually implanted with 3.0 mm or larger balloons, so burr sizes of up to 2.5 mm should pass through most stents, provided complete stent expansion is achieved. If a stent is compressed by plaque and will not allow a large burr, it does not appear to lead to a complication. Instead, ablation of the stent strut may occur, or the burr simply may not cross the lesion. In the BARASTER registry, 62% of cases were performed without IVUS guidance to ensure full stent expansion, yet no significant complications occurred in this cohort. A rarely seen complication is the development of a vessel rupture distal to a stented segment, which led to the only Rotablator-related death in the BARASTER study. Unlike the protected environment of the stented segment, the distal segment is subject to trauma from the large atherectomy burrs.

Results similar to those of the BARASTER registry were found by von Dahm and colleagues in 100 patients treated with rotational atherectomy (plus adjunctive balloon angioplasty in the majority, 92%).[38] These investigators also found a 97% acute clinical success rate and a 35% rate of subsequent follow-up events. Recurrent restenosis was predicted by longer lesion and stent lengths. In both this trial and the BARASTER registry, when target vessel revascularization was required, it was in the form of coronary artery bypass graft surgery in approximately 50% of cases, which highlights the aggressiveness of the restenosis found in patients treated with rotational atherectomy in these registries.

A European randomized trial between rotational atherectomy and balloon angioplasty for in-stent restenosis was recently presented at the European Congress of Cardiology meetings, the ARTIST (Angioplasty versus Rotational Atherectomy in the Treatment of In-STent restenosis) trial. Investigators for this trial randomized 300 patients with in-stent restenosis to rotational atherectomy with low-pressure balloon inflations (similar to the ROTA arm of the BARASTER registry) or stand-alone balloon angioplasty. There was no restenosis benefit using the strategy of rotational atherectomy with low-pressure balloon inflations, similar to the findings in the BARASTER registry comparing the ROTA to the balloon angioplasty arms.

Sharma and colleagues[44] have presented data from a small, single-center randomized study, the ROSTER (ROtational atherectomy versus balloon angioplasty for in-STEnt Restenosis) trial.[44] Twenty-six patients randomized to rotational atherectomy with adjunctive balloon angioplasty had similar acute results to 26 patients randomly assigned to receive high-pressure balloon angioplasty to 12 atmospheres; however, 50% of patients treated with plain balloon angioplasty required additional stents to cover dissections. The incidence of creatinine phosphokinase release was similar in the two groups (16% with rotational atherectomy versus 12% with balloon angioplasty; p not significant).

At clinical follow-up after a mean of 5 ± 3 months, patients treated with rotational atherectomy were less likely to have a clinical event (4% versus 27%; p = 0.03). The improved follow-up outcomes in this trial compared with the above trials may be partly explained by the short time to follow-up, as well as by the shorter lesion lengths (13.9 ± 4.7 mm as opposed to 21 mm in BARASTER and in the trial reported by von Dahm). Vessel diameter and previous therapy for in-stent restenosis are other variables that differ between studies and that are likely to be of clinical significance.[52,53]

DIRECTIONAL CORONARY ATHERECTOMY

Case reports exist of the use of other atherectomy devices to treat in-stent restenosis, including the transluminal extraction catheter (TEC), pull-back atherectomy, and directional coronary atherectomy (DCA) devices.[46,54–61] DCA in particular has been evaluated in the treatment of in-stent restenosis.[46,54,60,61] Early investigators noted a high incidence of complications, primarily dissections, using this device for in-stent restenosis.[3,54,62,63] Unintended removal of coil stents was also reported.[62,63]

More recently, Palacios and colleagues[46,60] performed a retrospective comparison between patients with in-stent restenosis treated with DCA and those treated with balloon angioplasty.[46,60] The 40 patients treated with DCA all had an acute success without complications and a 6–month clinical event rate (death, MI, or target vessel revascularization) of 22%. This was in contrast to the balloon group, in which acute clinical success was achieved in only 85% with a follow-up event rate of 60%. However, the two groups were not well matched for baseline characteristics.

Cattelaens and colleagues[61] attempted directional atherectomy in 30 patients with in-stent restenosis and were able to deliver the device in 28 of these. They achieved a < 20% residual stenosis in 82% before the use of adjunctive balloon angioplasty. In three patients balloon rupture occurred, possibly owing to a sharp metal edge created from the atherectomy cutter. Stent material was detected by histopathological siderin staining of the removed material in 89%, with macroscopically visible metal in 69%.

DCA probably removes more tissue than other atherectomy devices (*Fig. 22.8*). Therefore, if debulking proves to be clinically advantageous in treating in-stent restenosis, DCA may have the greatest impact when it can be successfully performed. However, the bulkiness of the currently available atherectomy device limits its application to larger vessels in non-tortuous arteries.

Whether the scaffolding ability of a stent is compromised by disruption of one or more metal struts by an atherectomy device is not known, nor is it known if continued scaffolding is required after therapy for in-stent restenosis. As noted above, parts of metal stents are routinely removed when using DCA for in-stent restenosis.[61] Rotational atherectomy for in-stent restenosis can also weaken metal struts and probably causes some distal embolization of metal particles. In vitro testing by SciMed Life Systems (Boston Scientific Corporation, Maple Grove, Minnesota) was performed using a burr-to-stent ratio of 0.9–1.1, followed by pulsatile fatigue testing to simulate 10 years of implantation. Scanning electron

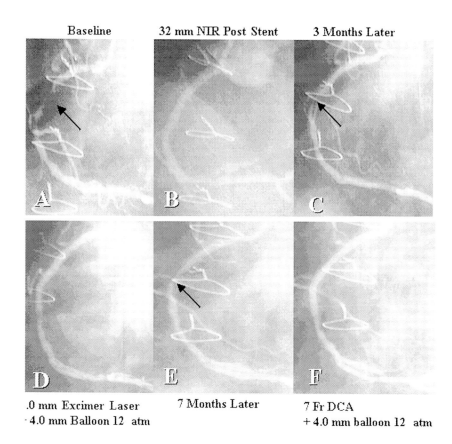

Baseline	32 mm NIR Post Stent	3 Months Later

.0 mm Excimer Laser — 7 Months Later — 7 Fr DCA
- 4.0 mm Balloon 12 atm — — + 4.0 mm balloon 12 atm

Figure 22.8 *Angiographic images of a stented lesion with recurrent in-stent restenosis treated with different atherectomy devices. (a) Baseline lesion in a right coronary artery. (b) Lesion after treatment with a 32 mm NIR stent. (c) In-stent restenosis (arrow) 3 months later. (d) Result after treatment with a 2.0 mm eccentric laser catheter followed by a 4.0 mm balloon inflated to 12 atmospheres. (e) Recurrent in-stent restenosis (arrow) 7 months later. (f) Result after treatment with a 7 Fr directional atherectomy (DCA) cutter followed by a 4.0 mm balloon inflation to 12 atmospheres. A larger lumen diameter is seen after the directional atherectomy than after the laser atherectomy procedure.*

microscopic analysis identified a single strut from one out of eight stents that had a crack but no loss of structural integrity.

Clinical events that suggest significant rapid collapse of stents, such as acute closure or MI, have not been described for any atherectomy device. It is not known if subsequent restenosis may occur as a result of inadequate scaffolding characteristics of a damaged stent, although, as noted above, loss of structural integrity was not seen despite aggressive ablation of stent metal.

CUTTING BALLOON

Strategies other than debulking devices have also been examined for the treatment of in-stent restenosis. The cutting balloon is an angioplasty balloon with three blades that incise the plaque slightly during balloon inflation. In theory, this modifies the plaque, allowing for improved efficacy of the angio-

plasty procedure. Recently, this device has been evaluated in 167 lesions with in-stent restenosis.[64] Acute success was achieved in all lesions. Angiographic follow-up was achieved in 72% at 5 months and demonstrated a 29% rate of restenosis, which appears favorable in this cohort of lesions with rather diffuse in-stent restenosis (mean length 17 ± 11 mm).

STENTING FOR IN-STENT RESTENOSIS

Placing a new stent to treat in-stent restenosis has several theoretic advantages and disadvantages. Investigators from the Washington Heart Center performed serial IVUS studies before, immediately after, and a further 45 minutes after treating in-stent restenosis. They noted an initial decrease in intrastent tissue; however, this was offset in certain cases by recurrent tissue in-growth after only a few minutes, which they termed 'instant' in-stent restenosis.[23]

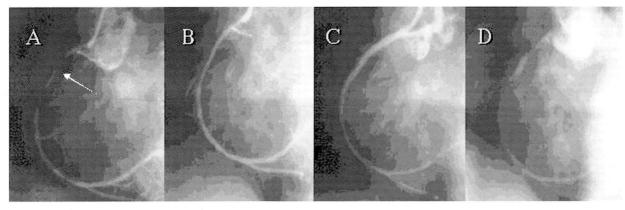

Restenosis 3 months   Balloon Dilatation   30 mm AVE Micro II   Recurrent Restenosis
Post 2-NIR stents   32 mm Crown   7 months later

Figure 22.9 *Treatment of in-stent restenosis with additional stent placement. (a) In-stent restenosis in an ostial/proximal right coronary artery. Two 16 mm NIR stents had been placed 3 months previously. The arrow points to lesion. (b) After treatment with balloon angioplasty of the in-stent restenotic lesion. (c) After placement of a 30 mm long AVE II Microstent and a 32 mm Crown stent, an improved angiographic appearance compared to after balloon angioplasty alone. (d) Recurrent in-stent restenosis 7 months later. Despite improving the initial angiographic appearance with the placement of additional stents, aggressive recurrent restenosis has occurred.*

Given the lack of clinical stent thrombosis or vascular closure occurring after therapy for in-stent restenosis, it is unlikely that platelet or thrombus deposition is the cause of this rapid increase in intrastent tissue. Since the mechanism of balloon angioplasty is extrusion of tissue through the stent struts, it is more likely that the extruded tissue subsequently falls back into the lumen due to vascular recoil. The placement of a new stent may then compress this tissue keeping it out of the lumen – at least temporarily.

Studies using QCA and IVUS[20,22,65] have shown that the lumen achieved with balloon angioplasty when treating in-stent restenosis is not as large as the lumen dimensions at the time of initial stent implantation. However, the implantation of a new stent allows for recovery of the initial luminal results, as identified by QCA and IVUS.[27,28] Under the hypothesis that 'bigger is better', these improved dimensions should translate into more favorable subsequent outcomes.

However, stented lesions that restenose have already demonstrated a predilection for the development of a hyperproliferative response to the acute and chronic injury of a foreign body. These lesions are therefore potentially more likely to mount an additional exuberant response to further injury and foreign body implantations (*Fig. 22.9*). This process may in fact be ongoing at the time of presentation with in-stent restenosis, and further stent implantation may actually be 'feeding a burning fire', although data obtained by atherectomy specimens at the time of in-stent restenosis are conflicting.[52,59] In a series of 57 in-stent restenotic lesions treated with additional stents at Centro Cuore Columbus, in Milan, Italy, recurrent clinical restenosis occurred in 40%.[27] Similar results have been reported by other centers, with rates ranging between 27% and 70%.[24–26,28–30] In some of these cases new stents were placed to cover dissections occurring during balloon angioplasty for in-stent restenosis and perhaps could not have been avoided. However, the relatively poor outcomes seen in these retrospective studies do not support the likelihood that additional stenting for in-stent restenosis is likely to be of any significant benefit unless it is combined with strategies to decrease the intimal proliferative response.

In contrast to the above studies, a subgroup analysis of 38 patients with in-stent restenosis who comprised part of the placebo group in the SCRIPPS (Scripps Coronary Radiation to Inhibit Proliferation Post Stenting) prospective, randomized trial of intravascular radiation therapy was performed by Russo and colleagues.[67] Twenty-five patients in this subgroup received new stents and 13 were treated with balloon angioplasty alone. The group receiving new stents had a larger minimum lumen diameter (MLD) at 6–month angiographic follow-up, although the need for target lesion revascularization was similar between the two groups.

INTRAVASCULAR BRACHYTHERAPY

As noted above, intrastent restenosis appears to be exclusively a hyperproliferative response. Therefore, therapy that minimizes this response has the potential to be particularly effective. This hypothesis was tested with the use of radiation therapy in the SCRIPPS trial, reported by Teirstein and colleagues,[68] in stented and non-stented restenotic lesions. In this study of 54 lesions with multiple episodes of restenosis, the incidence of subsequent restenosis was significantly reduced when intravascular therapy with gamma-irradiation was applied, from 54% to 17%. Radiation therapy was particularly beneficial in the cohort with in-stent restenosis.[67] Of lesions evaluated in this trial, 35 had in-stent restenosis, 18 were randomly assigned to irradiation and 17 were assigned to placebo. Those treated with adjunctive radiation therapy had a subsequent restenosis rate of only 11%, compared to 71% among those treated with balloon angioplasty alone ($p = 0.0001$). This lower rate of restenosis was due to a significant reduction in the late loss. (Late loss is the MLD at the end of the intervention minus the MLD at the 6–month follow-up angiogram.) In the SCRIPPS trial, the late loss was 1.19 mm in the placebo group but only 0.17 mm in the irradiated group ($p = 0.001$). These results are being confirmed with larger randomized trials.[69,70]

Future studies will evaluate other methods of brachytherapy, including the use of beta-radiation and possibly other sources of radiation. In evaluating the results of brachytherapy for in-stent restenosis, restenosis outside the stent boundaries must also be carefully analysed. As the radiation dose recedes longitudinally, an increase in proliferation theoretically may occur. However, in the SCRIPPS trial, a narrowing > 50% occurred outside the stent in only 9% of cases treated with radiation therapy versus 18% with placebo. Notably, at 1-year follow-up, new lesions were not seen to occur in other vessels after radiation therapy was applied focally to refractory lesions. This topic is covered more thoroughly in Chapter 23.

CONCLUSIONS

As the use of intracoronary stents rises, the problem of in-stent restenosis will continue to raise concern and will further increase the cost of health-care delivery. The identification of effective strategies to address this problem is an important challenge. The indication and use of such therapies will depend partly on their costs and ease of use. If the strategies are inexpensive, easy to administer, and associated with minimal risks, then it may be appropriate to include them at the time of initial stent implantation. If, however, the strategies are expensive, cumbersome, or associated with significant risks, then they should be selectively applied, either to de novo lesions at high risk of restenosis or to restenotic lesions at risk of severe or recurrent restenosis. The risk factors for such clinically severe restenosis would need to be identified.

The use of gamma-irradiation is an example of a technique that appears to be effective but cumbersome, and it is therefore probably most effective for selected lesions. Balloon angioplasty is safe and relatively inexpensive and appears to be reasonably effective for focal in-stent restenosis. Debulking devices and other tools, such as the cutting balloon, also appear to be safe and possibly somewhat more effective than balloon angioplasty, however, optimal strategies need to be defined. The role of these devices in the therapy of in-stent restenosis needs to be further clarified with randomized trials. Additional stents should be used to cover important dissections that occur in the therapy of in-stent restenosis. They may also be effective in reducing the problem of 'instant' restenosis, in combination with the use of antiproliferative strategies such as radiation therapy. However, the use of additional stents solely to optimize early angiographic results without their being combined with effective antiproliferative therapy cannot be recommended at this time owing to the high rate of recurrent restenosis. Finally, the majority of research in the management of in-stent restenosis has focused on the Palmaz–Schatz slotted tube stent. Whether in-stent restenosis behaves in the same way with other stent types is not known.

REFERENCES

1. Yokoi H, Kimura T, Nakagawa Y et al. Long-term clinical and quantitative angiographic follow-up after the

Palmaz–Schatz stent restenosis (abstract). *J Am Coll Cardiol* 1996; **27**: 224A.

2. Baim DS, Levine MJ, Leon MB et al. Management of restenosis within the Palmaz–Schatz coronary stent (the U.S. multicenter experience). *Am J Cardiol* 1993; **71**: 364–366.

3. Macander PJ, Roubin GS, Agrawal SK et al. Balloon angioplasty for treatment of in-stent restenosis: feasibility, safety, and efficacy. *Cathet Cardiovasc Diagn* 1994; **32**: 125–131.

4. Reimers B, Moussa I, Akiyama T et al A. Long-term clinical follow-up after successful repeat percutaneous intervention for stent restenosis. *J Am Coll Cardiol* 1997; **30**: 186–192.

5. Bauters C, Banos JL, Van Belle E et al. Six-month angiographic outcome after successful repeat percutaneous intervention for in-stent restenosis. *Circulation* 1998; **97**: 318–321.

6. Sridhar K, Teefy PlJ, Almond DG et al. Long-term clinical outcomes of patients with in-stent restenosis (abstract). *Circulation* 1996; **94 (suppl)**: I-454.

7. Tan HC, Sketch MH Jr, Tan ME et al. Is there an optimal treatment strategy for stent restenosis? (abstract). *Circulation* 1996; **94 (suppl)**: I-90.

8. Dussaillant GR, Mintz GS, Pichard AD et al. A serial volumetric intravascular ultrasound analysis of instent restenosis (abstract). *J Am Coll Cardiol* 1996; **27**: 362A.

9. Hoffman R, Mintz GS, Dussaillant GR et al. Patterns and mechanisms of in-stent restenosis. A serial intravascular ultrasound study. *Circulation* 1996; **94**: 1247–1254.

10. Dussaillant GR, Mintz GS, Pichard AD et al. Small stent size and intimal hyperplasia contribute to restenosis: a volumetric intravascular ultrasound analysis. *J Am Coll Cardiol* 1995; **26**: 720–724.

11. Mintz GS, Popma JJ, Pichard AD et al. Arterial remodeling after coronary angioplasty. A serial intravascular ultrasound study. *Circulation* 1996; **94**: 35–43.

12. Kimura T, Kaburagi S, Tamura T et al. Remodeling of human coronary arteries undergoing coronary angioplasty or atherectomy. *Circulation* 1997; **96**: 475–483.

13. Itoh A, Hall P, Maiello L et al. Acute recoil of Palmaz–Schatz stent: a rare cause of suboptimal stent implantation: report of two cases with intravascular ultrasound findings. *Cathet Cardiovasc Diagn* 1996; **37**: 334–338.

14. Fernandez-Aviles F, Alonso J, Duran JM et al. Clinical pattern and long-term behavior of significant angiographic restenosis after coronary stenting (abstract). *J Am Coll Cardiol* 1998; **31 (suppl)**: 141A.

15. Nibler N, Kastrati A, Elezi S et al. Angiographic and clinical follow-up of patients with asymptomatic restenosis after coronary stent implantation (abstract). *J Am Coll Cardiol* 1998; **31**: 65A.

16. Kimura T, Tamura T, Yokoi H, Nobuyoshi M. Long-term clinical and angiographic follow-up after placement of Palmaz–Schatz coronary stent: a single center experience. *J Interv.Cardiol* 1994; **7**: 129–139.

17. Hermiller JB, Fry ET, Peters TF et al. Late coronary artery stenosis regression within the Gianturco–Roubin intracoronary stent. *Am J Cardiol* 1996; **77**: 247–251.

18. Serruys PW, Sousa E, Belardi J et al. Benestent-II trial: subgroup analysis of patients assigned either to angiographic and clinical follow-up or clinical follow-up alone (abstract). *Circulation* 1997; **96 (suppl)**: I-653–I-654.

19. Cutlip DE, Ho KKL, Kuntz RE, Baim DS. Influence of routine angiographic follow-up on clinical restenosis

outcome in the ASCENT trial (abstract). *J Am Coll Cardiol* 1998; **31**: 139A.

20. Mehran R, Mintz GS, Popma JJ et al. Mechanisms and results of balloon angioplasty for the treatment of in-stent restenosis. *Am J Cardiol* 1996; **78**: 618–622.

21. Schiele F, Meneveau N, Vuillemenot A et al. Assessment of balloon angioplasty in intrastent restenosis with intracoronary ultrasound (abstract). *J Am Coll Cardiol* 1998; **31**: 495A-496A.

22. Gorge G, Konorza T, Voegele E et al. Incomplete restoration of luminal dimensions after PTCA in restenotic stented segments: an intravascular ultrasound analysis (abstract). *J Am Coll Cardiol* 1997; **29**: 311A.

23. Shiran A, Waksman R, Abizaid A et al. Is recurrent in-stent restenosis INSTANT restenosis? An intravascular ultrasound study (abstract). *Circulation* 1997; **96 (suppl)**: I-87–I-88.

24. Debbas N, Stauffer JC, Eeckhout E et al. Stenting within a stent: treatment for repeat in-stent restenosis in a venous graft. *Am Heart J* 1997; **133**: 460–463.

25. Cecena FA. Stenting the stent: alternative strategy for treating in-stent restenosis. *Cathet Cardiovasc Diagn* 1996; **39**: 377–382.

26. Moris C, Alfonso F, Lambert JL et al. Stenting for coronary dissection after balloon dilation of in-stent restenosis: stenting a previously stented site. *Am Heart J* 1996; **131**: 834–836.

27. Goldberg SL, Loussararian AH, di Mario C et al. Stenting for in-stent restenosis (abstract). *Circulation* 1997; **96**: I-88.

28. Mehran R, Abizaid AS, Mintz GS et al. Mechanisms and results of additional stent implantation to treat focal in-stent restenosis (abstract). *J Am Coll Cardiol* 1998; **31**: 455A.

29. Lefevre T, Louvard Y, Morice MC et al. In-stent restenosis: should we stent the stent? A single center prospective study (abstract). *Circulation* 1997; **96 (suppl)**: I-88.

30. Elezi S, Kastrati A, Schuhlen H et al. Stenting for restenosis of stented lesions: acute and 6 months clinical and angio-graphic follow-up (abstract). *Circulation* 1997; **96 (suppl)**: I-88.

31. Mehran R, Ito S, Abizaid A et al. Does lesion length affect late outcome of patients with in-stent restenosis? Results of the multicenter Laser Angioplasty for Stent Restenosis (LARS) registry (abstract). *J Am Coll Cardiol* 1998; **31 (suppl)**: 142A.

32. Sharma SK, Rjawat Y, Kakarala V et al. Angiographic pattern of in-stent restenosis after Palmaz–Schatz stent implantation (abstract). *J Am Coll Cardiol* 1997; **29 (suppl)**: 313A.

33. Ribichini F, Steffenino G, Dellavalle A et al. Plasma activity and insertion/deletion polymorphism of angiotensin I-converting enzyme: a major risk factor and a marker of risk for coronary stent restenosis. *Circulation.* 1998; **97**: 147–154.

34. Ribichini F, Steffenino G, Dellavalle A et al. The pattern (focal/diffuse) of angiographic in-stent restenosis is associated to the I/D polymorphism of the angiotensin converting enzyme gene (abstract). *Circulation* 1997; **96 (suppl)**: I-87.

35. Hamm CW, Simon R, Beabra Gomes RJ et al. Laser angioplasty for within stent restenosis: final results of the LARS surveillance study (abstract). *J Am Coll Cardiol* 1998; **31 (suppl):** 143A.

36. Buchbinder M, Goldberg SL, Fortuna R et al. Rotational atherectomy for intra-stent restenosis: initial experience (abstract). *Circulation* 1996; **94 (suppl)**: I-621.

37. Goldberg SL, Shawl F, Buchbinder M et al. Rotational atherectomy for in-stent restenosis: the BARASTER Registry (abstract). *Circulation* 1997; **96 (suppl)**: I-80.

38. Klues HG, Reffelmann T, vom Dahl J, Hanrath P. High-speed rotational coronary atherectomy for the treatment of restenosis in coronary stents (abstract). *J Am Coll Cardiol* 1997; **29**: 313A.

39. Mehran R, Mintz GS, Satler LF et al. Treatment of in-stent restenosis with excimer laser coronary angioplasty. Mechanisms and results compared to PTCA alone. *Circulation* 1997; **96**: 2183–2189.

40. Mehran R, Mintz GS, Popma JJ et al. Mechanisms of lumen enlargement during atheroablation of in-stent restenosis: a volumetric ultrasound analysis (abstract). *J Am Coll Cardiol* 1997; **29**: 497A.

41. Goldberg SL, Shawl F, Buchbinder M et al. The BARASTeR Registry Participants. Rotational atherectomy for in-stent restenosis: the BARASTER Registry (abstract). *Circulation* 1997; **96 (suppl)**: I-80.

42. Khanolkar UB. Percutaneous transluminal rotational atherectomy for treatment of in-stent restenosis. *Indian Heart J* 1996; **48**: 281–282.

43. Stone GW. Rotational atherectomy for treatment of in-stent restenosis: role of intracoronary ultrasound guidance. *Cathet Cardiovasc Diagn* 1996; **39 (suppl)**: 73–77.

44. Sharma SK, Kini A, Duvvuri S et al. Randomized trial of rotational atherectomy vs balloon angioplasty for in-stent restenosis (ROSTER) (abstract). *J Am Coll Cardiol* 1998; **31 (suppl)**: 142A.

45. Mehran R, Abizaid AS, Abizaid A et al. Rotational atherectomy for the treatment of in-stent restenosis: long-term outcome compared to balloon angioplasty alone (abstract). *Am J Cardiol* 1997; **80 (suppl)**: 23S.

46. Mahdi NA, Leon M, Mikulic M et al. PTCA, directional and rotational coronary atherectomy in the management of Palmaz–Schatz in-stent restenosis (abstract). *J Am Coll Cardiol* 1998; **31 (suppl)**: 275A.

47. Buttner HJ, Muller C, Hodgson JMcB et al. Rotational ablation with adjunctive low-pressure balloon dilatation in diffuse in-stent restenosis: immediate and follow-up results (abstract). *J Am Coll Cardiol* 1998; **31**: 141A.

48. Ellis SG, Popma JJ, Buchbinder M et al. Relation of clinical presentation, stenosis, morphology, and operator technique to the procedural results of rotational atherectomy and rotational atherectomy-facilitated angioplasty. *Circulation* 1998; **89**: 882–892.

49. Bass TA, Whitlow PL, Moses JW et al. Acute complications related to coronary rotational atherectomy strategy. A report from the STRATAS trial (abstract). *J Am Coll Cardiol* 1997; **29 (suppl)**: 68A.

50. Kuntz RE, Safian RD, Carrozza JP et al. The importance of acute luminal diameter in determining restenosis after coronary atherectomy or stenting. *Circulation* 1992; **86**: 1827–1835.

51. vom Dahl J, Klues HG, Radke P et al. Angiographic long-term results of coronary rotational atherectomy for treatment of diffuse in-stent restenosis are dependent on the length of the initial in-stent restenosis (abstract). *Eur Heart J* 1998; **19 (suppl)**: 114.

52. Mehran R, Abizaid AS, Mintz GS et al. Patterns of in-stent restenosis: classification and impact on subsequent target lesion revascularization (abstract). *J Am Coll Cardiol* 1998; **31**: 141A.

53. Jolly N, Ellis SG, Franco I et al. Determinants of recurrent in stent restenosis: insights from clinical follow-up (abstract). *Circulation* 1997; **96**: I-472.

54. Strauss BH, Umans VA, van Suylen RJ et al. Directional atherectomy for treatment of restenosis within coronary stents: clinical, angiographic and histologic results. *J Am Coll Cardiol* 1992; **20**: 1465–1473.

55. Ikari Y, Yamaguchi T, Tamura T et al. Transluminal extraction atherectomy and adjunctive balloon angioplasty for restenosis after Palmaz–Schatz coronary stent implantation. *Cathet Cardiovasc Diagn* 1993; **30**: 127–130.

56. Chow WH, Chan TF. Pullback atherectomy for the treatment of intrastent restenosis (letter). *Cathet Cardiovasc Diagn* 1997; **41**: 94–95.

57. Virk SJ, Bellamy CM, Perry RA. Transluminal extraction atherectomy for stent restenosis in a saphenous vein bypass graft (letter). *Eur.Heart J* 1997; **18**: 350–351.

58. Hara K, Ikari Y, Tamura T, Yamaguchi T. Transluminal extraction atherectomy for restenosis following Palmaz–Schatz stent implantation. *Am J Cardiol* 1997; **79**: 801–802.

59. Patel JJ, Meadaa R, Cohen M et al. Transluminal extraction atherectomy for aortosaphenous vein graft stent restenosis. *Cathet Cardiovasc Diagn* 1996; **38**: 320–324.

60. Pathan A, Butte A, Harrell L et al. Directional coronary atherectomy is superior to PTCA for the treatment of Palmaz–Schatz stent restenosis (abstract). *J Am Coll Cardiol* 1997; **29 (suppl)**: 68A.

61. Cattelaens N, Gerckens U, Mueller R et al. Directional atherectomy for treatment of stent restenosis: feasibility and histopathological findings in 28 patients (abstract). *J Am Coll Cardiol* 1998; **31**: 142A.

62. Meyer T, Schmidt T, Buchwald A, Wiegand V. Stent wire cutting during coronary directional atherectomy. *Clin Cardiol* 1993; **16**: 450–452.

63. Bowerman RE, Pinkerton CA, Kirk B, Waller BF. Disruption of a coronary stent during atherectomy for restenosis. *Cathet Cardiovasc Diagn* 1991; **24**: 248–251.

64. Nakamura M, Suzuki T, Matsubara T et al. Results of cutting balloon angioplasty for stent restenosis. Japanese multicenter registry (abstract). *J Am Coll Cardiol* 1998; **31**: 235A.

65. Mehran R, Mintz GS, Popma JJ et al. Treatment of in-stent restenosis: an intravascular ultrasound study of results in 159 stented lesions (abstract). *J Am Coll Cardiol* 1997; **29**: 77A.

66. Goldberg SL, Loussararian AH, di Mario C et al. Stenting for in-stent restenosis (abstract). *Circulation* 1997; **96**: I-88.

67. Russo RJ, Massullo V, Jani SK et al. Restenting versus PTCA for in-stent restenosis with or without intracoronary radiation therapy: an analysis of the SCRIPPS trial (abstract). *Circulation* 1997; **96 (suppl)**: I-219.

68. Teirstein PS, Massullo V, Jani S et al. Catheter-based radiotherapy to inhibit restenosis after coronary stenting. *N Engl J Med* 1997; **336**: 1697–1703.

69. Waksman R, White RL, Chan RC et al. Localized intracoronary radiation therapy for patients with in-stent restenosis: preliminary results from a randomized clinical study (abstract). *Circulation* 1997; **96**: I-219.

70. Waksman R, White RL, Chan RC et al. Intracoronary radiation therapy for patients with in-stent restenosis. Interim report from a randomized clinical study (abstract). *J Am Coll Cardiol* 1998; **31**: 222A.

Chapter 23 Coronary radiation therapy

Remo Albiero, Carlo Di Mario and Antonio Colombo

INTRODUCTION

Restenosis after coronary angioplasty is a major limitation of an otherwise highly effective and safe procedure for the treatment of atherosclerotic coronary artery disease. Although the advent of coronary stenting has significantly reduced restenosis rates by inhibiting elastic recoil, intimal proliferation as the second major mechanism for post-interventional restenosis has not been effectively suppressed, and an overall restenosis rate of 20–30% remains. Despite numerous trials, no effective pharmacologic therapy has been found. Intracoronary Radiation Therapy (IRT), or brachytherapy, a term derived from the Greek *brachy* meaning 'short', is an invasive procedure that delivers radiation over a small distance by placing the source adjacent to or within a lesion. It is a very promising strategy to prevent the intimal hyperplasia that leads to restenosis after percutaneous coronary interventions.[1-4] The rationale for using this new technique is that radiation has been shown to be highly effective and safe in treating benign vascular malformations and in preventing keloid formation.

Both IRT and external beam radiotherapy (also known as *teletherapy*, a term derived from the Greek *tele* meaning 'from afar'), which delivers radiation from an external radiation sources have been used to administer radiotherapy to a vascular lesion after angioplasty. However, external irradiation has the disadvantages that a higher dose rate than in IRT is used, treatment times are longer, the source is positioned far from the target, and radiation is delivered to a larger volume of tissue. For these reasons, external irradiation is presently not recommended.[5]

Two types of IRT are commonly used: one uses a catheter-based radiation delivery system; the other uses radioactive stent implantation. Catheter-based systems use either gamma-radiation (^{192}iridium (^{192}Ir)) or beta-radiation (^{90}strontium, (^{90}Sr), ^{90}yttrium (^{90}Y), ^{32}phosphorus (^{32}P), ^{188}rhenium (^{188}Re), or ^{186}rhenium (^{186}Re)) to deliver the prescribed dose at high- or low-dose rates. Stents use beta-radiation (^{32}P) at a very low dose rate.

Beta-particles and gamma-particles differ in both charge and mass. Beta-particles, which have the same mass as an electron, have a greater mass and charge than gamma-particles, which are photons. Thus, beta-particles have a greater degree of tissue attenuation than gamma-particles, and they are characterized by a sharp decline in dose rate within millimeters of the actual source. Thus, exposure to surrounding tissue as well as to the catheterization staff can be kept to a minimum. In contrast, gamma-particles deliver an appreciable dose even centimeters away from the source owing to greater tissue penetration than beta-particles and produce the most homogeneous dose distribution over the vessel wall, but require additional shielding in the catheter laboratory and deliver a relatively high dose to the myocardium.

The properties of radioisotopes used for IRT are shown in *Table 23.1*. None of the beta-emitters is ideal: ^{32}P and ^{188}Re have lower energy than desired, ^{90}Y, ^{188}Re, and ^{186}Re have a short half-life, and ^{90}Sr is difficult to fabricate. The only way to obtain a beta-isotope with both higher energy and longer half-life

Table 23.1

Properties of radioisotopes used for intracoronary radiation therapy

Element	Isotope	Emission	Half-life	Average energy (keV)
Iridium	^{192}Ir	gamma	74 days	375
Phosphorus	^{32}P	beta	14 days	600
Strontium	^{90}Sr	beta	28 years	970
Yttrium	^{90}Y	beta	64 hours	970
Rhenium	^{188}Re	beta	17 hours	780
Rhenium	^{186}Re	beta	89 hours	1070

is to use a parent–daughter combination of isotopes in radioactive equilibrium. The two isotope pairs thus far identified for use in intravascular brachytherapy are tungsten (W) with [188]Re and ^{90}Sr with [90]Y.

Using the same target treatment doses, both gamma- and beta-catheter-based systems have demonstrated similar results, despite differences in the isotope characteristics (e.g. penetration, activity, dose rate) in reducing neointimal proliferation after balloon angioplasty in porcine coronary arteries. Catheter-based systems seem more flexible for several reasons; on the other hand, they require a substantial amount of hardware.

Beta-emitting radioactive stents have also been of value, especially in large vessels, because of their low activity and their proximity to the vessel wall. Stents are implanted via a conventional stent delivery system with small modifications consisting of a lucite or plastic protector. However, stents emit a non-homogeneous radiation profile owing to the mesh-like structure. In addition, not every lesion can be reached by a stent, nor does every lesion require a stent solely to deliver radiation.

MECHANISM OF ACTION OF RADIATION IN REDUCING RESTENOSIS

Wilcox and colleagues[6] described the role of the adventitia in the arterial response to angioplasty. They found that the first major site of cell proliferation between 2–3 days after angioplasty was the adventitial (the proliferating cells were myofibroblasts) and not the medial wall. Seven days after angioplasty, cell proliferation was predominant in the neointima (adventitial myofibroblasts migrated into the neointima, which contributed to the mass of the restenosis lesion) and was reduced in the media and adventitia.

Waksman and colleagues[7] analysed the mechanism by which beta-([90]Sr–[90]Y) and gamma-(^{192}Ir) intravascular irradiation, designed to deliver 14 Gy or 28 Gy at a depth of 2 mm from the source, reduce vascular lesion formation after balloon overstretch injury of pig coronary arteries. Two weeks after injury, there were fewer alpha-actin-positive myofibroblasts in the adventitia of the irradiated vessels than in non-irradiated controls, and morphometric analysis indicated that the vessel perimeter of the irradiated vessels was significantly larger than in controls.

These animal studies demonstrated that:

(a) IRT inhibits development of the restenosis lesion by significantly reducing cell proliferation in the media and adventitia early after injury;
(b) alpha-actin staining of myofibroblasts in the adventitia was reduced in the irradiated vessels;
(c) adventitial myofibroblasts contribute to post-angioplasty restenosis by proliferating, forming a fibrotic scar surrounding the injury site, and migrating into the neointima; this might contribute to negative vascular remodeling associated with clinical restenosis.
(d) IRT inhibits the adventitial fibrosis that develops at the injury site.

Brenner and colleagues[8] analysed the radiobiology of intravascular irradiation. They considered various mechanistic interpretations of the experimental and clinical observations that doses of 12–20 Gy appear to be efficacious in preventing restenosis. Using in vitro models of human smooth muscle cells, they investigated the relative radiosensitivity of smooth muscle cells and endothelial cells, and measured the dose-dependent ability of smooth muscle cells to repopulate a denuded region in a confluent layer of cells. They found that doses > 20 Gy, which would be required to eliminate the smooth muscle cell population completely, are too large because of the unacceptable risk of late complications. However, doses that can be practically given in vascular irradiation (< 20 Gy) will certainly delay restenosis by 1–3 years, with larger doses producing longer delays. Whether such doses can avert restenosis permanently is unclear, since permanent prevention at realistic doses depends critically on the assumption that those smooth muscle cells which survive irradiation have a significantly limited capacity for proliferation. With regard to current animal model experiments, routine follow-up of < 1 year, which is standard practice, is probably too short to address some of the key mechanistic questions in intravascular radiation therapy.

CATHETER-BASED RADIATION DELIVERY SYSTEMS

ANIMAL MODELS

Gamma-radiation

Weinberger and colleagues[9] demonstrated that IRT before overstretch balloon angioplasty markedly reduces neointima formation in the pig model. They delivered 20 Gy, 15 Gy, or 10 Gy to the coronary artery wall of 10 pigs, using a 2 cm ribbon of ^{192}Ir positioned at the target segment. Subsequently, overdilatation balloon angioplasty was performed at the irradiated segment. In 10 control pigs, overdilatation balloon angioplasty was performed without previous irradiation. At 30 days, by histopathological analysis, neointimal area was decreased by 71.4% at 20 Gy and by 58.3% at 15 Gy compared with control animals ($p < 0.05$ for both). A stimulatory effect on smooth muscle cell proliferation was noted at 10 Gy, with a 123% increase in neointimal area compared with controls ($p < 0.05$). The effective therapeutic dose range for the prevention of restenosis in this model begins at approximately 15 Gy delivered to the vessel wall.

Waksman and colleagues[10] demonstrated that low-dose intracoronary gamma-irradiation using a high-activity ^{192}Ir source that delivered 3.5 Gy, 7.0 Gy, or 14.0 Gy to the site of coronary arterial overstretch balloon injury in pigs inhibited subsequent intimal thickening (hyperplasia) in a dose-related manner. At 14 days, all arteries treated with radiation demonstrated significantly decreased neointima formation compared with control arteries.

Mazur and colleagues[11] examined the effects of intracoronary gamma irradiation (^{192}Ir) delivered at a high dose rate on neointimal hyperplasia after injury induced by two methods: balloon overstretch injury (circumflex artery), and stent implantation (left anterior descending and right coronary artery) in a porcine model of coronary restenosis. They treated the coronary artery segments with doses of 10 Gy (in eight animals), 15 Gy (in nine animals), 25 Gy (in nine animals), or control (simulation wire only; in eight animals). After 28 days, histopathology showed a striking reduction in the amount of neointima in the irradiated arteries compared with control vessels.

BETA-RADIATION

Studies by Waksman and colleagues in pig coronary arteries demonstrated that:

(a) After coronary arterial overstretch balloon injury, low-dose intracoronary beta-irradiation, using [90]Sr–[90]Y with doses between 7 Gy and 56 Gy delivered to a depth of 2 mm, inhibits neointima formation at 14 days in a dose-related manner, and that no further inhibitory effect is seen beyond 28 Gy.[12]

(b) Intracoronary delivery of ^{90}Y at a dose of 18 Gy prescribed to treat the vessel wall 1 mm from the surface of a centering catheter balloon results in consistent homogeneous inhibition of neointima formation post-injury.[13]

(c) Intracoronary radiation with [90]Sr–[90]Y at a dose of 14 Gy reduces neointima formation at 28 days in segments of coronary vessels that were stented immediately after irradiation. The neo-intimal area was significantly reduced in the irradiated stented arteries compared with control arteries treated with stent only (1.98 mm² with ^{192}Ir and 2.53 mm² with [90]Sr–[90]Y versus 3.82 mm² in the control stented arteries, $p < 0.005$).[14]

CLINICAL STUDIES WITH GAMMA-IRT

Venezuela trial

Condado and colleagues[1,15] performed the first clinical trial utilizing gamma-radiation for prevention of restenoisis after percutaneous transluminal coronary angioplasty (PTCA). Radiation was hand-delivered using a 0.36 mm (0.014-inch) wire or a 0.46 mm (0.018-inch) wire with a 30 mm long segment of ^{192}Ir into a non-centered 4 Fr closed-end lumen catheter (AngioRad). Twenty-one patients (22 arteries) underwent standard PTCA followed by IRT with a prescribed dose of 18–25 Gy to 1.5 mm depth.

Angiographic complications included two cases of subacute thrombosis within 30 days and four aneurysms (two procedure-related and two occurring within 3 months), which (based on later recalculation) were possibly due to the administration of an actual dose up to 55 Gy in a short time.[16]

For this study a 3-year clinical and angiographic follow-up is available.[17] One aneurysm increased between 3 months and 2 years (from 27 mm² to 46 mm²), but all aneurysms remained unchanged at 3 years. No other angiographic complications were observed. The binary restenosis was 28.6% (n = 6) at 6 months and 23.8% (n = 5) at 2 and 3 years, owing to regression of stenosis in one lesion. At 8-month follow-up, loss index was 0.19 with a negative late loss (favorable vascular remodeling) in 10 out of 22 arteries treated. At 3-year follow-up, the late loss (0.29 mm) and loss index (0.25) remained low, total occlusion developed in three lesions (two early, and one at 2 years), two patients had repeat PTCA, and one patients had a non-target lesion myocardial infarction.

SCRIPPS trial

In the SCRIPPS (Scripps Coronary Radiation to Inhibit Proliferation Post Stenting) trial, Teirstein and colleagues[18] studied the safety and efficacy of catheter-based intracoronary gamma-radiation plus stenting to reduce coronary restenosis in 55 patients with previous restenosis. Radiation was manually delivered using a [192]Ir 0.76 mm (0.030-inch) nylon ribbon with seeds (Best Medical International, Springfield, Virginia, USA) into a closed-end lumen, non-centered 4.5 Fr catheter. Patients with restenosis underwent stenting in all non-stented lesions or repeated coronary stenting (restenting in > 80% of patients), as required per protocol, and were then randomly assigned (double-blind trial) to receive catheter-based irradiation with ^{192}Ir or placebo. Dosimetry was guided by intravenous ultrasound (IVUS) (8–30 Gy). Clinical follow-up was performed, with quantitative coronary angiographic and IVUS measurements at 6 months. Of the 55 patients enrolled, 26 were assigned to the ^{192}Ir group and 29 to the placebo group. Angiographic studies were performed in 53 patients (96%) at a mean of 6.7 ± 2.2 months. The mean minimal luminal diameter at follow-up was larger in the ^{192}Ir group than in the placebo group (2.43 ± 0.78 mm versus 1.85 ± 0.89 mm; $p = 0.02$). Late luminal loss was significantly lower in the ^{192}Ir group than in the placebo group (0.38 ± 1.06 mm versus 1.03 ± 0.97 mm; $p = 0.03$). Angiographically identified restenosis (≥ 50% reduction of the luminal diameter at follow-up) occurred in 17% of the patients in the ^{192}Ir group compared with 54% of those in the placebo group ($p = 0.01$, 69% reduction). IVUS detected a reduction of intimal hyperplasia volume and an increase in cross-sectional area in the ^{192}Ir group. There were no apparent complications of the treatment.

In the SCRIPPS trial,[19] a subanalysis was performed to quantitate the impact of patient, lesion and technical characteristics on late angiographic outcome. Late luminal loss and loss index were calculated for several patient subgroups, including patients with diabetes mellitus, in-stent restenosis, multiple previous PTCA procedures, longer lesion lengths, saphenous vein grafts, small vessel diameters, and minimum dose exposures of at least 8.00 Gy. In the treated group, late loss was particularly low in patients with diabetes mellitus (0.19 mm), in-stent restenosis (0.17 mm), reference vessel diameters < 3.0 mm (0.07 mm), and in patients who received a minimum radiation dose to the entire adventitial border of at least 8.00 Gy. By two-factor analysis of variance, used to test for an interaction between patient characteristics and treatment effect, a significant interaction between subgroup characteristics and treatment effect (late loss) was found in patients with in-stent restenosis ($p = 0.035$), and in patients receiving a minimum dose of 8.00 Gy to the adventitial border ($p = 0.009$).

This substudy of the SCRIPPS trial suggests that patient characteristics associated with a more aggressive proliferative response to injury appeared to confer an enhanced response to radiotherapy. Furthermore, a dose threshold response to ^{192}Ir was found, with an enhanced response occurring when the entire circumference of the adventitial border was exposed to at least 8.00 Gy.

At 3-year clinical follow-up,[20] treatment with ^{192}Ir in the SCRIPPS trial demonstrated a significant clinical benefit. All living patients were contacted at a mean of 34 ± 7.8 months in placebo versus 35 ± 3.4 months in the ^{192}Ir group (p not significant) after their index study procedure. They were assessed with respect to the need for target-lesion revascularization (TLR) or non-target-lesion revascularization (non-TLR), occurrence of MI, or death. TLR was significantly lower in the ^{192}Ir group (15.4% versus 52.2%; $p = 0.005$). Non-TLR was similar in ^{192}Ir and placebo patients (23.1% versus 24.1%; p not significant). There were three deaths in the placebo group and two deaths in the ^{192}Ir group (p not significant). The composite end-point of death, MI, or TLR was significantly lower in ^{192}Ir-treated patients than in the placebo-treated patients (30.1% versus 58.6%; $p = 0.038$). In this study of patients with previous coronary restenosis, coronary stenting followed by catheter-based IRT substantially reduced the rate of subsequent restenosis with significant clinical benefit at 3-year follow-up. This was the first study to demonstrate the potential clinical effectiveness of radiation and it caught the imagination of the interventional cardiology field.

WRIST trial

The WRIST trial (Washington Radiation for In-Stent Restenosis Trial)[21] is a double-blind randomized trial in patients with in-stent restenosis. One hundred and thirty patients with 130 episodes of in-stent restenosis (100 in native coronaries and 30 in vein grafts) underwent PTCA, laser ablation, or rotational atherectomy, and/or additional stenting (30%) followed by radiation, which was manually delivered using a high activity (300 mCi) [192]Ir 0.76 mm (0.030-inch) nylon ribbon with seeds (Best Medical

International, Springfield, Virginia, USA) into a non-centered 5 Fr closed-end lumen catheter (Medtronic, San Diego, California, USA). Patients were randomized to receive either ^{192}Ir or placebo. The prescribed dose was 15 Gy to a 2 mm radial distance from the center of the source. IVUS was not used for dosimetry. The calculated minimum dose delivered was 7.3 Gy and the maximum dose was 45 Gy. The mean dwell time was 21.8 minutes. Patients with in-stent restenosis at follow-up were eligible to receive radiation if initially randomized to placebo.

Radiation was delivered successfully to all lesions. There were no procedural, in-hospital, or 30-day major cardiac events. At 6-month angiographic follow-up, there was no evidence of coronary aneurysm or perforation. Fifty-one patients presented with clinical and angiographic in-stent restenosis at follow-up; of these, 12 were from the radiation group and 39 had received placebo (19% versus 58%; $p <$ 0.05, 67% reduction). Late loss index was 0.16 in the ^{192}Ir group and 0.69 in the placebo group. TLR was 14% versus 63% (79% reduction) and target vessel revascularization was 29% versus 68% (61% reduction). The 39 patients with restenosis in the placebo group were crossed over to receive radiation therapy. In this cross-over group, the 6-month angiographic follow-up, obtained in 35 out of 39 patients, demonstrated 29 patent vessels without restenosis (74.4%).[22] In the 12 patients (seven native vessels and five saphenous vein grafts) who had recurrent angina and angiographic restenosis (> 50 percentage diameter stenosis) despite radiation therapy, the predominant patterns of radiation failures were edge stenosis (n = 5) and total occlusions (n = 4). In the five patients with edge stenosis, the ratio of the radiation ribbon length to the lesion length was 1.05:1, supporting the hypothesis that inadequate coverage of the treated area by the radiation ribbon can lead to edge restenosis.[23]

GAMMA 1 trial

This multicenter double-blind randomized trial is the first industry-sponsored study (Cordis, Warren, New York, USA) in patients with in-stent restenosis in native coronaries with a diameter of 2.75–4.0 mm and a length ≤ 45 mm. Two hundred and fifty-two patients were enrolled in 12 centers between December 1997 and July 1998.[24] This trial used the same radiation system as that used in the SCRIPPS and WRIST trials. Dosimetry (the same as that used in the SCRIPPS trial) was guided by IVUS (8–30 Gy).

Patients were randomized to receive either [192]Ir (n = 133) or placebo (n = 119). Mean lesion length was 18.7 mm in the ^{192}Ir and 20.4 mm in the placebo group. Mean dwell time was 20.7 (10.8–39.2) minutes in the ^{192}Ir group and 20.6 (12.5–32.2) minutes in the placebo group. For the treatment of in-stent restenosis, rotational atherectomy was used in 11–13% of the lesions and stenting in 84–88%. Major adverse cardiac events at 30 days occurred in five (4.2%) patients in the ^{192}Ir group and in five (4.2%) patients, with one death, in the placebo group.

Six-month angiographic follow-up was performed in 86% of the patients. In-stent restenosis (≥ 50 percent diameter stenosis) occurred in 21.6% of the patients in the ^{192}Ir group, compared with 52% of those in the placebo group ($p <$ 0.0001, 58% reduction). In-lesion restenosis was 32.4% in the ^{192}Ir group and 56.4% in the placebo group ($p =$ 0.001, 43% reduction). However, in shorter lesions treated with a ribbon with six or 10 seeds, in-lesion restenosis was 24.4% in the ^{192}Ir group and 51.6% in the placebo group ($p =$ 0.002, 53% reduction). In addition, in-lesion restenosis in longer lesions treated using a ribbon with 14 seeds was 44.4% in the ^{192}Ir group and 64.1% in the placebo group ($p =$ 0.08). The higher in-lesion restenosis rate observed in this study compared with the SCRIPPS and WRIST trials was possibly due to the unfavorable results obtained in longer lesions as the consequence of a less homogeneous dose delivered (prescribed by IVUS) and of inadequate lesion coverage by the radiation ribbon.

ARTISTIC trial

The ARTISTIC (Angiorad Radiation Therapy for In-Stent resTenosis Intra Coronaries) trial[25] is a multicenter double-blind randomized study of 450 patients with in-stent restenosis using a high-activity (500 mCi) [192]Ir source, along 29 mm of a 0.36 mm (0.014-inch) wire (Angiorad gamma wire system, United States Surgical Corporation). The wire is delivered via a mechanical afterloader into a 3.2 Fr closed-end lumen balloon catheter positioned at the angioplasty site after intervention (Vascular Therapies). The prescription dose is 12 Gy for vessels of diameter 2.5–3.0 mm, 15 Gy for vessels of diameter 3.1–4.0 mm, and 18 Gy for vessels of diameter 4.1–5.0 mm. In the feasibility phase, two centers enrolled 26 patients who presented with a single in-stent restenotic lesion < 26 mm in length. Rotational ablation was used in eight out of 25 patients (32%), balloon angioplasty alone in 13 out of 25 (52%), and additional stents were placed in two of out 25 (8%). Radiation was delivered successfully to 25 out of 26 sites (96.2%). Mean dwell time was 10.30 ± 2.10 minutes and was tolerated by all patients. The maximum and minimum dose to the vessel wall, calculated by IVUS, was 45 Gy and 10 Gy, respectively. There were no procedural, in-hospital, or 30-day major adverse cardiac events. At 6 months, four out of 25 patients (16%) presented with clinical restenosis. This pilot trial confirms the results of the SCRIPPS and WRIST trials.

ARREST trial

The ARREST trial (Angiorad Radiation for REstenosiS Trial) uses the same radiation system as that used in the ARTISTIC trial. This is a multicenter, double-blind, randomized trial in 700 patients with de novo or restenotic lesions following PTCA or provisional stenting. The prescription dose to the media determined by IVUS is 8–35 Gy. In the feasibility phase (ARREST pilot study[26]), four centers enrolled 25 patients who presented with single native coronary lesions. Following determination of vessel size by IVUS, all patients underwent successful delivery of 12 Gy to the adventitial medial border with a maximum dose to the intima not to exceed 50 Gy. Mean radiation source dwell time was 9.7 ± 2.6 minutes. Total procedural success (angiographic success without complications) was 96% (24 out of 25 patients). There were no out-of-hospital adverse events in the first 30 days. At 6-month angiographic follow-up, binary in-lesion restenosis rate was 47% with a late loss index of 0.70. This trial used lower doses of radiation than the Venezuela trial, which may explain the difference in outcomes.

Other ongoing studies

The SVG WRIST is a multicenter, double-blind, randomized trial in 120 patients with in-stent restenosis in saphenous vein grafts using the same radiation system and methods used in the WRIST trial.

The LONG WRIST is a single-center, double-blind, randomized trial in 120 patients with long lesions (36–80 mm) of in-stent restenosis using the same radiation system and methods used in the WRIST trial.

SMARTS (SMall Artery Radiation Therapy Study) is a multicenter, double-blind, randomized study in 180 patients with small vessels (2.00–2.75 mm in diameter) treated with PTCA with provisional stenting. This trial uses the same radiation system as that used in the ARTISTIC and ARREST trials. The dose prescribed is 12 Gy at a distance of 2 mm from the vessel wall.

The R² (Rotablation Radiation) trial is a multicenter, double-blind, randomized study in 180 patients who undergo rotational atherectomy to a non-stented lesion, followed by radiation. This trial uses the same radiation system as that used in the ARTISTIC and ARREST trials and in SMARTS. The dose prescribed is 12 Gy, 15 Gy or 18 Gy at a distance of 2 mm from the vessel wall.

The GRANITE (Gamma Radiation to Atheromatous Neointima using Intracoronary Therapy in Europe) study is a prospective uncontrolled evaluation of the efficacy of low-dose ¹⁹²Ir in preventing in-stent restenosis in 120 patients. Recruitment will begin in May 1999. The primary end-points are angiographic outcomes at 6 months and 3 years.

CLINICAL STUDIES WITH BETA-IRT

Geneva trial

In this study, reported by Popowsky and colleagues[27] and Verin and colleagues,[28] 15 patients (six women and nine men, mean age 71 ± 5 years) underwent intracoronary beta-irradiation immediately after a conventional PTCA procedure. IRT was done using a titanium-coated pure ⁹⁰Y source wire via a segmented centering balloon 30 mm in length (Schneider, Bulach, Switzerland). A dose of 18 Gy was delivered to the surface of the balloon over 6.5 minutes, with a dose < 4 Gy calculated at 2 mm from the source. During the follow-up period of 178 ± 17 days, no complication occurred that could be attributed to radiation therapy. No aneurysm or angiographically detectable thrombus was observed in any of the irradiated arterial segments. Four out of 15 (27%) patients underwent further target lesion revascularization and six out of 15 (40%) had binary angiographic restenosis. These results did not suggest a marked impact on the expected restenosis rate, possibly owing to the insufficient dose administered to the adventitia.[29]

BETA WRIST

A ⁹⁰Y source on a 0.36 mm (0.014-inch) wire 29 mm in length, automatically loaded into a centering balloon, is the system made by Schneider Inc. and used in the following ongoing trials.

The BETA WRIST is a single-center registry of 49 patients with in-stent restenosis in native coronary arteries treated with angioplasty, laser atherectomy, rotational atherectomy, and/or additional stents, followed by a dose of 20.6 Gy prescribed at 1.0 mm from the surface of the balloon. As reported by Waksman and colleagues,[30] the dwell time was 3 ± 0.4 minutes and fractionation of the dose, owing to ischemia, was required in 11 patients (27%). In this trial, there were no major adverse cardiac events at 30 days. At 6-month follow-up, there was no difference in rate of death, MI, or coronary artery bypass grafts between the irradiated group and a control group of 50 non-irradiated patients. However, in the irradiated group there was a lower percentage of repeat PTCA (24.5% versus 56%; p = 0.001), any major adverse cardiac event (32.7% versus 72%; p = 0.001), and TLR (16.3% versus 66%; p = 0.001) compared with the control group.

A dose-finding European multicenter open label study in 160 patients after PTCA with doses of 9 Gy, 12 Gy and 18 Gy at 1 mm from the balloon surface is currently taking place. The interim results of this trial show a lower restenosis rate in the highest dose group.

BERT trial

In the BERT (Beta Energy Restenosis Trial) lesions were treated with balloon angioplasty followed by beta-radiation generated by a hydraulically hand-delivered train of a ^{90}Sr–^{90}Y source contained in 12 small canisters without a centering balloon (Novoste Corporation, Norcross, Georgia, USA). Doses of 12 Gy, 14 Gy and 16 Gy to 2 mm from the source were administered. This system was used in 23 patients in the initial BERT-1 trial,[31] in another 30 patients in the Canadian arm of the trial,[32] and in 31 patients in the European arm (BERT-1.5).[33] This trial showed that the beta-emitter ^{90}Sr–^{90}Y significantly reduced treatment time and operator exposure compared with previous trials with the gamma-emitter ^{192}Ir. In addition, most of the patients had a slightly larger minimum lumen diameter at follow-up than at the completion of the procedure (dramatic inhibition of the late loss after angioplasty), and no aneurysms were observed. The most updated results of this study[34] show that, of 85 patients enrolled, 78 were treated and completed the 6-month angiographic follow-up. There were no major radiation incidents. TLR was needed in 11 out of 78 patients (14.1%). The late loss index for the entire group (78

patients) was 0.08. The dichotomous restenosis rate (> 50%) was 16.7% (13 out of 78 lesions) at the lesion site and 7.7% (6 out of 78 lesions) at the edges, with a total restenosis of 24.7%. An increased lumen diameter at 6 months was recognized in 40 out of 78 treated vessels.

A serial IVUS analysis (pre-intervention, post-intervention and at 6-months) was performed in the Canadian and European arms of the trial. In the Canadian arm,[35] IVUS demonstrated that beta-radiation inhibits neointima formation, with no reduction of total vessel area at 6-month follow-up. In this IVUS study, there was no significant reduction in lumen area (from 5.69 ± 1.72 mm² after treatment to 6.04 ± 2.63 mm² at follow-up) and no significant change in external elastic membrane area (from 13.71 ± 4.54 mm² to 14.22 ± 4.71 mm²) over the 6-month follow-up. Intimal wall area (external elastic membrane area minus lumen area) was 8.01 ± 3.85 mm² after radiation therapy and 8.19 ± 3.44 mm² at follow-up (p not significant). No significant differences were noted between the different dose groups.

In the European arm,[36] in the first 17 patients (54%) with a complete 6-month follow-up, IVUS demonstrated a significant increase in plaque volume at follow-up (199.1 ± 59.3 mm³ versus 247.7 ± 67.7 mm³; p < 0.0004), without a significant change in luminal volume (227.6 ± 77.8 mm³ versus 228.2 ± 85.1 mm³; p not significant), owing to an increase in total vessel volume similar to that in plaque volume (426.7 ± 124.4 mm³ versus 476.0 ± 125.8 mm³; p < 0.001), suggesting that in irradiated segments after PTCA, the adaptive increase of the total vessel volume might be the major determinant of the luminal volume at follow-up.

Following the encouraging results of this pilot study, other trials are ongoing using the Novoste radiation Beta Cath System (^{90}Sr–^{90}Y):

(a) the BETA-CATH trial, a randomized, multicenter, double-blind study on prevention of restenosis after coronary balloon angioplasty with provisional stenting in 1100 patients, in which the dose delivered is 14 Gy or 18 Gy at 2 mm from the source;

(b) the START (STent And Radiation Therapy) trial, a randomized, multicenter, double-blind trial on treatment of in-stent restenosis in 386 patients, with a dose of 18–20 Gy at 2.0 mm from the source;

(c) the Beta Radiation In Europe (BRIE) study, a European registry multicenter open label study in 80 patients after PTCA or stenting in two vessels, with a dose of 16 Gy to 2 mm from the source.

PREVENT

The Proliferation REduction using Vascular ENergy Trial (PREVENT)[37] is a prospective, blinded, randomized trial of intracoronary brachytherapy using beta-emitting radiation (^{32}P) sealed in a 0.46 mm (0.018-inch) nitinol source wire 27 mm long, utilizing a helical centering balloon 30 mm long and a source delivery unit (IRT System, Guidant, Santa Clara, California, USA). Eligible candidates are those with successful angioplasty (PTCA alone or PTCA and stent) of single, native coronary artery lesions (de novo or restenotic). Patients are randomized to receive 0 Gy (control), 16 Gy, 20 Gy, or 24 Gy at 1.0 mm into the artery wall. Eighty-four patients have been enrolled. Treatment time is 2–8 minutes. There were no major adverse cardiac events during initial hospitalization or in those eligible for 12-month follow-up (44 patients). The 6-month follow-up results of this trial show a restenosis rate of 26% in the ^{32}P group compared with 44% in the control group, with a loss index of 0.05.

Intimal Hyperplasia Inhibition with Beta In-stent Trial (INHIBIT) is a multicenter trial for patients with in-stent restenosis that Guidant plans to conduct in 320 patients using the same radiation system used in PREVENT. The dose in this study will be 20 Gy ^{32}P at 1.0 mm from the source.

LIQUID-FILLED BALLOONS

Another possible catheter-based irradiation technique is the inflation of the balloon dilatation catheter with a radioactive solution. This has advantages over other proposed irradiation procedures in that it guarantees a homogeneous irradiation of the vessel wall, owing to self-centering of the inflated balloon. By adjusting inflation time of the balloon, it is possible to change the amount of radiation delivered to the vessel wall. The short penetration distance of the beta-particles (generally totally absorbed within 10 mm) simplifies radiation protection and avoids irradiation of more distant tissues or catheter personnel.

All three high-energy beta-emitters ^{90}Y, ^{32}P, and ^{188}Re are suitable for this application. However, the use of long-lived beta-emitters for this application carries significant risk for severe radio-intoxication if the balloon ruptures and releases the radionuclides into the bloodstream. To overcome this risk, a shorter-lived beta-emitter should be used. Since ^{68}gallium (^{68}Ga) combines efficacy, deep tissue penetration, availability, and a shorter half-life with superior safety, it is considered the most promising isotope for liquid-filled balloon brachytherapy. It has been calculated that 50 mCi ^{68}Ga inside a 3.0 mm × 30 mm balloon would deploy 25 Gy to a 1 mm deep prescription point within 3.7 minutes.[38] A whole-body dose of 5 REM (in the upper range of diagnostic X-ray procedures) would result from accidental systemic delivery of this activity.

Makkar and colleagues[39] demonstrated inhibition of restenosis in porcine coronaries in a randomized, operator-blinded protocol. They used a dose of 14 Gy at 0.5 mm tissue depth, which was delivered before stenting with balloons filled with ^{188}Re (which has a beta-emitting half-life of 17 hours), and a dose of 29 Gy at 0.5 mm depth after stenting. They found significant reductions in the percent diameter stenosis as assessed by angiography and in the percent area stenosis and the neointimal area as assessed by IVUS in the treated groups compared with the control groups. The results obtained in this study in which radiation was administered after stenting demonstrated that the stent struts do not prevent delivery of an effective radiation dosage.

Hoher and colleagues[40] designed a randomized trial that included 200 patients to test the effect of local ^{188}Re irradiation using a coronary balloon catheter (3.0 mm in diameter, 20 mm in length) to deliver 30 Gy at the vessel surface and 15 Gy at 0.5 mm depth within 10 minutes of local irradiation. No side effects occurred with the exception of angina during inflation. Follow-up results are pending.

Other ongoing trials using liquid-filled balloons are:

(a) The Columbia University Restenosis Elimination (CURE) trial,[41] a single-center open-label study at Columbia University, New York, USA. It includes 30 patients after PTCA and 30 patients after stenting using a solution of liquid ^{188}Re from a generator complexed with a renal perfusion isotope, which fills a perfusion coronary balloon, Lifestream™ (Guidant, Santa Clara, California, USA). The dose used in this trial is 20 Gy to the balloon surface. The trial started in October 1997.

(b) The MARS trial (Mallinckrodt Angioplasty Radiation multicenter international Study)[42] a feasibility study in 30 patients for native coronaries using the ^{186}Re liquid-filled balloon from Mallinckrodt.

(c) The Radiation Angioplasty Trial (RADIANT),[43] a feasibility trial for patients with in-stent restenosis using the liquid-filled balloon from Vascular

Therapies (Menlo Park, California, USA). The same system is used in an ongoing two-center randomized trial at Klinikum Rechts der Isar, Technische Universität, Munich, Germany and Cedars-Sinai Medical Center, Los Angeles, California, USA. The purpose of this trial is to evaluate the effectiveness for the prevention of recurrent restenosis after PTCA for treatment of in-stent restenosis. At the end of 1998, 21 patients had been randomized, with no reports of major adverse cardiac events at 4-week follow-up.

(d) The RadioCath trial[42] is a two-center pilot study at the University Hospital of Leuven, Belgium and the Academic Hospital of Utrecht, The Netherlands. The study aims to evaluate the safety and performance of the Mallinckrodt liquid-filled balloon for the treatment of de novo lesions after PTCA in 60 patients. The dose is 20 Gy delivered at 0.05 mm into the vessel wall.

(e) The only study using a [188]Re liquid-filled balloon with an almost complete angiographic follow-up is an Australian pilot study at the Royal Perth Hospital, Perth, Australia, which is being conducted in patients with coronary in-stent restenosis.[44] In this study, 26 patients with symptomatic and angiographic in-stent restenosis underwent conventional restenosis treatment (22 patients had rotational atherectomy, 26 patients had PTCA, and three patients had restenting) followed by a dose of 30 Gy at 0.5 mm into the vessel wall. Six-month follow-up angiography was obtained in 24 out of 26 patients (92%). Only one patient (4%) had restenosis in the irradiated segment, and four patients (17%) had restenosis at the irradiation border zone (edge effect).

RADIOACTIVE STENTS

Radiation delivered on an intravascular stent is an appealing approach to prevent neointimal hyperplasia. Surface activation in a cyclotron and ion implantation techniques are used to render commercially available vascular stents radioactive. Stents that emit beta-particles, most commonly ^{32}P, are employed because of the short half-life of beta-particles (14.3 days) and their limited range of tissue penetration (95% of the dose is delivered within 4 mm of the stent edge). The dose drops off rapidly to < 0.001 times the original dose at 5 months after implantation. Based on the characteristics of beta-emissions

(i.e. rapid drop-off, minimal leaching), radioisotope stents containing ^{32}P appear to be safe.

Whether the predominant mechanism by which radioactive stents prevent neointimal hyperplasia is inhibition of smooth muscle cell proliferation and migration or radiation-induced apoptosis is still unclear. Fischell and colleagues[45] demonstrated that very low doses of beta-particle emission from a ^{32}P-impregnated stent completely inhibited the growth and migration of both rat and human smooth muscle cells within a range of 5.5–10.6 mm from the wire. They proposed a mechanism of action of radioactive stents in preventing neointimal hyperplasia. A computer model was used to look at the radiation dose delivered as a function of distance from the stent. With very low-activity stents, it is presumed that DNA of the smooth muscle cells is damaged as they migrate through the 'electron fence' on the way to the neolumen, diminishing the population of myofibroblasts and reducing hyperplasia. Catheter-based radiation therapies may disable these cells before they migrate, although such an approach may not inhibit early recoil or late contraction.

Data supporting radiation-induced apoptosis as the mechanism of intimal hyperplasia inhibition come from Hehrlein and colleagues.[47] They found that in the early phase of vascular injury (up to 1 week after stent implantation), the arterial media contained more apoptotic cells when the stents were radioactive.

The effectiveness of ^{32}P radioactive beta-particle-emitting stents with varying activities (range 0.14–23 µCi) in inhibiting neointimal proliferation has been evaluated in several animal models and recently in humans.

ANIMAL MODELS

Animal studies in pig iliac and coronary arteries and in rabbit iliac arteries have shown the efficacy of a beta-particle-emitting radioactive stent in the inhibition of subsequent neointimal cell proliferation. Laird and colleagues[48] demonstrated a significant reduction at 28 days in neointimal area (1.76 ± 0.37 mm^2 versus 2.81 ± 1.22 mm^2; $p = 0.05$) and percentage area stenosis ($24.6 \pm 2.9\%$ versus $36.0 \pm 10.7\%$; $p = 0.02$) within very low-activity beta-particle-emitting stents (^{32}P, activity level 0.14 µCi) implanted in seven porcine iliac arteries compared with seven control stents (^{31}P, non-radioactive).

Alt and colleagues[49] investigated the effect of different doses of [198]gold ([198]Au)-coated stents on neointimal proliferation in the coronary arteries of 18 small pigs. [198]Au which had a half-life of 2.7 days (energy 0.96 MeV) might be useful as a source of beta-particles since it may interact less with endothelial cell regrowth owing to its short half-life. Au-coated stainless steel stents of 5 μm in diameter (InFlow Dynamics, Munich, Germany) were activated in the neutron beam of a nuclear reactor. Stent activities were produced to fall into six dose categories ranging from 0 Gy to 20 Gy. Thirty-six stents were randomly implanted. IVUS was performed at 4 weeks. The blinded IVUS investigation at 4 weeks indicated a dose-dependent inhibition of neointimal proliferation.

Waksman and colleagues[50] demonstrated a significant dose-dependent increase in vessel area and lumen area (favorable effect in reducing in-stent restenosis) in 41 porcine coronary arteries using a beta-emitting radioactive stent with activities of 0 μCi, 3 μCi, 10 μCi or 20 μCi, which were implanted 30 days after a non-radioactive 7.5 mm (half Palmaz–Schatz) stent had been implanted.

Hehrlein and colleagues[51] analysed the effects of a ^{32}P radioactive beta-particle-emitting Palmaz–Schatz stent (7.5 mm in length) in a rabbit model on the inhibition of neointimal hyperplasia compared with conventional stents. Stent activity levels of 4 μCi and 13 μCi were chosen for the study. At 4 weeks and at 12 weeks after placement of conventional stents and ^{32}P-implanted stents in rabbit iliac arteries, neointima formation was potentially inhibited by radioactive stents only at an activity level of 13 μCi. Radioactive stents were endothelialized after 4 weeks, but endothelialization was less dense than in conventional stents. Incomplete endothelialization at 3 months after ^{32}P radioactive stent implantation has also been observed in rabbit iliac[52] and in normal dog coronary arteries.[53]

In some circumstances, radioactive stents can stimulate rather than inhibit intimal hyperplasia. Carter and colleagues[54] evaluated the dose-related effects of ^{32}P beta-particle-emitting radioactive stents in a porcine coronary restenosis model. Thirty-seven pigs underwent placement of 35 non-radioactive and 39 radioactive stents with activity levels of 0.15 μCi, 0.5 μCi, 1 μCi, 3 μCi, 6 μCi, 14 μCi, and 23 μCi. At 28 days, neointimal and medial smooth muscle cell density were inversely related to increasing stent activity. At low (0.15 μCi and 0.5 μCi) and high (3–23 μCi) stent activities, there was a reduction in neointimal area (low: 1.63 ± 0.67 mm²; and high: 1.73 ± 0.97 mm² versus control: 2.40 ± 0.87 mm²) and in percentage area stenosis (low: $26 \pm 7\%$; high: $26 \pm 12\%$) versus control: $37 \pm 12\%$; $p \leq 0.01$). The 1 μCi stents, however, had greater neointimal formation

(4.67 ± 1.50 mm²) and more luminal narrowing ($64 \pm 16\%$) than the control stents ($p < 0.0001$).

Carter and colleagues[55] also evaluated the dose rate and cumulative dose effects of 0–58 μCi ^{32}P radioactive stents at 3 months after implant in a porcine model of restenosis. By quantitative coronary angiography they demonstrated a lower percentage diameter stenosis in the body ($13 \pm 13\%$) but not the margins ($48 \pm 8\%$) of the stent compared with non-radioactive stents ($25 \pm 15\%$; $p < 0.001$). In this study, a cumulative dose of more than 75 Gy promoted the formation of a hypocellular matrix rich neointima.

The effect of radiation delivered by a stent on the extracellular matrix deposition has also been evaluated by Hehrlein and colleagues[47] in the rabbit model. They demonstrated, by immunocytochemical analysis, an increase in the expression of collagen type I after radioactive stent implantation, whereas the production of collagen type III and type IV was unchanged.

In a proliferative double-injury cholesterol-fed porcine model, Carter and colleagues[56] showed that there was an increase in the neointimal area 6 months after coronary placement of ^{32}P beta-emitting radioactive stents with increasing radiation activities of 0 μCi to 12 μCi. They created fibrocellular coronary arterial lesions by feeding the pigs with cholesterol 2 weeks before coronary artery overstretch balloon injury (balloon-to-artery ratio 1.2–1.5:1). Animals were maintained on a cholesterol diet for 4 weeks and were then stented (balloon-to-artery ratio 1:1). The animals were fed a normal diet until they were killed at 6-months. A dose-dependent increase in the late lumen loss was observed by quantitative coronary angiography (r = 0.72, $p < 0.001$), and a corresponding dose-dependent increase in mean neointimal area and in-stent percentage diameter stenosis on histology (r = 0.64, $p < 0.001$). The results of this study indicate that radiation at low-dose rates, as delivered by a stent, stimulates intimal hyperplasia in lesions 1 month after angioplasty when the treated plaque is probably still in the healing phase.

Schulz and colleagues[57] demonstrated in the pig overstretch model that beta-particle-emitting radioactive [198]Au stents with activity levels of 55.4 μCi, 35.8 μCi, 22.8 μCi, 14.9 μCi, and 10.4 μCi induce neointimal proliferation rather than inhibit it. Eleven non-radioactive and 33 beta-particle-emitting stents were implanted. Three months after stent implantation, significantly lower neointimal formation and less luminal narrowing was seen the control group compared with the group that had beta-particle-emitting stents ($p < 0.001$).

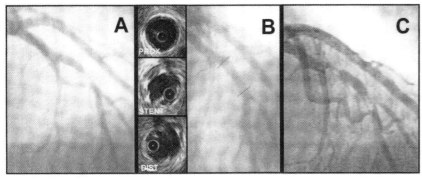

Baseline   Post Stent   6 month Follow-up

Figure 23.1 *Representative patient with the 'candy wrapper' pattern of restenosis after implantation of a radioactive* ^{32}*P beta-emitting stent. (A) Baseline angiography demonstrates a tight stenosis in the mid-left anterior descending coronary artery. (B) After implantation of a 15 mm BX IsoStent with an activity of 8.14 µCi, IVUS images show very little plaque burden of the contiguous proximal and distal reference segment. (C) At 4-month follow-up, there is absence of late loss inside the stent, but a tight stenosis is present just beyond*

CLINICAL STUDIES

The safety and feasibility of ^{32}P radioactive beta-emitting stent implantation in patients with symptomatic de novo or restenotic native coronary lesions has been evaluated in the low-dose IRIS 1A trial (IsoStents for Restenosis Intervention Study),[58] using 0.5–1.0 µCi (mean 0.69 µCi) in 32 patients and in the IRIS 1B trial[60] using 0.75–1.5 µCi (mean 1.14 µCi) in 25 patients. These pilot clinical trials[60] have found that radioactive ^{32}P Palmaz–Schatz stents can be safely implanted with a high acute success rate. However, coronary angiography, performed in 52 out of 57 patients (92.9%) at 6-month follow-up, showed a binary intralesion restenosis, both within the stent and at the edges, in 21 out of 52 patients (40.4%), which was no different from the rate seen with currently available non-radioactive stents.

A dose-finding study to evaluate the safety and efficacy at 6-month follow-up of implanting ^{32}P radioactive stents in patients with coronary artery disease started in Milan in October 1997.[61-63] Two types of slotted tubular stents (both 15 mm long) manufactured by Isostent (San Carlo, California, USA) were implanted; first the Palmaz–Schatz 153 stents, with an initial activity level of 0.75–3.0 µCi, and later the BX stent with initial activity levels of 3–6 µCi, and 6–12 µCi were used.

The results of this dose-finding study demonstrate that the use of ^{32}P beta-emitting stents is feasible and safe. At 6-month follow-up, no deaths had occurred and only one patient had stent thrombosis with a Q-wave myocardial infarction caused by discontinuation of both ticlopidine and aspirin 3 months after the procedure. In addition, radioactive beta-emitting stents with an initial activity level between 3.0 µCi

and 12.0 µCi almost completely inhibited intimal hyperplasia within the stent with a pure intrastent restenosis rate of 16%, 3% and 0% in the 0.75–3.0 µCi, the 3–6 µCi and the 6–12 µCi groups, respectively.

However, a high intralesion restenosis rate of 41–52% (average 47%) was observed, owing to an increased late loss and restenosis in the first 1–3 mm proximal and distal to the stent edges: the 'candy wrapper' pattern of restenosis (*Fig. 23.1*). The precise mechanism by which this phenomenon occurs remains poorly understood. One possible and simple explanation is that the low dose of radiation at the stent edges, caused by a sharp decline of the dose rate within millimeters of the stent margins,[64] combined with balloon trauma in the segments adjacent to the stent (especially with an aggressive stent implantation strategy), could exaggerate the proliferative response at the stent margins.

This dose-finding study is continuing in Milan to determine if a future increase in the overall stent radioactivity level (12–20 µCi) combined with a different approach to radioactive stent implantation will solve the problem of edge restenosis. The stent implantation technique currently used is more conservative than our usual recommendations for stent deployment: the balloon selected to pre-dilate the lesion is smaller than usual, and the stent is deployed using a balloon with a diameter closely matching the angiographic reference diameter and inflated at a nominal pressure of 8 atmospheres. In addition, post-dilation is done with a shorter balloon with a balloon-to-artery ratio of 1:1. This ratio is chosen so that the ends do not extend outside the stent struts, in order to diminish any trauma to the proximal and distal reference segments.

OTHER ONGOING CLINICAL STUDIES USING ³²P RADIOACTIVE STENTS

A small safety study using 15 mm ³²P Palmaz–Schatz coronary stents with an activity level of 1.5–3 µCi started in June 1997 in Heidelberg, Germany. At 30 days, there were no major clinical events in 11 patients who had restenosis after conventional PTCA.[65] At 6-month follow-up, the clinically driven target vessel revascularization rate was 36% (4/11). Restenosis was at the articulation of the stents and, at a lower rate, at the proximal and distal edges.[47]

Another small study was started in Rotterdam, The Netherlands in November 1997 using ³²P radioactive stents with an activity level of 0.75–1.5 µCi. At 6-month follow-up, in 26 patients with de novo or restenotic lesions in whom 26 ³²P Isostents (five Palmaz–Schatz and 21 BX stents) were implanted, there were no cases of death or myocardial infarction. In addition, in the first 16 patients who returned for angiographic follow-up, there were three target segment restenoses (19%).

The preliminary results from these two small clinical studies using ³²P radioactive stents have shown that clinical or angiographic restenosis was not lower compared with contemporary stent trials using non-radioactive stents.

UNRESOLVED ISSUES

A number of important issues remain unresolved, such as defining which component of the arterial wall serves as the target tissue for radiation, the minimal effective dose, the maximum tolerable dose, the therapeutic window, the timing of irradiation, and possible late complications.

Although the initial and the 3-year follow-up results of the SCRIPPS and Venezuela trials are convincing, little is known about the longer-term results. It has to be considered that perivascular fibrosis, which may occur with a delay of 5–10 years depending on the dosage, could curtail the initial success. In addition, radiation therapy may be associated with malignancy that could develop after years. For example, in patients with Hodgkin's lymphoma, the time of maximum risk of death from another tumor following radiotherapy is 10–12 years. Nevertheless, intracoronary irradiation is a promising method for the prevention of restenosis and remains high on the priority list in combatting this phenomenon.

REFERENCES

1. Serruys PW, Levendag PC. Intracoronary brachytherapy: the death knell of restenosis or just another episode of a never-ending story? *Circulation* 1997; **96**: 709–712.
2. Teirstein PS. Radiotherapy to inhibit coronary restenosis: kind of a light at the end of the tunnel? *Eur Heart J* 1998; **19**: 3–6.
3. King SB 3rd. Intravascular radiation for restenosis prevention: could it be the holy grail? *Heart* 1996; **76**: 99–100.
4. King SB 3rd. Radiation for restenosis: watchful waiting. *Circulation* 1999; **99**: 192–194.
5. Koh WJ, Mayberg MR, Chambers J et al. The potential role of external beam radiation in preventing restenosis after coronary angioplasty. *Int J Radiat Oncol Biol Phys* 1996; **36**: 829–834.
6. Wilcox JN, Waksman R, King SB, Scott NA. The role of the adventitia in the arterial response to angioplasty: the effect of intravascular radiation. *Int J Radiat Oncol Biol Phys* 1996; **36**: 789–796.
7. Waksman R, Rodriguez JC, Robinson KA et al. Effect of intravascular irradiation on cell proliferation, apoptosis, and vascular remodeling after balloon overstretch injury of porcine coronary arteries. *Circulation* 1997; **96**: 1944–1952.
8. Brenner DJ, Miller RC, Hall EJ. The radiobiology of intravascular irradiation. *Int J Radiat Oncol Biol Phys* 1996; **36**: 805–810.
9. Weinberger J, Amols H, Ennis RD et al. Intracoronary irradiation: dose response for the prevention of restenosis in swine. *Int J Radiat Oncol Biol Phys* 1996; **36**: 767–775.
10. Waksman R, Robinson KA, Crocker IR et al. Endovascular low-dose irradiation inhibits neointima formation after coronary artery balloon injury in swine. A possible role of radiation therapy in restenosis prevention. *Circulation* 1995; **91**: 1533–1539.
11. Mazur W, Ali MN, Khan MM et al. High dose rate intracoronary radiation for inhibition of neointimal formation in the stented and balloon-injured porcine models of restenosis: angiographic, morphometric, and histopathologic analyses. *Int J Radiat Oncol Biol Phys* 1996; **36**: 777–788.
12. Waksman R, Robinson KA, Crocker IR et al. Intracoronary low-dose beta-irradiation inhibits neointima formation after coronary artery balloon injury in swine restenosis model. *Circulation* 1995; **92**: 3025–3031.
13. Waksman R, Saucedo J, Chan R et al. Yttrium-90 delivered via a centering ctheter and remote afterloader, uniformly inhibits neointima formation after balloon injury or stenting in swine coronary arteries (abstract). *J Am Coll Cardiol* 1998; **31**: 278A.
14. Waksman R, Robinson KA, Crocker IR et al. Intracoronary radiation before stent implantation inhibits neointima formation in stented porcine coronary arteries. *Circulation* 1995; **92**: 1383–1386.
15. Condado JA, Waksman R, Gurdiel O et al. Long-term angiographic and clinical outcome after percutaneous transluminal coronary angioplasty and intracoronary radiation therapy in humans. *Circulation* 1997; **96**: 727–732.
16. Waksman R. Local catheter-based intracoronary radiation therapy for restenosis. *Am J Cardiol* 1996; **78**: 23–28.

17. Condado JA, Lansky AJ, Saucedo JF et al. Three year clinical and angiographic follow-up after intracoronary 192-iridium radiation therapy (abstract). *Circulation* 1998; **98**: I-651.

18. Teirstein PS, Massullo V, Jani S et al. Catheter-based radiotherapy to inhibit restenosis after coronary stenting. *N Engl J Med* 1997; **336**: 1697–1703.

19. Teirstein PS, Massullo V, Jani S et al. A subgroup analysis of the Scripps Coronary Radiation to Inhibit Proliferation Poststenting Trial. *Int J Radiat Oncol Biol Phys* 1998; **42**: 1097–1104.

20. Teirstein PS, Massullo V, Jani S et al. Three-year clinical and angiographic follow-up after catheter-based intracoronary radiotherapy (abstract). *J Am Coll Cardiol* 1999; **33**: 56A.

21. Waksman R, White LR, Chan RC et al. Intracoronary radiation therapy for patients with in-stent restenosis: 6 month follow-up of a randomized clinical study (abstract). *Circulation* 1998; **98**: I-651.

22. Waksman R, White RL, Chan RC et al. Clinical and angiographic outcomes of patients with in-stent restenosis crossing over from placebo to radiation therapy (abstract). *J Am Coll Cardiol* 1999; **33**: 57A.

23. Waksman R, White RL, Chan RC et al. Angiographic patterns of in-stent restenosis lesions that failed radiation therapy (abstract). *J Am Coll Cardiol* 1999; **33**: 63A.

24. Leon MB, Teirstein PS, Lansky AJ et al. Intracoronary gamma radiation to reduce in-stent restenosis: the multicenter gamma randomized clinical trial (abstract). *J Am Coll Cardiol* 1999; **33**: 19A.

25. Waksman R, Porrazzo MS, Chan RC et al. Results from the ARTISTIC feasibility study of 192-iridium gamma radiation to prevent recurrence of in-stent restenosis (abstract). *Circulation* 1998; **98**: I-442.

26. Faxon DP, Buchbinder Cleman MW et al. Intracoronary radiation to prevent restenosis in native coronary lesions: the results of the pilot phase of the ARREST trial (abstract). *J Am Coll Cardiol* 1999; **33**: 56A.

27. Popowski Y, Verin V, Urban P. Endovascular beta-irradiation after percutaneous transluminal coronary balloon angioplasty. *Int J Radiat Oncol Biol Phys* 1996; **36**: 841–845.

28. Verin V, Urban P, Popowski Y et al. Feasibility of intracoronary beta-irradiation to reduce restenosis after balloon angioplasty. A clinical pilot study. *Circulation* 1997; **95**: 1138–1144.

29. Teirstein P. Beta-radiation to reduce restenosis. Too little, too soon? *Circulation* 1997; **95**: 1095–1097.

30. Waksman R, White RL, Chan RC et al. Intracoronary beta radiation therapy for in-stent restenosis: preliminary report from a single center clinical study (abstract). *J Am Coll Cardiol* 1999; **33**: 19A

31. King SB 3rd, Williams DO, Chougule P et al. Endovascular beta-radiation to reduce restenosis after coronary balloon angioplasty: results of the beta energy restenosis trial (BERT). *Circulation.* 1998; **97**: 2025–2030.

32. Bonan R, Arsenault A, Tardif JC et al. Beta energy restenosis trial, Canadian Arm (abstract). *Circulation.* 1997; **96**: I-219.

33. Coen V, van der Giessen WJ, Gijzel A et al. Beta energy radiation trial (BERT-1.5): experience of Rotterdam (abstract). In: *Syllabus, Cardiovascular Radiation Therapy.* Sponsored by the Cardiology Research Foundation, Washington, DC. 17–19 February 1999.

34. King SB 3rd, Klein JL, Williams DO et al. The Beta Energy Restenosis Trial: updated results and subgroup analysis (abstract). *Circulation* 1998; **98**: I-651.

35. Meerkin D, Tardiff JC, Crocker IR et al. Effects of intracoronary beta-radiation therapy after coronary angioplasty: an intravascular ultrasound study. *Circulation* 1999; **99**: 1660–1665.

36. Sabate M, Serruys PW, van der Giessen et al. Beta Energy Restenosis Trial (BERT-1.5): quantitative volumetric assessment by three-dimensional intravascular ultrasound imaging (abstract). *Circulation* 1998; **98**: I-508.

37. Raizner AE, Oesterle S, Waksman R et al. The PREVENT trial, a feasibility study of intracoronary brachytherapy in the prevention of restenosis: an interim report (abstract). *Circulation* 1998; **98**: I-651.

38. Stoll HP, Hutchins GD, Winkle WL et al. Gallium-68 positron radiation combines biological efficacy, deep tissue penetration, generator availability and superior safety for liquid-filled balloon brachytherapy (abstract). *Circulation* 1998; **98**: I-709.

39. Makkar R, Honda H, Li A et al. Brachytherapy with β-emitting rhenium-188 balloon following stent implantation inhibits restenosis (abstract). *Circulation* 1998; **98**: I-778.

40. Hoher M, Wohrle J, Schutte C et al. Intracoronary radiotherapy with liquid rhenium-188 to prevent restenosis following balloon angioplasty: first results from a randomized trial (abstract). *Circulation* 1998; **98**: I-651.

41. Weinberger J, Amols HI, Schiff PB et al. Initial results of the CURE safety trial: coronary brachytherapy with radioactive-liquid-filled balloons (abstract). *J Am Coll Cardiol* 1999; **33**: 94A.

42. De Scheerder I, Coussement P, Vanbilloen H et al. The Mallinckrodt ¹⁸⁶Re liquid approach (abstract). In: *Syllabus, Cardiovascular Radiation Therapy.* Sponsored by the Cardiology Research Foundation, Washington, DC. 17–19 February 1999.

43. Schuhlen H, Haubner R, Eigler N et al. Intracoronary brachytherapy with a ¹⁸⁸Re liquid-filled balloon. A randomized trial with the Radiant Beta System for treatment of in-stent restenosis (abstract). In: *Syllabus, Cardiovascular Radiation Therapy.* Sponsored by the Cardiology Research Foundation, Washington, DC. 17–19 February 1999.

44. Mews GC, Fox R, Cope G et al. Rhenium 188 liquid filled balloon for the treatment of intracoronary instent restenosis: a 26 patient pilot study (abstract). In: *Syllabus, Cardiovascular Radiation Therapy.* Sponsored by the Cardiology Research Foundation, Washington, DC. 17–19 February 1999.

45. Fischell TA, Kharma BK, Fischell DR et al. Low-dose, beta-particle emission from 'stent' wire results in complete, localized inhibition of smooth muscle cell proliferation. *Circulation* 1994; **90**: 2956–2963.

46. Fischell TA, Carter AJ, Laird JR. The beta-particle-emitting radioisotope stent (isostent): animal studies and planned clinical trials. *Am J Cardiol* 1996; **78**: 45–50.

47. Hehrlein C. Radioactive stents: the European experience. In: Waksman R, ed. *Vascular Brachytherapy* 2nd edn. Armonk, New York: Futura Publishing, 1999, 333–342.

48. Laird JR, Carter AJ, Kufs WM et al. Inhibition of neointimal proliferation with low-dose irradiation from a beta-particle-emitting stent. *Circulation* 1996; **93**: 529–536.

49. Alt E, Herrmann RA, Rybnikar A et al. Reduction of neointimal proliferation after implantation of a beta particle

emitting gold Au 198 coated stent (abstract). *J Am Coll Cardiol* 1998; **31**: 350A.

50. Waksman R, Kim WH, Chan RC et al. Effectiveness of a β-emitting radioactive stent for the treatment of in-stent restenosis in porcine coronaries (abstract). *Circulation* 1998; **98**: I-779.

51. Hehrlein C, Stintz M, Kinscherf R et al. Pure beta-particle-emitting stents inhibit neointima formation in rabbits. *Circulation* 1996; **93**: 641–645.

52. Farb A, Tang AL, Virmani R. Neointima is reduced but endo-thelialization is incomplete 3 months after ^{32}P β-emitting stent placement (abstract). *Circulation* 1998; **98**: I-779.

53. Taylor AJ, Gorman PD, Farb A et al. Differential effect of ^{32}P β particle-emitting stents on the intima and adventitia in the dog model (abstract). *Circulation* 1998; **98**: I-779.

54. Carter AJ, Laird JR, Bailey LR et al. Effects of endovascular radiation from a beta-particle-emitting stent in a porcine coronary restenosis model. A dose-response study. *Circulation* 1996; **94**: 2364–2368.

55. Carter AJ, Jenkins JS, Bailey LR et al. Dose rate and cumulative dose effects of P-32 radioactive stents (abstract). *J Am Coll Cardiol* 1999; **33**: 20A.

56. Carter AJ, Scott D, Bailey LR et al. High activity 32P stents promote development of atherosclerosis at six months in a porcine model (abstract). *Circulation* 1997; **96**: I-607.

57. Schulz C, Niederer C, Andres C et al. Intracoronary radiation using a β-particle-emitting gold stent increases neointima formation in a porcine coronary restenosis model (abstract). *J Am Coll Cardiol* 1999; **33**: 21A.

58. Fischell TA, Carter A, Foster M et al. Lessons from the feasibility radioactive (IRIS) stent trials. In: Waksman R, ed. *Vascular Brachytherapy* 2nd edn. Armonk, New York: Futura Publishing, 1999, 475–481.

59. Moses J, Ellis S, Bailey S et al. Short-term (1 month) results of the dose response IRIS feasibility study of a beta-particle emitting radioisotope stent (abstract). *J Am Coll Cardiol* 1998; **31**: 350A.

60. Moses J. U.S. IRIS trials low-activity ^{32}P stent (abstract). In: *Syllabus, Cardiovascular Radiation Therapy.* Sponsored by the Cardiology Research Foundation, Washington, DC. 17–19 February 1999.

61. Albiero R, Di Mario C, De Cregorio J et al. Intravascular ultrasound (IVUS) analysis of β-particle emitting radioactive stent implantation in human coronary arteries. Preliminary immediate and intermediate-term results of the Milan study. *Circulation* 1998; **98**: I–780.

62. Albiero R, Wardeh AJ, Di Mario C et al. Acute and 30 day results of ^{32}P β-particle emitting radioactive stent implantation in patients with CAD: The European experience (abstract). *Circulation* 1998; **98**: I-778.

63. Albiero R, De Gregorio J, Kobayashi N et al. Acute and 6-month follow-up results of ^{32}P radioactive β-emitting stent implantation in patients with CAD. The Milan BX dose-response study (abstract). *J Am Coll Cardiol* 1999; **33**: 20A.

64. Janicki C, Duggan DM, Coffey CW et al. Radiation dose from a phosphorus-32 impregnated wire mesh vascular stent. *Med Phys* 1997; **24**: 437–445.

65. Hehrlein C, Brachmann J, Hardt S et al. P-32 stents for prevention of restenosis: results of the Heidelberg safety trial using the Palmaz–Schatz stent design at moderate activity levels in patients with restenosis after PTCA (abstract). *Circulation* 1998; **98**: I-780.

66. Wardeh AJ, Gijzel AL, van der Giessen WJ et al. β-particle emitting radioactive stent to prevent restenosis (abstract). *J Am Coll Cardiol* 1999; **33**: 21A.

Chapter 24 Platelet glycoprotein IIB/IIIA antagonists in coronary angioplasty and stenting

George D Dangas and Antonio Colombo

Dissections and thrombosis are the most important determinants of acute and subacute complications occurring during coronary interventions. Stents effectively treat dissections.[1] To prevent intracoronary thrombosis, most percutaneous coronary interventions have been performed during intense short-term anticoagulation with a combination of unfractionated heparin plus aspirin. Compelling data on the central role of platelets in arterial thrombosis[2-5] have clarified the need for more potent antiplatelet agents for the treatment of patients undergoing coronary interventions.

PLATELET GLYCOPROTEIN IIB–IIIA RECEPTOR ACTIVATION

Vessel wall injury during coronary intervention exposes the deep arterial wall components to the circulation. This exposure activates blood coagulation and leads to platelet thrombus formation and thrombin generation. Several pathways lead to platelet aggregation, including release of chemical mediators (adenosine diphosphate (ADP), serotonin, thromboxane A_2) with platelet degranulation, translocation of the adhesion mediator P-selectin to the platelet membrane, and structural changes of the platelet surface to a spiny spherical shape, which is more efficient for increased interplatelet adhesion and platelet factor X contact.[4,6] These interactions ultimately lead to thrombin generation, which provides a potent positive feedback to the entire process. Additionally, rheologic parameters, such as high shear stress, further promote platelet thrombus formation.[7] Despite the existence of multiple mediators of platelet activation, the final common pathway

for platelet aggregation depends on activation of the glycoprotein (GP) IIb/IIIa receptor.[8]

The molecule of the GP IIb/IIIa receptor is a heterodimer consisting of two transmembrane proteins, which are non-covalently bound to each other: a 136 KDa alpha-subunit, which consists of a heavy chain and a light chain, and a 92 KDa beta-subunit. Calcium is required for the structural integrity of the complex. The surface of one resting platelet contains approximately 50,000–80,000 randomly distributed GPIIb/IIIa receptors.[8,9] Platelet activation renders this receptor available to bind with ligands such as fibrinogen, vitronectin, fibronectin, or von Willebrand factor, all of which contain the peptide sequence arginine–glycine–aspartic acid (RGD).[10-13] The RGD sequence is abundant in many proteins involved in cell adhesion interactions, including the platelet–GPIIb/IIIa receptor activation. Fibrinogen is the most important ligand for platelet aggregation because it exists in high concentration in the blood, and it can simultaneously bind to GPIIb/IIIa receptors on two platelets because it is a divalent molecule; hence its direct contribution to interplatelet bridge formation.

Antiplatelet therapy has been thus far aimed at specific pathways of platelet activation: aspirin is an inhibitor of thromboxane A_2-mediated platelet aggregation,[15,16] and ticlopidine and clopidogrel inhibit ADP-mediated platelet aggregation (P_{2T}-type receptor).[17] However, despite inhibition of a specific pathway, platelet aggregation may still occur through alternative pathways. Since GPIIb/IIIa activation is the final common pathway for platelet aggregation, its inhibitors may potentially abolish platelet aggregation completely regardless of the initial thrombogenic stimuli.[8,18] The initial GPIIb/IIIa antagonist was the chimeric (human–mouse) monoclonal antibody, abciximab (c7E3 Fab). A series of peptide inhibitors (eptifibatide)

Table 24.1

Concomitant anticoagulation and dosage and approved indications of intravenous GPIIb/IIIa inhibitors in the USA

GPIIb/IIIa inhibitor	FDA approval		Clinical trials	GPIIb/IIIa dosage			Duration	Initial heparin dose	Target anticoagulation
	Indications	Recommended dose		Bolus	Timing of bolus	Infusion			
Abciximab	PCI	As in EPIC	EPIC	0.25 mg/kg over 5 minutes	10–60 minutes pre-PCI	10 µg/minute	12 hours	10000–12000 units bolus	ACT > 300 seconds PTT twice control
	Refractory unstable angina plus planned PCI within 24 hours	As in CAPTURE	EPILOG	0.25 mg/kg over 5 minutes	10–60 minutes pre-PCI	0.125 µg/kg per minute	12 hours	70 units/kg bolus 100 units/kg bolus	ACT > 200 seconds ACT > 300 seconds
			CAPTURE	0.25 mg/kg over 5 minutes	Unstable angina, planned PCI	10 µg/minute	18–24 hours pre-PCI until 1 hour post-PCI	≤ 100 units/kg bolus	PTT 60–85 seconds ACT 300 seconds
			EPISTENT	0.25 mg/kg over 5 minutes	20 minutes pre-PCI	0.125 µg/kg per minute	12 hours	70 units/kg bolus	ACT > 200 seconds
Eptifibatide	PCI	As in IMPACT II (the low dose)	IMPACT II	135 µg/kg 135 µg/kg	20 minutes pre-PCI	0.50 µg/kg per minute 0.75 µg/kg per minute	20–24 hours	100 units/kg bolus	ACT 300–350 seconds
	Unstable angina, non-Q-wave MI	As in PURSUIT (the high dose)	PURSUIT*	180 µg/kg	Unstable angina, non-Q-wave MI	1.3 µg/kg per minute 2.0 µg/kg per minute	72 hours + 24 hours post-PCI (total < 96 hours)	5000 units bolus + 1000 U/hr	PTT 50–70 seconds
Tirofiban	Unstable angina, non-Q-wave MI	As in PRISM-PLUS	RESTORE	10 µg/kg over 3 minutes	Immediately pre-PCI	0.15 µg/kg per minute	36 hours	150 units/kg	ACT 300–400 seconds
	Unstable angina, non-Q-wave MI		PRISM-PLUS†	0.4 µg/kg per minute	Unstable angina, non-Q-wave MI	0.10 µg/kg per minute	Total 48–108 hours, 12–24 hours post-PCI	5000 units bolus + 1000 units/hour	PTT twice control

ACT, activated clotting time; FDA, Food and Drug Administration; PCI, percutaneous coronary intervention; PTT, activated partial thromboplastin time.

* After interim analysis showing the safety of the high dose, the low dose arm was discontinued.

† The tirofiban alone arm (dose 0.6 µg/kg per minute for 30 minutes plus 0.15 µg/kg per minute) was discontinued owing to excess 7-day mortality compared to the heparin alone arm.

and non-peptide inhibitors (tirofiban) of the RGD sequence of the GPIIb/IIIa receptors have also been developed and studied during coronary interventions. Abciximab has a very high affinity for the receptor, whereas the newer agents competitively antagonize the RGD-containing ligands, binding with relatively low affinity. Additionally, abciximab has a longer biological half-life and also binds to the vitronectin receptor.[19] These pharmacologic differences between the various antiplatelet agents may explain some of the differences observed in clinical trials during coronary interventions.

GPIIB/IIIA INHIBITORS IN ANGIOPLASTY

Several large trials[20-27] have evaluated the efficacy of GPIIb/IIIa antagonists in reducing ischemic complications during coronary interventions (*Tables 24.1* and *24.2*). All trials have evaluated GPIIb/IIIa inhibitor therapy versus placebo in addition to heparin plus aspirin. A treatment arm of GPIIb/IIIa inhibitor without heparin (n = 345) was evaluated only in PRISM-PLUS (Platelet Receptor Inhibition in Ischemic Syndrome Management in Patients Limited by Unstable Signs and Symptoms); the GPIIb/IIIa-alone arm was interrupted after an interim analysis showing excessive 7-day mortality compared to the heparin arm (4.6% versus 1.1%).[25]

In the EPIC (Evaluation of c7E3 in Preventing Ischemic Complications) trial[20,21] (n = 2099), patients undergoing high-risk angioplasty were randomized to abciximab bolus plus 12-hour infusion, abciximab bolus only, or placebo. All the patients were treated with heparin and aspirin. Abciximab bolus plus infusion produced a 35% reduction in the 30-day primary end-point compared to placebo, but this benefit was accompanied by a 14% incidence of major bleeding complications and a 16.9% incidence of minor bleeding complications. Subgroup analyses showed that the treatment benefit was greater in patients with angina at rest,[28] evolving myocardial infarction (MI)[29] or in patients undergoing directional coronary atherectomy.[30] The high bleeding rate with abciximab was attributed to the large heparin dose and the target activated clotting time (ACT) of > 300 seconds. For this reason, subsequent trials reduced the heparin dose administered in the GPIIb/IIIa arms (see *Table 24.1*). The bolus-only arm produced results similar to placebo at all study points, indicating the importance of sustained platelet receptor blockade after the coronary intervention for achievement of clinically significant benefit.

Table 24.2

Safety and efficacy of intravenous GPIIb/IIIa platelet receptor antagonists during percutaneous coronary interventions

Trial	Agent	Major bleeding (%) GPIIb/IIIa	Placebo	30-day events (%)* GPIIb/IIIa	Placebo	6-month events (%)† GPIIb/IIIa	Placebo
EPIC	Abciximab	14.0[‖]	7.0	8.3[‖]	12.8	27.0[‖]	35.1
EPILOG†	Abciximab	2.0 / 3.5	3.1	5.2[‖] / 5.4[‖]	11.7	22.8[‖] / 22.3[‖]	25.8
CAPTURE	Abciximab	3.8[‖]	1.9	11.3[‖]	15.9	3.6	30.8
EPISTENT≠	Abciximab	1.5; 1.4	2.2	5.3[‖] / 6.9[‖]	10.8	5.6[‖] / 7.8[‖]	11.4
IMPACT II≠	Eptifibatide	5.1 / 5.2	4.8	9.2 / 9.9	11.4	10.5 / 10.1	11.6
PURSUIT§¶	Eptifibatide	10.6[‖]	9.1	11.5[‖]	16.40	NA	NA
RESTORE	Tirofiban	5.3	3.7	8.0	10.5	NA	NA
PRISM-PLUS§	Tirofiban	4.0	3.0	8.8[‖]	13.10	12.3[‖]	15.3§

* Death, MI, or urgent revascularization, except PRISM-PLUS, PURSUIT (only death or MI).
† Death, MI, or any revascularization, except IMPACT II, EPISTENT, PRISM-PLUS (only death or MI).
§ PURSUIT and PRISM-PLUS 30-day and 6-month results are only in patients who underwent interventions.
¶ In PURSUIT, GPIIb/IIIa results are for the 180 μg/kg + 2.0 μg/kg/minute eptifibatide dose.
≠ GPIIb/IIIa results in EPILOG are for low (top line) and high heparin dose arms, in EPISTENT for stent (top line) and angioplasty arms, and in IMPACT-II for low (top line) and high eptifibatide dose arms.
[‖] p < 0.05 GPIIb/IIIa inhibitor versus placebo.

The EPILOG (Evaluation of PTCA to Improve Long-term Outcome by c7E3 GPIIb/IIIa receptor blockade) trial[22] (n = 2792) tested abciximab in patients undergoing elective coronary intervention, in combination with two heparin doses: reduced dose versus standard dose, both weight-adjusted. This study was terminated prematurely because patients treated with abciximab had a 57% reduction in the 30-day composite end-point compared to the combination of heparin plus aspirin alone (see *Table 24.1*). The lower adjustment of the heparin dose in EPILOG in comparison to EPIC was accompanied by lower bleeding rates both in the GPIIb/IIIa and the placebo arms. Thus, EPILOG demonstrated that abciximab could be administered with low-dose weight-adjusted heparin and a target ACT of 250 seconds during coronary intervention and produce a low incidence of bleeding complications while still maintaining strong efficacy against ischemic complications.

In both the EPIC and EPILOG trials, abciximab was administered at the time of the coronary intervention in the cardiac catheterization laboratory with the initial bolus given 20 minutes before the procedure. In the CAPTURE (c7E3 Fab AntiPlatelet Therapy in Unstable REfractory angina) trial[23] (n = 1265), the efficacy of prolonged pre-intervention treatment with abciximab was evaluated. Patients treated with heparin and aspirin were randomized into treatment with abciximab or placebo for 18–24 hours before an anticipated coronary intervention and until 1 hour after completion of the coronary intervention. Patients treated with abciximab had a lower complication rate at 30-day follow-up, but they also showed significantly lower rates of progression to MI before the coronary intervention (0.6% in the abciximab group versus 2.1% in the placebo group; $p < 0.03$). The significantly higher bleeding rate in the abciximab group compared to the placebo group could be due to arterial puncture after prolonged pre-intervention treatment with abciximab and also due to the very low major bleeding rate in the placebo arm of the CAPTURE trial (1.9%) compared to the other trials (see *Table 24.1*).

Although the EPIC, EPILOG, and CAPTURE trials have provided strong evidence for the efficacy of the addition of abciximab to heparin and aspirin during coronary intervention in preventing ischemic complications, the long-term benefits implied in the EPIC trial population have not been as strong in the other two studies. At 6-month follow-up in the EPIC trial,[31] the rate of death, MI, or revascularization was 27% with abciximab (bolus plus infusion) and 35% with placebo ($p = 0.001$); the rate of death or MI was 8.9% versus 12.8% ($p = 0.02$). Furthermore, long-term

follow-up of the same population showed that the benefit from abciximab therapy was sustained even at 3 years:[32] the rate of death, MI, or revascularization was 41.1% with abciximab bolus plus infusion, 47.4% for abciximab bolus only, and 47.2% for placebo ($p = 0.009$). On the other hand, the CAPTURE trial showed no difference in the 6-month rate of death, MI, or revascularization between the abciximab group and the placebo group (31% versus 30.8%). The 6–month follow-up in the EPILOG trial showed a rate of death, MI, or revascularization of 22.8% with abciximab versus 25.8% with placebo ($p = 0.07$), and a rate of death or MI of 5.8% with abciximab versus 11.1% with placebo ($p < 0.0001$).

Explanations for these differential long-term effects of abciximab include:

(a) a decrease in relative risk reduction provided by abciximab when tested in the more stable population of the EPILOG trial compared to that of the EPIC trial;

(b) the very brief (1 hour) post-coronary intervention administration of abciximab in the CAPTURE trial compared to the 12-hour infusion in the EPIC and EPILOG trials; and

(c) the relatively low efficacy of abciximab in reducing the long-term target lesion revascularization rate.

The data provided by another study[33] that tested the hypothesis that abciximab could decrease the restenosis rate after stenting seem not to support a role for these agents in preventing restenosis.

The non-peptide RGD inhibitor, tirofiban, was tested in the RESTORE (Randomized Efficacy Study of Tirofiban for Outcomes and REstenosis) trial[24] (n = 2139) during high-risk coronary intervention. The RESTORE population (patients with unstable angina or MI) and the heparin dosage were similar to those of the EPIC trial. Tirofiban produced a remarkable reduction in the rate of death, MI, or revascularization of 38% at 48 hours and of 27% at 7 days, but the reduction was limited to only 16% (which is statistically insignificant) at the pre-specified time point of 30 days (see *Table 24.1*). For the end-points of death, MI, and urgent revascularization, the respective relative risk rate reductions for tirofiban versus placebo were 40%, 30% and 24%, respectively.

Tirofiban has also been evaluated in the context of the management of unstable angina and non-Q-wave MI with medical, interventional, or surgical therapy.[25] In the PRISM-PLUS trial (n = 1915), the tirofiban dosage was different from that used in the RESTORE trial, and it was administered for longer and mostly pre-intervention. Both dosages have been reported to achieve a > 80% inhibition of platelet aggregation at 30 minutes of infusion.[24,25] In the PRISM-PLUS trial, there was a significant reduction in the pre-specified composite end-point of death, MI, or refractory ischemia at 30 days with tirofiban compared to placebo (18.5% versus 22.3%; p = 0.03). With respect to the subgroup of patients who underwent coronary intervention (n = 475), there was a marginal benefit in the rate of death or MI at 30 days (8.8% with tirofiban versus 13.1% with placebo, relative risk 0.30, confidence interval 0.38–1.14) as well as at 6 months (see *Table 24.1*).

The peptide RGD inhibitor, eptifibatide, was studied during coronary intervention in the IMPACT-II (Integrilin to Minimize Platelet Aggregation and Prevent Coronary Thrombosis II) trial[26] (n = 4010). The 30-day primary end-point was not statistically significant compared to placebo in the high-dose arm, but there was a trend towards improved outcome in the group treated with low-dose eptifibatide (see *Table 24.1*). The superior efficacy of the low dose of eptifibatide over the high dose is difficult to explain. Additionally, the identical 30-day event rate (11.5%) between high and low risk patients in this trial was also unexpected. The different platelet aggregation results after eptifibatide treatment when PPACK (D-phenyl-alanyl-prolyl-arginine chloromethyl-ketone) and sodium citrate coated tubes were used is explained in part by the marginal benefit from the agent in IMPACT-II but the investigators give no explanation of why the lower dose was more effective. Phillips and colleagues showed the importance of ionized calcium concentration in the blood specimen for the accurate estimation of the drug-induced reduction in platelet aggregation. Whether the observed discrepancy with different collecting tubes affects only integrilin or other GPIIb/IIIa inhibitors as well has not been evaluated.

Eptifibatide in unstable angina and non-Q-wave MI has been evaluated in the Platelet Glycoprotein IIb/IIIa in Unstable Angina: Receptor Suppression Using Integrilin Therapy trial (PURSUIT)[27] (n = 10,948), with a protocol similar to that of the PRISM-PLUS trial. The dosage of eptifibatide used in the PURSUIT trial managed to achieve a > 80% ex vivo inhibition of platelet aggregation in specimens collected in PPACK. The primary end-point of the PURSUIT trial was the rate of death or MI at 30 days: it was 14.2% with eptifibatide versus 15.7% with placebo (relative reduction 9.6%; p = 0.04). In the PURSUIT trial, the selected subgroup of patients who underwent interventions within 72 hours of randomization had a significant reduction in the pre-intervention incidence of death or

MI: 1.7% with eptifibatide versus 5.5% with placebo (p < 0.001). However, the 17.7% relative reduction in the rate of death or MI at 30 days with eptifibatide compared to placebo (10.2% versus 12.4%) was not statistically significant.

Thrombocytopenia has been reported with GPIIb/IIIa inhibitors. It usually presents shortly after the bolus is given but the etiology is still unclear. An abrupt drop of the platelet count to < 100,000/ml has been observed in 1–2% of patients and < 50,000/ml in 0.5% of patients. The incidence of thrombocytopenia is similar with all GPIIb/IIIa inhibitors, but the platelet count recovers to normal within a few days of cessation of the agent.

One element common to all the studies mentioned above is that coronary stenting was used very

Table 24.3

Percutaneous transluminal coronary angioplasty (PTCA) results in Benestent II and EPILOG studies

	Benestent II (PTCA)	EPILOG (abciximab plus low-dose heparin)	EPILOG (placebo)
Patients (n)	410	935	939
1-month events (%)			
Death	0.2	0.3	0.8
Q-wave myocardial infarction	1.0	0.4	0.8
Non-Q-wave myocardial infarction	2.2	3.2	7.9
Repeat revascularization	1.7	1.6	5.2
Any event	5.1	5.2	11.7
Stenting (%)	13.4	11.0	13.0
6-month events (%)			
Death	0.5	1.1	1.7
Q-wave myocardial infarction	1.2	1.3	1.6
Non-Q-wave myocardial infarction	2.4	3.9	8.4
Repeat revascularization	13.2	19	19.4
Any event	19.3	22.8	25.8

sparingly. Stents were placed in 1.7% of the patients treated with the bolus of abciximab and in 0.6% of the placebo and of the bolus plus infusion patients in the EPIC study. In the EPILOG trial, stents were used in 15% of the patients. This practice pre-dates current standards and therefore all of the results must be viewed with this in mind. *Table 24.3* is a side-by-side comparison of the results of the EPILOG study with the percutaneous transluminal coronary angioplasty (PTCA) arm of the Benestent (BElgium NEtherlands Stent) II trial.[35] Two possible conclusions can be hypothesized:

(a) the Benestent II population was more clinically stable and therefore less likely to develop complications provided dissections were promptly treated by stenting; or

(b) stenting was performed at an earlier time of the intervention when some of the consequences of vessel occlusion were not yet in place.

The first hypothesis appears to be more likely when we consider the results of the more recent EPISTENT (Evaluation of Platelet IIb/IIIa Inhibitor for STENTing) study.[36]

GPIIB/IIIA INHIBITORS IN STENTING

The impact of abciximab on the rate of unplanned stenting during angioplasty or atherectomy has been evaluated in secondary analysis of the EPILOG trial. Among the 326 patients who required 'bail-out' stenting, the rate was 9.1% in the patients receiving the combination of abciximab plus low-dose heparin, compared to 14.7% with placebo ($p < 0.01$). The benefit was more pronounced in the treatment of eccentric or American Heart Association–American College of Cardiology type B2 or C lesions, and it was not associated with an increase in bleeding complications.[37] Additionally, among the PURSUIT patients who underwent coronary interventions, the effect of eptifibatide was similar in patients who had stents and in those who had non-stent coronary interventions.[27]

The major study that evaluated the efficacy of abciximab in stenting was the EPISTENT trial[36] (n = 2399). One-half of the patients had rest pain within 48 hours or MI within 1 week before the coronary intervention. Only a single treated lesion was acceptable for inclusion in the EPISTENT trial, and patients had to have lesions that could be revascularized with balloon angioplasty alone. Thus, patients with multivessel or complex, multidevice coronary interventions were excluded. Only the Palmaz–Schatz stent was used (with more than 1 stent used in 30% of cases). The protocol provided three treatment arms: stent plus placebo, stent plus abciximab, or PTCA plus abciximab. The angioplasty group had a 19% rate of stenting. The primary end-point of death, MI, or early revascularization at 30 days was 10.8%, 5.3% and 6.9% for these groups respectively ($p = 0.02$). The bleeding rate was low in both abciximab arms (1.5%), in fact even lower than in the heparin alone arm (2.2%). At 6-month follow-up, the respective incidence of death or MI was 11.4% (stent plus placebo) versus 5.6% (stent plus abciximab) versus 7.8% (PTCA plus abciximab) ($p < 0.001$); among the stent patients, only 13% of the abciximab group suffered death, MI, or revascularization compared to 18.3% in the placebo group ($p = 0.003$ (Topol EJ, oral presentation at the XXth European Congress of Cardiology, Vienna, Austria, August 1998).

These results strongly support the belief that the efficacy of abciximab in coronary interventions is independent of the benefit provided by stenting. Moreover, there was a lower rate of death or MI with balloon angioplasty plus abciximab than with stenting alone. On the other hand, the composite end-point results of the EPISTENT trial have been driven mainly by the marked reduction in the rate of in-hospital non-Q-wave MI. Stenting, by aggressive vessel stretch, plaque extrusion, or side-branch compromise, appears to be associated with a high rate of non-Q-wave MI, which is at least in part inhibited by abciximab. These periprocedural events have not been linked etiologically to unfavorable long-term outcome. Limited, predominantly asymptomatic, myocardial necrosis after successful stenting may have clinical significance only in small patient subgroups, such as those with decreased baseline ventricular function or diabetes mellitus. However, these issues remain controversial.

GPIIB/IIIA INHIBITORS IN ACUTE MI INTERVENTIONS

Since the prothrombotic effects of thrombolysis in acute MI have been mainly attributed to platelet activation, a potent antiplatelet strategy is considered a valuable approach for both primary or rescue angioplasty. The combination of GPIIb/IIIa inhibitors with fibrin-specific thrombolytic agents (recombinant plasminogen activator molecules) for primary pharmacologic reperfusion is being evaluated in ongoing trials.

In the EPIC trial,[20] 64 patients had primary angioplasty for acute MI; in this subgroup, abciximab bolus plus infusion therapy significantly decreased recurrent events at 30 days and 6 months. Based on these preliminary data, the RAPPORT (Reopro And Primary PTCA Organization and Randomized Trial) trial[38] (n = 483) evaluated abciximab in primary angioplasty. Abciximab was administered in the standard dosage, and the heparin dose was 100 units/kg, with subsequent boluses to maintain ACT > 300 seconds. The heparin dosage was higher than in the EPILOG trial and was associated with high major bleeding rates in both arms, though the rate was significantly higher in the abciximab arm than in the placebo arm (16.6% versus 9.5%; p = 0.02). There was significant reduction in the rate of death, MI, or urgent revascularization at 7 days, 30 days, and 6 months with abciximab compared to placebo: relative risk reduction was 67% at 7 days, 48% at 30 days, and 35% at 6 months. However, there was no difference with respect to the primary end-point of death, MI, or any revascularization at 6 months (28.2% versus 28.1%).

The combination of abciximab and lower heparin dose and stenting during acute MI is under evaluation (in prospective trials). Preliminary results from a smaller study[39] have indicated that GPIIb/IIIa inhibition is beneficial with acute MI stenting: the abciximab group had an improved wall motion index score at 14 days compared to placebo, and the 30-day rate of death, MI, or urgent revascularization rate was 2% with abciximab and 9% with placebo (p = 0.03).

APPROPRIATE DOSING, RELATIVE EFFICACY AND COST REDUCTION ARE THE QUESTS FOR THE FUTURE

All the trials discussed above provide strong evidence of benefits from the use of GPIIb/IIIa inhibitors during coronary interventions. These agents have now entered clinical practice. However, many logistic questions are yet to be clarified. First of all is the issue of the differential efficacy of the various agents. Abciximab differs from all other agents in many ways, and it is unclear which of its special properties may be responsible for the greater efficacy of the drug. If the winning property is its prolonged biolog-

ical half-life, then a combination of other intravenous and oral GPIIb/IIIa inhibitors may produce equivalent results at a lower cost. On the other hand, if the winning property is the lower dissociation constant of the receptor–monoclonal antibody complex, then the previously mentioned alternatives may still not be equivalent to abciximab.

The potential antigenicity of abciximab limits its readministration for the time being.[40] It is hoped that the ongoing R[3] (Reopro Readministration Registry) trial studying the complications of repeat abciximab administration will answer this question. In addition, the antiplatelet effect of abciximab wears off gradually over a 2-week period and is not easily reversed if a bleeding complication occurs or if the patient needs to undergo surgery. These are important drawbacks to be considered. The effect of abciximab can be reversed only with platelet transfusions that 'dilute' the antibody in a larger pool of platelet receptors, thereby decreasing its inhibitory activity on GPIIb/IIIa. Synthetic RGD inhibitors have a much faster elimination time (platelet function normalizes in 2–4 hours), but platelet transfusion is not effective for acute reversal of their action.

The problem of appropriate dosing of both the GPIIb/IIIa inhibitors and the adjunct antithrombosis regimen is a major issue that has not been resolved for any of the GPIIb/IIIa inhibitors. The availability of monitoring the percentage of fibrinogen-induced platelet aggregation[41] may favorably affect this problem. The test will provide a means of adjusting the dose of the GPIIb/IIIa inhibitor to optimize the therapeutic result.

Finally, GPIIb/IIIa inhibitors have a debatable effect on clinical restenosis. A positive effect on restenosis was documented only in the EPIC population. Despite the negative results of the Evaluation of ReoPro And Stenting to Eliminate Restenosis (ERASER) trial,[33] final judgement about angiographic restenosis should be withheld until after appropriate evaluation of long-term GPIIb/IIIa inhibition, possibly with an oral agent.

The optimal antithrombotic therapy in combination with a GPIIb/IIIa inhibitor has not been settled either. Higher doses of heparin have been associated with both higher bleeding rates and more ischemic events (see *Table 24.2*). GPIIb/IIIa inhibition has enabled the use of remarkably low heparin doses even in patients with acute syndromes. The possibility that very high heparin doses in complicated interventional procedures may actually *activate* platelets has emerged from the results of GPIIb/IIIa inhibitor plus low-dose heparin trials. In a recent study, ex vivo

Table 24.4

Percutaneous transluminal coronary angioplasty (PTCA) and stent results in Benestent II and EPISTENT trials

| | Benestent II | | EPISTENT | | |
	PTCA (n = 410)	Stent (n = 413)	Stent plus placebo (n = 809)	Stent plus abciximab (n = 794)	PTCA plus abciximab (n = 796)
Age (years)	59	50	59	59	60
Diabetes mellitus (%)	11	13	21.4	20.4	19.6
Previous myocardial infarction (%)	28	25	38.6	32.7	32.4
Unstable angina (%)	40	45	60	56.4	54.8
Recent unstable angina, < 48 hours (%)	–	–	16.2	16.9	16.1
Left anterior descending artery lesions (%)	52	50			
Bail-out stenting (%)	13.4	NA	NA	NA	19
30 days events (%)					
Death	0.2	0	0.6	0.3	0.8
Q MI	1.0	1.2	1.4	0.9	1.5
Non-Q MI	2.2	1.5	8.0	3.5	3.7
CABG	0.5	0.7	1.1	0.8	0.6
Repeat PTCA	1.2	0.5	2.1	1.3	1.9
Any MACE	5.1	3.9	10.8	5.3	6.9

NA, not applicable; MACE, major adverse cardiac events.

thrombosis under dynamic flow conditions was studied in patients with or without abciximab treatment during coronary intervention. The observed efficacy of abciximab in reducing the fibrin thrombus in addition to platelet aggregates implies an anticoagulant effect of this potent antiplatelet agent. Furthermore, the observed marginal increase in both thrombus components (a 28% increase in fibrin deposition and a 15% increase in platelet aggregates) after coronary intervention despite an ACT of 300–350 seconds underlines the potential stimulation of platelets by heparin.[42] The performance of coronary interventions with GPIIb/IIIa inhibition and very low heparin dosage is an important question for future investigations. Preliminary experience has shown that after successful stenting, heparin reversal can be done safely with protamine.[43,44]

Given the significant cost that GPIIb/IIIa inhibitor therapy adds to the already high economic burden of coronary intervention, especially with stents, there is wide skepticism with respect to the necessity of their universal use. Although an economic analysis of the EPIC trial[45] indicated that the long-term benefit from abciximab compensates for a large part of its initial cost, similar analyses with multidevice coronary interventions and stents have not been performed yet in other patient populations. Accordingly, the 'rescue' use of GPIIb/IIIa during coronary intervention has been developed, without any clinical data in clear support of this use. It is not known whether GPIIb/IIIa doses should be the same regardless of the clinical syndrome, or whether the benefits demonstrated in the clinical trials with pre-intervention administration remain valid with rescue use of GPIIb/IIIa. A clinical assessment of provisional GPIIb/IIIa use is warranted and may provide insight into the required duration and level of platelet inhibition for achievement of clinically significant benefits.

The results of the EPISTENT trial suggest that provisional stenting may be performed safely. This may be a means to reduce the cost of coronary intervention. The cross-over rate to placement of a stent was only 19%, the lowest observed in a balloon angioplasty arm of a clinical trial.

Examination of the recently published Benestent II Trial (see *Table 24.3*) shows that interventions can be performed safely in stable patients whose lesions do not have complex anatomy but have angiographic characteristics suitable for stenting. This population could be treated without the additional use of new antiplatelet drugs which could be reserved for more unstable clinical and anatomic settings.

Similar conclusions can be drawn from a comparison between the Benestent II and the EPISTENT results (*Table 24.4*). The patient population treated in the EPISTENT study represents an unselected group of patients and lesions, with the inclusion of patients with Braunwald class III unstable angina (not included in Benestent II). This fact may partially explain the good results obtained in the Benestent II patients despite the lack of any GPIIb/IIIa inhibitor therapy. In patients with clinical characteristics similar to the ones enrolled in the Benestent II study, additional treatment with GPIIb/IIIa inhibitors will probably add only minimal advantages because of the already low incidence of ischemic events.

In conclusion, GPIIb/IIIa inhibitor use during coronary interventions has produced a remarkable reduction in ischemic complications. Several issues remain to be resolved with respect to their exact dose, their differences in efficacy and side effects, and their use with special interventional devices, such as stents, which have significantly lower complication rates than angioplasty.

REFERENCES

1. Roubin GS, Cannon AD, Agrawal SK et al. Intracoronary stenting for acute and threatened closure complicating percutaneuos transluminal coronary angioplasty. *Circulation* 1992; **85**: 916–927.

2. Theroux P, Fuster V. Acute coronary syndromes. Unstable angina and non-Q-wave myocardial infarction. *Circulation* 1998; **97**: 1195–1206.

3. Davies MJ, Thomas AC. Plaque fissuring – the cause of acute myocardial infarction, sudden ischemic death, and crescendo angina. *Br Heart J* 1985; **53**: 363–373.

4. Vorchheimer DA, Badimon JJ, Fuster V. Platelet glycoprotein IIb/IIIa inhibitors and their antagonists in cardiovascular disease. *JAMA* 1999; **281**: 1407–1414.

5. Mizuno K, Satomura K, Miyamoto A et al. Angioscopic evaluation of coronary artery thrombi in acute coronary syndromes. *N Engl J Med* 1992; **326**: 287–291.

6. Ruggeri ZM. Mechanisms of shear-induced platelet adhesion and aggregation. *Thromb Haemost* 1993; **70**: 119–123.

7. Falk E, Shah PK, Fuster V. Coronary plaque disruption. *Circulation* 1995; **92**: 657–671.

8. Coller BS. The role of platelets in arterial thrombosis and the rationale for blockade of platelet GP IIb/IIIa receptors as antithrombotic therapy. *Eur Heart J* 1995; **16 (suppl L)**: 11–15.

9. Hynes RO. Integrins: versatility, modulation and signaling in cell adhesion. *Cell* 1992; **69**: 11–25.

10. Lefkovits J, Plow EF, Topol EJ. Platelet glycoprotein IIb/IIIa receptors in cardiovascular medicine. *N Engl J Med* 1995; **332**: 1553–1559.

11. Plow EF, McEver RP, Coller BS et al. Related binding mechanisms for fibrinogen, fibronectin, von Willebrand factor, and thrombospondin on thrombin-stimulated human platelets. *Blood* 1985; **66**: 724–727.

12. Pytela R, Pierschbacher MD, Ginsberg MH et al. Platelet membrane glycoprotein IIb/IIIa: member of a family of Arg–Gly–Asp-specific adhesion receptors. *Science* 1986; **231**: 1559–1562.

13. Ruoslahti E, Piersbacher MD. New perspectives in cell adhesion: RGD and integrins. *Science* 1987; **238**: 491–497.

14. Plow EF, Marguerie G, Ginsberg M. Fibrinogen, fibrinogen receptors, and the peptides that inhibit these interactions. *Biochem Pharmacol* 1987; **36**: 4035–4040.

15. Cairns JA, Lewis Jr D, Meade TW et al. Antithrombotic agents in coronary artery disease. *Chest* 1995; **108 (suppl I)**: 380S–400S.

16. Barnathan ES, Schwartz JS, Taylor et al. Aspirin and dipyridamole in the prevention of acute coronary thrombosis complicating coronary angioplasty. *Circulation* 1987; **76**: 125–134.

17. Schror K. The basic pharmacology of ticlopidine and clopidogrel. *Platelets* 1993; **4**: 252.

18. Coller BS. Blockade of platelet GPIIb/IIIa receptors as an antithrombotic strategy. *Circulation* 1995; **92**: 2373–2380.

19. Felding-Habermann B, Cheresh DA. Vitronectin and its receptors. *Curr Opin Cell Biol* 1993; **5**: 864–868.

20. The EPIC Investigators. Use of a monoclonal antibody directed against the platelet glycoprotein IIb/IIIa receptor in high-risk coronary angioplasty. *N Engl J Med* 1994; **330**: 956–961.

21. Aguirre FV, Topol EJ, Ferguson JJ et al. Bleeding complications with the chimeric antibody to platelet glycoprotein IIb/IIIa integrin in patients undergoing percutaneous coronary intervention. *Circulation* 1995; **91**: 2882–2890.

22. The EPILOG Investigators. Platelet glycoprotein IIb/IIIa receptor blockade and low-dose heparin during percutaneous coronary revascularization. *N Engl J Med* 1997; **336**: 1689.

23. The CAPTURE investigators. Randomised placebo-controlled trial of abciximab before and during coronary intervention in refractory unstable angina: the CAPTURE study. *Lancet* 1997; **349**: 1429–1435.

24. The RESTORE investigators. Effects of platelet glycoprotein IIb/IIIa blockade with tirofiban on adverse cardaic events in patients with unstable angina or acute myocardial infarction undergoing coronary angioplasty. *Circulation* 1997; **96**: 1445–1453.

25. The PRISM-PLUS investigators. Inhibition of the platelet glycoprotein IIb/IIIa receptor with tirofiban in unstable angina and non-Q-wave myocardial infarction. *N Engl J Med* 1998; **338**: 1488–1497.

26. The IMPACT-II investigators. Randomised placebo-controlled trial of effect of eptifibatide on complications of percutaneous coronary intervention: the IMPACT-II trial. *Lancet* 1997; **349**: 1422–1428.

27. The PURSUIT trial investigators. Inhibition of platelet glycoprotein IIb/IIIa with eptifibatide in patients with acute coronary syndromes. *N Engl J Med* 1998; **339**: 436–443

28. Lincoff AM, Califf RM, Anderson KM et al. Evidence for prevention of death and myocardial infarction with platelet membrane glycoprotein IIb/IIIa receptor blockade by abciximab (c7E3 Fab) among patients with unstable angina undergoing percutaneuos coronary revascularization. EPIC

Investigators. Evaluation of 7E3 in Preventing Ischemic Complications. *J Am Coll Cardiol* 1997; **30**: 149–156.

29. Lefkovits J, Ivanhoe RJ, Califf RM et al. Effects of platelet glycoprotein IIb/IIIa receptor blockade by a chimeric monoclonal antibody (abciximab) on acute and six-month outcomes after percutaneuos transluminal coronary angioplasty for acute myocardial infarction. EPIC investigators. *Am J Cardiol* 1996; **77**: 1045–1051.

30. Lefkovits J, Blankenship JC, Anderson KM et al. Increased risk of non-Q wave myocardial infarction after directional atherectomy is platelet dependent: evidence from the EPIC trial. Evaluation of 7E3 for the Prevention of Ischemic Complications. *J Am Coll Cardiol* 1996; **28**: 849–855.

31. Topol EJ, Califf RM, Weisman HF et al. Randomised trial of coronary intervention with antibody against platelet IIb/IIIa integrin for reduction of clinical restenosis: results at six months. *Lancet* 1994; **323**: 881–886.

32. Topol EJ, Ferguson JJ, Weisman HF et al. Long-term protection from myocardial ischemic events in a randomized trial of brief integrin IIb/IIIa blockade with percutaneous coronary intervention. *JAMA* 1997; **278**: 479–484.

33. ERASER Investigators. Acute platelet inhibition with abciximab does not reduce in-stent restenosis. *Circulation* 1999; **100**: 799–806.

34. Phillips DR, Teng W, Arfsten A et al. Effect of Ca^{2+} on GP IIb–IIIa interactions with integrilin; enhanced GP IIb–IIIa binding and inhibition of platelet aggregation by reductions in the concentration of ionized calcium in plasma anticoagulated with citrate. *Circulation* 1997; **96**: 1488–1494.

35. Serruys PW, van Hout B, Bonnier H et al, for the Benestent Study Group. Randomised comparison of implantation of heparin-coated stents with balloon angioplasty in selected patients with coronary artery disease (Benestent II). *Lancet* 1998; **352**: 673–681.

36. The EPISTENT investigators. Randomised placebo-controlled trial and balloon angioplasty-controlled trial to assess safety of coronary stenting with use of platelet glycoprotein-IIb/IIIa blockade. *Lancet* 1998; **352**: 87–92.

37. Kereiakes DJ, Lincoff AM, Miller DP et al. Abciximab therapy and unplanned coronary stent deployment; favorable effects on stent use, clinical outcomes, and bleeding complications. *Circulation* 1998; **97**: 857–864.

38. Brener SJ, Barr LA, Burchenal JEB et al, for the RAPPORT investigators. Randomized, placebo-controlled trial of platelet glycoprotein IIb/IIIa blockade with primary angioplasty for acute myocardial infarction. *Circulation* 1998; **98**: 734–741.

39. Neumann FJ, Blasini R, Schmitt C et al. Effect of glycoprotein IIb/IIIa receptor blockade on recovery of coronary flow and left ventricular function after the placement of coronary artery stents in acute myocardial infarction. *Circulation* 1998; **98**: 2695–2701.

40. Tcheng JE, Kereiakes DJ, Braden GA et al. Readministration of abciximab: interim report of the ReoPro readministration registry. *Am Heart J* 1999; **138**: S33–S38.

41. Coller BS, Lang D, Scudders L. Monitoring platelet GP IIb/IIIa antagonist therapy. *Circulation* 1997; **96**: 3828–3832.

42. Dangas G, Badimon JJ, Coller BS et al. Administration of abciximab during percutaneous coronary interventions decreases ex vivo platelet aggregates and fibrin deposition; implications for an anticoagulant effect of abciximab. *Arterioscler Thromb Vasc Biol* 1998; **18**: 1342–1349.

43. Colombo A, Hall PAX, Nakamura S et al. Preliminary experience using protamine to reverse heparin immediately following a successful coronary stent implantation. *J Am Coll Cardiol* 1995; **182A**: 741–744.

44. Pan M, Suarez de Lezo J, Medina A et al. In-laboratory removal of femoral sheath following protamine administration in patients having intracoronary stent implantation. *Am J Cardiol* 1997; **15**: 1336–1338

45. Mark DB, Talley JD, Topol EJ et al for the EPIC investigators. Economic assessment of platelet glycoprotein IIb/IIIa inhibition for prevention of ischemic complications of high-risk coronary angioplasty. *Circulation* 1996; **94**: 629–635.

Index